BECKER-SHAFFER'S

Diagnosis and Therapy of the Glaucomas

BECKER-SHAFFER'S
Diagnosis and Therapy of the Glaucomas

Seventh Edition

Robert L. Stamper, M.D.

Professor of Clinical Ophthalmology;
Director, Glaucoma Service,
University of California, San Francisco;
Chairman Emeritus,
Department of Ophthalmology,
California Pacific Medical Center,
San Francisco, California

Marc F. Lieberman, M.D.

Director of Glaucoma Services,
California Pacific Medical Center;
Clinical Professor of Ophthalmology,
University of California, San Francisco,
San Francisco, California

Michael V. Drake, M.D.

Steven P. Shearing Professor and Vice Chairman,
Department of Ophthalmology;
Senior Associate Dean,
School of Medicine,
University of California, San Francisco,
San Francisco, California

with 525 illustrations

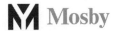 Mosby

St. Louis Baltimore Boston Carlsbad Chicago Minneapolis New York Philadelphia Portland
London Milan Sydney Tokyo Toronto

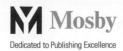

Developmental Editor: Wendy Buckwalter
Project Manager: Carol Sullivan Weis
Senior Production Editor: Karen M. Rehwinkel
Designer: Bill Drone

SEVENTH EDITION

Composition by Top Graphics
Printing/binding by Quebecor

Mosby, Inc.
11830 Westline Industrial Drive
St. Louis, Missouri 64146

International Standard Book Number   0-8016-7726-2

99 00 01 02 03 / 9 8 / 8 3 4 3 2 1

We dedicate this book to our families, whose love, devotion, support, and sacrifice made this multi-year project, as well as most of our other accomplishments, possible: to the memory of Maurice R. Stamper and Alfred and Netsy Lieberman, and to our parents Lionel and Viviane Paradise and Carl and Beatrice Drake; to our spouses Naomi Stamper and Brenda Drake; and to our children Juliet and Alison Stamper, Marjorie Stamper-Kurn, Michael Lieberman, and Christopher and Sean Drake.

And to our teachers, especially Drs. Becker and Shaffer, whose wisdom and encouragement have been a source of inspiration and strength; to our students, who help us continue learning; and to our patients, who constantly stimulate our search for better ways of managing their glaucoma.

Foreword

Writing a foreword for the seventh edition of *Diagnosis and Therapy of the Glaucomas* provides an opportunity for us to reminisce about our working together on the first two editions. In retrospect we were able to discuss and summarize the consequences of emerging research and clinical developments that promised to contribute to our knowledge about the glaucomas, their pathogenesis, diagnosis, and treatment. We have followed with interest and excitement the NIH-stimulated research, the changing concepts, the technological developments, and the newer methods of diagnosis and therapy. These have appeared in succeeding editions by Allan E. Kolker and John Hetherington, Jr., followed by H. Dunbar Hoskins, Jr. and Michael A. Kass, and in the present volume by Robert L. Stamper, Marc F. Lieberman, and Michael V. Drake.

A number of unresolved problems we faced 40 years ago continue to challenge current-day researchers, including the precise site and nature of obstruction to outflow in primary open-angle glaucoma, vascular versus mechanical effects of intraocular pressure on the optic nerve, the nature of genetic defects and their relationship to corticosteroid responsiveness, and the susceptibility to damage, as well as the possibilities for neuroprotection of the optic nerve in spite of the disordered pathophysiology.

We know from first-hand experience the time and effort that goes into library research in writing and rewriting a book such as this. We want to take this opportunity to express our appreciation to our students for revising and updating our early efforts in each of the subsequent editions. They have not only corrected our errors but have added the newest and timeliest concepts of research and practice to both diagnosis and therapy of the glaucomas. The present volume continues this tradition and once again offers the key references and provocative ideas to stimulate laboratory and clinical research. In addition, it provides in a single volume a practical approach to clinical problems, which should prove useful to students and residents, as well as practicing clinicians.

Bernard Becker, M.D.
Robert N. Shaffer, M.D.

Preface

This book has a proud history. It has served as a guide for treating patients with glaucoma to ophthalmologists throughout the world for almost four decades. The book was conceived and written by Bernard Becker and Robert N. Shaffer. It was later revised through multiple editions by Allan Kolker and John Hetherington, Jr. and, most recently, by H. Dunbar Hoskins, Jr. and Michael A. Kass. The current edition is the product of a third generation of glaucoma specialists who trained and/or practice in St. Louis and San Francisco.

We have followed the lead of our mentors in using the book to summarize our clinical experience with glaucoma and to interpret in a practical way the current literature and thinking about glaucoma and its management. Our understanding of glaucoma and its treatment has undergone significant change in the last decade. The book has been extensively rewritten, with new illustrations, many in color, and an extensive up-to-date bibliography. The classification of the glaucomas has been revised to reflect new findings in genetics and pathophysiology of both trabecular dysfunction and optic nerve damage. In addition, the classification of the infantile and pediatric glaucomas has been updated. In just the last few years, several new medications and operations have been added to our armamentarium. The sections on management not only review up-to-date information but also provide some guidance to the practitioner in individualizing the expanded and expanding choices for treatment. Glimpses into the possible treatments of the future are given. We hope the readers will be able to understand what we do know and what we still don't know about the glaucomas.

The format for this seventh edition has been updated to make reading, studying, and finding relevant information easier. As in previous editions, the emphasis is on providing, in one volume, the information necessary to allow the individual involved in or wishing to become involved in the management of the glaucomas to do so effectively and with understanding. Ultimately, the goal is to reduce vision loss and improve the quality of life for our patients at risk for glaucomatous disease.

Robert L. Stamper
Marc F. Lieberman
Michael V. Drake

Acknowledgments

First and foremost, we would like to thank our mentors, Drs. Bernard Becker and Robert N. Shaffer. They, of course, provided the first editions of this text. Perhaps more importantly, their clinical acumen, intellect, dedication to teaching, and integrity have inspired us in our careers. They have served as role models not only for us but for a half-century of ophthalmologists around the world.

We would also like to acknowledge with thanks the contributions of the following ophthalmolgists:
- Michael Berlin, M.D., for his contributions to the chapters on laser surgery.
- M. Roy Wilson, M.D., for his contributions on the epidemiology of open-angle glaucoma.
- Jacob A. Dan, M.D., Ph.D., and James Heltzer, M.D., for contributions to the chapters on medical therapy.
- Maurice Mosseri, M.D., for his contributions to the chapter on angle-closure glaucoma.

We also thank William H. Spencer, M.D., for his inspiration, encouragement, and support for this as well as so many other academic endeavors.

Every book has authors and editors. It is the editors who are the unsung heroes of a book. They wheedle, cajole, nag, suggest, help create, and, in the end, edit. It is the wheedling and the nagging that actually move a book toward its publication. The authors would like to thank Wendy Buckwalter, Laurel Craven, Susie Coladonato, Karen Rehwinkel, Carol Sullivan Weis, Bill Drone, and the staff at Mosby for their good work, as well as their good nature, patience, persistence, professionalism, and skills. We also extend our appreciation to our talented illustrator for this edition, Terry Toyama, as well as our illustrator for past editions, Nadine Sokol.

Behind the authors were a string of supporters. They include our families, the Departments of Ophthalmology at the University of California San Francisco and at California Pacific Medical Center, Pacific Vision Foundation, That Man May See, and The Glaucoma Research Foundation, all of San Francisco, and the Tibet Vision Project of the Public Health Institute of Santa Cruz, California. We are most appreciative of their encouragement and support.

Robert L. Stamper, M.D.

Marc F. Lieberman, M.D.

Michael V. Drake, M.D.

Contents

Section III
The Optic Nerve

Part IV
Clinical Entities, 215

Part V
Medical Treatment, 413

Part VI
Laser Therapy, 521
with Michael Berlin, M.D.

Part VII
Surgical Principles, 555

Part VIII

Surgical Procedures and Techniques, 581

Part IX

Present Status and Future Approaches, 677

BECKER-SHAFFER'S

Diagnosis and Therapy of the Glaucomas

PART I

Introduction

1

Introduction and Classification of the Glaucomas

DEFINITIONS

The concepts and definitions of glaucoma have evolved in the past 100 years,[1] but still they remain imprecise and subject to technical qualifications. The word *glaucoma* originally meant "clouded" in Greek; as such, it may have referred both to a mature cataract and to corneal edema that might result from chronic elevated pressure. Today the term does not refer to a single disease entity, but rather to a group of diseases that differ in their clinical presentation, pathophysiology, and treatment. These diseases are grouped together because they share certain features, including cupping and atrophy of the optic nerve head, which has attendant visual field loss and is frequently related to the level of intraocular pressure (IOP).

In this text, glaucoma is defined as a disturbance of the structural or functional integrity of the optic nerve that can usually be arrested or diminished by adequate lowering of IOP. An important distinction must be noted in the criteria currently used to define primary open-angle glaucoma (POAG), in contrast to all other forms of glaucoma. POAG is explicitly characterized as a "multifactorial optic neuropathy [with] a characteristic acquired loss of optic nerve fibers,"[2] developing in the presence of open anterior chamber angles and manifesting characteristic visual field abnormalities, in the absence of other known causes of the disease. In contrast, all other types of glaucoma—from primary angle-closure[3] to the secondary glaucomas—are defined first and foremost by the presence of elevated IOP, and not in reference to the optic neuropathy that follows sustained elevated IOPs.

Classically the primary glaucomas are not associated with known ocular or systemic disorders that account for the increased resistance to aqueous outflow; the primary diseases are usually bilateral and probably reflect genetic predispositions. Conversely, the secondary glaucomas are associated with ocular or systemic abnormalities responsible for the alteration in aqueous outflow; these diseases are often unilateral and acquired. Some have argued that the distinctions between "primary" and "secondary" simply reflect our imperfect understanding of pathophysiologic events that converge in the common final pathway of optic atrophy and visual field loss.[4] Although many risk factors have been associated with the development of POAG (Table 1-1), elevated IOP remains the most prominent factor—shared among the primary and secondary glaucomas—and the only factor contemporary ophthalmic intervention can reliably affect.

IOP is determined by the balance between the rate of aqueous humor production of the ciliary body, the resistance to aqueous outflow at the angle of the anterior chamber, and the level of episcleral venous pressure (Fig. 1-1). In most cases elevated IOP is caused by increased resistance to aqueous humor outflow. The optic nerve and visual field changes of glaucoma are determined by the resistance to damage of the optic nerve axons.

In most cases of glaucoma, progressive changes in the visual field and optic nerve are related to increased IOP; in some instances even "normal" levels of IOP are too high for proper functioning of the optic nerve axons. Although there may be absolutely no "safe" pressure that guarantees the absence of POAG,[5] lowering IOP to the low-normal range usually arrests or slows the progress of glaucoma.[6,6a] If this is not true, it can be postulated that (1) the IOP is not low enough to stabilize the disease; (2) the optic nerve is so damaged that even the normal age-related loss of axons produces further visual deterioration; or (3) there is a non–pressure-dependent element to the visual loss. If the third situation exists, it is not currently distinguishable from glaucoma.

Table 1-1 ——————————————————————————————

Risk Factors in Primary Open-Angle Glaucoma

Factor	Quality of Evidence	Remarks
Ocular Risk Factors		
Intraocular pressure	Excellent	Most important
Myopia	Good	Related to IOP and to optic nerve?
Increased cup/disc ratio	Equivocal	May represent early POAG
Asymmetric cupping	Equivocal	May represent early POAG
Disc hemorrhage	Equivocal	Prognostically important
Nonocular Risk Factors		
Age	Excellent	Causal mechanisms unknown
Race (e.g., African ancestry)	Excellent	Causal mechanisms unknown
Family history	Good	Multifactorial genetic factors
Adult onset diabetes	Good	Vasculopathy related?
Systemic hypertension	Fair	Biologically plausible
Migraine and peripheral vasospasm	Equivocal	More relevant in "low tension" disease?
Gender	Inadequate	Contradictory reports
Alcohol consumption	Inadequate	Requires confirmation
Cigarette smoking	Inadequate	Requires confirmation

Data from References 18, 20, 32-35 and Wilson MR: *Glaucoma: epidemiology and risk factors.* In Higginbotham EJ, Lee DA: *Management of difficult glaucomas,* Boston, 1994, Blackwell.

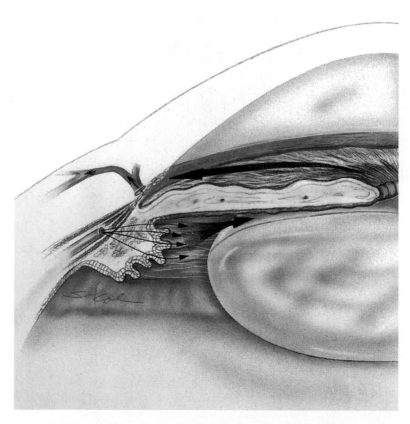

Figure 1-1 Anterior segment of the eye. Aqueous humor is formed by the ciliary epithelium, passes between the iris and lens to enter the anterior chamber, and leaves the eye through the trabecular meshwork and Schlemm's canal.

EPIDEMIOLOGIC AND SOCIOECONOMIC ASPECTS OF THE GLAUCOMAS

Whether manifesting as POAG, primary angle-closure, or congenital disease, glaucoma is among the leading causes of blindness in the developing world[7,8] and a major health problem in the developed world. In the United States, glaucoma of all types is the second leading cause of legal blindness, affecting more than 80,000 Americans.[2] Among white and black populations POAG accounts for nearly two thirds of all reported glaucoma cases.[9,10] Among some Asian populations, however, primary angle-closure glaucoma is the more common disease.[11,12]

It is estimated that 2.25 million people in the United States over the age of 40 years have POAG,[13] half of whom are unaware of their disease despite demonstrable visual field loss.[14] Another 10 million Americans are estimated to have IOPs greater than 21; approximately 10% of these eyes will convert to POAG over the course of a decade.[15] The relationship between IOP and glaucomatous optic neuropathy is complex. On the one hand, the higher the IOP, the likelier the risk of POAG; conversely, one out of six eyes with POAG never demonstrates IOP higher than the age-appropriate normal range.[16,17]

An enormous amount of superb epidemiologic information has been forthcoming in the past decade, characterized by comprehensive population-based studies with rigorous criteria for pressure measurements, angle evaluation, and disc and visual field assessment.[18-21] These studies consistently report a prevalence rate for POAG in 1% to 2% of white adults. However, significant racial differences exist. Among blacks, the prevalence is nearly 4 times higher.[14] These patients are twice as likely to be blind as their white counterparts, and they have the disease nearly 27% longer.[10,22] These facts reflect neither the supply of ophthalmologists nor the patient's personal income.[23] Even higher rates have been reported among some Caribbean populations,[24-26] although there are lower and more variable prevalence rates among the genetically heterogeneous African populations from whom these New World populations descended.[27]

A major development in applying the epidemiologic evidence to clinical use is the concept of risk factors (see Chapter 2). Table 1-1 lists those factors that have demonstrated to a greater or lesser extent statistical correlation with either the development or the progression of POAG.

With the basic medical resources available in the developed world,[17] nearly all cases of blindness from glaucoma are preventable if the disease is detected early and proper treatment is implemented. Detection depends on education—educating the public about the importance of routine examinations, and training fellow health professionals to recognize the signs and symptoms of glaucoma. Screening strategies that rely only on IOP measures and that neglect disc and visual field assessment are inadequate;[28] and even when full testing is performed, it may not be cost effective.[29] Only through a massive public health effort of education and outreach can this scourge of preventable, unnecessary glaucoma blindness be addressed.

CLASSIFICATION OF THE GLAUCOMAS

The most widely used classification system of the glaucomas separates angle-closure glaucoma from open-angle glaucoma. In angle-closure glaucoma, resistance to outflow is increased because the peripheral iris is blocking the trabecular meshwork—that is, the angle or periphery of the anterior chamber is closed (Fig. 1-2). In open-angle glaucoma, there is impaired flow of aqueous humor through the trabecular meshwork–Schlemm's canal–venous system (Fig. 1-3).

This classification scheme continues to be helpful because it clarifies pathogenetic mechanisms and therapeutic approaches. The four major divisions within this system are (1) angle-closure glaucoma; (2) open-angle glaucoma; (3) combined-mechanism glaucoma, in which two or more forms of glaucoma are present; and (4) developmental glaucoma, in which some anomaly of the anterior segment is present at birth. All four major divisions are subdivided into primary and secondary categories.

A similar classification system divides glaucoma into conditions that affect the internal flow, and conditions that affect the outflow of aqueous humor. Internal-flow block is caused by pupillary block or cilio-vitreo-lenticular block. Outflow block occurs with diseases of the trabecular meshwork, Schlemm's canal, collector channels, and the venous system.

Alternative classification systems[4] are based on other features of the diseases, including (1) the site of the outflow obstruction, which is divided into diseases that affect the pretrabecular passage of aqueous humor (e.g., posterior synechiae to the lens after ocular inflammation), the trabecular flow (e.g., glaucoma after administration of α-chymotrypsin), and the posttrabecular move-

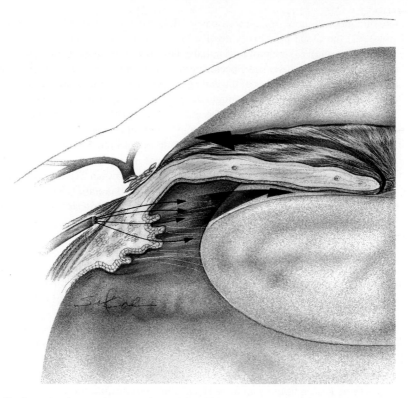

Figure 1-2 In angle-closure glaucoma, the peripheral iris covers the trabecular meshwork, obstructing aqueous humor outflow.

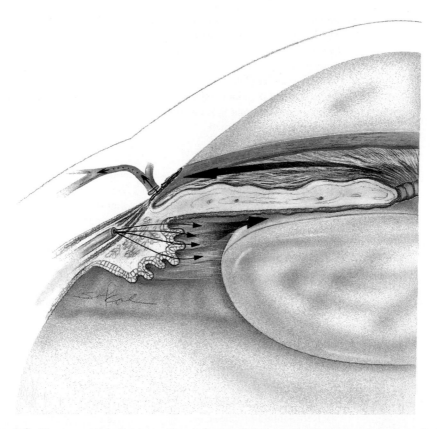

Figure 1-3 In open-angle glaucoma, there is impaired flow of aqueous humor through the trabecular meshwork–Schlemm's canal–venous system.

ment of aqueous humor (e.g., increased episcleral venous pressure from a carotid–cavernous sinus fistula); (2) the tissue principally involved (e.g., glaucoma caused by diseases of the lens or diseases of the retina); (3) the proximal initial events (e.g., steroid glaucoma); and (4) the age of the patient (e.g., congenital, juvenile). Specific diseases have also been subclassified, such as POAG types, based on various appearances of the damaged optic nerve,[30] or the angle-closure glaucomas, based on IOP levels and gonioscopic configurations as correlated with ultrasonic biomicroscopy.[31]

The reader is cautioned that all classification schemes are arbitrary and limited. Some cases do not fit neatly into one category or another. The classification that follows is not meant to be all-inclusive, but to be an aid in thinking about pathogenesis and treatment.

I. Angle-closure glaucoma

   A. With pupillary block

      Aqueous humor is restricted in moving from the posterior to the anterior chamber. The increased pressure in the posterior chamber bows the peripheral iris into contact with the trabecular meshwork.

      1. Primary angle-closure with pupillary block

         a. Acute

         b. Subacute (asymptomatic or intermittent)

         c. Chronic

      2. Secondary angle-closure with pupillary block

         a. Miotic induced

         b. Swollen lens

         c. Mobile lens syndromes (e.g., ectopia lentis, microspherophakia)

         d. Synechiae to lens, vitreous, or pseudophakia

   B. Without pupillary block

      In these conditions pupillary block is not responsible for holding the iris against the trabecular meshwork.

      1. Primary angle-closure without pupillary block (plateau iris)

         The angle is mechanically blocked by the peripheral iris, particularly when the pupil is dilated.

      2. Secondary angle-closure without pupillary block

         a. Anterior "pulling mechanism"

            The iris is pulled forward by some process in the angle, often by the contraction of a membrane.

            (1) Neovascular glaucoma

            (2) Iridocorneal endothelial syndromes (e.g., Chandler's syndrome)

            (3) Posterior polymorphous dystrophy

            (4) Epithelial downgrowth

            (5) Fibrous ingrowth

            (6) Flat anterior chamber

            (7) Inflammation

            (8) Penetrating keratoplasty

            (9) Aniridia

         b. Posterior "pushing mechanism"

            The iris is pushed forward by some condition in the posterior segment. Often the ciliary body is rotated anteriorly, allowing the lens to come forward also.

            (1) Ciliary-block glaucoma (malignant glaucoma)

            (2) Cysts of the iris and ciliary body

            (3) Intraocular tumors

            (4) Nanophthalmos

            (5) Suprachoroidal hemorrhage

            (6) Intravitreal air injection (e.g., retinal pneumopexy)

            (7) Ciliochoroidal effusions (e.g., panretinal photocoagulation)

               (a) Inflammation (e.g., posterior scleritis)

               (b) Central retinal vein occlusion

            (8) Scleral buckling procedure

            (9) Retrolental fibroplasia

II. Open-angle glaucoma
  A. Primary open-angle glaucoma
    1. IOPs higher than "normal range"
    2. IOPs within "normal range" (low tension glaucoma)
  B. Secondary open-angle glaucoma
    1. Pigmentary glaucoma
    2. Pseudoexfoliation glaucoma
    3. Steroid glaucoma
    4. Lens-induced glaucoma
      a. Phacolytic glaucoma
      b. Lens-particle glaucoma
      c. Phacoanaphylaxis
    5. Glaucoma after cataract surgery
      a. α-Chymotrypsin glaucoma
      b. Glaucoma with viscoelastics
      c. Glaucoma with pigment dispersion and intraocular lens
      d. UGH syndrome (uveitis + glaucoma + hyphema)
      e. Glaucoma after neodymium:yttrium-aluminum-garnet (Nd:YAG) laser posterior capsulotomy
      f. Glaucoma with vitreous in anterior chamber
    6. Glaucoma after trauma
      a. Chemical burns
      b. Electric shock
      c. Radiation
      d. Penetrating injury
      e. Contusion injury
    7. Glaucoma associated with intraocular hemorrhage
      a. Ghost cell glaucoma
      b. Hemolytic glaucoma
      c. Hemosiderosis
    8. Glaucoma associated with retinal detachment
    9. Glaucoma after vitrectomy
      a. Intraocular gas
      b. Intraocular silicone oil
    10. Glaucoma with uveitis
      a. Fuchs' heterochromic iridocyclitis
      b. Glaucomatocyclitic crisis (Posner-Schlossman)
      c. Precipitates on trabecular meshwork (trabeculitis)
      d. Herpes simplex
      e. Herpes zoster
      f. Sarcoidosis
      g. Juvenile rheumatoid arthritis
      h. Syphilis
      i. Human immunodeficiency virus (HIV) infection
    11. Glaucoma with intraocular tumors
      a. Malignant melanoma
      b. Metastatic lesions
      c. Leukemia and lymphoma
      d. Benign lesions (e.g., juvenile xanthogranuloma, neurofibromatosis)
    12. Amyloidosis
    13. Increased episcleral venous pressure
      a. Obstruction of venous drainage (e.g., superior vena cava obstruction)
      b. Arteriovenous fistula (e.g., carotid cavernous)
      c. Ocular episcleral venous anomalies (e.g., Sturge-Weber syndrome)
III. Combined-mechanism glaucoma
  Includes entities with a combination of two or more forms of glaucoma.

A. Open-angle glaucoma complicated by angle-closure glaucoma
1. Coincidental occurrence (e.g., trauma to eye predisposed to POAG)
2. Miotic induced
3. Swelling of the lens with age or disease
4. Flat anterior chamber following intraocular surgery
5. Peripheral anterior synechiae after laser trabeculoplasty
6. Peripheral anterior synechiae from inflammation
7. Neovascular glaucoma after central retinal vein occlusion

B. Mixed-mechanism angle-closure glaucoma with trabecular damage
Despite a patent iridectomy, previous iridotrabecular contact may damage the trabecular meshwork in the absence of peripheral anterior synechiae.

IV. Developmental glaucoma
Anomalies of the anterior segment are present at birth. Glaucoma may be present at birth or may appear in first decades of life (see Chapter 20 for detailed classification of pediatric glaucoma diseases).

A. Primary congenital (infantile) glaucoma
1. Congenital glaucoma
2. Autosomal dominant juvenile glaucoma
3. Glaucoma associated with systemic abnormalities
4. Glaucoma associated with ocular abnormalities

B. Secondary glaucoma
1. Traumatic glaucoma
2. Glaucoma with intraocular neoplasm
3. Uveitis glaucoma
4. Lens-induced glaucoma
5. Glaucoma after congenital cataract surgery
6. Steroid-induced glaucoma
7. Neovascular glaucoma
8. Secondary angle-closure glaucoma
9. Glaucoma with elevated episcleral venous pressure
10. Glaucoma secondary to intraocular infection

REFERENCES

1. Drance SM: *The changing concept of glaucoma in the 20th century.* In van Buskirk EM, Shields MB, editors: *100 years of progress in glaucoma,* Philadelphia, 1997, Lippincott-Raven.
2. American Academy of Ophthalmology: *Primary open-angle glaucoma: preferred practice pattern,* San Francisco, 1996, The Academy.
3. American Academy of Ophthalmology: *Primary angle-closure glaucoma: preferred practice pattern,* San Francisco, 1996, The Academy.
4. Shields MB, Ritch R, Krupin T: *Classifications of the glaucomas.* In Ritch R, Shields MB, Krupin T, editors: *The glaucomas,* ed 2, St Louis, 1996, Mosby.
5. Sommer A: Doyne Lecture. Glaucoma: facts and fancies, *Eye* 10:295, 1996.
6. Grant MW, Morton W, Burton JF: Why do some people go blind after glaucoma? *Ophthalmology* 89:991, 1982.
6a. Collaborative Normal-Tension Glaucoma Study Group: The effectiveness of intraocular pressure reduction in the treatment of normal-tension glaucoma, *Am J Ophthalmol* 126:498, 1998.
7. Quigley HA: Number of people with glaucoma worldwide, *Br J Ophthalmol* 80:389, 1996.

8. Thylefors B, Negrel AD: The global impact of glaucoma, *Bull World Health Organ* 72:323, 1994.
9. Teikari JM, O'Donnell J: Epidemiologic data on adult glaucomas: data from the Hospital Discharge Registry and the Registry of Right to Free Medication, *Acta Ophthalmol Scand Suppl* 67:184, 1989.
10. Tielsch JM, and others: Blindness and visual impairment in an American urban population. The Baltimore Eye Survey, *Arch Ophthalmol* 108:286, 1990.
11. Congdon NG, and others: Biometry and primary angle-closure glaucoma among Chinese, white, and black populations, *Ophthalmology* 104:1489, 1997.
12. Shiose Y, and others: Epidemiology of glaucoma in Japan: a nationwide glaucoma survey, *Jpn J Ophthalmol* 35:133, 1991.
13. Wilson RS: *Epidemiology of glaucoma.* In Epstein DL, Allingham RR, Schuman JS, editors: *Chandler and Grant's glaucoma,* ed 4, Baltimore, 1997, Williams & Wilkins.
14. Tielsch JM, and others: Racial variations in the prevalence of primary open-angle glaucoma. The Baltimore Eye Survey, *JAMA* 266:369, 1991.

15. Quigley HA, and others: Risk factors for the development of glaucomatous visual field loss in ocular hypertension, *Arch Ophthalmol* 112:644, 1994.
16. Sommer A, and others: Relationship between intraocular pressure and primary open angle glaucoma among white and black Americans, *Arch Ophthalmol* 109:1090, 1991.
17. Sommer A: Diagnosis and treatment of the glaucomas, *Community Eye Health* 9:17, 1996.
18. Klein BE, and others: Prevalence of glaucoma. The Beaver Dam Eye Study, *Ophthalmology* 99:1499, 1992.
19. Coffey MA, and others: Prevalence of glaucoma in the west of Ireland, *Br J Ophthalmol* 77:17, 1993.
20. Dielemans I, and others: The prevalence of primary open-angle glaucoma in a population-based study in The Netherlands. The Rotterdam Study, *Ophthalmology* 101:1851, 1994.
21. Tielsch JM: The epidemiology and control of open angle glaucoma: a population-based perspective, *Annu Rev Public Health* 17:121, 1996.

22. Quigley HA, Vitale S: Models of open-angle glaucoma prevalence and incidence in the United States, *Invest Ophthalmol Vis Sci* 38:83, 1997.

23. Javitt JC: Preventing blindness in Americans: the need for eye health education, *Surv Ophthalmol* 40:41, 1995.

24. Mason RP, and others: National survey of the prevalence and risk factors of glaucoma in St Lucia, West Indies. Part I. Prevalence findings, *Ophthalmology* 96:1363, 1989.

25. Leske MC, and others: The Barbados Eye Study: prevalence of open angle glaucoma, *Arch Ophthalmol* 112:821, 1994.

26. Leske MC, and others: Risk factors for open-angle glaucoma. The Barbados Eye Study, *Arch Ophthalmol* 113:918, 1995.

27. Broadway D, Murdocj I: *Glaucoma in blacks.* In El Sayyad F, and others, editors: *The refractory glaucomas,* New York, 1995, Igaku-Shoin.

28. Sommer A: Epidemiology as it relates to screening for glaucoma, *Surv Ophthalmol* 33:441, 1989.

29. Boivin JF, McGregor M, Archer C: Cost effectiveness of screening for primary open angle glaucoma, *J Med Screen* 3:154, 1996.

30. Spaeth GL: A new classification of glaucoma including focal glaucoma, *Surv Ophthalmol* 38:S9, 1994.

31. Kim YY, Jung HR: Clarifying the nomenclature for primary angle-closure glaucoma, *Surv Ophthalmol* 42:125, 1997.

32. Klein BE, Klein R, Jensen SC: Open-angle glaucoma and older-onset diabetes. The Beaver Dam Eye Study, *Ophthalmology* 101:1173, 1994.

33. Klein BE, Klein R, Ritter LL: Relationship of drinking alcohol and smoking to prevalence of open-angle glaucoma. The Beaver Dam Eye Study, *Ophthalmology* 100:1609, 1993.

34. Dielemans I, and others: Primary open-angle glaucoma, intraocular pressure, and diabetes mellitus in the general elderly population. The Rotterdam Study, *Ophthalmology* 103:1271, 1996.

35. Dielemans I, and others: Primary open-angle glaucoma, intraocular pressure, and systemic blood pressure in the general elderly population. The Rotterdam Study, *Ophthalmology* 102:54, 1995.

2

Patient Management

Throughout this text, many aspects of different types of glaucoma, tests, and results are discussed, including comments regarding diagnosis and treatment. However, it is useful to generalize some aspects of the management of glaucoma patients. The concepts presented here represent a few of the many possible ways to care for glaucoma patients and are the result of years of experience. Nevertheless, they are only recommendations, which must be modified to the requirements of each patient and physician.

SYMPTOMS AND HISTORICAL INFORMATION RELATED TO THE GLAUCOMAS

Many factors in the patient's history bear on the diagnosis and treatment of glaucoma. Most patients with glaucoma, especially primary open-angle glaucoma (POAG), are asymptomatic until late in the course of the disease. However, certain patients may have symptoms such as pain, redness, halo vision, blurred vision, and a change in the appearance of the eye. Pain associated with glaucoma is related to the height of the intraocular pressure (IOP) and the rapidity with which it rises to that level. Conditions that cause rapid and sustained rises of IOP to high levels, such as acute angle-closure glaucoma, are often accompanied by pain. Conditions such as POAG that cause less dramatic changes in IOP to moderate levels are usually not associated with pain. Occasionally young patients with open-angle glaucoma (e.g., pigmentary glaucoma) may experience discomfort when IOP rises rapidly to high levels. Other mechanisms for pain in glaucoma include inflammation, bullous keratopathy, and drug-induced side effects (e.g., miotic-induced ciliary and orbicularis muscle spasm). In angle-closure glaucoma or glaucoma associated with acute iritis, conjunctival injection may take the form of a ciliary flush. Other causes of red eyes in glaucoma patients include neovascular glaucoma, hyphema, subconjunctival hemorrhage, bullous keratopathy, drug reactions, and increased episcleral venous pressure.

When IOP rises rapidly, the corneal endothelium may not be able to adequately pump fluid from the cornea—resulting in edema of the epithelium and, sometimes, the stroma. This condition may produce a visual sensation of colored halos around incandescent lights. Episodic blurring of vision is often noted when rapid elevations of IOP cause corneal edema. It is important to remember that many patients refer to uncolored semicircular or radiating images as halos. This distortion in vision may be caused by opacities in the media, uncorrected refractive errors, and alterations in the tear film. In these latter conditions the ophthalmologist can often elicit "halo" vision in the office while the IOP is normal and the cornea is clear.

Glaucoma can alter vision in a number of other ways. Occasionally a patient may note a diminished visual field during some activity that requires monocular vision (e.g., aiming a rifle, looking through a camera). Patients with asymmetric vision loss may not be aware of their defect until they close the better eye. Loss of Snellen visual acuity usually occurs late in the course of glaucoma unless some other problem occurs, such as central retinal vein occlusion.

A few patients may complain of a change in the appearance of the eye. This includes exophthalmos, ocular displacement, haziness of the cornea, and an alteration in pupil size, shape, or position.

A careful medical history may provide important information related to glaucoma. The medical history should include the following points:

1. Ocular history should include queries about amblyopia, trauma, inflammation, surgery,

cataract, retinal detachment, and inflammation. If not questioned directly, patients may not remember a "trivial" eye injury that may have occurred many years ago.

2. General medical history should focus on obtaining information about vascular diseases (e.g., hypertension, diabetes, cardiac problems, hypotensive episodes) that might affect ocular perfusion, or other conditions that could mimic or aggravate glaucomatous visual field loss (e.g., demyelinating diseases, central nervous system tumors, or aneurysms). A history of migraine or other vasospastic disorders is important particularly for "normal pressure" glaucoma. The clinician must know about the patient's general health before prescribing medication or considering surgery. For example, topical β-blocker agents can exacerbate asthma or congestive heart failure.

3. The patient's medication history and allergies should also be documented. Many drugs (e.g., corticosteroids or anticholinergic agents) can alter IOP and affect the course of glaucoma. Conversely, many ocular medications can induce or aggravate systemic medical problems. Frequent exchange of information between the ophthalmologist and the family physician is important. A history of sulfa allergy may make the use of carbonic anhydrase inhibitor therapy unwise unless no other alternative is available.

4. The presence of a family history of ocular diseases—especially glaucoma, but also including cataract, strabismus, amblyopia, and retinal problems—should be determined. Many glaucoma conditions are familial, and information about family members may aid diagnosis and treatment.

Furthermore, now that certain kinds of glaucoma have been related to specific gene abnormalities, elicitation of the family history and even pedigree may be very important for the patient and his or her siblings and offspring.

The ocular examination should include measurement of best visual acuity; an evaluation of the adnexa for exophthalmos, signs of trauma, or inflammation; and assessment of motility for signs of restriction or paresis. The pupil should be evaluated for size, shape, and reactivity. The slit lamp should be used for assessment of the cornea for epithelial, stromal, and endothelial abnormalities, and for anterior synechiae. The slit lamp should also be used to assess the iris for atrophy, growths, or blood vessels; the anterior chamber for depth and clarity; and the lens and vitreous for clarity. The IOP should be measured before dilation or gonioscopy. The examination should also include a careful evaluation of the retina and its vessels, the macula, and the optic nerve. The status of the optic nerve should be documented periodically, preferably by an objective method such as photography or another imaging technique. Careful descriptions or drawings are acceptable if photography or digital imaging is not available. The nerve fiber layer should be evaluated both for generalized thinning and for localized defects. Gonioscopy is indicated whenever the diagnosis of any kind of glaucoma is suspected. A visual field examination should also be undertaken either for baseline or for follow-up.

DIAGNOSIS

Several risk factors are known to contribute to the development of glaucoma, its progression or lack thereof, and its extent. The known factors include heredity, race, the size of the eye (small for angle-closure, large for open-angle), the presence or absence of systemic vascular disease, vasospastic disorders including migraine, and the size and shape of the optic cup (see Table 1-1). Although elevated IOP is a major risk factor, it is not the only one and is not, in and of itself, enough to account for all of the damage unless it is very elevated.

If glaucoma is thought of as a disease that damages the structural and/or functional integrity of the eye and can often be slowed or arrested by lowering IOP, then decisions are simplified. Those patients who have structural or functional damage either caused by pressure or affected by pressure should be treated. In most instances the damage is fairly obvious, in the form of visual field loss, classic disc cupping, nerve fiber layer defects, corneal edema, arterial pulsations, or sometimes pain. Usually IOP is above the statistically normal range, so glaucoma is easy to diagnose. Once the disease is diagnosed, the decision to treat is simplified.

In other situations, things are not quite so simple. There may be questionable damage with normal pressure, or there may be elevated pressure without damage. These patients are glaucoma suspects and can be divided into four categories, depending on the level of IOP, the evidence of damage, and the presence of other risk factors.[1]

IDENTIFYING GLAUCOMA SUSPECTS

The purpose of identifying someone as a glaucoma suspect is to detect the earliest sign of damage and, by intervening at that point, to prevent any visually significant damage from occurring in that person's lifetime. This approach has the advantage of withholding treatment from those who may never need it.

Although some patients have progressive glaucomatous damage with no recorded IOPs above 21 mm Hg, other patients have IOPs frequently above 21 mm Hg without exhibiting glaucomatous damage. The 21 mm Hg mark remains useful for classifying glaucoma suspects for two reasons. First, 21 mm Hg represents 2 standard deviations above the mean IOP of 16 mm Hg in white populations. Pressure above this would occur in only 2.5% of normal cases if IOPs were indeed distributed normally in the population. Actually, the distribution of IOP is skewed to the right, so that 4% to 5% of "normal" patients may have pressures higher than 21 mm Hg. Although this is a small percentage of the normal patients, the actual number of patients with elevated IOP who never develop damage far exceeds the number of those who do develop damage. Therefore the chance of requiring treatment when only elevated IOP is present (<30 mm Hg), with no other risk factors, is probably less than 10%.[2] Second, elevated pressure can cause glaucomatous damage. This is certainly true in experimental animals. The higher the pressure, the more rapidly the damage progresses. If the damage has not progressed too far, it can be arrested in many cases by adequate lowering of the IOP. Thus elevated IOP is an important risk factor and must be taken seriously.

Anatomic signs may also make someone suspicious for glaucoma. Signs include the presence of narrow angles, an enlarged but not definitely pathologic optic cup, and thinning of or defects in the nerve fiber layer. Functional signs such as early but not definite visual field changes could also place someone in the suspect category. Color vision deficits may also herald the onset of glaucomatous damage. Finally, hereditary or genetic information—such as a strong family history of glaucoma or possession of a gene associated with glaucoma, as well as other high risk factors such as race or high myopia, even in the absence of elevated IOP or increased cupping—warrants closer observation than the general population. Table 1-1 lists the risk factors for primary open-angle glaucoma.

Damage to the optic nerve is central to the diagnosis of glaucoma. Damage to the functional or structural integrity of the eye that is typical of glaucoma may be absent, questionably present, or present. If it is present, the patient either has or has had glaucoma or some disease that mimics it. If it is absent or questionably present, the patient may have glaucoma. Usually, the dilemma arises when trying to recognize early optic nerve or visual function damage typical of POAG.

If a patient is a glaucoma suspect, the ophthalmologist must decide whether to treat or to observe the patient. That decision is usually based on both the physician's judgment of the amount of risk to the patient if left untreated and the patient's anxiety about the condition (or about medications). Boxes 2-1 through 2-4 list some examples of various types of glaucoma suspects and their management. Signs indicative of disc or field damage are listed in Box 2-5. The purpose of observing the glaucoma suspect is to recognize any evidence of early damage. If damage progresses, then the presence of glaucoma (or other optic neuropathy) has been proven, and treatment must commence or be escalated.

Box 2-1
Glaucoma Suspect Type I

Normal Intraocular Pressure, No Damage
Strong family history of glaucoma
Retinal vascular occlusion
Exfoliative syndrome
Angle recession
Pigmentary dispersion syndrome
Narrow angles
Uveitis
History of halos
Management: Monitor periodically and inform patient of need for follow-up.

Box 2-2
Glaucoma Suspect Type II

Normal Intraocular Pressure, Possible Damage

Suspicious optic disc
Suspicious nerve fiber layer defects
Suspicious visual field
Reduced psychophysical function
Management: Confirm the finding by repeat testing if needed, as with suspicious visual fields. Demonstrate a normal variant, another cause of damage, or an elevated intraocular pressure (IOP) expressed at other times. If the patient demonstrates increased IOP, then treat for glaucoma. Otherwise, treat any other existing disease or conduct annual or semi-annual examinations depending on risk factors.

Box 2-3
Glaucoma Suspect Type III

High Intraocular Pressure, No Damage
Management
1. Pressure >35 mm Hg (some authorities choose >30 mm Hg): Risk of damage is great. Treat.
2. Pressure 25-30 mm Hg: Treat if (1) other eye has damage, (2) patient is elderly or has siblings or parents with glaucoma, (3) patient has other risk factors, (4) patient has complicating ocular or vascular disease, or (5) there is poor patient follow-up or poor compliance. If treatment is poorly tolerated, treatment may be stopped and the patient observed at least every 4 months for progression of the disease.
3. Pressure 21-24 mm Hg: Treat if other eye has damage. Otherwise, observe. Some authorities would treat if the risk factor(s) above exist.
4. Pressure ≥25 mm Hg and very narrow angles: consider laser iridotomy.

Box 2-4
Glaucoma Suspect Type IV

High Intraocular Pressure, Possible Damage

Peripheral anterior synechiae and narrow angles
Notch or local rim narrowing of optic nerve
Early arcuate scotoma or paracentral scotoma
Management: Generally, treat such eyes, especially if the other eye has damage, the patient has a strong family history, or the patient has a complicating ocular disease.

Box 2-5
Possible Glaucomatous Damage

Visual field
  Generalized depression
  Baring of blind spot
  Nasal step <10°
  Relative scotoma <5°
  Statistical field loss index P = 0.05-0.10
Visual function
  Reduced color vision
  Reduced temporal contrast sensitivity
  Abnormal pattern electroretinogram

Optic nerve head
  Cup:disc ratio >0.5
  Asymmetry of disc cups >0.2 cup:disc ratio
  Disc hemorrhage
  Disc pit
  Rim area <1.10 mm^2
  Vertically oval cup
  Diffuse or localized nerve fiber layer defect
Chamber angle
  Peripheral anterior synechiae

DETERMINING ADEQUACY OF TREATMENT

If the patient is treated, how does the ophthalmologist determine whether adequate treatment has been provided? In the future it may be possible to make the optic nerve more resistant to either pressure-related damage or non–pressure-related damage, or to treat directly the causes of non–pressure-related damage. Presently, our therapeutic tools only lower the patient's IOP. The real object, though, is to prevent or slow further structural or functional damage. Hence the first test of successful therapy is whether IOP has been lowered, but the ultimate test is whether progressive structural or functional damage has been prevented. Another issue of great importance is the patient's quality of life. If the natural course of the disease has been for the cupping to progress but not to interfere with the patient's important activities, then this must be weighed against any treatment plan that may seriously impair the patient's quality of life—whether through functional interference or financial drain.

IOP and its measurement are discussed in Chapter 5. One must remember, however, that it is difficult to know the patient's true pressure. In reality, it is measured infrequently—almost never at night or on Sunday, rarely after vigorous exercise or emotional upset, and never when the patient is sleeping. Thus the sample size of IOPs is quite small. For example, if pressure is measured for a period of 5 seconds once every 3 months, the sample is for only 5 seconds out of 7,776,000 seconds, giving a sample frequency of 0.0000643%. To make matters worse, the physician introduces bias into the sample by telling patients that they are going to be tested for the effect of the treatment prescribed by measuring their IOP when they return. Most patients want good test results, so naturally they use the medication on the day they are tested—even though they may not use it regularly at other times.[3,4]

The effect a given treatment has on IOP when only one eye is treated can be determined with reasonable certainty (see Chapter 22). The other eye acts as a control, although a modest "crossover" effect may be seen. Most glaucoma medications have some effect within 2 hours after administration, and this can be determined easily in a single office visit. Some medications take longer to be effective. Epinephrine derivatives may take as long as a month to show full effect, but their use is declining. β-blockers can produce a large immediate effect that diminishes over 4 to 6 weeks or, conversely, may require as much as a month for their full effect to develop. The effects on IOP of the α-adrenergic agonist, prostaglandins, topical carbonic anhydrase inhibitors, and cholinergic agents can usually be assessed within a few hours of using a drop. Laser trabeculoplasty typically necessitates 4 to 5 weeks to reach maximum effect. Surgically lowering pressure rarely produces stabilized effects before 1 month, so it may take a month or more to determine the treatment's effect on pressure. With medications, the physician can only assume that the pressure measured reflects what the medication can do to the IOP. It should never be assumed that the medications are being used regularly by the glaucoma patient.

A reasonable first goal in a younger patient with little damage is to lower the pressure at least 20% from the baseline IOP. Baseline pressure should be derived from at least two, and preferably more, measurements taken hours or days apart. Pressures can vary from hour to hour and day to day. The authors have seen patients with POAG undergoing baseline examinations before drug trials demonstrate a pressure variation of as much as 10 mm Hg within 1 hour. Thus pressure can fluctuate markedly just as with measurement of any biologic function. If feasible, a trial in one eye is useful. If after the appropriate period there is little effect on IOP in the treated eye as compared with the untreated eye, then either the treatment is not sufficient or the patient is not using it. Either way, the treatment is not successful.

It is not enough to lower IOP into the statistically normal range. Many patients continue to progress despite IOPs under 21 or 22 mm Hg. The physician should set a *target pressure* for each patient. The target pressure is a "best guess" level of IOP, below which further damage is unlikely to occur. The estimate is based on the initial level of IOP, degree of existing damage, age, and presence of other risk factors (see Chapter 22). Clinical experience and some statistical data support the concept that the more severe the existing optic nerve damage, the lower the IOP must be to prevent further deterioration.[5-8] Thus a patient with early damage may tolerate a pressure around 20 mm Hg, whereas a patient with advanced cupping and field loss may deteriorate unless the pressure is consistently below 16 mm Hg. Moreover, 20 mm Hg is considered "good" control for a patient with early damage and initial pressures of 30 mm Hg, but it is considered "poor" control for a patient with a cup:disc ratio of 0.9 and advanced visual field loss and whose pressures have never exceeded 23 mm Hg. The more risk factors and the greater the damage at the time of diagnosis, the lower the target pressure should be set. *As time goes on, the target pressure should be reassessed and lowered if progression of damage occurs.*

TREATMENT FOLLOW-UP

The initial efficacy of therapy is determined by its effect on IOP, but long-term efficacy must be determined by analysis of damage. Therefore it is essential to have good baseline studies of the factors to be followed, which most often are the visual field and the optic nerve head (Table 2-1). Careful and rigorous documentation of the initial status of these factors is essential to ensure accurate decisions regarding future therapy. Analysis of both is discussed in detail in subsequent chapters.

Once a therapy has been determined effective, how should the treatment be followed? Determining follow-up procedures depends on two factors—amount of damage and adequacy of pressure control. Guidelines for pressure control for long-term management of chronic open-angle glaucoma are presented in Table 2-2. These guidelines may not be applicable in all situations, and the physician must individualize each case. One must also remember that the IOP measured in the office is a minute sample size of the patient's pressure; the ultimate decisions affecting therapy rest on changes in the visual field or the optic nerve head.

DOCUMENTATION OF PROGRESS

Like any psychophysical test, visual fields fluctuate. Computerized perimetry quantifies this fluctuation, thereby offering advantages over manual techniques. Recognition of change in the visual field, however, is confounded by this fluctuation. To minimize confusion introduced by this fluctuation, a newly diagnosed glaucoma patient may require two or three field examinations in the first year of diagnosis to establish a firm baseline for future comparison. This concept is discussed in Chapter 10.

Table 2-1

Levels of Damage

	Disc	Visual Field
Mild	0.0-0.5 with uniform pink rim	None, mild depression, or slight defect
Moderate	0.6-0.7 with some local narrowing of rim	General depression, arcuate defect, or paracentral scotoma
Advanced	0.8-0.9 with rim narrowing or notching	Large arcuate, double arcuate, hemifield loss, or fixation threatened

Table 2-2

Guidelines for Level of Intraocular Pressure (mm Hg) Control Related to Damage Level*

| Control | Level of Damage | | |
	Mild	Moderate	Advanced
Good	<21	<18	<16
Uncertain	21-24	19-22	16-18
Uncontrolled	>25	>21	>18

*These guidelines are only estimates. The target pressures should be individualized. The more advanced the glaucoma, the older the patient, the greater the number of risk factors, and the greater the vascular component, the lower the target pressure should be. The more advanced the damage and the poorer the control, the more frequent the reevaluations must be. The fewer the number of risk factors and the less advanced the glaucoma, the more tolerant the optic nerve is likely to be of slightly elevated pressures. The better the control, the earlier the disease, and the fewer the number of risk factors, the less frequently the patient can be evaluated.

Table 2-3

Recommended Frequency of Visual Field Evaluation

Target Intraocular Pressure Achieved?	Progression of Damage	Duration of Control (Months)	Follow-Up Visual Field Interval (Months)
Yes	No	<6	4-12
Yes	No	>6	6-24
Yes	Yes	N/A	2-6
No	No	N/A	2-6
No	Yes	N/A	1-6

Modified from American Academy of Ophthalmology: *Primary open-angle glaucoma, preferred practice pattern,* San Francisco, American Academy of Ophthalmology, 1996.
N/A, Not applicable.

Photographs or other forms of imaging of the optic nerve are also invaluable in evaluating progression of the disease and should be taken at the initial examination and subsequently whenever change is suspected. Careful examination of the disc should be performed at least every 6 months and more frequently if the pressure is uncontrolled. Repeat photographs or imaging should occur every 1 to 3 years even if there does not appear to be any clinical change. Usually photographs or imaging techniques detect subtle changes before the clinician can do so. The frequency of IOP measurements should be related to the adequacy of control of the disease. If the disease has been stable for several years and the pressure constant, then follow-up examinations can be performed safely 1 to 3 times a year. If the pressure is high or the disease is newly diagnosed and the physician is unsure of the response to medications, visits may be scheduled weekly or monthly until the physician is certain that rapid worsening of damage will not occur. If the pressure is very high then more frequent visits may be necessary.

Pressure measurements are at best a guideline for the effectiveness of therapy. It is necessary to measure the visual field and/or fundus to know if the disease is truly controlled. In advanced disease with fixation threatened, it is reasonable to perform visual field examinations every 3 to 6 months, perhaps using a high-resolution test pattern, to detect the earliest sign of progression and start more aggressive therapy. Indeed, examinations less often than this make it difficult, if not impossible, to distinguish normal fluctuation of the test from pathologic change. In a patient with less severe damage whose IOP is well controlled, field examination once a year or so is sufficient. In glaucoma suspects, or in glaucoma patients with no visual field loss and well-controlled pressures, field examinations may be performed annually. One suggested schedule for the frequency of visual field follow-up is proposed by the American Academy of Ophthalmology's Preferred Practice Pattern for primary open-angle glaucoma (Table 2-3).

Newer tests such as red-free photography and laser-assisted imaging of the nerve fiber layer and image analysis of the optic nerve head also may be helpful in recognizing progression of the disease. The clinician can still provide sensitive and accurate determination of progression using a carefully performed clinical field examination supplemented with a clinical and photographic evaluation of the nerve head.

PATIENT EDUCATION

Because glaucoma is a chronic, lifelong condition with few debilitating symptoms, patient cooperation with follow-up and treatment is crucial to the success of management. Patients must be educated about their disease initially, then frequently during follow-up. Poor compliance with treatment is correlated with poor understanding of glaucoma and its long-term dangers.[4] Even with good patient education, compliance may be inadequate in as high as one third of patients.[4] Many brochures are now available that help the physician to describe glaucoma, treatment alternatives, and the advantages and disadvantages of such alternatives. Patients can also find information on the Internet, but the reliability of that information cannot always be confirmed. The physician should supplement any outside information with open discussion. Glaucoma support groups, where patients share their experiences, exist in some places and may be helpful.

Questions should be welcome. Many patients need constant encouragement and reeducation over the years. Patients should also be included in the therapeutic decision process because sometimes the major negative effect of glaucoma (especially early in the disease) may be from the treatment rather than the condition. Therapeutic goals and potential side effects and complications of each alternative of treatment should be discussed. Patient preferences should be sought.

Patients should be taught how to use eyedrops and about punctal occlusion and eyelid closure to minimize side effects. The treating physician should encourage each patient to discuss possible side effects and effects on quality of life. Patients may not associate systemic side effects with eyedrop therapy or may be reluctant to mention such delicate issues as impotence or decreased libido with a busy eye doctor. An atmosphere of openness and partnership should be established from the beginning.

EFFECTIVE JUDGMENT

Society is demanding more of physicians than ever before. In these days of cost containment and spiraling utilization of newer and better medical techniques, it is the physician's responsibility to provide excellent and efficient care for each patient. The pressures of outside influences, such as managed care organizations, should not prevent the most effective care—cost and efficiency are important but not the only considerations. By reducing the use of medical resources for those patients whose disease is well controlled and slowly (if at all) progressive, more resources can be directed toward patients whose conditions are uncontrolled or who face an imminent threat to their vision. It is a challenging but rewarding effort to tailor care to fit the patient's needs.

REFERENCES

1. Hoskins HD Jr: *Definition, classification and management of the glaucoma suspect. Proceedings from the New Orleans Academy of Ophthalmology Glaucoma Symposium,* St Louis, 1980, Mosby.
2. Sommer A, and others: Relationship between intraocular pressure and primary open angle glaucoma among white and black Americans. The Baltimore Eye Survey, *Arch Ophthalmol* 109:1090, 1991.
3. Kass MA: Compliance and prognosis in glaucoma, *Arch Ophthalmol* 103:504, 1985 (editorial).
4. Kass MA, and others: Compliance with topical timolol treatment, *Am J Ophthalmol* 103:188, 1987.
5. Richardson JT: *Medical and surgical decisions in chronic glaucomas.* In Heilman K, editor: *Glaucoma: conceptions of a disease,* Stuttgart, 1976, Thieme.
6. Chandler PA: Long-term results in glaucoma therapy, *Am J Ophthalmol* 49:221, 1960.
7. Abedin S, Simmons RJ, Grant WM: Progressive low-tension glaucoma: treatment to stop glaucomatous cupping and field loss when these progress despite normal intraocular pressure, *Ophthalmology* 89:1, 1982.
8. Glaucoma Laser Trial Research Group: The Glaucoma Laser Trial (GLT) and Glaucoma Laser Trial Follow-up Study: 7. Results, *Am J Ophthalmol* 120:718, 1995.

PART II

Aqueous Humor Dynamics

3

Aqueous Humor Formation

FUNCTION OF AQUEOUS HUMOR

Several risk factors probably contribute to damaging the optic nerve and concomitant visual loss in glaucoma. Intraocular pressure (IOP) that is too high for the continued health of the nerve is universally accepted as one of the most important of those risk factors. Therefore the study of those elements that contribute to the creation, maintenance, and variation of IOP is material to the understanding of the pathophysiology of this disease. Aqueous formation (F), facility of outflow (C), and episcleral venous pressure (P_v) are the major intraocular determinants of IOP. These factors are related to one another by the Goldmann equation,

$$P_0 = F/C + P_v$$

in which P_0 is the IOP in the undisturbed eye in mm Hg, aqueous formation is in μl/min, the facility of outflow is in μl/min/mm Hg, and the episcleral venous pressure is in mm Hg. From the equation it is evident that IOP will increase when the aqueous formation rate increases, the episcleral venous pressure increases, or the outflow facility decreases.

Aqueous humor was originally thought to be stagnant. It was not until 1921 that Seidel proved that the aqueous was, indeed, circulating. Using a needle, Seidel connected a reservoir containing a blue dye to a rabbit eye. When the reservoir was lowered, clear fluid from the anterior chamber entered the tubing; when the reservoir was raised, the dye entered the eye and eventually appeared in the blood of the episcleral venous plexus.[1,2] Seidel concluded that aqueous humor must be continuously formed and drained. Two decades later, Ascher showed that aqueous humor enters the venous system at the limbus through the aqueous veins and first flows alongside the blood stream in a laminar fashion before mixing completely with the blood in the veins.[3] Ashton studied neoprene casts of Schlemm's canal and the aqueous veins and demonstrated a direct connection between these two structures.[4] From the work of the last half century it is clear that aqueous humor is a relatively cell-free, protein-free fluid that is formed by the ciliary body epithelium in the posterior chamber. It then passes between the iris and the lens, enters the anterior chamber through the pupil, and exits the eye at the anterior chamber angle through the trabecular meshwork, Schlemm's canal, and the aqueous veins. In the anterior chamber, the aqueous humor is subject to thermal currents because of the temperature difference between the iris and the cornea.

During its passage through the eye, the aqueous humor serves a number of important functions. It serves in lieu of a vascular system for the avascular structures of the eye, including the cornea, lens, and trabecular meshwork. It brings to the eye essential nutrients, such as oxygen, glucose, and amino acids,[5] and removes metabolites and potentially toxic substances, such as lactic acid and carbon dioxide.[6,7] It inflates the globe and maintains IOP, both of which are important for the structural and optical integrity of the eye. In many species, including humans, aqueous humor contains a very high concentration of ascorbate, which may act to scavenge free radicals and protect the eye against the effects of ultraviolet and other radiation. Under adverse conditions (e.g., inflammation, infection), it facilitates cellular and humoral immune responses. During inflammation, the rate of aqueous humor formation decreases, and its composition is altered to permit accumulation of immune mediators. Aqueous humor provides the proper chemical environment for the tissues of the eye and provides an optically clear medium to allow good visual function.

ANATOMY OF THE CILIARY BODY

Structure

The ciliary body is the portion of the uveal tract that lies between the iris and the choroid (Fig. 3-1). On cross-section the ciliary body has the shape of a right triangle. It is attached anteriorly to the scleral spur, creating a potential space (supraciliary space) between itself and the sclera. The iris inserts into the short anterior side of the ciliary body, leaving a narrow width of ciliary face visible on gonioscopy between the peripheral iris and the scleral spur. The lens is attached to the ciliary body by the zonules, which separate the vitreous compartment posteriorly from the aqueous compartment anteriorly (Fig. 3-2). The iris in turn divides the aqueous space into the posterior and anterior chambers. The junction of the iris, sclera, and cornea is called the anterior chamber angle.

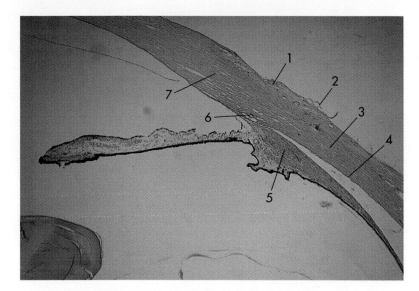

Figure 3-1 Light micrograph of the anterior segment of the eye showing *1,* Tenon's capsule; *2,* episclera; *3,* sclera; *4,* lamina fusca; *5,* ciliary body; *6,* Schlemm's canal; and *7,* peripheral cornea. (Courtesy of William H. Spencer, M.D.)

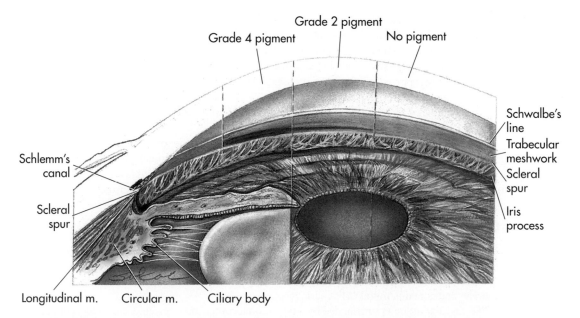

Figure 3-2 Schematic view of the zonules separating the vitreous cavity from the posterior chamber and the iris separating the anterior and posterior chambers.

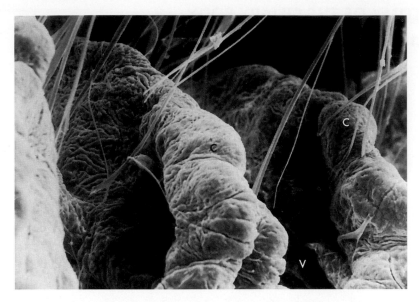

Figure 3-3   Scanning electron micrograph of the ciliary processes *(C)* showing the valleys *(V)* and the zonular insertions (× 155). (From Tripathi RC, Tripathi BJ: *Anatomy of the human eye, orbit, and adnexa.* In Davson H, editor: *The eye, vegetative physiology and biochemistry,* vol 1A, ed 3, New York, 1984, Academic Press.)

The ciliary body is composed of muscle, vascular tissue, and epithelium. The ciliary muscle consists of three separate muscles—the longitudinal (meridional), the oblique (radial or intermediate), and the circular (sphincteric). The longitudinal muscle attaches anteriorly to the scleral spur and trabecular meshwork and posteriorly to the suprachoroidal lamina, with some fibers connecting to the choroid and sclera as far posteriorly as the equator of the globe. When the longitudinal muscle contracts, it pulls open the trabecular meshwork and Schlemm's canal. The circular muscle fibers run parallel to the limbus. When these fibers contract they relax the zonules, allowing the lens to change shape. The radial muscle connects the longitudinal and circular muscles. The function of the radial muscle is not entirely clear, but it is postulated that contraction of the radial fibers may widen the uveal trabecular spaces.

The ciliary body runs from the scleral spur to the ora serrata, a distance of approximately 6 mm (see Fig. 3-1). The posterior portion of the ciliary body has a relatively flat inner surface and is named the pars plana. The anterior portion of the ciliary body has approximately 70 to 80 radial ridges (the ciliary processes) on its inner surface and is named the pars plicata (Fig. 3-3). The ciliary processes are approximately 2 mm in length, 0.5 mm in width, and 0.9 mm in height.[8] The surface area of the pars plicata is estimated to be 5.7 cm² in rabbits[9] and 6 cm² in humans.[10] Thus the pars plicata has a large surface area (approximately 5 times the surface area of the corneal endothelium) for both active fluid transport and ultrafiltration.

Because of the invagination of the embryonic optic vesicle, the inner surfaces of both the pars plana and the pars plicata are lined by two layers of epithelium—an outer pigmented layer that is continuous with the retinal pigment epithelium, and an inner nonpigmented layer that is continuous with the retina (Fig. 3-4). The two layers of the epithelium have their apical surfaces in apposition.

Ultrastructure of the Ciliary Processes

Each ciliary process is composed of a central core of stroma and capillaries covered by a double layer of epithelium (Fig. 3-4, *B*).[11] The capillary endothelium is thin and has tiny fenestrae that face toward the pigmented ciliary epithelium. The capillary endothelium is surrounded by a basement membrane that contains mural cells (pericytes).

The vascular tissue is surrounded by a thin stroma composed of ground substance, collagen fibrils, and occasional wandering cells. The ground substance contains mucopolysaccharides, protein, and a solute of plasma.

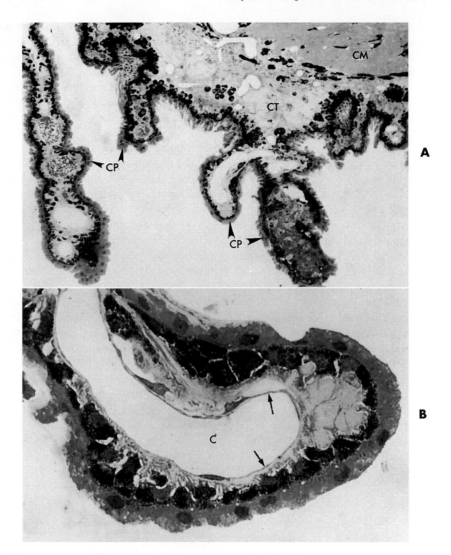

Figure 3-4 **A,** Light micrograph of the ciliary processes *(CP),* with connective tissue stroma *(CT)* between the ciliary muscle *(CM)* and the two epithelial layers. The vessels extend into the processes, and the stroma also contains melanocytes and fibroblasts. (× 197.) **B,** Extension of the vessel layer into the ciliary process. The beaded appearance *(arrows)* of the thin endothelial lining of the capillary *(C)* is due to ultramicroscopic fenestrations increasing capillary permeability for the formation of aqueous humor. (Photomicrograph; × 800.) The pigmented and nonpigmented epithelial layers are demonstrated. (From Tripathi RC, Tripathi BJ: *Anatomy of the human eye, orbit, and adnexa.* In Davson H, editor: *The eye, vegetative physiology and biochemistry,* vol 1A, ed 3, New York, 1984, Academic Press.)

The pigmented epithelium is composed of low cuboidal cells with numerous cytoplasmic melanin granules (Fig. 3-5). This layer is separated from the stroma by an atypical basement membrane, a continuation of Bruch's membrane containing collagen and elastic fibers. The function of the pigmented epithelium is not entirely clear. The basal portion of this layer has a great number of infoldings and mitochondria, suggesting a role in active metabolic processes. The cytoplasm and cell membrane of the pigmented epithelial cells stain for the presence of carbonic anhydrase.[12]

The nonpigmented epithelial layer is composed of columnar cells, which are separated from the aqueous humor by a basement membrane. The nonpigmented ciliary epithelium has the morphologic features of a tissue involved in fluid transport, including extensive infoldings in the basal and lateral membranes, numerous mitochondria, well-developed rough endoplasmic reticulum, and tight junctions connecting adjacent apical cell membranes (see Fig. 3-5). In addition, sodium potassium adenosine triphosphatase (Na^+K^+ ATPase) is found near the lateral infoldings of the membranes. Rows of vesicles are seen near the free surface of the epithelium and were called pinocytotic vesicles in the past. It now appears that these vesicles are a fixation artifact.[13]

The potential space between the two epithelial layers is called the ciliary channel. One group of investigators postulates that aqueous humor is secreted into this space, particularly after stimulation of the system with various agents, such as β-adrenergic agonists.[14] This theory requires further study.

Adjacent cells within each epithelial layer and the apical surfaces of the two layers are connected by gap junctions, puncta adherentia, and desmosomes.[15-17] Gap junctions are low-resistance pathways that provide electrical coupling of cells and facilitate transport of ions from one cell to another.[15,16] Puncta adherentia and desmosomes are structural supports between cell membranes. The nonpigmented ciliary epithelial cells are also joined at their apical membranes by tight junctions (zonulae occludentae), which are thought to be an important component of the blood–aqueous barrier.[18-25] Tracers injected into the ciliary body pass through the stroma and the clefts between the pigmented epithelial cells until they reach the apical cell membranes of the nonpigmented ciliary epithelium, where they are restricted by the tight junctions. However, these tight junctions are permeable to low molecular weight polar solutes.

There is considerable evidence that aqueous humor is produced in the anterior portion of the ciliary processes. The anterior portion of the nonpigmented ciliary epithelium has morphologic features that indicate active fluid transport, including increased basal and lateral interdigitations, numerous mitochondria, and a well-developed rough endoplasmic reticulum. The epithelium is supplied by a rich capillary network with numerous fenestrations.[15] With a gonioprism, systemically administered fluorescein can be observed entering the posterior chamber at the tips of the ciliary processes.[26] Finally, the nonpigmented ciliary epithelium, especially in the region of the lateral interdigitations, shows evidence of abundant Na^+K^+ ATPase, considerable activity for glycolytic enzymes,[27] and a high rate of incorporation of labeled sulfate into macromolecules, such as glycolipids and glycoproteins.[28,29]

Many nerve terminals are seen in the connective tissue adjacent to the pigmented epithelium,[30]

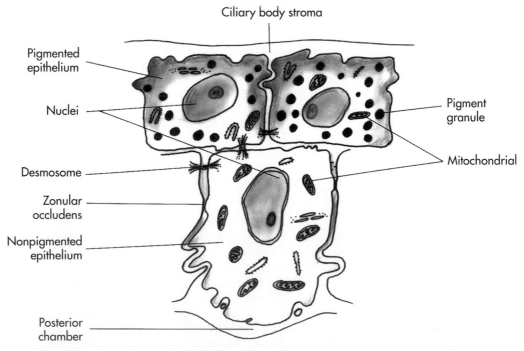

Figure 3-5   Schematic view of nonpigmented and pigmented ciliary epithelium. (Modified from Shields MB: *Textbook of glaucoma,* ed 2, Baltimore, 1987, Williams & Wilkins.)

but they do not appear to penetrate the basal lamina and reach the nonpigmented epithelium. These terminals appear to arise from sympathetic and parasympathetic fibers. In addition, the nonpigmented ciliary epithelial cells have β-adrenergic and cholinergic receptors.[31,32] The function of these receptors and nerve terminals is not clear.

Vascular Supply

The long posterior ciliary arteries arise as trunks from the ophthalmic artery, pierce the globe near the optic nerve, and run forward to the ciliary body, where they anastomose to form the major arterial circle (Fig. 3-6). The anterior ciliary arteries also contribute to the major circle, but to a lesser extent than the long posterior ciliary arteries.[33] Several precapillary arterioles branch from the major arterial circle to supply each ciliary process. These arterioles have sphincters that may play a role in regulating blood supply and aqueous humor formation. The precapillary arterioles break up into plexuses of tortuous vessels within each ciliary process. The vessels collect and flow into choroidal and pars plana veins, which then flow into the vortex system. Some drainage also occurs via the intrascleral veins to the episcleral veins.

The ciliary body has a very high blood flow, estimated to be 81 μl/min in the monkey eye and, by calculation, 154 μl/min in humans.[34,35] In cats, venous blood from the anterior uvea is only 4% to 5% less saturated with oxygen than is arterial blood.[36] This indicates that oxygen consumption is not a limiting factor in aqueous humor formation under normal conditions. The rate of plasma flow to the ciliary processes in rabbits is at least 50 μl/min.[37] If the rate of aqueous production is assumed to be 2 to 4 μl/min, the formation of aqueous humor removes only 4% to 8% of the volume of plasma available to the ciliary processes.[38] Thus a modest reduction in the rate of plasma flow to the ciliary processes would not be expected to decrease aqueous humor formation substantially. However, it is probable that profound vasoconstriction would have an effect on aqueous production.

The ciliary processes of many species, including primates, appear to have limited autoregulation of their blood supply. In general, the vascular responses of the ciliary processes are similar to

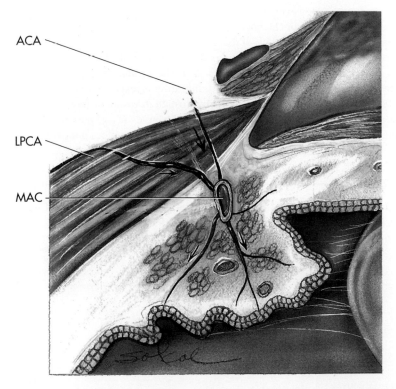

Figure 3-6 Blood supply to anterior segment of the eye. *LPCA,* Long posterior ciliary artery; *ACA,* anterior ciliary artery; *MAC,* major arterial circle.

those of the choroid but dissimilar to those of the iris and retina.[38,39] Vasodilation of the ciliary blood vessels is seen following administration of carbon dioxide,[40,41] application of prostaglandins,[42-45] paracentesis,[46,47] and parasympathetic stimulation.[34] Vasoconstriction in the anterior uveal tract vessels occurs after stimulation of α-adrenergic nerves.[48-50]

MECHANISM OF AQUEOUS FORMATION

The formation of aqueous humor is a complex process that involves ultrafiltration and diffusional exchange of water and solutes with the plasma from blood flowing through the ciliary processes. Active transport of substances from this dialysate of plasma into the posterior chamber then occurs. The fluid is further changed by diffusional exchange and active transport of substances out of the eye as it bathes other tissues, such as the lens, cornea, iris, and trabecular meshwork. It has been known for a long time that aqueous humor is not a simple dialysate of plasma; the concentrations of many of the elements of the aqueous humor differ from those that would be expected if ultrafiltration and passive diffusion were the only processes. The Gibbs-Donnan equilibrium describes the concentration of substances in a dialysate; Table 3-1 contrasts the actual concentration of various solutes in the aqueous humor with that found in a simple dialysate.[51] Each of the processes involved in aqueous formation is discussed.

Ultrafiltration

More than twice the weight of the ciliary processes themselves (or about 150 ml) of blood flows through the ciliary processes each minute.[35] As blood passes through the capillaries of the ciliary processes, about 4% of the plasma filters through the fenestrations in the capillary wall into the interstitial spaces between the capillaries and the ciliary epithelium.[38] The process by which a fluid and its solutes cross a semipermeable membrane under a pressure gradient (e.g., capillary blood pressure) is called ultrafiltration. In the case of the ciliary body, fluid movement is favored by the hydrostatic pressure difference between the capillary pressure and the interstitial fluid pressure (IOP) and is resisted by the difference between the oncotic pressure of the plasma and the aqueous humor. The rate of protein leakage through the vessel walls into the tissue space of the ciliary processes is relatively low.[38,52] However, the ciliary epithelial layers are even less permeable to the passage of colloids into the posterior chamber. Thus the colloid concentration in the tissue space of the ciliary processes is approximately 75% of that in plasma.[52-55] The high concentration of colloids in the tissue space of the ciliary processes favors the movement of water from the plasma into the ciliary stroma but retards the movement of water from the stroma into the posterior chamber. Although a few investigators have postulated that ultrafiltration is responsible for the majority of aqueous humor formation,[56-59] is it unlikely that the hydrostatic pressure difference between the ciliary capillaries and the posterior chamber can overcome the large oncotic pressure differential. Furthermore, a theory that proposes a predominant role for ultrafiltration does not explain why active ion trans-

Table 3-1 ─────────────────────────────────

**Actual Concentration of Various Solutes in Aqueous Humor of Rabbit
As Compared With Values of Dialysate of Plasma**

Substance	Aqueous Humor Concentration / Plasma Concentration	Concentration in Dialysate / Concentration in Plasma
Na^+	0.96	0.945
K^+	0.955	0.96
Mg^{++}	0.78	0.80
Ca^{++}	0.58	0.65
Cl^-	1.015	1.04
HCO_3^-	1.26	1.04
Glucose	0.86	0.97

Modified from Davson H: *Physiology of the ocular and cerebrospinal fluids*, London, 1966, J & A Churchill

port inhibitors such as ouabain are capable of reducing aqueous humor formation by 70% to 80%. Thus ultrafiltration helps to move fluid out of the capillaries into the stroma but alone is insufficient to account for the volume of fluid moved into the posterior chamber. The latter step requires an active metabolic process. Ultrafiltration and active secretion occur in tandem.[60]

Active Transport

Active transport (secretion) is an energy-dependent process that selectively moves a substance against its electrochemical gradient across a cell membrane. It is postulated that the majority of aqueous humor formation depends on an ion or ions being actively secreted into the intercellular clefts of the non-pigmented ciliary epithelium beyond the tight junctions (Fig. 3-7). This process is accomplished by about a million nonpigmented epithelial cells, each of which secretes aqueous humor equal to about one third of its own intracellular volume per minute.[35] In the small spaces between the epithelial cells, the secreted ion or ions create sufficient osmotic forces to attract water. By the time the newly secreted fluid reaches the posterior chamber, the osmotic driving force has been nearly dissipated.[18,61,62]

It is not clear which ion or ions are actively transported across the nonpigmented ciliary epithelium, though most theories include sodium, chloride, or bicarbonate (Table 3-2). Electrophysiologic studies of the isolated ciliary epithelium indicate that the transepithelial potential difference and the short circuit current, indicators of ion transport across membranes, are dependent on Na^+ and HCO_3^-.[63,64] A number of investigators postulate that the active transport of the sodium ion is the key process in aqueous humor formation.[7,65,66] This theory is supported by the observation that membrane-bound ouabain-sensitive Na^+K^+ ATPase (the enzyme that facilitates transport of potassium into, and sodium out of, cells) is found in the nonpigmented ciliary epithelium of many different species.[19,24,67-69] Furthermore, ouabain inhibition of Na^+K^+ ATPase decreases aqueous humor formation by 70% to 80%.[70] Enough Na^+ and K^+ ATPase activity is present in the ciliary nonpigmented epithelium to drive aqueous humor formation mainly by the sodium gradient.[67]

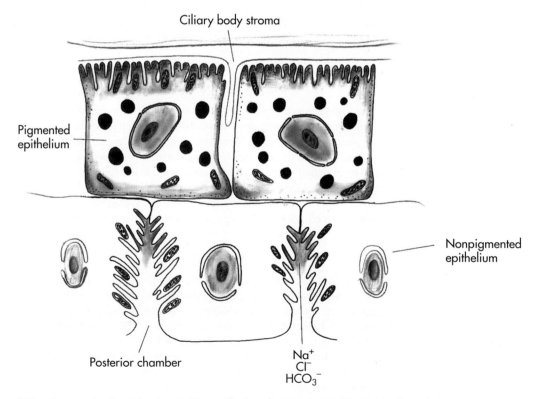

Figure 3-7 Pigmented and nonpigmented ciliary epithelium. Ions are secreted into intercellular clefts of the nonpigmented epithelial cells. The ions create sufficient osmotic force to attract water. (Modified from Lutjen-Drecoll E: *Morphologic basis for aqueous humor formation.* In Drance SM, Neufeld AH: *Glaucoma: applied pharmacology in medical treatment,* New York, 1984, Grune & Stratton.)

Table 3-2

Composition of Anterior and Posterior Chamber Aqueous Humor In Rabbit and Man

Substance (nM/kg H_2O)	Rabbits*			Humans†	
	Anterior Chamber Aqueous Humor	Posterior Chamber Aqueous Humor	Plasma	Anterior Chamber Aqueous Humor	Plasma
Na^+	145	144	146	163	176
Cl^-	105	105	112	126	117
HCO_3^-	28	34	24	22	26
pH	7.60	7.57	7.40	7.21	7.40
Ascorbate	0.96	1.30	0.02	0.92	0.06

*Modified from Kinsey VE, Reddy DVN: *Chemistry and dynamics of aqueous humor.* In Prince JH, editor: *The rabbit in eye research,* Springfield, Ill, 1966, Charles C Thomas.

†Modified from Becker B: Chemical composition of human aqueous humor: effects of acetazolamide, *Arch Ophthalmol* 57:793, 1957, American Medical Association.

Table 3-3

Effect of Acetazolamide on Composition of Anterior Chamber Aqueous Humor*

Substance	Human		Rabbit	
	Before	After	Before	After
Cl^-	1.08	1.02	0.94	0.96
H^+	1.52	1.30	0.70	0.89
HCO_3^-	0.83	0.94	1.35	1.11
Ascorbate	15	18	44	52

Modified from Becker B: Chemical composition of human aqueous humor: effects of acetazolamide, *Arch Ophthalmol* 57:793, 1957, American Medical Association.

*Expressed as a ratio of anterior chamber concentration to plasma concentration.

For many years investigators believed that the bicarbonate ion could not be actively secreted into the aqueous humor of the primate eye because the posterior chamber bicarbonate concentration is lower than the plasma concentration. However, more recent investigations indicate that bicarbonate is actually present in excess in newly formed posterior chamber aqueous humor.[71] Bicarbonate appears to be in deficit in the aqueous humor because the fluid that is usually sampled has undergone metabolism and diffusional exchange with surrounding tissue. Carbonic anhydrase type II (isoenzyme C)[72,73] is present in the cell membrane and cytoplasm of the nonpigmented and pigmented epithelium of the ciliary body. This enzyme catalyzes the following reaction:

$$\overset{C.A.}{CO_2 + OH^- \leftrightharpoons HCO_3^-}$$

Drugs that inhibit carbonic anhydrase, such as acetazolamide and methazolamide, decrease both the rate of entry of bicarbonate into newly formed aqueous humor[74] and the rate of entry of water into the posterior chamber. The carbonic anhydrase inhibitors, when given orally or parenterally, also produce systemic acidosis, which further decreases aqueous formation.[75] Following carbonic anhydrase inhibition, anterior chamber concentrations of Cl^-, H^+, and HCO_3^- more closely resemble plasma values (Table 3-3). On the other hand, the concentration of ascorbate rises with carbonic anhydrase inhibition because its active pump is not linked to carbonic anhydrase and because the rate of aqueous formation is diminished. Some investigators have postulated that carbonic anhydrase plays an indirect role in aqueous humor formation by providing hydrogen or bicarbonate ions for an intracellular buffering system.[76] Although this theory has been discussed widely, it has not been substantiated directly (Table 3-3). There is also evidence that the chloride ion is actively transported into the posterior chamber. Chloride secretion is affected by pH and the concentration of Na^+.[77,78] It is quite possible that the active transport of sodium, chloride, and bicarbonate ions is linked in some way.

Diffusion

Diffusion is the movement of a substance across a membrane along its concentration gradient. As the aqueous humor passes from the posterior chamber to Schlemm's canal, it is in contact with the ciliary body, iris, lens, vitreous, cornea, and trabecular meshwork. There is sufficient diffusional exchange with the surrounding tissues, so that the anterior chamber aqueous humor resembles plasma more closely than does the posterior chamber aqueous humor (see Table 3-2).[79] Aqueous humor provides glucose, amino acids, oxygen, and potassium to surrounding tissues and removes carbon dioxide, lactate, and pyruvate.

CHEMICAL COMPOSITION OF THE AQUEOUS HUMOR

It is difficult to obtain aqueous humor samples, particularly posterior chamber samples, from human eyes. Accordingly, most of our knowledge about the composition of the aqueous humor is based on animal studies, particularly studies of the rabbit. It is important to emphasize that there are substantial differences among species, as indicated in Table 3-2. For example, the aqueous humor concentration of ascorbate in the rabbit eye is 18 times higher than the plasma concentration. In contrast, there is no substantial accumulation of ascorbate in the aqueous humor of the rat.

The entry of various substances into the eye depends on a number of factors, including molecular size, electrical charge, and lipid solubility. Large molecules, such as proteins, penetrate the eye poorly. The capillaries of the ciliary body are permeable to proteins, but the nonpigmented ciliary epithelium and the capillaries of the iris are not. Thus the overall entry of protein into the aqueous humor is rather low. The concentration of protein in the aqueous humor of the human eye is approximately 0.02%, whereas protein concentration in plasma is 7%. Smaller proteins, such as albumin, are present in higher concentration than the larger proteins, such as IgD, IgA, and IgM.[80] The concentration of protein leaving the eye via Schlemm's canal is quite low, suggesting that a substantial portion of the protein must exit with the uveoscleral flow.[38,55,81 84]

Smaller, water-soluble molecules (e.g., creatinine, sucrose, urea) are not restricted by the capillaries of the ciliary body but are somewhat limited by the nonpigmented ciliary epithelium. The entry of these molecules is inversely related to their size and electrical charge.

Lipid-soluble molecules (e.g., ethanol) pass readily through the nonpigmented ciliary epithelium. It is thought that lipid-soluble molecules pass through lipid portions of membranes in proportion to the concentration gradient across the membrane. Thus lipid-soluble substances move primarily by diffusion, whereas water-soluble molecules move by ultrafiltration and secretion.

A number of substances enter the eye by facilitated transport. In the previous section it was established that Na^+, Cl^-, and HCO_3^- are thought to be actively transported into the intercellular clefts of the nonpigmented ciliary epithelium, resulting in osmotic-driven fluid flow. In addition, a number of other water-soluble substances of larger size or greater electrical charge are thought to be actively transported into the eye, including some sugars, ascorbate, and some amino acids.

Moreover, a number of transport systems actively move substances out of the eye. One system is similar to the organic anion transport mechanism of the renal tubule. This system transports large anions—such as paraminohippurate (PAH), phenolsulfonphthalein, fluorescein, penicillin, prostaglandins, glucuronides, and sulfates—out of the posterior chamber. The system is inhibited by probenecid and bromcresol green.[85-87] A second system transports iodide compounds out of the posterior chamber. This system is inhibited by perchlorate and thiocyanate.[88-90] There is some disagreement about whether there is a third transport system for iodipamide and related compounds.[91-93] These systems all demonstrate the common properties of facilitated transport, including saturation, Michaelis Menten kinetics, and competitive inhibition. It is postulated that these ocular transport systems prevent the accumulation of toxic substances in the eye. For example, ocular tissues have limited ability to metabolize prostaglandins, so an active transport system in the ciliary body and retina is necessary to prevent accumulation of these potentially toxic compounds.[94,95] The aqueous humor concentrations of many important substances are given in Table 3-2.

Sodium. Most of the sodium in the aqueous humor enters the eye by active transport either primarily or linked to bicarbonate.[96,97] This is an energy-dependent process that is facilitated by Na^+K^+ ATPase.[64,98] A lesser amount of sodium enters the eye by ultrafiltration or diffusion. The aqueous humor sodium concentration is not closely linked to the plasma sodium concentration.[99]

Chloride. Chloride is actively transported into the aqueous humor. This process seems to depend on pH and the concentration of sodium.[77,78]

Potassium. Potassium enters the eye by active secretion and diffusion.[100] Some potassium is taken up by the lens.

Ascorbic acid. Ascorbic acid is actively transported into the eye against a large concentration gradient.[79,101]

Amino acids. Some amino acids are present in the aqueous humor in low concentration and some in high concentration when compared with plasma.[102] It is thought that there are at least three different active transport mechanisms for neutral, basic, and acidic (dicarboxylic) amino acids.[5]

Bicarbonate. Bicarbonate is actively transported into the posterior chamber of the human eye[71] either primarily or linked to sodium. It is thought that some bicarbonate is lost by diffusion to the vitreous and some is decomposed into carbon dioxide.

Glucose. The concentration of glucose in the aqueous humor is relatively low because most of it is lost to the vitreous or taken up by the lens and cornea.[87]

Phosphate. The concentration of phosphate in the aqueous humor is relatively low because it is incorporated into a number of active molecules.

Pyruvate and lactate. The concentrations of pyruvate and lactate are relatively high, presumably because of glycolytic activity by avascular tissues such as the lens and the cornea.[103]

THE BLOOD–AQUEOUS BARRIER

The blood–aqueous barrier consists of all of the barriers to the movement of substances from the plasma to the aqueous humor. For example, in the ciliary body the barriers include the vascular endothelium, basement membrane, stroma, and pigmented and nonpigmented epithelium. Although all of the structures participate in the blood–aqueous barrier, the tight junctions (zonae occludentes) connecting the apical portions of adjacent nonpigmented epithelial cells in the ciliary processes have been most often implicated as the actual site of the barrier.[58,104] These junctions are not as "tight" as their name would imply—in that they do allow passage of some small ions and water.[105] The blood–aqueous barrier is responsible for maintaining the differences in chemical composition between the plasma and the aqueous humor.

Many endogenous and exogenous stimuli increase the permeability of the epithelia and vascular endothelium (i.e., break the blood–aqueous barrier), producing an increase in aqueous humor protein concentration (Box 3-1). In some cases this increase is accompanied by pupillary miosis and an accumulation of white blood cells. The breach of the barrier often is accompanied by a transient rise in IOP, which is then followed by a period of prolonged hypotonia.

Box 3-1
Stimuli That Break Down the Blood–Aqueous Barrier

Trauma
  Mechanical injury of iris or lens
  Contusion
  Paracentesis
Chemical irritants
  Nitrogen mustard
  Formaldehyde
  Acid
  Alkali
Neural activity
  Stimulation of trigeminal nerve
Immunogenic activity
  Bovine serum albumin

Endogenous mediators
  Histamine
  Bradykinin
  Prostaglandins and other eicosanoids
  Serotonin
  Acetylcholine
Miscellaneous
  Bacterial endotoxins
  X radiation
  Infrared radiations
  Laser energy
  Alpha melanocyte-stimulating hormone

Modified from Eakins KE: Prostaglandin and non-prostaglandin mediated breakdown of the blood–aqueous barrier, *Exp Eye Res* 25(suppl):483, 1977.

In some situations (e.g., intraocular infection) a breakdown of the blood–aqueous barrier is clearly therapeutic because it brings mediators of cellular and humoral immunity to the interior of the eye. In other situations (e.g., some forms of uveitis and following trauma) the breakdown of the barrier is inappropriate and favors the development of complications, such as cataract and synechia formation.

There appear to be multiple mechanisms for compromise of the blood–aqueous barrier. One important mechanism is mediated by prostaglandins. This system is activated by a variety of stimuli, including paracentesis, and is blocked by nonsteroidal antiinflammatory agents such as aspirin and indomethacin. Another important mechanism is mediated by sensory innervation and neural peptides, including substance P. This system is activated by a variety of stimuli (e.g., topical nitrogen mustard) and is blocked by retrobulbar lidocaine and capsaicin.[106]

When the blood–aqueous barrier is broken, protein-rich fluid collects in cysts beneath and between the epithelial cells of the ciliary body. The contents of these cysts eventually burst into the posterior chamber.[104,107,108] Protein-rich fluid also enters the eye via reflux from Schlemm's canal in some situations.[109,110]

RATE OF AQUEOUS HUMOR FORMATION AND MEASUREMENT TECHNIQUES

Many investigators have measured the rate of aqueous humor formation in humans with a variety of techniques. Despite the different techniques used, the majority of studies find a rate of aqueous humor formation of 2 to 3 μl/min (Table 3-4). The techniques for measuring aqueous humor formation can be divided into two major categories: (1) pressure-dependent methods that use volumetric analysis of the eye and (2) tracer methods that monitor the rate of appearance or disappearance of various substances from the eye.

Pressure-Dependent Techniques

The theoretical background of the pressure-dependent methods is considered in more detail in the next chapter, but it can be summarized briefly as follows. When fluid is introduced into a closed system, there is an immediate rise in the pressure within the system. In the case of the eye, if fluid is injected into the globe, there is a rise in IOP, the magnitude of which depends on many factors, including the distensibility of the ocular coats. If the relationship between the volume of fluid injected and the change in IOP is known, it is possible to consider the reverse situation—that is, the relationship between the decline in IOP and the volume of fluid leaving the eye. If IOP is elevated by artificial means (e.g., placing a weight on the eye), the decline in IOP over time is a measure of the loss of fluid (e.g., egress of aqueous humor) from the eye under the condition of increased pressure. This is a measure of the facility of outflow, and after an assumption about the level of the episcleral venous pressure, the rate of aqueous humor formation can be calculated from the Goldmann equation. It should be stressed that all of the pressure-dependent methods calculate the rate of aqueous formation rather than measure it directly. On the other hand, most of them have the advantage of being able to be performed on the eye *in vivo* without significant risk.

Table 3-4

Rate of Aqueous Humor Flow in Human Eyes

Investigator	Subjects (n)	Mean ± SD Aqueous Flow (μl/min)	Technique
Bloom and others[137]	19	2.8 ± 0.6	Fluorescein iontophoresis
Coakes and Brubaker[141]	20	2.9 ± 0.4	Fluorescein iontophoresis
Brubaker and others*	113	2.4 ± 0.6	Fluorescein iontophoresis
McLaren and Brubaker†	300	2.8 ± 0.6	Fluorescein iontophoresis

*From Brubaker RF, and others: The effect of age on aqueous humor formation in man, *Ophthalmology* 88:283, 1981.
†From McLaren JW, Brubaker RF: A scanning ocular fluorophotometer, *Invest Ophthalmol Vis Sci* 29:1285, 1988.

Tonography

The most commonly used pressure-dependent method is tonography, which is based on the old observation that IOP declines when the eye is massaged. For this technique a weight such as a Schiotz tonometer is placed on the cornea to produce a sudden rise in IOP, which then declines over time. The rate at which the IOP declines over time is related to the facility of outflow. This value and the IOP in the undisturbed eye can be used to calculate the rate of aqueous formation.[111-113]

There are a number of problems inherent to tonography, such as difficulties in performing the technique and in calibrating the equipment. Furthermore, a number of assumptions must be made about the response of the eye to an acute elevation in IOP, including the displacement of fluid, the elastic properties of the eye, the ocular blood volume, the rate of aqueous humor formation, and the level of episcleral venous pressure. Despite these problems tonography has been used widely to estimate the rate of aqueous humor formation and seems to correlate reasonably well with other techniques. A full discussion of tonography and the other pressure-dependent methods is included in Chapter 4.

Suction Cup

One pressure-dependent method uses a suction cup, which is applied to the sclera with a vacuum 50 mm Hg below atmospheric pressure.[114-117] This occludes intrascleral and episcleral venous drainage and raises IOP. The rate of aqueous humor formation is then calculated from the rise in IOP following occlusion or from the rate of fall in IOP after the device is removed from the eye. This method suffers from many of the same problems as tonography.

Perfusion

It is possible to estimate aqueous humor production by measuring outflow facility with a perfusion apparatus.[118] This technique has its greatest use in animal eyes and enucleated human eyes but can be done preoperatively. After a needle is inserted into the eye, the pressure-flow relationships are determined by perfusing the anterior chamber at a known rate and measuring the resultant IOP. Alternatively, the anterior chamber can be perfused at a known pressure to determine the flow through the eye. When the rate of fluid inflow from the apparatus is plotted against the perfusion pressure (pressure in the perfusion line minus IOP), the facility of outflow can be determined, and the rate of aqueous humor formation can be calculated. Obviously, this technique is only suitable for eyes that are going to be operated on or enucleated anyway and are therefore not normal eyes.

Tracer Methods

There are a number of techniques described for measuring aqueous humor flow that do not alter IOP. Generally these approaches measure the rate of appearance or disappearance of various tracers from the anterior chamber. Thus these techniques actually measure the rate of aqueous humor flow through the anterior chamber rather than the rate of aqueous formation. Any aqueous humor formed in the posterior chamber and passing posteriorly to the vitreous and retina would not be detected by these approaches. Despite this limitation it is thought that the tracer techniques are more accurate than the pressure-dependent techniques because the globe and IOP are not altered.

Photogrammetry

The anterior-chamber aqueous humor is stained with fluorescein applied topically or using iontophoresis. Newly formed aqueous humor appears as a clear bubble emerging from the posterior chamber into the fluorescein-stained anterior chamber. The volume of the bubble can be estimated by projecting a series of light stripes onto the bubble and photographing them. By mathematically integrating the area under the stripes, a reasonably accurate measure of the volume may be obtained. The rate of change in the size of the bubble is estimated from sequential photographs and is a measure of the rate of aqueous humor formation.[119,120] This is an accurate technique but necessitates the administration of parasympathomimetic drugs to produce a miotic pupil. It is argued that the parasympathetic agent may alter the normal aqueous dynamics and may skew the results.

Radiolabeled Isotopes

There have been a number of attempts to measure the accumulation of isotopes in the anterior chamber or the decay of isotopes after intracameral injection.[121] O'Rourke and co-workers[121,122] injected radiolabeled albumin into the anterior chamber and measured the rate of disappearance of radioactivity using an external gamma counter. This technique requires the assumption that all loss of radioactivity is due to the flow of aqueous humor. Other problems with the method include leakage of fluid around the needle, breakdown of the blood–aqueous barrier, and elevation of IOP.[123] Infusion into the anterior chamber must be done slowly, and the tracer must be allowed to mix adequately with the aqueous humor. A push-pull apparatus is used so that fluid is injected and removed at the same time and rate to avoid disturbing IOP.[124] Similarly, a radiolabeled protein can be injected into the vitreous, and its disappearance can be measured using an external scintillation counter. Clearly this technique is not applicable to human eyes.[125] It is also possible to measure aqueous humor flow by injecting a tracer into the anterior chamber and measuring its appearance in the general circulation.[126] Another method is to inject intravenously a radiolabeled substance that circulates to the eye from the blood stream and that is rapidly cleared by the kidney. Once the agent is cleared by the kidney, its rate of disappearance from the eye can be measured. This rate of disappearance is dependent on the rate of aqueous flow.[127,128]

Fluorescein

Following oral administration of fluorescein, the dye appears in the anterior chamber. The rate of appearance can be measured with optical techniques, allowing for the calculation of aqueous humor flow.[37,129-131] Fluorescein administered intravenously appears in the anterior chamber much like oral fluorescein as described above.[132-135] The rate of appearance of the dye allows for the calculation of the rate of aqueous humor flow. In a related technique the eye is exposed to infrared radiation for 2 to 3 minutes, leading to a rapid reversible breakdown of the blood–aqueous barrier and an influx of fluorescein from the plasma. When the infrared radiation is stopped, the barrier is reestablished rapidly. The subsequent rate of decrease of fluorescein in the anterior chamber is related to aqueous humor flow.[136]

Fluorescein is administered topically as multiple eye drops or by iontophoresis. After a suitable period of time the rate of decay of the fluorescein concentration is taken as a measure of aqueous humor flow through the anterior chamber. This necessitates a mathematical analysis that considers the volume of the anterior chamber and the effect of the fluorescein depot in the cornea.[9,35,137-155] This technique is now used widely to measure aqueous humor flow in clinical situations.

Fluoresceinated Dextrans

Large fluorescein-labeled molecules are injected intravitreally. The loss of fluorescein over time is measured by optical techniques and is related to aqueous humor flow through the anterior chamber.[156] However, because the eye must be entered, disturbance of the normal physiology would seem inevitable, and the results of this kind of analysis would be suspect.

Paraminohippurate

PAH is injected intravenously, leading to a high plasma PAH concentration and penetration of the substance into the aqueous humor. When the intravenous infusion is stopped, there is rapid renal clearance of PAH, which leads to a low plasma concentration. Since PAH in the posterior chamber is transported out of the eye, the anterior-chamber PAH concentration over time reflects aqueous humor flow. Aqueous humor is sampled in one eye and then 1 to 2 hours later in the other eye. The difference in the PAH concentrations between the two eyes reflects the aqueous flow rate. The obvious problem with this technique is that it necessitates bilateral paracentesis for chemical analysis.[157]

Iodide

The iodide technique is similar to the PAH technique described above. When large doses of iodide are administered, the substance diffuses into the anterior chamber from the plasma but is actively transported out of the eye behind the iris. Labeled iodide and nonlabeled iodide are administered at different times, and the concentrations are measured after paracentesis. The relative concentrations in the aqueous humor reflect flow through the anterior chamber.[158]

FACTORS AFFECTING AQUEOUS HUMOR FORMATION

As noted previously, aqueous humor formation averages about 2.6 to 2.8 μl/min in normal humans during the daytime. The rate of formation at any given time is similar between the two eyes of the

Table 3-5

Factors That Affect Aqueous Humor Production

Condition	Effect on Aqueous Humor Flow
Hypothermia[96,175]	Decrease
Hyperthermia[199]	Increase
Acidosis[75]	Decrease
Alkalosis[75]	Increase
Third ventricle injection of	
Prostaglandins	Increase
Arachidonic acid	Increase
Hyperosmotic solutions	Decrease
Hypoosmotic solutions	Increase
Calcium[180]	Increase
Diabetes mellitus	Decrease
Retinal detachment	Decrease
Ocular inflammation	Decrease
Cyclodestructive procedures	Decrease
Choroidal detachment	Decrease
Cyclodialysis	Decrease?

same individual (coefficient of variation = 15%).[35] Like most physiologic functions, the production of aqueous humor is not static; rather, it varies. The flow does not seem to vary much from day to day in normal young individuals (coefficient of variation = 23%). Table 3-5 summarizes some of the known factors that influence the rate of aqueous formation. The important ones are discussed below.

Diurnal Variation

IOP fluctuates over the course of the day. The most common diurnal variation has the maximum pressure in the morning hours and the minimum pressure late at night or early in the morning. Some individuals reach their peak IOPs in the afternoon or evening. Other individuals follow no consistent pattern. Most authorities attribute the diurnal fluctuation of IOP to diurnal variations in aqueous humor formation.[114] However, some believe there is a diurnal fluctuation in outflow facility as well (see Chapter 4). Aqueous flow is higher in the morning than in the afternoon.[159] The rate of aqueous formation during sleep is approximately one half the rate upon first awakening.[160] It is postulated that the reduction in flow is the result of decreased stimulation of the ciliary epithelium by circulating catecholamines.[150,160]

Age and Sex

Aqueous humor formation appears to be similar in males and females.[60] There is a reduction in aqueous formation with age,[9,132,133,161-163] particularly after age 60.[9,161] However, the decline with age is less than was previously thought.[161] Brubaker and co-workers,[35] in a study of over 300 normal volunteers, showed a decline in aqueous production of about 3.2% per decade in adults; this represents a reduction in aqueous production of about 25% over a lifetime. Therefore age appears to have less effect on aqueous humor production than it does on IOP and anterior chamber volume.[9] The reason(s) for the decrease in the rate of aqueous formation with age are not clear. One study suggests that the decrease could be due to changes in the ultrastructure of aging ciliary epithelial cells.[164]

Intraocular Pressure/Pseudofacility

Many investigators have postulated a feedback mechanism whereby aqueous humor formation increases or decreases to compensate for changes in IOP. One proposed example of this phenomenon

Table 3-6

Rate of Aqueous Humor Flow in Human Eyes With Glaucoma or Elevated Intraocular Pressure

Abnormality	Subjects (n)	Affected Eyes Mean ± SD	Unaffected Fellow Eyes (Normal) Mean ± SD	Comments
Open-angle glaucoma[55]	6	2.4 ± 0.5	—	
Exfoliative syndrome with glaucoma[101]	9	2.3 ± 0.8	2.9 ± 0.9	Flow significantly lower in affected eyes; blood–aqueous barrier leaky to fluorescein
Fuchs' heterochromic iridocyclitis with increased IOP[102]	10	3.2 ± 1.3	3.4 ± 0.7	Blood–aqueous barrier leaky to fluorescein
Pigmentary glaucoma[55]	5	2.9 ± 0.6	—	
Corticosteroid-induced glaucoma[51]	5	—	—	Ratio of flow in treated eye to untreated eye: 1.01 ± 0.14
Elevated episcleral venous pressure[51]	1	1.7	—	
Sturge-Weber syndrome with elevated IOP[51]	1	3.4	2.9	
Progressive low-tension glaucoma[51]	1	2.2 ± 0.4	—	
Argon laser trabeculoplasty[53]				
Before	9	1.5 ± 0.5	1.9 ± 0.9	No effect on flow from lowering IOP with laser treatment
After	9	1.4 ± 0.6	1.9 ± 1.0	

Modified from Brubaker RF: *The physiology of aqueous humor formation.* In Drance SM, Neufeld AH, editors: *Glaucoma: applied pharmacology in medical treatment,* New York, 1984, Grune & Stratton.

is the apparent decrease in aqueous formation that occurs during tonography. This decrease could be misinterpreted as an increase in outflow facility, so this phenomenon has been termed pseudo-facility. However, more recent studies suggest that pseudofacility, or the feedback control of aqueous formation, has been greatly overstated. Carlson and co-workers[139] altered IOP by changing body position and found only slight changes in aqueous formation. In addition, prolonged alterations of IOP do not seem to affect aqueous humor formation.[165] For example, when topical corticosteroids are administered to sensitive patients for several weeks, IOP rises, but there is no corresponding fall in aqueous humor formation.[166] Conversely, laser trabeculoplasty lowers IOP in glaucomatous eyes without a concomitant increase in aqueous formation.[167-169] Another piece of evidence suggesting the lack of a negative feedback system is that fluorophotometric studies demonstrate a normal rate of aqueous formation in patients with glaucoma or ocular hypertension (Table 3-6). Furthermore, in patients with unilateral pigmentary dispersion glaucoma, the aqueous flow is equivalent in both eyes.[170] Finally, in patients with myotonic dystrophy in which IOPs are frequently under 10 mm Hg, no difference in aqueous flow rates were seen compared with normal eyes.[171] Thus increased IOP is unlikely to affect aqueous humor production in any major way. These observations suggest one further important implication—the increased IOP in glaucoma is the result of decreased outflow facility and not increased aqueous formation.

Blood Flow to the Ciliary Body

A modest reduction of plasma flow to the ciliary processes does not reduce aqueous humor production substantially. However, a profound vasoconstriction does diminish the rate of aqueous flow. Acute experimental carotid artery occlusion in rabbits and monkeys reduces aqueous humor production.[172-175] However, this effect appears to be transient, and aqueous production rises to near normal levels in a few weeks.[176] In humans with unilateral carotid artery occlusion, aqueous humor production is normal and equal in both eyes.[60]

Neural Control

There has been considerable interest in the neural control of aqueous humor formation. As mentioned, stimulation of the cervical sympathetic chain decreases aqueous humor production.[48,49] Furthermore, stimulation of hypothalamic centers[177-179] or injection of a number of substances—such as calcium, hyperosmotic and hypoosmotic solutions, and prostaglandins—into the third ventricle can alter IOP.[180] Studies on the transection of the optic nerve in humans and experimental animals suggest some form of central regulatory mechanism for IOP using the optic nerve as the pathway.[181,182] In rabbits, the circadian rhythm of aqueous flow is tied to the light:dark cycle.[183] Using the technique of ventriculocisternal perfusion, Liu and Neufeld found interaction between the brain and IOP that was not easy to explain by any simple theory.

The sympathetic system seems to be an important pathway for signals from the brain that influence the rate of aqueous formation. In fact, the sympathetic system may be involved in the circadian rhythms of aqueous production and IOP.[184] However, unilateral Horner's syndrome does not appear to affect the aqueous formation rate, the IOP, or the response of the eye to the commonly used adrenergic agonists and antagonists.[155,185] Thus central nervous system mechanisms do influence aqueous secretory rates, but the mechanisms are unclear at this time.

Hormonal Effects

Although several circulating hormones (e.g., corticosteroids) may have a significant effect on IOP, few have been studied for their effect on aqueous humor formation.[186] Brubaker and co-workers studied melatonin, progesterone, and desmopressin for their possible effects on aqueous formation rates; none were found to affect aqueous formation in any significant way. Levene[187] has suggested that systemic variations in corticosteroid levels may account for the circadian changes in IOP. A low-dose epinephrine infusion will increase nocturnal aqueous secretion in humans by about 27%.[188] Using a selective β_2-adrenergic agonist, terbutaline, Gharagozloo and co-workers[189] showed that exogenously administered β-agonists exert their maximum effect of increasing aqueous secretion during sleep and had little or no effect during waking hours. Since endogenous epinephrine secretion is at its minimum during sleep, some correlation may be inferred from the reduced nocturnal aqueous formation and the status of circulating β-adrenergic agonists.

Intracellular Regulators

Cyclic adenosine monophosphate plays an important role in the intracellular secretory processes of rabbit ciliary body.[190-192] Perhaps cyclic guanosine monophosphate is a secondary messenger for regulation of aqueous secretion.[193] As Brubaker points out, the challenge is to determine how to link what happens on the cellular and tissue levels with the observed phenomena in the intact eye.[35]

Cherksey and co-workers[194,195] have found an anion-selective channel in cultured human non-pigmented ciliary epithelial cells. Although aqueous humor formation appears normal in eyes of patients with cystic fibrosis (a disease with defective adrenergically-regulated chloride channels), it is possible that some endogenous humoral or neural factor regulates the activity of this channel and thus is responsible for diurnal variation and the effect of adrenergic agents on aqueous flow.[196]

CLINICAL ASPECTS OF AQUEOUS HUMOR FORMATION

Clinical Conditions

Many conditions affect the rate of aqueous humor production, including ocular and systemic conditions. The known conditions are summarized in Tables 3-5 and 3-6. Although Goldmann calculated from tonographic data that eyes with primary open-angle glaucoma (POAG) had decreased aqueous formation rates, subsequent data strongly suggest that aqueous formation is unaffected by POAG and by pigmentary and exfoliative glaucoma.[35] Aqueous flow was not significantly reduced by Fuchs' heterochromic iridocyclitis.[107] Similarly, some conditions with low IOP, such as low-tension glaucoma or myotonic dystrophy, do not affect aqueous formation.[60,171] A long-held assumption has been that retinal detachment, cyclodialysis, and ocular inflammation are conditions that reduce the rate of aqueous formation. Many of these assumptions are based on tonographic evidence.[198] However, no studies using modern techniques have been published to confirm them.

As might be expected, systemic conditions that slow metabolism also reduce aqueous formation. Hypothermia and systemic acidosis decrease aqueous production.[75,96,175] Conversely, hyperthermia and alkalosis increase the rate of aqueous formation.[75,199] Insulin-dependent diabetes mellitus also seems to decrease aqueous flow.[200]

Pharmacologic Agents

Many drugs have an effect on aqueous humor formation. Some stimulate secretion, others inhibit it. Only two classes of drugs have any significant role in stimulating aqueous secretion. They are β-adrenergic agents and endogenously administered corticosteroids. Contrary to early conceptions based on tonographic data that epinephrine reduces aqueous formation, acutely administered β-adrenergic agents seem to increase aqueous formation rates, especially during sleep, as noted above.[35] This effect may diminish with chronic administration. Topical corticosteroids do not seem to have any effect on aqueous secretion. However, systemically administered hydrocortisone may significantly increase aqueous flow.[201] Pilocarpine may increase aqueous formation, but only slightly and not enough to be clinically significant.[49] Intracameral atrial natriuretic factor also increases aqueous flow, but only transiently.[202]

Although only a small number of agents increase aqueous production, over a dozen have been shown to decrease the rate of production. These are listed in Table 3-7. Because of toxicity or route of administration, most of these agents have not been found to be useful therapeutically in humans. Systemically administered carbonic anhydrase inhibitors reduce aqueous formation by approximately 40%. These agents decrease the rate of appearance of bicarbonate and water in newly formed posterior-chamber aqueous humor.[33,74] Topically applied carbonic anhydrase inhibitors lower IOP and also cause a small reduction in aqueous humor formation. Their mechanism of action seems similar to that of the systemic carbonic anhydrase inhibitors.[203]

The β-adrenergic antagonists are also known to reduce aqueous humor formation. Fluorophotometric studies demonstrate a 16% to 47% decrease in aqueous formation after the administration

Table 3-7

Agents That Affect Aqueous Humor Formation

Agent	Effect on Aqueous Flow
β-Adrenergic agonists	Increase
Systemically administered corticosteroids	Increase
Pilocarpine	Slight increase
Ouabain	Decrease
Cyclic guanosine monophosphate	Decrease
Atrial natriuretic peptide	Decrease
Vanadate	Decrease
Cholera toxin	Decrease
Prazosin	Decrease
Metyrapone	Decrease
Vasopressin	Decrease
Halothane	Decrease (clinically important)
Barbiturates	Decrease (clinically important)
Ketamine	Decrease (clinically important)
Forskolin	Decrease
δ-9-Tetrahydrocannabinol	Decrease
β-Adrenergic blocking agents	Decrease (clinically useful)
α-Adrenergic agonists	Decrease (clinically useful)
Carbonic anhydrase inhibitors	Decrease (clinically useful)

of topical timolol, betaxolol, bupranolol, or levobunolol.[130,140,149,204] Other agents are also effective. Although both carbonic anhydrase inhibitors and α-adrenergic agonists decrease aqueous formation during sleep, the β-adrenergic antagonists do not.[205]. An adaptation to the ability of timolol and other β-antagonists to reduce aqueous formation may occur after chronic use, but this effect seems not to be clinically significant.[35] The effect of β-adrenergic antagonists may last for 1 or more weeks after cessation of administration.[206]

The α-adrenergic agonist clonidine, a drug used as an antihypertensive agent, was found to reduce aqueous flow in the human eye.[79] A derivative of clonidine, apraclonidine, was later found to be a better-tolerated clinical agent and to lower IOP by reducing aqueous formation.[207]

It was believed that topical epinephrine preparations reduced aqueous humor formation.[208-210] Recent studies are somewhat contradictory but suggest that aqueous humor formation is either slightly increased or relatively unchanged by topical epinephrine.[147,151,153,211] Na^+K^+ ATPase inhibitors, such as ouabain, decrease aqueous formation in rabbits,[65] cats,[70] and humans.[70] Unfortunately, these drugs are ineffective topically and must be administered systemically or intravitreally, which is not clinically feasible. Vanadate, an inhibitor of Na^+K^+ ATPase, reduces aqueous humor formation and IOP in rabbits and monkeys, but this drug appears to act by a mechanism distinct from its effect on this enzyme.[212-214] A variety of other drugs, including sedatives, anesthetic agents, and hormones, depress aqueous humor production.[215,216]

Surgery

A number of surgical procedures, including cyclocryotherapy and cyclodiathermy, reduce aqueous humor formation (Table 3-5). It is not clear whether these procedures act on the ciliary epithelium or the ciliary body vasculature. There is considerable controversy about whether cyclodialysis decreases aqueous humor flow.[60,132]

REFERENCES

1. Seidel E: Weitere experimentelle untersuchengen uber die quelle und den verlauf der intraokularen saftstromung IX Mitterlung Uber den abfluss des kammerwasser aus der vorderen augenkammers, *Graefes Arch* 104:537, 1921.
2. Seidel E: Weitere experimentelle untersuchengen uber die quelle und den verlauf der intraokularen saftstromung. XII Mitterlung uber den manometrischen nachweis des physiologeschen druckgefalles zwischen vorderkammer und Schlemmscher kanal, *Graefes Arch* 107: 101, 1921.
3. Ascher KW: The aqueous veins. I. Physiological importance of the visible elimination of intra-ocular fluid, *Am J Ophthalmol* 25:1174, 1942.
4. Ashton N: Anatomical study of Schlemm's canal and aqueous veins by means of neoprene casts: part I. Aqueous veins, *Br J Ophthalmol* 35:921, 1951.
5. Reddy DVN: Dynamics of transport systems in the eye, *Invest Ophthalmol Vis Sci* 18:1000, 1979.
6. Cole DF: Aqueous humor formation, *Doc Ophthalmol* 21:116, 1965.
7. Cole DF: Secretion of aqueous humor, *Exp Eye Res* 25(suppl):161, 1977.
8. Hogan MJ, Alvarado JA, Weddell JE: *Histology of the human eye: an atlas textbook,* Philadelphia, 1971, WB Saunders.
9. Brubaker RF, and others: The effect of age on aqueous humor formation in man, *Ophthalmology* 88:283, 1981.
10. Bauermann M: Uber das Ciliafortsatzgeflusssjstem Den Zusammen Kunft Dtsch Opthal Ges 48:364, 1930.

11. Smelser GK: Electron microscopy of a typical epithelial cell and of the normal human ciliary process, *Trans Am Acad Ophthalmol Otolaryngol* 70:738, 1966.
12. Lutjen-Decoll E, Lonnerholm G, Eichhorn M: Carbonic anhydrase distribution in the human and monkey eye by light and electron microscopy, *Graefes Arch Clin Exp Ophthalmol* 220:285, 1983.
13. Tormey JM: The ciliary epithelium: an attempt to correlate structure and function, *Trans Am Acad Ophthalmol Otolaryngol* 70:755, 1966.
14. Fujita H, Konko K, Sears M: Eine neue funktion der nicht pigmentierten epithels der ziliarkorperfortsatze bei der kammerwasserproduktion, *Klin Mbl Augenheilk* 185:28, 1984.
15. Hara K, and others: Structural differences between regions of the ciliary body of primates, *Invest Ophthalmol Vis Sci* 16:912, 1977.
16. Ober M, Rohen JW: Regional differences in the fine structure of the ciliary epithelium related to accommodation, *Invest Ophthalmol Vis Sci* 18:655, 1979.
17. Raviola G, Raviola E: Intercellular injections in the ciliary epithelium, *Invest Ophthalmol Vis Sci* 17:958, 1978.
18. Bairati A, Orzalesi N: The ultrastructure of the epithelium of the ciliary body: a study of the function complexes and the changes associated with the production of plasmoid aqueous humor, *Z Zellforsch Mikrosk Anat* 69:635, 1966.
19. Cole DF: Location of ouabain-sensitive adenosinetriphosphatase in ciliary epithelium, *Exp Eye Res* 3:72, 1964.

20. Shiose Y: Electron microscopic studies on blood retinal and blood–aqueous barriers, *Jpn J Ophthalmol* 14:73, 1970.
21. Smith RS: Ultrastructural studies of the blood aqueous barrier. I. Transport of an electron-dense tracer in the iris and ciliary body of the mouse, *Am J Ophthalmol* 71:1066, 1971.
22. Smith RS, Rudt LA: Ultrastructural studies of the blood aqueous barrier. II. The barrier to horseradish peroxidase in primates, *Am J Ophthalmol* 76:937, 1973.
23. Smith RS, Rudt LA: Ocular, vascular and epithelial barriers to microperoxidase, *Invest Ophthalmol Vis Sci* 14:556, 1975.
24. Ustitalo R, Palkama A: Localization of sodium-potassium stimulated adenosine triphosphatase activity in the rabbit ciliary body using light and electron microscopy, *Ann Exp Fenn* 48:84, 1970.
25. Vegge T: An epithelial blood-aqueous barrier to horseradish peroxidase in the processes of the vervet monkey *Ceropithecus aethips, Z Zellforsch Mikrosk Anat* 114:309, 1971.
26. Mizuno K, Asoka M: Cycloscopy and fluorescein cycloscopy, *Invest Ophthalmol* 15:561, 1976.
27. Russmann W: Levels of glycolytic enzyme activity in the ciliary epithelium prepared from bovine eyes, *Ophthalmic Res* 2:205, 1971.
28. Feeney L, Mixon R: Localization of 35 sulfated macromolecules at the site of active transport in the ciliary processes, *Invest Ophthalmol* 13:882, 1974.

29. Feeney L, Mixon R: Sulfate and galactose metabolism in differentiating ciliary body and iris epithelia: autoradiographic and ultrastructural studies, *Invest Ophthalmol* 14:364, 1975.

30. Ruskell GL: *Innervation of the anterior segment of the eye.* In Lutjen-Drecoll E, editor: *Basic aspects of glaucoma research,* Stuttgart, 1982, Schattauer.

31. Bloom JN, and others: Cholinergic and adrenergic receptors in freshly isolated ciliary epithelium, *Invest Ophthalmol Vis Sci* 24(suppl):89, 1983.

32. Neufeld A, Bartels SP: Receptor mechanisms for epinephrine and timolol. In Lutjen-Drecoll, editor: *Basic aspects of glaucoma research,* Stuttgart, 1982, Schattauer.

33. Woodlief NF: Initial observations on the ocular microcirculation in man. I. The anterior segment and extraocular muscles, *Arch Ophthalmol* 98:1268, 1980.

34. Alm A, Bill A, Young FA: The effects of pilocarpine and neostigmine on the blood flow through the anterior uvea in monkeys: a study with radioactively labelled microspheres, *Exp Eye Res* 15:31, 1973.

35. Brubaker RF: Flow of aqueous humor in humans, *Invest Ophthalmol Vis Sci* 32:3145, 1991.

36. Alm A, Bill A: The oxygen supply to the retina. I. Effects of changes in intraocular and arterial blood pressures, and in arterial PO_2 and PCO_2 on the oxygen tension in the vitreous body of the cat, *Acta Physiol Scand* 84:261, 1972.

37. Lindner K: Zur Untersuchung des Flussigkeitswechsels in Auge, *Dtsch Ophthalmol* 42:33, 1920.

38. Bill A: Blood circulation and fluid dynamics in the eye, *Physiol Rev* 55:383, 1975.

39. Bill A, Nilsson S: *The blood supply of the eye and its regulation.* In Lutjen-Drecoll E, editor: *Basic aspects of glaucoma research,* Stuttgart, 1982, Schattauer.

40. Alm A, Bill A: The oxygen supply to the retina. II. Effects of high intraocular pressure and of increased arterial carbon dioxide tension on uveal and retinal blood flow in cats, *Acta Physiol Scand* 84:306, 1972.

41. Alm A, Bill A: The effect of stimulation of the cervical sympathetic chain on retinal oxygen tension and on uveal, retinal and cerebral blood flow in cats, *Acta Physiol Scand* 88:84, 1973.

42. Cole DF, Unger WG: Prostaglandins as mediators for the responses of the eye to trauma, *Exp Eye Res* 17:357, 1973.

43. Neufeld AH, Sears ML: Prostaglandin and eye, *Prostaglandins* 4:157, 1973.

44. Podos SM, Becker B, Kass MA: Prostaglandin synthesis, inhibition and intraocular pressure, *Invest Ophthalmol Vis Sci* 12:426, 1973.

45. Whitelock RAF, Eakins KE: Vascular changes in the anterior uvea of the rabbit produced by prostaglandins, *Arch Ophthalmol* 89:495, 1973.

46. Neufeld AH, Jampol LM, Sears ML: Aspirin prevents the disruption of the blood aqueous barrier in the rabbit eye, *Nature* 238:158, 1972.

47. Perkins ES, Unger WG, Bass M: The role of prostaglandin in the ocular responses to laser irradiation of the iris, *Exp Eye Res* 17:394, 1973.

48. Bill A: Autonomic nervous control of uveal blood flow, *Acta Physiol Scand* 56:70, 1962.

49. Langham ME, Rosenthal AR: The role of cervical sympathetic nerve in regulation of the intraocular pressure and circulation, *J Physiol* 210:786, 1966.

50. Langham ME, Taylor CB: The influence of superior cervical ganglionectomy on intraocular dynamics, *J Physiol* 152:447, 1960.

51. Davson H: *Physiology of the ocular and cerebrospinal fluids,* London, 1956, J & A Churchill.

52. Bill A: Capillary permeability to and extravascular dynamics of myoglobin, albumin and gamma globulin in the uvea, *Acta Physiol Scand* 73:204, 1968.

53. Allansmith M, Newman L, Whitney C: The distribution of immunoglobulin in the rabbit eye, *Arch Ophthalmol* 86:60, 1971.

54. Allansmith MR, and others: Immunoglobulins in the human eye, *Arch Ophthalmol* 89:36, 1973.

55. Bill A: A method to determine osmotically effective albumin and gamma globulin concentrations in tissue fluids, its application to the uvea and a note on the effects of capillary "leaks" on tissue fluid dynamics, *Acta Physiol Scand* 73:511, 1968.

56. Green K, Pederson E: Contribution of secretion and filtration to aqueous humor formation, *Am J Physiol* 222:1218, 1972.

57. Pederson JE, Green K: Aqueous humor dynamics: a mathematical approach to measurement of facility, pseudofacility, capillary pressure, active secretion and X_c, *Exp Eye Res* 15:265, 1973.

58. Pederson JE, Green K: Aqueous humor dynamics: experimental studies, *Exp Eye Res* 15:277, 1973.

59. Weinbaum S, Langham ME, Goldgrabben JR: The role of secretion and pressure-dependent flow in aqueous humor formation, *Exp Eye Res* 13:266, 1972.

60. Brubaker RF: *The physiology of aqueous humor formation.* In Drance SM, Neufeld AH, editors: *Glaucoma: applied pharmacology in medical treatment,* New York, 1984, Grune & Stratton.

61. Curran PF, Macintosh JR: A model system for biological water transport, *Nature* 193:347, 1962.

62. Diamond JM, Bossert WH: Standing-gradient osmotic flow, *J Gen Physiol* 50:2061, 1967.

63. Kishida S, and others: Electric characteristics of ciliary body, *Jpn J Ophthalmol* 25:407, 1981.

64. Krupin T, and others: Transepithelial electrical measurements on isolated rabbit iris–ciliary body, *Invest Ophthalmol Vis Sci* 22(suppl):100, 1982.

65. Becker B: Ouabain and aqueous humor dynamics in the rabbit eye, *Invest Ophthalmol* 2:325, 1963.

66. Cole DF: Effects of some metabolic inhibitors upon the formation of the aqueous humour in rabbits, *Br J Ophthalmol* 44:739, 1960.

67. Riley MV, Kishida K: ATPases of ciliary epithelium: cellular and subcellular distribution and probable role in secretion of aqueous humor, *Exp Eye Res* 42:559, 1986.

68. Shiose Y, Sears ML: Localization and other aspects of the histochemistry of nucleoside phosphatase in the ciliary epithelium of albino rabbits, *Invest Ophthalmol* 4:64, 1965.

69. Shiose Y, Sears ML: Fine structural localization of nucleoside phosphatase activity in the ciliary epithelium of albino rabbits, *Invest Ophthalmol* 5:152, 1966.

70. Simon KA, Bonting SL, Hawkins NM: Studies on sodium-potassium–activated adenosine triphosphatase. II. Formation of aqueous humor, *Exp Eye Res* 1:253, 1962.

71. Zimmerman TJ, and others: The effects of acetazolamide on the movement of sodium into the posterior chamber of the dog eye, *J Pharmacol* 199:510, 1976.

72. Dobbs PD, Epstein DL, Anderson PJ: Identification of isoenzyme C as the principal carbonic anhydrase in human ciliary processes, *Invest Ophthalmol Vis Sci* 18:867, 1979.

73. Kumpulainen T: Immunohistochemical demonstration of carbonic anhydrase isoenzyme C in the epithelium of the human ciliary processes, *Histochemistry* 77:281, 1983.

74. Maren TH, and others: The rates of ion movement from plasma to aqueous humor in the dogfish, *Squalus acanthias,* *Invest Ophthalmol* 14:662, 1975.

75. Krupin T, and others: Acidosis, alkalosis and aqueous humor dynamics in rabbits, *Invest Ophthalmol Vis Sci* 16:997, 1977.

76. Cotlier E: Bicarbonate ATP-ase in ciliary body and a theory of Diamox effect on aqueous humour production, *Int Ophthalmol* 1:123, 1979.

77. Holland MG: Chloride ion transport in the isolated ciliary body. II. Ion substitution experiments, *Invest Ophthalmol* 9:30, 1970.

78. Holland MG, Gipson CC: Chloride ion transport in the isolated ciliary body, *Invest Ophthalmol* 9:20, 1970.

79. Kinsey VE, Reddy DVN: *Chemistry and dynamics of aqueous humor.* In Prince JH, editor: *The rabbit in eye research,* Springfield, Ill, 1966, Charles C Thomas.

80. Sen DK, Sarin GS, Saha K: Immunoglobulins in human aqueous humor, *Br J Ophthalmol* 61:216, 1977.

81. Bill A: Intraocular pressure and blood flow through the uvea, *Arch Ophthalmol* 67:336, 1962.

82. Bill A: The aqueous humor drainage mechanism in the cynomolgus monkey *Macaca irus* with evidence for unconventional routes, *Invest Ophthalmol* 4:911, 1965.

83. Bill A: Movement of albumin and dextran through the sclera, *Arch Ophthalmol* 74:248, 1965.

84. Bill A, Phillips CI: Uveoscleral drainage of aqueous humor in human eyes, *Exp Eye Res* 12:275, 1971.

85. Becker B: The transport of organic anions by the rabbit eye. I. In vitro iodopyracet (Diodrast) accumulation by ciliary body–iris preparations, *Am J Ophthalmol* 50:862, 1960.

86. Bito LZ, Davson H, Salvador EV: Inhibition of in vitro concentrative prostaglandin accumulation by prostaglandins, prostaglandin analogues and by some inhibitors of organic anion transport, *J Physiol* 256:257, 1976.

87. Bito LZ, Salvador EV: Intraocular fluid dynamics. II. Post mortem changes in solute concentrations, *Exp Eye Res* 10:273, 1970.

88. Becker B: Iodide transport by the rabbit eye, *Am J Physiol* 200:804, 1961.

89. Forbes M, Becker B: The transport of organic anions by the rabbit eye. II. In vitro transport of iodopyracet (Diodrast), *Am J Ophthalmol* 50:867, 1960.

90. Forbes M, Becker B: The transport of organic anions by the rabbit ciliary body. IV. Acetazolamide and rate of aqueous flow, *Am J Ophthalmol* 51:1047, 1961.

91. Barany EH: Inhibition by hippurate and probenecid of in vitro uptake of iodipamide and *o*-iodohippurate: a composite uptake system for iodipamide in choroid plexus, kidney cortex, and anterior uvea of several species, *Acta Physiol Scand* 86:12, 1972.

92. Barany EH: The liver-like anion transport system in rabbit kidney, uvea and choroid plexus. I. Selectivity of some inhibitors, direction of transport, possible physiological substrates, *Acta Physiol Scand* 88:412, 1973.

93. Barany EH: The liver-like anion transport system in rabbit kidney, uvea and choroid plexus. II. Efficiency of acidic drugs and other anions as inhibitors, *Acta Physiol Scand* 88:491, 1973.

94. Bito LZ, Salvador EV: Intraocular fluid dynamics. III. The site and mechanism of prostaglandin transfer across the blood intra-ocular fluid barriers, *Exp Eye Res* 14:233, 1972.

95. Bito LZ, Wallenstein MC, Baroody R: *The role of transport processes in the distribution and disposition of prostaglandins.* In Samuelsson B, Paoletti R, editors: *Prostaglandins and thromboxane research,* vol 1, New York, 1976, Lippincott-Raven.

96. Becker B: The effect of hypothermia on aqueous humor dynamics. III. Turnover of ascorbate and sodium, *Am J Ophthalmol* 51:1032, 1961.

97. Berggren L: Effect of composition of medium and of metabolic inhibitors on secretion in vitro by the ciliary processes of the rabbit eye, *Invest Ophthalmol* 4:83, 1965.

98. Bonting SL, Becker B: Studies on sodium-potassium activated adenosinetriphosphatase. XIV. Inhibition of enzyme activity and aqueous humor flow in the rabbit eye after injection of ouabain, *Invest Ophthalmol* 3:523, 1964.

99. Cole DF: Some effects of decreased plasma sodium concentration on the composition and tension of the aqueous humor, *Br J Ophthalmol* 43:268, 1959.

100. Bito LZ, Davson H: Steady-state concentrations of potassium in the ocular fluids, *Exp Eye Res* 3:283, 1964.

101. Becker B: Chemical composition of human aqueous humor: effects of acetazolamide, *Arch Ophthalmol* 57:793, 1957.

102. Dickinson JC, Durham DC, Hamilton PB: Ion exchange chromatography of free amino acids in aqueous fluid and lens of the human eye, *Invest Ophthalmol* 7:551, 1968.

103. de Berardinis E, and others: The chemical composition of the human aqueous humour in normal and pathological conditions, *Exp Eye Res* 4:179, 1965.

104. Poos F: Uber den histologischen und klinischen Erscheinungen bei akuten lokalen Capillarkreislaufstorungen am Auge, *Graefes Arch* 127:489, 1931.

105. Raviola G: Structural basis of the blood-ocular barriers, *Exp Eye Res* 25(suppl):27, 1977.

106. Eakins KE: Prostaglandin and non-prostaglandin mediated breakdown of the blood-aqueous barrier, *Exp Eye Res* 25(suppl):483, 1977.

107. Greeff R: Befund am Corpus Ciliare nacht Punktion der vorderen Kammer: ein beitrag zur Lehre vom Flussigkeitswechsel im Auge und der Fibrinbildung im Kammerwasser, *Arch Augenheilk* 28:178, 1894.

108. Rohen J: Morphologische Beitrage zum Problem der Kammerwasserbildung. I. Die Gestalt der Blutkammerwasserschranke beim Kaninchen in Ruhe und nacht funktioneller Belastung, *Ber Dtsch Ophthalmol Gest* 58:65, 1953.

109. Okisaka S: Effects of paracentesis on the blood–aqueous barrier: a light and electron microscopic study on the cynomolgus monkey, *Invest Ophthalmol* 15:824, 1976.

110. Raviola G: Effects of paracentesis on the blood-aqueous barrier: an electron microscope study on *Macaca mulatta* using horseradish peroxidase as a tracer, *Invest Ophthalmol* 13:828, 1974.

111. Grant WM: A tonographic method for measuring the facility and rate of aqueous flow in human eyes, *Arch Ophthalmol* 44:204, 1950.

112. Grant WM: Clinical measurements of aqueous outflow, *Arch Ophthalmol* 46:11, 1951.

113. Moses RL: Theory and calibration of the Schiøtz tonometer, *Invest Ophthalmol* 10:534, 1971.

114. Ericson LA: Twenty-four hourly variations on the aqueous flow: examination with perilimbal suction cup, *Acta Ophthalmol Scand Suppl* 50:1, 1958.

115. Langham ME, Maumenee AE: The diagnosis and treatment of glaucoma based on a new procedure for the measurement of ocular dynamics, *Trans Am Acad Ophthalmol Otolaryngol* 68:227, 1964.

116. Rosengren B: A method for producing intraocular rise in tension, *Acta Ophthalmol Scand Suppl* 12:403, 1934.

117. Rosengren B: Rise in the ocular tension produced by circumlimbal pressure on the sclera, *Trans Ophthalmol Soc UK* 76:65, 1956.

118. Langham ME, Eisenlohr JE: A manometric study of the rate of fall of the intraocular pressure in the living and dead eyes of human subjects, *Invest Ophthalmol* 2:72, 1963.

119. Holm O: A photogrammetric method for estimation of the pupillary aqueous flow in the living human eye, I. *Acta Ophthalmol* 46:254, 1968.

120. Holm O, Wiebert O: A photogrammetric method for estimation of the pupillary aqueous flow in the living human eye. II. Statistical evaluation of pupillary flow measurements, *Acta Ophthalmol* 46:1230, 1968.

121. Macri RJ, O'Rourke J: Measurements of aqueous humor turnover rates using a gamma probe, *Arch Ophthalmol* 83:741, 1970.

122. O'Rourke J: *Nuclear ophthalmology: dynamic function studies in intraocular disease,* Philadelphia, 1976, WB Saunders.

123. Davson H, Spaziani E: The fate of substances injected into the anterior chamber of the eye, *J Physiol* 151:202, 1960.

124. Sperber GO, Bill A: A method of near-continuous determination of aqueous humor flow; effects of anesthetics, temperature and indomethacin, *Exp Eye Res* 39:435, 1984.

125. Maurice DM: Protein dynamics in the eye studied with labelled proteins, *Am J Ophthalmol* 47:361, 1959.

126. Bill A, Hellsing K: Production and drainage of aqueous humour in the cynomolgus monkey *Macaca irus* with evidence for unconventional routes, *Invest Ophthalmol* 4:920, 1965.

127. Barany EH, Kinsey VE: The rate of flow of aqueous humor: I. The rate of disappearance of para-aminopuric acid, radioactive Rayopake and radioactive Diodrast from the aqueous humor of rabbits, *Am J Ophthalmol* 32:177, 1949.

128. Kinsey VE, Barany EH: The rate of flow of aqueous humor: II. Derivation of rate of flow and its physiologic significance, *Am J Ophthalmol* 32:189, 1949.

129. Amsler H, Huber A: Methodik and urste klinische Ergebnisse einer Functionsprufund der Blut-Kammerwasser-Schranke, *Ophthalmologica* 111:155, 1946.

130. Araie M, Takase M: Effects of various drugs on aqueous humor dynamics in man, *Jpn J Ophthalmol* 25:91, 1981.

131. Araie M, and others: Aqueous humor dynamics in man as studied by oral fluorescein, *Jpn J Ophthalmol* 24:346, 1980.

132. Goldmann H: Uber Fluorescein in der menschlichen Vorderkammer: Das Kammerwasser-Minutenvolumen des Menschen, *Ophthalmologica* 119:65, 1950.

133. Goldmann H: Abflussdruck, Minutenvolumen und Widerstand der Kammerwasserstromung des Menschen, *Doc Ophthalmol* 5-6:278, 1951.

134. Nagataki S: Aqueous humor dynamics of human eyes as studied using fluorescein, *Jpn J Opthalmol* 19:235, 1975.

135. Nagataki S, Mishima S: Aqueous humor dynamics in glaucomato-cyclitic crisis, *Invest Ophthalmol* 15:365, 1976.

136. Dyster-Aas K, Krakau CET: Aqueous flow determination in the rabbit by means of a minimal eye trauma, *Invest Ophthalmol* 3:127, 1964.

137. Bloom JN, and others: Fluorophotometry and the rate of aqueous flow in man. I. Instrumentation and normal values, *Arch Ophthalmol* 94:435, 1976.

138. Brubaker RF, Gaasterland D: The effect of isoproterenol on aqueous humor formation in humans, *Invest Ophthalmol Vis Sci* 25:357, 1984.

139. Carlson KH, McLaren JW, Brubaker RF: The effect of body position on intraocular pressure and aqueous flow, *Invest Ophthalmol Vis Sci* 28:1346, 1987.

140. Coakes RL, Brubaker RF: The mechanism of timolol in lowering intraocular pressure, *Arch Ophthalmol* 96:2045, 1978.

141. Coakes RL, Brubaker RF: Method of measuring aqueous humor flow and corneal endothelial permeability using a fluorophotometry nomogram, *Invest Ophthalmol Vis Sci* 18:288, 1979.

142. Dailey RA, Brubaker RF, Bourne WM: The effects of timolol maleate and acetazolamide on the rate of aqueous formation in normal human subjects, *Am J Ophthalmol* 93:232, 1982.

143. Jones RF, Maurice DM: New methods for measuring the rate of aqueous flow in man with fluorescein, *Exp Eye Res* 5:208, 1966.

144. Langley D, MacDonald RK: Clinical method of observing changes in the rate of flow of aqueous humor in the human eye. I. Normal eyes, *Br J Ophthalmol* 36:432, 1952.

145. Lee DA, Brubaker RF, Nagataki S: Effect of thymoxamine on aqueous humor formation in the normal human eye as measured by fluorophotometry, *Invest Ophthalmol Vis Sci* 21:805, 1981.

146. Lee DA, Topper JE, Brubaker RF: Effects of clonidine on aqueous humor flow in normal human eyes, *Exp Eye Res* 38:239, 1984.

147. Nagataki S, Brubaker RF: Early effects of epinephrine on aqueous formation in the normal human eye, *Ophthalmology* 88:278, 1981.

148. Nagataki S, Brubaker RF: Effect of pilocarpine on aqueous humor formation in human beings, *Arch Ophthalmol* 100:818, 1982.

149. Reiss GR, Brubaker RF: The mechanism of betaxolol, a new ocular hypotensive agent, *Ophthalmology* 90:1369, 1983.

150. Reiss GR, and others: Aqueous humor flow during sleep, *Invest Ophthalmol Vis Sci* 25:776, 1984.

151. Schenker HI, and others: Fluorophotometric study of epinephrine and timolol in human subjects, *Arch Ophthalmol* 99:1212, 1981.

152. Starr PAJ: Changes in aqueous flow determined by fluorophotometry, *Trans Ophthalmol Soc UK* 86:639, 1966.

153. Townsend DJ, Brubaker RF: Intermediate effect of epinephrine on aqueous formation in the normal human eye as measured by fluorophotometry, *Invest Ophthalmol Vis Sci* 19:256, 1980.

154. Weekers R, Delmarcelle Y: Hypotonie oculaire par reduction du debit de l'humeur aqueuse, *Ophthalmologica* 125:425, 1953.

155. Wentworth WO, Brubaker RF: Aqueous humor dynamics in a series of patients with third neuron Horner's syndrome, *Am J Ophthalmol* 92:407, 1981.

156. Johnson F, Maurice D: A simple method of measuring aqueous humor flow with intravitreal fluoresceinated dextrans, *Exp Eye Res* 39:791, 1984.

157. Oppelt WW: Measurement of aqueous humor formation rates by posterioranterior chamber perfusion with inulin: normal values and the effect of carbonic anhydrase inhibition, *Invest Ophthalmol* 6:76, 1967.

158. Becker B: The measurement of rate of aqueous flow with iodide, *Invest Ophthalmol* 1:52, 1962.

159. McLaren JW, Brubaker RF: A scanning ocular fluorophotometer, *Invest Ophthalmol Vis Sci* 29:1285, 1988.

160. Topper JE, Brubaker RF: Effects of timolol, epinephrine and acetazolamide on aqueous flow during sleep, *Invest Ophthalmol Vis Sci* 26:1315, 1985.

161. Becker B: The decline in aqueous secretion and outflow facility with age, *Am J Ophthalmol* 46:731, 1958.

162. Gaasterland D, and others: Studies of aqueous humor dynamics in man. VI. Effect of age on parameters of intraocular pressure in normal human eyes, *Exp Eye Res* 26:651, 1978.

163. Kupfer C: Clinical significance of pseudofacility, *Am J Ophthalmol* 75:193, 1973.

164. Lutjen-Drecoll E: *Functional morphology of the ciliary epithelium*. In Lutjen-Drecoll E, editor: *Basic aspects of glaucoma research*, Stuttgart, 1982, Schattauer.

165. Bill A: The effect of ocular hypertension caused by red cells on the rate of formation of aqueous humor, *Invest Ophthalmol* 7:162, 1968.

166. Anselmi P, Bron AJ, Maurice DM: Action of drugs on the aqueous flow in man measured by fluorophotometry, *Exp Eye Res* 7:487, 1968.

167. Araie M, and others: Effects of laser trabeculoplasty on the human aqueous humor dynamics: a fluorophotometric study, *Am J Ophthalmol* 16:540, 1984.

168. Brubaker RF, Liesegang TJ: Effect of trabecular photocoagulation on the aqueous dynamics of the human eye, *Am J Ophthalmol* 96:139, 1983.

169. Yablonski ME, Cook DJ, Gray J: A fluorophotometric study of the effect of argon laser trabeculoplasty on aqueous humor dynamics, *Am J Ophthalmol* 99:579, 1985.

170. Brown JD, Brubaker RF: A study of the relation between intraocular pressure and aqueous humor flow in the pigment dispersion syndrome, *Ophthalmology* 96:1468, 1989.

171. Walker SD, Brubaker RF, Nagataki S: Hypotony and aqueous humor dynamics in myotonic dystrophy, *Invest Ophthalmol Vis Sci* 22:744, 1982.

172. Bill A: Effects of acetazolamide and carotid occlusion on the aqueous blood flow in unanesthetized rabbits, *Invest Ophthalmol* 13:954, 1974.

173. Kornbluth W, Linner E: Experimental tonography in rabbits: effect of unilateral ligation of a common carotid artery on aqueous humor dynamics as studied by means of tonography and fluorescein appearance time, *Arch Ophthalmol* 54:717, 1955.

174. Linner E: Ascorbic acid as a test substance for measuring relative changes in the rate of plasma flow through the ciliary processes. IV. The effect of carotid ligation and cervical sympathectomy in guinea pigs on the ascorbic acid content of the aqueous humor at varying plasma levels, *Acta Physiol Scand* 26:130, 1952.

175. Pollack IP, Becker B: The effect of hypothermia on aqueous humor dynamics. IV. Carotid artery ligation and blood flow, *Am J Ophthalmol* 51:1039, 1961.

176. Ross KS, Macri RJ, Kupfer C: The effect of carotid artery ligation on aqueous humor formation in the rhesus monkey *Macaca mulatta*, *Exp Eye Res* 27:687, 1978.

177. Gloster J, Greaves DP: Effect of diencephalic stimulation upon intra-ocular pressure, *Br J Ophthalmol* 41:513, 1957.

178. Schmerl E, Steinberg B: Separation of diencephalic centers concerned with pupillary motility and ocular tension, *Am J Ophthalmol* 33:1379, 1950.

179. von Sallmann L, Lowenstein O: Responses of intraocular pressure, blood pressure, and cutaneous vessels to electrical stimulation in the diencephalon, *Am J Ophthalmol* 39:11, 1955.

180. Krupin T, and others: Increased intraocular pressure and hypothermia following injection of calcium into the rabbit third ventricle, *Exp Eye Res* 27:129, 1978.

181. Podos SM, Krupin T, Becker B: Mechanism of intraocular pressure response after optic nerve transection, *Am J Ophthalmol* 72:79, 1971.

182. Riise D, Simonsen E: Intraocular pressure in unilateral optic nerve lesions, *Acta Ophthalmolol Scand Suppl* 47:750, 1969.

183. Smith SD, Gregory DS: A circadian rhythm of aqueous flow underlies the circadian rhythm of IOP in NZW rabbits, *Invest Ophthalmol Vis Sci* 30:775, 1989.

184. Belmonte C, and others: Effects of stimulation of the ocular sympathetic nerves on the IOP and aqueous humor flow, *Invest Ophthalmol Vis Sci* 28:1649, 1987.

185. Bron AJ: Sympathetic control of aqueous secretion in man, *Br J Ophthalmol* 53:37, 1969.

186. Kass MA, Sears ML: Hormonal regulation of intraocular pressure, *Surv Ophthalmol* 22:153, 1977.

187. Levene RZ, Schwartz B: Depression of plasma cortisol and the steroid ocular pressure response, *Arch Ophthalmol* 80:461, 1968.

188. Kacere RD, Dolan JW, Brubaker RF: Intravenous epinephrine stimulates aqueous formation in the human eye, *Invest Ophthalmol Vis Sci* 33:2861, 1992.

189. Gharagozloo NZ, and others: Terbutaline stimulates aqueous flow in humans during sleep, *Arch Ophthalmol* 106:1218, 1988.

190. Caprioli J, Sears ML: The adenyl cyclase receptor complex and aqueous humor formation, *Yale J Biol Med* 57:283, 1984.

191. Sears ML: Regulation of aqueous flow by the adenylate cyclase receptor complex in the ciliary epithelium, *Am J Ophthalmol* 110:194, 1985.

192. Waitzman M, Woods W: Some characteristics of an adenyl cyclase preparation, *Exp Eye Res* 12:99, 1971.

193. Nathanson JA: Atriopeptin-activated guanylate cyclase in the anterior segment: identification, localization, and effects of atriopeptins on IOP, *Invest Ophthalmol Vis Sci* 28:1357, 1987.

194. Cherksey BD, Alvarado JA, Polansky JR: Ion channel activity of ciliary process epithelium vesicles reconstituted into planar bilayers, *Invest Ophthalmol Vis Sci* 29(suppl):175, 1988.

195. Polansky JR, Cherksey BR, Alvarado JA: *Update on beta adrenergic drug therapy.* In Drance SM, van Buskirk AM, Neufeld AH, editors: *Applied pharmacology of the glaucomas,* Philadelphia, 1991, Williams & Wilkins.

196. McCannel CA, and others: A study of aqueous humor formation in patients with cystic fibrosis, *Invest Ophthalmol Vis Sci* 33:160, 1992.

197. Johnson D, Liesegang TJ, Brubaker RF: Aqueous humor dynamics in Fuchs' uveitis syndrome, *Am J Ophthalmol* 95:783, 1983.

198. Pederson JE: Ocular hypotony, *Trans Ophthalmol Soc UK* 105:220, 1986.

199. Krupin T, and others: The effect of hyperthermia on aqueous humor dynamics in rabbits, *Am J Ophthalmol* 83:561, 1977.

200. Hayashi M, and others: Decreased formation of aqueous humor in insulin-dependent diabetic patients, *Br J Ophthalmol* 73:621, 1989.

201. Kimura R, Honda M: Effect of orally administered hydrocortisone on the rate of aqueous flow in man, *Acta Ophthalmol Scand Suppl* 60:582, 1982.

202. Samuelsson-Almen M, and others: Effects of atrial natriuretic factor (ANF) on intraocular pressure and aqueous humor flow in the cynomolgus monkey, *Exp Eye Res* 53:253, 1991.

203. Kalina PH, and others: 6-amino-2-benzothiazolesulfonamide: the effect of a topical carbonic anhydrase inhibitor on aqueous humor formation in the normal human eye, *Ophthalmology* 95:772, 1988.

204. Yablonski ME, and others: A fluorophotometric study of the effect of topical timolol on aqueous humor dynamics, *Exp Eye Res* 27:135, 1978.

205. McCannel CA, Heinrich SR, Brubaker RF: Acetazolamide but not timolol lowers aqueous humor flow in sleeping humans, *Graefes Arch Clin Exp Ophthalmol* 230:518, 1992.

206. Schlecht LP, Brubaker RF: The effects of withdrawal of timolol in chronically treated glaucoma patients, *Ophthalmology* 95:1212, 1988.

207. Gharagozloo NZ, Relf SJ, Brubaker RF: Aqueous flow is reduced by the alpha-adrenergic agonist, apraclonidine hydrochloride (ALO 2145), *Ophthalmology* 95:1217, 1988.

208. Becker B, Ley AP: Epinephrine and acetazolamide in the therapy of the glaucomas, *Am J Ophthalmol* 45:639, 1958.

209. Garner LL, and others: Effect of 2% levo-rotary epinephrine on the intraocular pressure of the glaucomatous eye, *Arch Ophthalmol* 62:230, 1959.

210. Weekers R, Delmarcelle Y, Gustin J: Treatment of ocular hypertension by adrenaline and diverse sympathomimetic amines, *Am J Ophthalmol* 40:660, 1955.

211. Higgins RG, Brubaker RF: Acute effect of epinephrine on aqueous humor formation in the timolol-treated eye as measured by fluorophotometry, *Invest Ophthalmol Vis Sci* 19:420, 1980.

212. Becker B: Vanadate and aqueous humor dynamics: Proctor Lecture, *Invest Ophthalmol Vis Sci* 19:1150, 1980.

213. Krupin T, Becker B, Podos SM: Topical vanadate lowers intraocular pressure in rabbits, *Invest Ophthalmol Vis Sci* 19:1 360, 1980.

214. Mittag TW, and others: Vanadate effects on ocular pressure, $(Na^+ K^+)$ ATPase and adenylate cyclase in rabbit eyes, *Invest Ophthalmol Vis Sci* 25:1335, 1984.

215. Krupin T, and others: Halothane anesthesia and aqueous humor dynamics in laboratory animals, *Invest Ophthalmol Vis Sci* 19:518, 1980.

216. Schutten WH, Van Horn DL: The effects of ketamine sedation and ketamine-pentobarbital anesthesia upon the intraocular pressure of the rabbit, *Invest Ophthalmol Vis Sci* 16:531, 1977.

4

Aqueous Humor Outflow

There is a constant flow of aqueous humor through the anterior segment of the eye. The aqueous humor is formed by the ciliary processes, passes from the posterior chamber to the anterior chamber through the pupil, and exits the eye at the angle. Most of the fluid enters the venous system by way of the trabecular meshwork and Schlemm's canal; this fluid movement is referred to as *conventional* or *canalicular* (in reference to Schlemm's canal) outflow. A lesser amount of aqueous humor passes through other structures in the anterior segment, including the anterior ciliary muscle, and the iris to reach the supraciliary and suprachoroidal spaces. From here the fluid passes through the sclera or through the loose connective tissue around the penetrating nerves and vessels; this fluid movement is referred to as *uveoscleral, unconventional,* or *extracanalicular outflow.*

FACILITY OF OUTFLOW

The Goldmann equation can be rearranged to give a simplified view of the factors that determine the ease with which aqueous humor leaves the eye by conventional outflow.

$$C = \frac{F}{P_O - P_V}$$

In this equation, C is the facility of outflow (μl/min/mm Hg), F is the aqueous humor production (μl/min), P_O is the intraocular pressure (IOP) in the undisturbed eye (mm Hg), and P_V is the episcleral venous pressure (mm Hg). The factor referred to as C is often expressed as its reciprocal, R, which is the resistance to outflow (mm Hg $\times$ min $\times$ μl^{-1}).

It is generally accepted that the juxtacanalicular trabecular meshwork and the inner wall of Schlemm's canal provide the major portion of the normal resistance to outflow. Furthermore, it is postulated that these tissues are the sites of the abnormal resistance to outflow found in most cases of open-angle glaucoma. (Open-angle glaucoma is rarely caused by elevated episcleral venous pressure.) Because aqueous humor outflow and open-angle glaucoma are so closely associated, it is important to understand the anatomy and physiology of the angle structures in some detail.

ANATOMY OF OUTFLOW SYSTEM

The major pathway from the anterior chamber to the venous system includes the trabecular meshwork, the juxtacanalicular tissue, the endothelium of Schlemm's canal, and the collector channels. Each of these tissues is described in some detail.

Trabecular Meshwork

In meridional section, the trabecular meshwork has a triangular shape, with its apex at Schwalbe's line and its base at the scleral spur (Fig. 4-1). The meshwork consists of a stack of flattened, interconnected, perforated sheets, which run in meridional fashion from the peripheral cornea and Descemet's membrane anteriorly to the scleral spur posteriorly. The sheets are fused in such a manner that only two or three layers are seen anteriorly, whereas 12 to 20 layers are detectable posteriorly. The inner layers of the trabecular meshwork border the anterior chamber and are referred to as the uveal meshwork. The outer layers, the corneoscleral meshwork, are separated from the endothelium of Schlemm's canal by a thin strip of connective tissue called the juxtacanalicular tissue (Fig. 4-2).

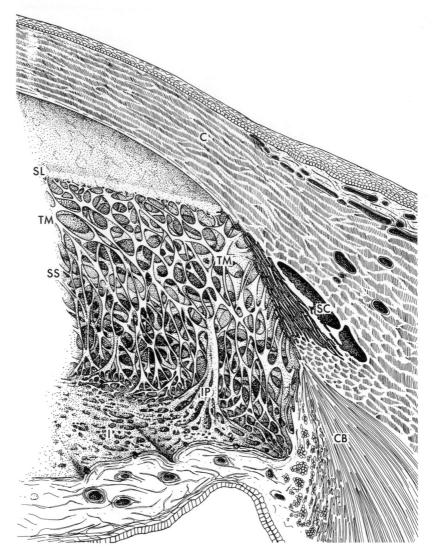

Figure 4-1 Semidiagrammatic representation of structures of the angle of the anterior chamber. Note the superimposed trabecular sheets with intratrabecular and intertrabecular spaces, through which aqueous humor percolates to reach Schlemm's canal. *SL*, Schwalbe's line; *SS*, scleral spur; *IP*, iris process; *TM*, trabecular meshwork; *C*, cornea; *I*, iris; *SC*, Schlemm's canal; *CB*, ciliary body. (From Tripathi RC, Tripathi BJ: *Functional anatomy of the anterior chamber angle.* In Duane TD, Jaeger EA, editors: *Biomedical foundations of ophthalmology,* vol 1, New York, 1982, Harper & Row.)

In many eyes the innermost layers of the uveal meshwork take the form of fine strands that arise from the anterior surface of the iris, bridge the angle recess, and insert into the deeper uveal trabeculae or Schwalbe's line (see Fig. 4-1). These strands are a normal variant and have been given a variety of names, including *iris processes, pectinate fibers, uveal trabeculae, ciliary fibers, ciliocorneal fibers,* and *uveocorneal fibers.* The deeper layers of the uveal meshwork have the more typical appearance of flattened sheets with wide perforations. The sheets branch and interconnect in multiple planes. The inner layers are oriented radially, whereas the deeper layers are oriented circumferentially.

The corneoscleral meshwork consists of 8 to 15 perforated sheets, each 5 to 12 μm thick.[1] The perforations are elliptic in shape and become progressively smaller from the superficial layers of the uveal meshwork to the deep layers of the corneoscleral meshwork (Fig. 4-2).[1-3] The perforations are not aligned, so aqueous humor must follow a circuitous route to reach Schlemm's canal (Fig. 4-3).

The ultrastructure of the trabecular meshwork is similar to that of other highly compliant and

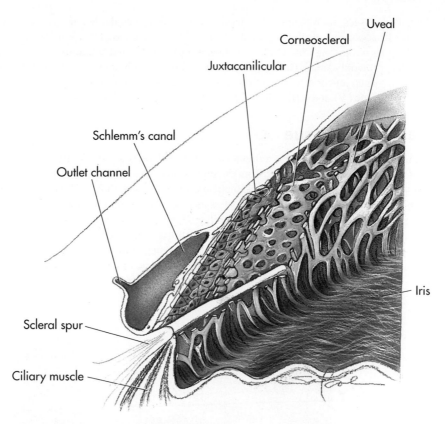

Figure 4-2 Schematic view of different layers of the outflow system. (Modified from Shields MB: *Textbook of glaucoma,* Baltimore, 1987, Williams & Wilkins.)

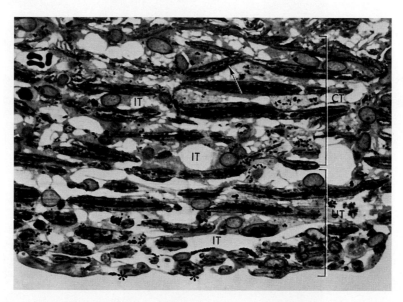

Figure 4-3 Light micrograph of trabecular meshwork in 70-year-old human eye. Meridional section shows morphology of uveal trabeculae *(UT)* and corneoscleral trabeculae *(CT)*. Note the rounded profile of inner uveal trabecular sheets *(asterisks)* compared with flattened profile of outer uveal and corneoscleral sheets, and a progressive narrowing of intertrabecular spaces *(IT)* in the latter region. *Arrow* denotes branching of a trabecular sheet. (Original magnification × 760.) (From Tripathi RC, Tripathi BJ: *Functional anatomy of the anterior chamber angle.* In Duane TD, Jaeger EA, editors: *Biomedical foundations of ophthalmology,* vol 1, New York, 1982, Harper & Row.)

resilient tissues, such as lung and blood vessels.[4] The trabecular beams have a central core of types I and III collagen and elastin (Fig. 4-4).[4] The core is surrounded by a cortical zone (also referred to as a *glass membrane*) that contains collagen types III, IV, and V; laminin; fibronectin; and heparin sulfate proteoglycan.[4,5] The beams are covered by a continuous layer of endothelial cells that are joined by gap junctions and tight junctions.[6,7] The endothelial cells have microfilaments, including actin.[8,9] Types VI and VIII collagen have also been identified in trabecular meshwork tissues.[10-15]

Juxtacanalicular Tissue

The juxtacanalicular tissue is a thin layer of tissue, 2 to 20 μm thick, that separates the outer layers of the corneoscleral meshwork from the inner wall of Schlemm's canal. This tissue has been called a variety of names, including pericanalicular tissue, endothelial meshwork, cribriform tissue, and pore tissue. The tissue has a ground substance of glycosaminoglycans and glycoproteins[5,16,17] that contain types III, IV, and V collagen; curly collagen; fibronectin; fibroblasts; and star-shaped cells that have been referred to as subendothelial, cribriform, and juxtacanalicular cells.[7,18,19] Fibronectin content is increased in elderly patients and in patients with glaucoma.[20] Some investigators have noted that the juxtacanalicular tissue contains a network of elastic fibers that may provide support for the inner wall of Schlemm's canal. This network is attached to some of the tendons of the ciliary muscle.[21,22]

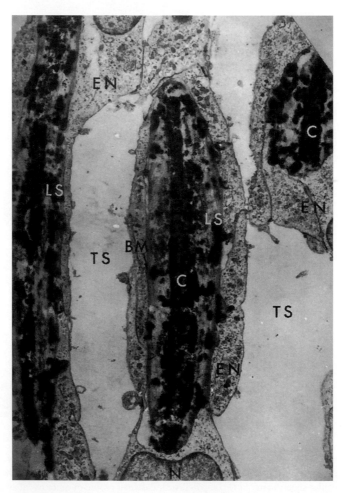

Figure 4-4   Electron micrograph of a meridional section of human corneoscleral trabecular meshwork. (× 11,000.) *TS*, Trabecular space; *EN*, endothelial cell; *N*, nucleus of endothelial cell; *BM*, basement membrane; *LS*, long-spacing collagen; *C*, collagen. (Courtesy of L. Feeney, San Francisco.)

Schlemm's Canal

Schlemm's canal is an endothelial-lined circular channel that runs circumferentially around the globe. The canal resembles a lymphatic channel in its structure. The endothelium is derived from a vascular origin, and it retains some of the properties of a blood vessel into adult life.[23] It is surrounded by sclera, trabecular meshwork, and the scleral spur. Generally Schlemm's canal has a single slitlike lumen that is 190 to 370 μm in diameter.[24] However, in some eyes the lumen is irregular and can even become a plexiform channel with multiple branches. Septae run from the external walls to the internal walls and may provide some support for the canal. The septae have dense collagenous cores that resemble sclera. The outer wall of Schlemm's canal has a single layer of endothelium that lacks pores or vacuoles.[25]

Inner Wall of Schlemm's Canal

The endothelium lining the inner wall of Schlemm's canal consists of a monolayer of spindle-shaped cells (see Fig. 4-2). There is some debate about whether these endothelial cells sit directly on the juxtacanalicular tissue or are separated from it by an incomplete basement membrane. The overall structure of the junctions between endothelial cells of Schlemm's canal is quite complex and variable.[26] The nuclei of the endothelial cells and a series of large or giant vacuoles form projections into the lumen of Schlemm's canal (Fig. 4-5).[16,27,28] Some authorities believe these giant vacuoles

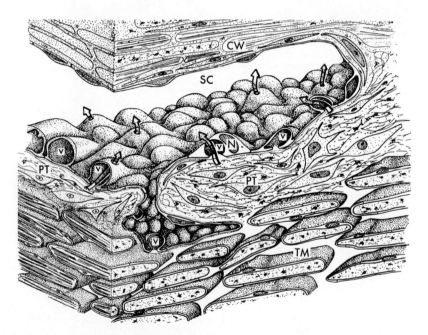

Figure 4-5 The walls of Schlemm's canal *(SC)* and adjacent trabecular meshwork in a composite sectional and three-dimensional view. The endothelial lining of the trabecular wall of Schlemm's canal is very irregular, and the cells show luminal bulges corresponding to cell nuclei *(N)* and macrovacuolar configurations *(v)*. The latter may represent cellular invaginations occurring from the basal aspect and eventually opening on the apical aspect of the cell to form transcellular channels *(arrows),* through which aqueous humor flows down a pressure gradient. The endothelial lining of the trabecular wall is supported by an interrupted, irregular basement membrane and a zone of pericanalicular connective tissue *(PT)* of variable thickness. The cellular element predominates in this zone, and the fibrous elements, especially elastic fibers, are irregularly arranged in a netlike fashion. Here the open spaces are narrower than those of the trabecular meshwork *(TM).* The corneoscleral trabecular sheets show frequent branching, and the endothelial covering may be shared between adjacent sheets. The corneoscleral wall *(CW)* of Schlemm's canal is more compact than the trabecular wall, with a predominance of lamellar arrangement of collagen and elastic tissue. (From Tripathi RC, Tripathi BJ: *Functional anatomy of the anterior chamber angle.* In Duane TD, Jaeger EA, editors: *Biomedical foundations of ophthalmology,* vol 1, New York, 1982, Harper & Row.)

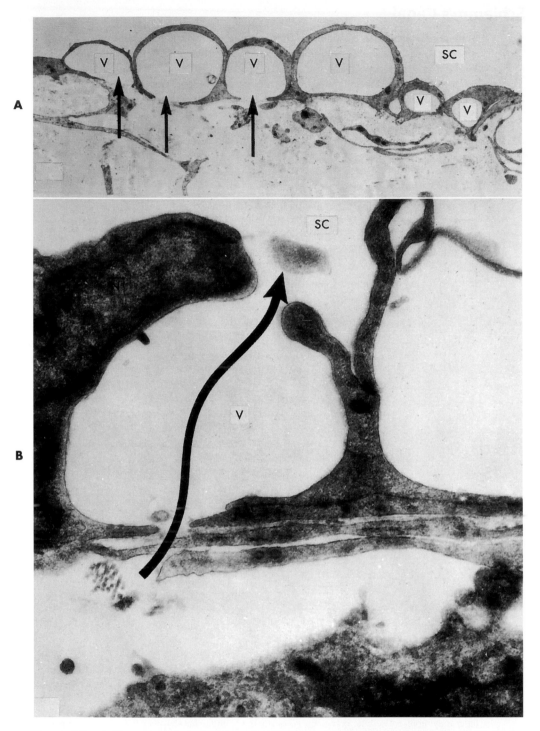

Figure 4-6   **A,** Electron micrograph of the endothelial lining of Schlemm's canal *(SC),* showing the majority of the vacuolar configurations *(V)* at this level of section having direct communication *(arrows)* with the subendothelial extracellular spaces, which contain aqueous humor in life. (Original magnification × 3970.) **B,** Electron micrograph of a vacuolar structure that at this level of section shows both basal and apical openings, thus constituting a vacuolar transcellular channel *(long arrow).* In this way the fluid-containing extracellular space on the basal aspect of the cell is temporarily connected with the lumen of Schlemm's canal *(SC),* allowing bulk outflow of aqueous humor. *N,* indented nucleus of the cell. (Original magnification × 23,825.) (From Tripathi RC, Tripathi BJ: *Functional anatomy of the anterior chamber angle.* In Duane TD, Jaeger EA, editors: *Biomedical foundations of ophthalmology,* vol 1, New York, 1982, Harper & Row.)

form and recede in cyclic fashion and serve as a pathway for fluid movement (Fig. 4-6).* In some cases apparent giant vacuoles are not actually intracellular vacuoles but rather dilations of the paracellular spaces that may vary under different conditions of pressure and flow.[37]

Collector Channels

Schlemm's canal is drained by a series of collector channels that in turn drain into a complex system of intrascleral, episcleral, and subconjunctival venous plexuses.[38-40] The collector channels arise from the outer wall of Schlemm's canal at irregular intervals of 0.3 to 2.8 mm. A few vessels proceed directly from Schlemm's canal to the episcleral and conjunctival veins. These vessels have a characteristic laminar flow of aqueous humor and blood that can be seen on slit-lamp examination a few millimeters posterior to the limbus.[41-43]

Scleral Spur

The scleral spur is a fibrous ring that, on meridional section, appears as a wedge that projects from the inner aspect of the anterior sclera (see Figs. 4-1 and 4-2). The spur is attached anteriorly to the trabecular meshwork and posteriorly to the sclera and the longitudinal portion of the ciliary muscle. When the ciliary muscle contracts, it pulls the scleral spur posteriorly, which increases the width of the intertrabecular spaces and prevents Schlemm's canal from collapsing. The spur consists of collagen types I and III and elastic tissue oriented in circular fashion.[4,44,45]

Schwalbe's Line

Schwalbe's line (composed of collagen and elastic tissue)[46] is an irregular elevation 50 to 150 μm wide that runs circumferentially around the globe. This line or zone marks the transition from trabecular to corneal endothelium, the termination of Descemet's membrane, and the insertion of the trabecular meshwork into the corneal stroma.

PHYSIOLOGY OF THE OUTFLOW SYSTEM

The trabecular meshwork and the outflow channels perform a number of important functions, the most obvious of which is to allow the egress of aqueous humor. In addition, the trabecular endothelial cells phagocytize particulate matter and debris, thus serving as the reticuloendothelial system of the anterior segment of the eye. Finally, the scleral spur, trabecular meshwork, and ciliary muscle provide structural support to prevent the collapse of Schlemm's canal.

At one time there was considerable controversy over whether aqueous humor circulates or is a stagnant fluid. The latter concept was supported by studies that found a higher pressure in Schlemm's canal than in the eye itself. However, this finding was incorrect because it is technically difficult to measure pressure in small channels. Not until many years later was it established that the pressure in Schlemm's canal is actually lower than IOP. Classic studies of the aqueous outflow system by Ascher[41] and earlier work by Goldmann[47] confirmed that aqueous humor circulates through the eye and then enters the extraocular venous system. There are a number of potential pathways for aqueous humor to leave the eye, including the trabeculocanalicular, uveoscleral, transcorneal, and postiridial routes. The trabeculocanalicular and uveoscleral routes account for most of the aqueous elimination, and they are discussed in detail later in this section.

Some aqueous humor passes from the anterior chamber into the tear film through the cornea. The total volume of fluid transferred by this route is limited by the high hydraulic resistance of the cornea. The best example of the functioning of this pathway is the slight fall in IOP that occurs in the fellow eye during tonography. If the fellow eye is anesthetized and uncovered, and if blinking is suppressed, enough aqueous humor moves across the cornea to lower IOP slightly.[48]

The volume of aqueous humor that flows through the angle of the anterior chamber is approximately equal to the volume of fluid that flows through the pupil. Most of the aqueous humor and its constituents leave the eye by bulk fluid flow—that is, fluid flows along the normal pressure gra-

*Refs: 1-3, 18, 22, 24, 29-36.

dients in a non–energy-dependent process. However, certain substances in the aqueous humor leave the eye by different processes than bulk flow. For example, substances soluble in both aqueous solutions and lipids leave the eye faster than water, which in turn leaves the eye 4 times faster than sodium.[49] These different turnover rates reflect the fact that the aqueous humor and its constituents are influenced by contact with many different tissues, as well as by diffusion, active transport, and metabolism.

Trabeculocanalicular Flow

Most of the aqueous humor passes into Schlemm's canal by traversing the uveal meshwork, corneoscleral meshwork, juxtacanalicular tissue, and endothelial lining of the canal (Fig. 4-7). From the canal the fluid is transferred by 20 to 30 collector channels to an intrascleral venous plexus, which in turn communicates with an episcleral venous plexus and the anterior ciliary veins. Some of the aqueous humor is carried directly from Schlemm's canal to the episcleral plexus by the aqueous veins.[41]

The trabecular meshwork–Schlemm's canal system has been compared with a spongelike, one-way valve for the egress of aqueous humor.[4] Because the eye contains so many avascular tissues, a continuous circulation of aqueous humor is necessary to supply nutrients and remove waste products. Under normal circumstances the trabecular meshwork permits aqueous humor to leave the eye while maintaining IOP within a fairly narrow range. This is crucial for the structural integrity and optical functioning of the eye. The trabecular meshwork has the anatomic appearance of a compliant and resilient tissue capable of serving its major function despite different rates of aqueous humor formation, different levels of IOP, and different amounts of ciliary muscle tone. The trabecular meshwork seems compliant enough to respond to functional changes in the eye and yet resilient enough to return to its normal state when these changes are no longer present.[4]

It is important to stress that the trabecular meshwork functions as a one-way valve—that is, it permits bulk flow out of the eye but restricts flow in the other direction. The trabecular meshwork is a crucial part of the normal blood–aqueous barrier. When IOP is low, the trabecular meshwork is compressed, which prevents red blood cells and plasma proteins from entering the anterior chamber (Fig. 4-8).[50-52] This is important for the optical properties of the eye and limits the entrance of potentially noxious substances.

Another important function of the trabecular meshwork is that the trabecular endothelial cells actively phagocytize foreign material and debris—that is, the endothelium acts as the reticuloen-

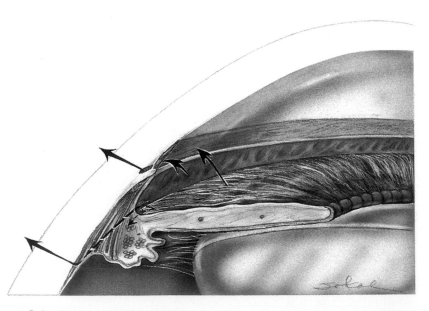

Figure 4-7   Aqueous humor leaving the eye by trabeculocanalicular flow and uveoscleral flow.

dothelial system of the anterior segment of the eye. Because of this property, Bill[49] has compared the meshwork with a self-cleaning filter. If the trabecular endothelial cells become engorged with foreign material, they may be destroyed or may become wandering cells.

A number of authorities have raised the question of whether the trabecular meshwork directly regulates IOP.[35,46,53,54] These authorities have postulated the existence of a receptor in the trabecu-

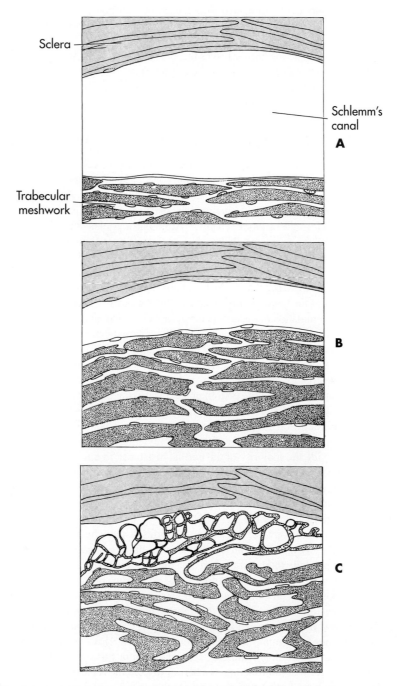

Figure 4-8 Schematic drawing of the trabecular meshwork and Schlemm's canal at different levels of intraocular pressure (IOP). **A,** IOP less than episcleral venous pressure, so the meshwork is collapsed. **B,** IOP equal to episcleral venous pressure. **C,** IOP 30 to 40 mm Hg greater than episcleral venous pressure. The meshwork is distended into the lumen of Schlemm's canal. (Modified from Johnstone MA, Grant WM: *Am J Ophthalmol* 75:380, 1973. Published with permission from the American Journal of Ophthalmology. Copyright by the Ophthalmic Publishing Company.)

lar meshwork that responds to pressure or tissue distention and then provides feedback to modulate some process, such as aqueous humor formation,[51] ciliary muscle tone, or glycosaminoglycan synthesis.[17,54,55] Although this concept remains intriguing, there is no evidence to support that such a feedback system exists. In fact, in the studies done to date elevations or depressions of IOP are not accompanied by substantial changes in the rate of aqueous humor formation[56,57] (see Chapter 3).

Because of the absence of clotting factors under physiologic conditions, the outflow channels appear to be protected from obstruction caused by clotting. In addition, fibrinolytic activity, including tissue plasminogen activator, is present in the trabecular meshwork and the endothelium of Schlemm's canal.[8,59]

Even though aqueous humor leaves the eye mainly by bulk flow, the trabecular meshwork is a living tissue that must expend energy for normal functioning. Studies using tissue culture of excised animal trabecular meshwork indicate that the tissue has moderate glycolysis and respiration[60] and an active pentose shunt system.[61]

Normal Resistance to Aqueous Humor Outflow

It is generally accepted that the major portion of the normal resistance to outflow lies between the anterior chamber and Schlemm's canal. This concept is supported by the studies of Grant,[62] who found a 75% decrease in the resistance to outflow when he incised the entire trabecular meshwork in enucleated human eyes. The reduction in resistance was even more striking when similar experiments were performed in monkey eyes.[63] Although it is clear that the trabecular meshwork, the endothelium of Schlemm's canal, and the canal itself contribute to the normal resistance to outflow, there is great controversy about which of these tissues constitutes the major barrier to bulk flow of aqueous humor.[64-66]

There is some evidence that the endothelium of Schlemm's canal, a monolayer connected by tight junctions, serves as the major barrier to aqueous humor egress.[2] This theory is supported by tracer studies that show accumulation of material at the inner wall of Schlemm's canal.[2,18,29] Further support comes from the improvement in outflow facility that follows experimental infusion of certain substances, such as iodoacetic acid,[67] N-ethylmaleimide,[68] cytochalasin B or D,[69-72] EDTA,[73,74] and colchicine.[75] Histologic studies suggest that these agents alter the inner wall of Schlemm's canal.[69,72-74]

Many investigators currently believe that aqueous humor enters Schlemm's canal by traversing transcellular channels in the endothelial cells.[34] Tripathi[2,33,34] has suggested that these channels form and recede in cyclic fashion. The cycle begins with an invagination on the trabecular side of the endothelial cell and progresses to a transcellular channel with a small pore opening into Schlemm's canal. Only a small fraction of the invaginations open into the canal at any one time, which may provide the majority of the normal resistance to outflow.

The number and size of the pores increase with increasing levels of IOP.[50,51] At low levels of IOP the invaginations and the pores disappear. The formation of the vacuoles continues in enucleated eyes and is not inhibited by hypothermia, which suggests a mechanical rather than an active metabolic rearrangement of the cell.[76]

It is important to point out that some authorities dispute this theory of aqueous egress and question whether the invaginations are really part of a fluid transport system or are merely artifacts.[18] Bill[49] has estimated the total number and area of the pores and believes they are too numerous to account for the normal resistance to outflow. Some authorities postulate that aqueous humor passes between the endothelial cells, opening and closing the cell junctions in some unknown fashion.

Other investigators believe that the trabecular meshwork itself is the site of the normal resistance to outflow. If the trabecular spaces were empty, it is clear that the channels would be too large and too numerous to account for the resistance to outflow. However, the channels are filled with glycosaminoglycans, including hyaluronic acid, chondroitin sulfate, and dermatan sulfate,[32,77-84] which in polymerized form could function as a barrier to fluid movement.[18,54,85,86] The highly polymerized complexes also have strong negative charges that may affect fluid and ion movement. It has been further suggested that the resistance to fluid movement in these channels could be modulated by lysosomal enzymes that catabolize the glycosaminoglycans.[55] This theory is supported by perfusion studies of nonprimate eyes in which hyaluronidase decreases resistance.[62,87] Furthermore, prolonged perfusion without hyaluronidase leads to a gradual reduction in resistance caused by the washout of a hyaluronidase-sensitive factor.[88,89] However, these phenomena are not seen in primate eyes, and perfusion studies in monkeys suggest that the glycosaminoglycans constitute only a small portion of the normal resistance to outflow.[90]

Some investigators propose alternative mechanisms by which the trabecular meshwork could control normal aqueous humor egress. It has been noted that glucocorticoid receptors are present in the meshwork.[91-93] It is possible that these receptors may affect collagen or glycosaminoglycan synthesis and thus control aqueous outflow.[91,92,94] Trabecular endothelial cells also synthesize prostaglandins, which may modulate outflow.[95]

A few researchers have suggested that Schlemm's canal is the site of the normal resistance to outflow. However, the structure of the canal suggests it provides little resistance to fluid flow unless it collapses. Although the canal may collapse at very high levels of IOP, there is no evidence to support that it does so at normal levels of pressure (see Fig. 4-8). Whether aqueous humor flows circumferentially in the canal or whether each section of the canal is drained exclusively by one or two collector channels is controversial. Van Buskirk and Grant[96] found that aqueous humor did not flow more than 10° around the canal of enucleated human eyes. In contrast, Moses and co-workers[97] noted that refluxed blood flowed circumferentially around the canal in living subjects.

The collector channels provide a small resistance to fluid flow.[98] However, there is no reason to believe that this resistance is a major factor controlling normal aqueous humor egress.

Uveoscleral Flow

A lesser amount of the aqueous humor exits the eye by an alternate route through the ciliary muscle, the iris, the sclera, and other structures of the anterior segment (see Fig. 4-7). This alternate pathway is known by a number of terms, including *uveoscleral, unconventional, extracanalicular, secondary,* and *uveovortex flow.* As Bill[49] pointed out, flow through the trabecular meshwork and Schlemm's canal seems to involve a well-designed system. In contrast, uveoscleral flow seems more primitive and resembles a leak more than a well-designed fluid transport system.[99]

Aqueous humor enters the ciliary muscle through the uveal trabecular meshwork, the ciliary body face, and the iris root. The fluid passes posteriorly between the bundles of the ciliary muscle until it reaches the supraciliary and suprachoroidal spaces. Aqueous humor leaves the eye through the spaces around the penetrating nerves and blood vessels and through the sclera.[18,100-104] Even large molecules such as horseradish peroxidase and albumin can pass through intact sclera.[49,105,106]

A few investigators have questioned whether aqueous humor can exit the eye by entering the uveal vascular system. Tracer studies indicate that there is some exchange of substances between the aqueous humor and the plasma in the uveal blood vessels. However, the net fluid flow into the uveal vascular system is quite low for a number of reasons. First, the iris capillaries have thick walls that restrict movement of water and ions.[49] Furthermore, pressure in the uveal capillaries is higher than IOP. This pressure difference partially offsets the difference in oncotic pressure between the plasma and the tissue fluid of the uveal tract. Thus there is little driving force for fluid to cross the capillary walls.

Uveoscleral flow seems to be present in most species, but the portion of the aqueous humor transported by this system varies considerably. For example, unconventional flow constitutes about 3% of the total outflow in rabbit eyes but represents more than 50% of the total outflow in some species of monkeys. In human eyes the unconventional pathway is estimated to carry 5% to 25% of the total aqueous outflow. It should be pointed out that direct measurements of uveoscleral flow in humans have been limited to a few eyes, many of which were scheduled for enucleation because of intraocular tumors.[105] It is possible that such eyes are atypical and that the results are not representative of normal eyes. Calculations based on noninvasive measurements indicate that uveoscleral outflow may constitute as much as 35% of the outflow.[40,99,107] Furthermore, in primate and human studies, uveoscleral outflow increases up to fourfold when the anterior segment is inflamed.[106,108]

Uveoscleral flow has been studied with a variety of tracer substances, including fluorescein, radiolabeled molecules, and small plastic spheres.[101,109,110] In human experiments ^{131}I-albumin can be traced by autoradiography from the anterior uveal tract to the posterior pole.[105]

Uveoscleral flow increases when IOP is raised from atmospheric pressure to the level of episcleral venous pressure. However, above this pressure level uveoscleral flow is largely independent of IOP. An increased IOP provides a greater driving force for uveoscleral flow, but it also compacts the anterior ciliary muscle bundles.[100,111] These two factors must nearly offset one another because in the uninflamed eye the facility of uveoscleral flow is quite low at 0.02 to 0.052 μl/min/mm Hg.[103,106]

The main resistance to uveoscleral flow is the tone of the ciliary muscle. Factors that contract the ciliary muscle (such as pilocarpine) lower uveoscleral flow, whereas factors that relax the ciliary muscle (such as atropine) raise uveoscleral flow.[112,113] Uveoscleral outflow is increased significantly by prostaglandins.[114-118] Prostaglandins in low dose are among the most potent IOP-lowering agents available.[119-128]

As mentioned above, pilocarpine decreases and atropine increases uveoscleral flow.[112,113] This is consistent with a large body of work indicating that the therapeutic effect of pilocarpine in most glaucoma patients reflects increased trabecular outflow (caused by contraction of the iris sphincter and ciliary muscle)[129-137] over the decreased uveoscleral flow following muscarinic stimulation. Some studies have shown that pilocarpine antagonizes therapeutic prostaglandin agents,[138] but clinical experience is mixed in this area.[139,140] A few studies indicate that epinephrine may lower IOP, in large part by increasing uveoscleral flow.[107,141,142] Cyclodialysis is an operation designed to lower IOP by detaching a portion of the ciliary body from the scleral spur. There is evidence that cyclodialysis acts to increase uveoscleral flow.[57,107]

METHODS FOR MEASURING FACILITY OF OUTFLOW

There are three common methods used to measure facility of outflow—tonography, perfusion, and suction cup. It is also possible to calculate the resistance to outflow from the Goldmann equation by measuring aqueous humor formation and IOP as discussed in Chapter 3.

Tonography

Tonography has been the most widely used clinical technique for measuring facility of outflow. Although most clinicians no longer use tonography as a routine clinical test, it is appropriate to discuss this technique in some detail because it has taught us much about the pathophysiology of glaucoma and the mechanism of action of various treatment modalities.

During tonography a Schiøtz tonometer is placed on the cornea for a few minutes. The weight of the tonometer increases IOP and also increases the outflow of aqueous humor above its normal rate. The tonometer is usually connected to a continuous recording device that measures the subsequent decline of IOP over time. Using the Friedenwald tables, the change in the IOP readings allows the clinician to infer the volume of aqueous humor displaced from the eye.[143] If the assumption is made that the displacement of fluid from the eye, ΔV, is the only factor involved in the fall of IOP during the test, then the following equation is true:

$$\frac{\Delta V}{t} = \text{rate of fluid outflow}$$

If the weight of the tonometer raises IOP from its initial level of P_O to an average value of P_t, then the outflow facility, C, is calculated from Grant's equation[144] as follows:

$$C = \frac{\dfrac{\Delta V}{t}}{P_t - P_O}$$

Tonography rests on a number of assumptions that can be debated, including those that follow:
1. An acute elevation of IOP alters nothing besides the rate of aqueous humor outflow. In fact, raising IOP with a Schiøtz tonometer compresses the eye and affects outflow facility itself.[145] In addition, tonography raises episcleral venous pressure by approximately 1.25 mm Hg.[146] Some clinicians correct for this effect by adding this number to P_O. Finally, acutely raising IOP may reduce aqueous humor formation.[147-149] A drop in aqueous humor production would create the impression of an increased outflow facility, so this phenomenon has been termed *pseudofacility*. Recently the concept of pseudofacility has been questioned because chronic changes in IOP are not accompanied by corresponding changes in aqueous humor formation.[57,150,151] Even acute alterations of IOP do not appear to be accompanied by major changes in aqueous humor formation.[148,152]

2. All eyes respond with similar distention of the ocular coats to the acute increase in IOP. In fact, the distensibility (usually expressed as its reciprocal term, ocular rigidity) varies considerably—that is, ocular rigidity is low in myopic eyes with thin sclera and high in some hyperopic eyes with thick sclera. The ophthalmologist can estimate ocular rigidity by comparing applanation and Schiøtz pressure readings or by measuring IOP using a Schiøtz tonometer with two or three different weights.

3. Raising IOP does not affect the ocular blood volume. In fact, when IOP is raised, blood is expelled from the eye. This means that the decline in IOP during tonography is not caused solely by aqueous humor leaving the eye.[153]

Tonography is also subject to a number of errors, including those that follow:

1. *Operator errors.* The test results are affected by improper cleaning, calibration, and positioning of the instrument.

2. *Patient errors.* If patients blink, squeeze, move, hold their breath, or lose fixation, the test results are less valid.

3. *Instrument errors.* Inaccuracies arise from the assumption that the cornea is perfectly spherical. In the electronic tonometers, the space between the plunger and the wall of the tonometer is large enough to allow corneal molding.[154] This phenomenon may give a false high facility reading. Finally, if a voltage regulator is not used, variations in line voltage may lead to a drift in the IOP measurement.

4. *Reading errors.* It takes considerable experience to decide which tracings are acceptable.

There have been a number of attempts to improve tonography by altering the technique. One approach has been to lengthen the test to 7 to 10 minutes and to disregard the initial portion of the tracing.[155] Another approach has been to use constant area tonography, in which a 5- to 6-mm zone of the cornea is flattened for a few minutes. During this period IOP declines, as does the force necessary to flatten the cornea.[156,157] Yet another approach has been constant pressure tonography, in which the force applanating the eye is varied to maintain a constant IOP.[158]

Perfusion

It is also possible to measure facility of outflow with a perfusion apparatus. This technique is used most often in animal eyes and enucleated human eyes, but it can also be used in living human eyes in an operative situation. With a needle in the anterior chamber, the pressure-flow relationships through the eye can be calculated by one of two methods. In the first method, known as constant-flow perfusion, IOP is measured after fluid is driven into the eye at a constant rate by a mechanical syringe. This process is repeated at two or more flow rates, and outflow facility, C, is calculated from the formula below, in which F_2 and F_1 are the flow rates and P_2 and P_1 are the corresponding IOP readings.[159,160]

$$C = \frac{F_2 - F_1}{P_2 - P_1}$$

In the second method, known as constant-pressure perfusion, a reservoir of fluid is placed at a known height above the eye, thereby fixing IOP. The amount of fluid entering the eye is calculated from the change in the weight of the reservoir over time. If this is done at two or more heights above the eye, outflow facility is calculated from the preceding formula.[150,161]

Suction Cup

The final method used to determine outflow facility is the suction cup. This device is applied to the sclera with a vacuum 50 mm Hg below atmospheric pressure. The vacuum occludes intrascleral and episcleral venous drainage and raises IOP. The facility of outflow is calculated from the decline in IOP after the suction cup is removed. The suction cup technique usually gives lower values for outflow facility than does tonography.[162]

FACILITY OF OUTFLOW AND ITS CLINICAL IMPLICATIONS

At one time tonography was considered a crucial part of the work-up for every patient suspected of having glaucoma. Sometimes tonography was performed 30 to 60 minutes after the ingestion of a liter of water, which served as a type of stress test for the outflow system.[163] It was also common to divide the IOP, P_O, by the outflow facility, C, to better separate glaucomatous eyes from normal eyes. The mean outflow facility in normal eyes ranged from 0.22 to 0.28 µl/min/mm Hg in various studies, and the mean P_O/C ratio ranged from 55 to 60.[163,164] Unfortunately, outflow facility and P_O/C are not distributed in a normal or Gaussian fashion, and there is considerable overlap between glaucomatous eyes and normal eyes (Table 4-1). When one considers this overlap and the lack of reproducibility of tonographic measurements, it is clear why clinicians no longer diagnose glaucoma on the basis of outflow facility. Tonography is neither sufficiently sensitive nor specific to make the diagnosis of glaucoma. Furthermore, tonography measurement necessitates a skilled technician and a fair amount of time to set up and clean the apparatus, prepare and test the patient, and dismantle and store the apparatus. In the overwhelming majority of cases tonography served only to confirm the diagnosis. If the tonography test gave results contrary to the clinical impression, the quality of the test was called into question more often than the presumptive diagnosis. Thus clinicians abandoned tonography because the added value of the test was minimal when compared with the time and effort it took to obtain quality results.

Some investigators have claimed other uses for tonography, including those that follow:

1. *To predict the development of primary open-angle glaucoma (POAG).* Some investigators have found tonography to be useful in predicting which ocular hypertensive individuals will develop glaucomatous visual field loss.[163,165] However, other investigators have come to the opposite conclusion.[166] It seems fair to conclude that a poor facility of outflow correlates with higher pressures, and that higher pressures correlate with an increased risk of developing glaucoma, but because pressure measurement is easier and more reliable than tonography, it is perhaps more reasonable to base predictions on the pressure directly.

2. *To assess the adequacy of antiglaucoma therapy.* A few studies have shown that glaucomatous eyes with outflow facilities in the normal range under treatment are less likely to suffer progressive visual field loss.[163] Again, outflow facility is probably acting as a surrogate for pressure.

3. *To detect wide diurnal swings in IOP.* Eyes with low outflow facilities are probably more likely to suffer wide diurnal swings in IOP. However, in one study the C value did not correlate as well as a single IOP reading with the diurnal fluctuation in IOP.[167]

4. *To help diagnose angle-closure glaucoma.* Some clinicians add tonography to provocative tests for primary angle-closure glaucoma. A test is considered positive if C falls 25% to 30% and the angle is closed on gonioscopy. This was more important when a positive test exposed the patient to the risks of incisional surgery, but with the ready accessibility of laser peripheral iridotomy, there is usually little reason not to perform iridotomy in the presence of a gonioscopically closed angle.

5. *To determine the mechanism of action of ocular hypotension medications and different glaucoma operations.* Tonography may be unnecessary or redundant in many clinical settings, but it still has an important role in laboratory and clinical research. The role of tonography in determining the mechanism of action of new drugs and other therapeutic interventions remains essential.

Table 4-1

Tonographic Results in Glaucomatous Eyes

	Normal Eyes (n = 909)(%)	Glaucomatous Eyes (n = 250)(%)
C value		
< 0.18	2.5	65
< 0.13	0.15	43
P_O/C ratio		
> 100	2.5	73
> 138	0.15	50
P_O/C ratio after H_2O		
> 100	2.5	95

Modified from Becker B: *Trans Am Acad Ophthalmol Otolaryngol* 65:156, 1961.

FACTORS AFFECTING THE FACILITY OF OUTFLOW

Many factors influence the facility of outflow (Table 4-2), including those discussed here.

Age

There is a modest decline in outflow facility with age.[168-170] This decline appears to counterbalance a similar decrease in aqueous humor formation. Histologic studies indicate a number of age-related changes in the trabecular meshwork, including thickening and fusion of the trabecular sheets, degeneration of collagen and elastic fibrils, accumulation of wide-spacing collagen, loss of endothelial cells, hyperpigmentation of the endothelial cells, accumulation of intracellular organelles, accumulation and alteration of extracellular matrix, and decrease in the number of giant vacuoles.[22,171-173]

Hormones

A number of investigators have postulated that endogenous glucocorticoids regulate aqueous humor outflow.[174] Corticosteroids administered topically, systemically, or periocularly are capable of re-

Table 4-2

Factors Affecting Aqueous Humor Outflow

Factor	Effect	Comments
Age	Decrease	
Hormones		
Corticosteroids	Decrease	
Progesterone	Increase	
Relaxin	Increase	
Chorionic gonadotropin	Increase	
Thyroxin	Increase	Questionable
Ciliary muscle tone	Increase	
Anterior chamber depth	Increase	Increases with increasing depth
Drugs		
Parasympathomimetic agents	Increase	
Parasympatholytic agents	Decrease	
Ganglionic blocking agents	Decrease	
Bradykinin	Increase	
Cyclic adenosine monophosphate	Increase	
Substance P	Decrease	
Surgery		
Argon laser trabeculoplasty	Increase	
Filtering surgery	Increase	
Cyclodialysis	Increase	
Cataract extraction	Decrease	Temporary effect
Penetrating keratoplasty	Decrease	Temporary effect
Water ingestion	Decrease	
Neural regulation		
III nerve stimulation	Increase	
III nerve ablation	Decrease	
Sympathetic stimulation	Increase	
Sympathectomy	Increase	Temporary effect
Particulate matter		
Red blood cells	Decrease	
White blood cells	Decrease	
Pigment	Decrease	
Heavy molecular weight protein	Decrease	
Hyaluronic acid	Decrease	
α-Chymotrypsin	Decrease	
Macrophages with foreign material	Decrease	

ducing outflow facility. The response to corticosteroids appears to be genetic in part and is greater in certain groups, including patients with POAG and their first-degree relatives, myopic patients, and diabetic patients. This subject is reviewed at length in Chapter 18. Other hormones, such as progesterone,[175,176] thyroxin,[177] relaxin, and chorionic gonadotropin,[177] have been postulated to influence outflow facility in physiologic or pharmacologic doses. Other active substances, such as prostaglandins, substance P, and angiotensin, may affect aqueous outflow.[95,178]

Ciliary Muscle Tone

Increased tone of the ciliary muscle increases total outflow facility. The increased tone can be the result of accommodation,[179,180] electrical stimulation of the oculomotor nerve, posterior depression of the lens,[50,51,96] or administration of parasympathomimetic drugs such as pilocarpine.[113] The increased muscle tone pulls the scleral spur posteriorly and internally, which opens the intertrabecular spaces and Schlemm's canal (Fig. 4-9).

Drugs

Pilocarpine and other cholinergic agents increase outflow facility.[113] Epinephrine and dipivefrin and other β-adrenergic agonists increase both conventional and unconventional outflow.[141,142,181,182] The parasympatholytic agents and the ganglionic blocking agents reduce outflow facility. Prostaglandins increase uveoscleral outflow.* Alpha agonists decrease aqueous production and increase uveoscleral outflow.[183,184] Bradykinin was noted to increase outflow facility in one study.[185]

Surgical Therapy

Filtering operations and argon laser trabeculoplasty improve outflow facility. Cataract extraction and penetrating keratoplasty reduce outflow facility temporarily, perhaps by deforming the trabecular meshwork and reducing its support.[186] Cyclodialysis, as mentioned previously, increases uveoscleral outflow.[49,57]

Diurnal Fluctuation

There is considerable controversy about whether or not there is a diurnal fluctuation of outflow facility.[174,187,188]

Glaucoma

Outflow facility is reduced in most forms of glaucoma. This can occur through a variety of mechanisms, depending on the type of glaucoma. In primary infantile glaucoma the outflow structures develop improperly (see Chapter 20). In angle-closure glaucoma the peripheral iris is pushed or pulled against the trabecular meshwork, preventing aqueous humor from reaching the outflow channels (see Chapters 15 and 16). The trabecular meshwork can also be covered by a membrane, as in epithelial downgrowth, neovascular glaucoma, or the iridocorneal endothelial syndrome.

In the secondary open-angle glaucomas the trabecular meshwork can be obstructed by a variety of particulate matter, including red blood cells, white blood cells, tumor cells, ghost cells, zonular fragments (after α-chymotrypsin), pigment particles, and lens particles (see Chapter 18). The meshwork can also be obstructed by nonparticulate foreign matter, such as lens protein and viscoelastic substances.

There is great controversy about the fundamental defect of the outflow channels in POAG. A variety of theories have been proposed to explain the decreased outflow facility of this disease, including (1) an accumulation of foreign material in the trabecular meshwork, (2) a loss of trabecular endothelial cells, (3) a collapse of Schlemm's canal, and (4) an obstruction of the collector channels. This subject is discussed at length in Chapter 17.

---

*Refs: 118, 121, 125, 126, 135, 136.

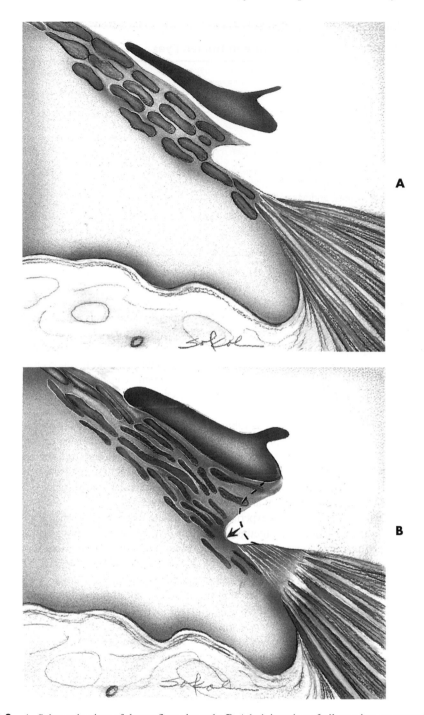

Figure 4-9   **A,** Schematic view of the outflow channels. **B,** Administration of pilocarpine contracts the ciliary muscle, which pulls the scleral spur posteriorly and internally, opening the intertrabecular spaces and Schlemm's canal.

EPISCLERAL VENOUS PRESSURE

Aqueous humor leaving the eye by trabeculocanalicular outflow eventually passes into the venous system. The pressure in the veins that receive the aqueous humor is referred to as episcleral venous pressure.

Episcleral venous pressure can be measured by a variety of techniques, including pressure chambers,[42,146,189-193] torsion balance devices,[189,194] force displacement transducers, air jets,[42] and

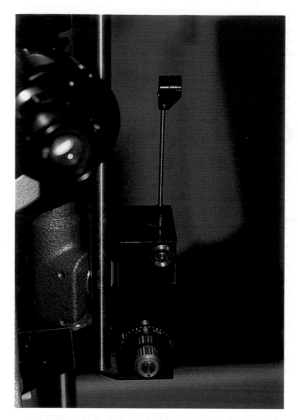

Figure 5-1   Goldmann tonometer.

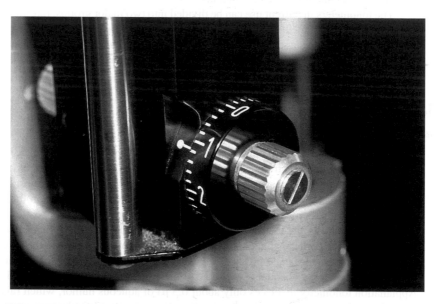

Figure 5-2   Goldmann applanation tonometer. Dial indicates force applied to applanate cornea; this number multiplied by 10 equals intraocular pressure in millimeters of mercury.

the clinician looks through the split prism in contact with the eye, he or she sees a central blue circle, the flattened cornea, surrounded by two yellow-green semicircles. When the inner margins of the two semicircles are aligned in a smooth S curve at the midpoint of their pulsations, the proper degree of applanation has been achieved.

Goldmann tonometry is quite accurate and reproducible if the proper technique is used. Interobserver variability is in the range of 0 to 3 mm Hg,[5] which is less than the diurnal variation of IOP. The technique of Goldmann tonometry is as follows:

1. The patient is asked not to drink alcoholic beverages for 12 hours. Food and liquid in usual quantities are permitted, although large amounts of fluid (e.g., 500 ml or more) should be avoided for 2 hours before the test.

2. The patient is told the purpose of the test and is reassured that the measurement is not painful. The patient is instructed to relax, maintain position, and hold the eyes open wide.

3. One drop of a topical anesthetic, such as 0.5% proparacaine, is placed in each eye, and the tip of a moistened fluorescein strip is touched to the tear layer on the inner surface of each lower lid. Alternatively, one drop of a combined anesthetic-fluorescein solution can be instilled in each eye.

4. The tonometer tip is cleaned with a sterilizing solution,[2,7-10] and the tip and prism are set in correct position on the slit lamp. Sterile tonometer tip covers may be used rather than a disinfecting solution, if preferred.[11]

5. The tension knob is set at 1 g. If the knob is set at 0, the prism head may vibrate when it touches the eye and damage the corneal epithelium. The 1 g position is used before each measurement. As a rule, it is more accurate to measure IOP by increasing rather than decreasing the force of applanation.

6. The 0 graduation mark of the prism is set at the white line on the prism holder. If the patient has more than 3 D of corneal astigmatism, the area of contact between the cornea and the prism is elliptic rather than circular. In this situation the prism should be rotated to about 45° from the long axis of the ellipse—that is, the prism graduation corresponding to the least curved meridian of the cornea should be set at the red mark on the prism holder.[12] An alternative approach is to average the IOP readings obtained with the axis of the prism horizontal and then vertical.[13,14]

7. The cobalt filter is used with the slit beam opened maximally. The angle between the illumination and the microscope should be approximately 60°. The room illumination is reduced.

8. The patient is seated in a comfortable position on an adjustable stool or examining chair facing the slit lamp. The heights of the slit lamp, chair, and chin rest are adjusted until the patient is comfortable and in the correct position for the measurement. The patient's chin is supported by the chin rest, and the forehead by the forehead bar. The forehead bar should be well above the patient's eyebrows, so the frontalis muscle can be used to open the eyes wide. The patient's collar should be loosened if necessary. The patient should breathe normally during the test to avoid Valsalva's maneuver.

9. The palpebral fissure is a little wider if the patient looks up. However, the gaze should be no more than 15° above the horizontal to prevent an elevation of IOP that is especially marked in the presence of restrictive neuromuscular disease such as dysthyroid ophthalmopathy.[15,16] A fixation light may be placed in front of the fellow eye. The patient should blink the eyes once or twice to spread the fluorescein-stained tear film over the cornea, and then should keep the eyes open wide. In some patients it is necessary for the examiner to hold the eyelids open with the thumb and forefinger of one hand. Care must be taken not to place any pressure on the globe because this raises IOP. Resting the thumb and forefinger against the orbital rim while retracting the lids may help the examiner avoid putting pressure on the globe.

10. The operator sits opposite the patient in position to look through the microscope and moves the assembly toward the subject. When the black circle near the tip of the prism moves slightly, it indicates contact between the prism and the globe. Alternatively, the assembly is advanced toward the patient until the limbal zone has a bluish hue. The biprism should not touch the lids or lashes because this stimulates blinking and squeezing. If the tonometer tip touches the lids, the fluorescein rings will thicken, which may cause an overestimation of IOP.

11. The clinician observes the applanation through the biprism at low power. A monocular view is obtained of the central applanated zone and the surrounding fluorescein-stained tear film. Using the control stick, the observer raises, lowers, and centers the assembly until two equal semicircles are seen in the center of the field of view. If the two semicircles are not equal in size, IOP is overestimated. The clinician turns the tension knob in both

directions to ensure that the instrument is in good position. If the semicircles cannot be made "too small," the instruments is too far forward. If the semicircles cannot be made "too large," the instrument is too far from the eye.

12. The fluorescein rings should be approximately 0.25 to 0.3 mm in thickness—or about one tenth the diameter of the flattened area. If the rings are too narrow, the patient should blink two or three times to replenish the fluorescein; additional fluorescein may be added if necessary. If the fluorescein rings are too narrow, IOP is underestimated. If the fluorescein rings are too wide, the patient's eyelids should be blotted carefully with a tissue, and the front surface of the prism should be dried with lint-free material. An excessively wide fluorescein ring is less of a problem than a very narrow ring but can cause IOP to be overestimated.

13. The fluorescein rings normally undergo a rhythmic movement in response to the cardiac cycle. The tension knob is rotated until the inner borders of the fluorescein rings touch each other at the midpoint of their pulsations.

14. IOP is measured in the right eye until three successive readings are within 1 mm Hg. IOP is then measured in the left eye.

15. The reading obtained in grams is multiplied by 10 to give the IOP in millimeters of mercury. This value is recorded along with the date, time of day, list of ocular medications, and time of last instillation of ocular medication.

16. It is possible to transfer bacteria, viruses, and other infectious agents with the tonometer head,[17] including such potentially serious infections as epidemic keratoconjunctivitis, hepatitis B, and, theoretically, acquired immunodeficiency syndrome. The biprism should be rinsed and dried immediately after use. Between uses, the prism head should be soaked in a solution such as diluted bleach or 3% hydrogen peroxide. Seventy-percent ethanol and 70% isopropanol are effective as sterilizing solutions but were shown in one study to cause mild damage to the tonometer tip after one month of immersion.[18,19]

17. The Goldmann tonometer should be calibrated at least once a month. If the Goldmann tonometer is not within 0.1 g of the correct calibration, the instrument must be repaired.

Although the Goldmann tonometer is reliable and accurate through a wide range of IOPs, errors in measurement can arise from a number of factors, including those that follow:

1. Inadequate fluorescein staining of the tear film causes an underestimation of IOP. This commonly occurs when too much time elapses between the instillation of the fluorescein and the measurement of the pressure. To avoid this problem the IOP should be measured within the first minute or so after instilling the fluorescein.

2. Elevating the eyes more than 15° above the horizontal causes an overestimation of IOP.

3. Widening the lid fissure excessively causes an overestimation of IOP.[20]

4. Repeated tonometry reduces IOP, causing an underestimation of the true level.[21,22] This effect is greatest between the first and second readings, but the trend continues through a number of repetitions.[6]

5. A scarred, irregular cornea distorts the fluorescein rings and makes it difficult to estimate IOP.

6. The thickness of the cornea affects IOP readings.[23] If the cornea is thick because of edema, IOP is underestimated.[23] If the cornea is thick because of additional tissue, IOP is overestimated.[23,24] The Goldmann tonometer is accurate after epikeratophakia.[25] Central corneal pressures have been shown to be lower than peripheral corneal readings following photorefractive keratectomy.[26]

7. If the examiner presses on the globe, or if the patient squeezes his eyelids, IOP is overestimated. Taking time to reassure the patient and taking care to avoid causing pressure against the globe can help guard against these problems.

8. If corneal astigmatism is greater than 3 D, IOP is underestimated for with-the-rule astigmatism and overestimated for against-the-rule astigmatism.[13] The IOP reading is inaccurate 1 mm Hg for every 3 D of astigmatism.[27]

Perkins Tonometer

The Perkins tonometer is similar to the Goldmann tonometer except that it is portable and counterbalanced, so it can be used in any position.[28] This instrument is useful in a number of situations, including in the operating room, at bedside, and with patients who are obese or for other reasons cannot be examined at the slit lamp. The light comes from batteries, and the force comes from a spring varied manually by the operator. Because the Perkins tonometer is portable, it is useful in circumstances in which the patients or subjects do not have access to an examination room, such as in community or remote pressure screening sessions.

Draeger Tonometer

The Draeger tonometer is similar to the Goldmann and Perkins tonometers except that it uses a different biprism. The force for applanation is supplied by an electric motor.[29,30] Like the Perkins instrument, the Draeger tonometer is portable and counterbalanced, so it can be used in a variety of positions and locations.

MacKay-Marg Tonometer

The MacKay-Marg tonometer consists of a movable plunger, 1.5 mm in diameter, that protrudes slightly from a surrounding footplate or sleeve. The movements of the plunger are measured by a transducer and recorded on a paper strip. When the instrument touches the cornea, the plunger and its supporting spring are opposed by the IOP and the corneal bending pressure (Fig. 5-3, *A*). As the instrument is advanced, the corneal bending pressure is transferred to the footplate, and a notch is seen in the pressure tracing (Fig. 5-3, *B*). The height of the notch is the measure of IOP. When the instrument is advanced farther, the cornea is indented farther, and IOP rises (Fig. 5-3, *C*).[31-33] The

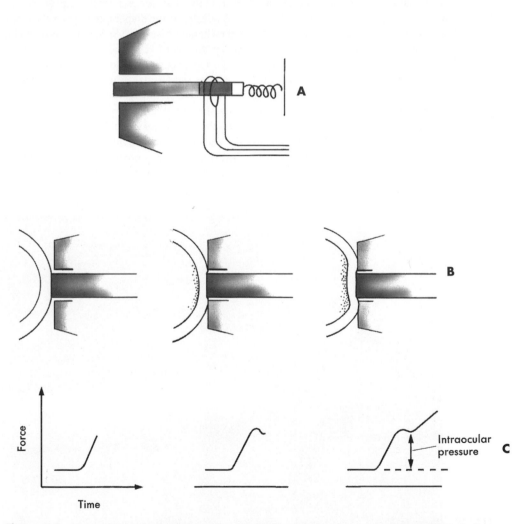

Figure 5-3 Intraocular pressure (IOP) tracing with MacKay-Marg tonometer. **A,** Advancing plunger is opposed by IOP and corneal bending pressure. **B,** Notch indicates corneal bending pressure has been transferred to footplate. Height of notch corresponds to IOP. **C,** With continued advancement of plunger, cornea is indented, and IOP rises. (Modified from Moses RA: *Tonometry.* In Cairns JE, editor: *Glaucoma,* vol 1, London, 1986, Grune & Stratton.)

transfer of the corneal bending force occurs at an applanation area 6 mm in diameter. Applanation over this area displaces approximately 8 μl of aqueous humor and raises IOP about 6 to 7 mm Hg—P_t is 6 or 7 mm Hg higher than P_O.

The MacKay-Marg tonometer measures IOP over a brief interval, so several readings should be averaged to reduce the effects of the cardiac and respiratory cycles. This instrument is useful for measuring IOP in eyes with scarred, irregular, or edematous corneas because the end point does not depend on the evaluation of a light reflex sensitive to optical irregularity, as does the Goldmann tonometer. The tip of the instrument is covered with a plastic film to prevent transfer of infection. The tonometer is calibrated by comparing the plunger displacement with gravity to a fixed number of units on the tonometer recording paper. The MacKay-Marg tonometer is also fairly accurate when used over therapeutic soft contact lenses.[34]

Recently a number of small portable applanation tonometers have been marketed that work on the same principle as the MacKay-Marg tonometer (Fig. 5-4). They appear to be accurate in common clinical situations.[35] We have found them particularly useful in community health fairs, on ward rounds, and in other circumstances in which rapid portable tonometry is indicated.

Pneumatic Tonometer

The pneumatic tonometer has a sensing device that consists of a gas chamber covered by a polymeric silicone diaphragm. A transducer converts the gas pressure in the chamber into an electrical signal that is recorded on a paper strip. The gas in the chamber escapes through an exhaust vent between the diaphragm and the tip of the support nozzle. As the diaphragm touches the cornea, the gas vent is reduced in size, and the pressure in the chamber rises.[36-38] Some models of this instrument use a digital display, and some a paper tracing, to record IOP. The instrument emits a whistling sound when it is placed properly on the cornea. The pneumatic tonometer was designed originally as an applanation instrument. However, as Moses and Grodzki[39] have indicated, the device currently marketed has some properties that are more like an indentation tonometer.

The pneumatic tonometer is useful for measuring IOP in eyes with scarred, irregular, or edematous corneas. The small applanation tip makes the instrument useful in laboratory settings in which some other tonometers can prove unwieldy.[40] The instrument provides a good measurement of IOP, although it overestimates pressure at low levels and underestimates pressure at high levels. Calibration of the instrument is empirical. The pneumatic tonometer can be used for tonography if it is

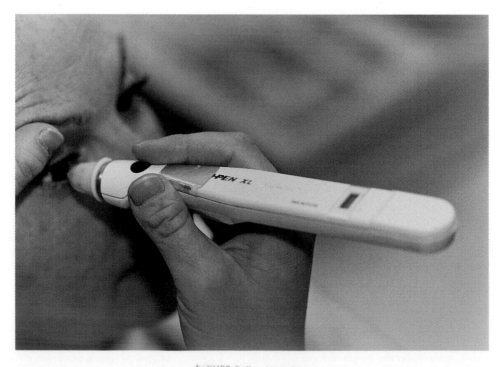

Figure 5-4   Tono-Pen.

fitted with weights and used in a continuous recording mode. The pneumatic tonometer is fairly accurate when used over therapeutic soft contact lenses.[41]

Noncontact Tonometer

The noncontact tonometer applanates the cornea by a jet of air, so there is no direct contact between the device and the surface of the eye. This theoretically avoids the need to sterilize the instrument, but a recent study found the air puff produces a tear film aerosol that could potentially contain infectious material.[42] The force of the air jet increases rapidly and linearly with time. The instrument also emits a collimated beam of light that is reflected from the central cornea and then received by a photocell. When an area of the cornea 3.6 mm in diameter is flattened, the light reflected to the photocell is at a maximum. The time required to produce the peak reflection is directly related to the force of the air jet and thus to the counterbalancing IOP.[43-45]

The noncontact tonometer is useful for screening programs because it can be operated by nonmedical personnel and there is no direct contact between the instrument and the eye. The IOP readings obtained with the noncontact tonometer correlate fairly well with readings taken by Goldmann tonometry, but differences of several millimeters of mercury are not unusual, particularly with pressures higher than the low 20s.[46-49] The tonometer can be used without topical anesthesia, but it is more accurate with anesthesia. The patient should be warned that the air puff can be startling, even after topical anesthetic.[50] The noncontact tonometer measures IOP over very short intervals, so it is important to average a series of readings.[51] The instrument has an internal calibration system.

Maklakow Tonometer

The Maklakow (also spelled Maklakov) tonometer differs from the other applanation instruments in that a known force is applied to the eye, and the area of applanation is measured—a technique known as constant-force rather than constant-area applanation.[52] The instrument consists of a wire holder into which a flat-bottom weight, ranging from 5 to 15 g, is inserted. The surface of the weight is painted with a dye, such as mild silver protein (Argyrol) mixed with glycerin, and then the weight is lowered onto the cornea. During the procedure the patient is supine, and the cornea is anesthetized. The weight is lifted from the cornea, and the area of applanation is taken to be the area of missing dye, which is measured either directly or indirectly from an imprint on test paper. IOP is inferred from the weight (W) and the diameter of the area of applanation (d) by using the following formula:

$$P_t = \frac{W}{\pi(d/2)^2}$$

IOP is measured in grams per square centimeter and is converted to millimeters of mercury by dividing by 1.36.

The Maklakow tonometer is used widely in Russia and China but has never achieved great popularity in Western Europe or the United States. This instrument displaces a greater volume of aqueous humor than the other applanation devices (but less than a Schiøtz tonometer), which means that the IOP readings are more influenced by ocular rigidity.[53] Attempts have been made to overcome this problem by measuring IOP with two different weights. The Maklakow tonometer does not correct for corneal bending, capillary attraction, or tear encroachment on the layer of dye.

Many instruments similar to the Maklakow device have been described, including the Applanometer, Tonomat, Halberg tonometer,[54] and GlaucoTest.[55]

Indentation Instruments

In indentation tonometry a known weight is placed on the cornea, and the IOP is estimated by measuring the deformation or indentation of the globe. The Schiøtz tonometer is the prototype for this class of instruments.

Schiøtz Tonometer

The Schiøtz tonometer consists of a metal plunger that slides through a hole in a concave metal footplate (Figs. 5-5 and 5-6). The plunger supports a hammer device connected to a needle that crosses a scale. The plunger, hammer, and needle weigh 5.5 g. This can be increased to 7.5, 10, or

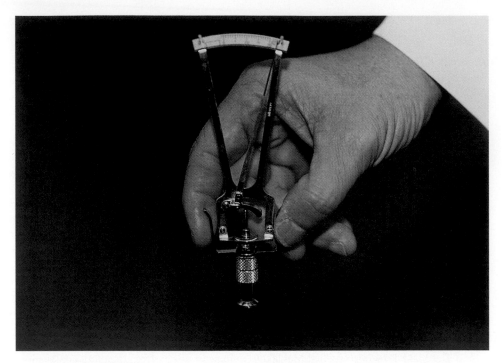

Figure 5-5   Shiøtz tonometer.

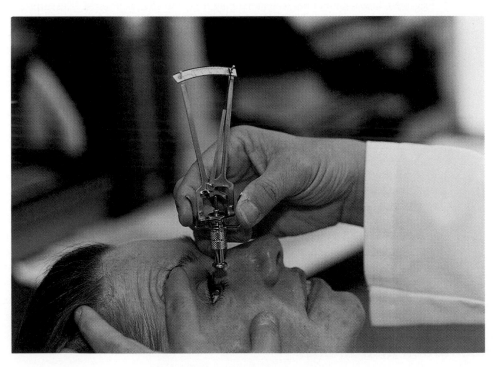

Figure 5-6   Shiøtz tonometry technique.

15 g by the addition of appropriate weights. The more the plunger indents the cornea, the higher the scale reading—that is, the lower the IOP, the higher the scale reading. Each scale unit represents a 0.05-mm protrusion of the plunger.[56]

The technique of Schiøtz tonometry is summarized as follows:

1. The patient lies supine and fixates on an overhead target, such as a light or a mark on the ceiling. Alternatively, the examiner may place the patient's thumb in the appropriate po-

sition to serve as a fixation target. This is useful in patients with limited vision in the fellow eye.

2. The examiner explains the nature of the test and reassures the patient that the measurement is painless. The patient is told to relax, breathe normally, fixate on the target, and open the eyes wide.

3. A drop of topical anesthetic, such as 0.5% proparacaine, is instilled in each eye.

4. The tonometer tip and footplate are wiped carefully with an alcohol swab and allowed to air dry. If the tonometer has been stored disassembled in its case, it should be wiped with the alcohol swab before assembly. The alcohol must be allowed to evaporate before the instrument touches the eye.

5. The examiner retracts the patient's lids without placing tension on the globe. The tonometer is placed directly over the eye, and when the patient relaxes, it is lowered gently onto the cornea (Fig. 5-6). The tonometer should be perpendicular to the corneal apex. The examiner must be careful not to press the tonometer against the globe.

6. The measurement is noted to the nearest 0.25 scale units. If a wide pulse pressure is present, the center point of the fluctuation is chosen as the end point. If the scale reading is less than 3 units, additional weight is added to the plunger.

7. The IOP measurement is repeated until three consecutive readings agree within 0.5 scale units.

8. The average scale reading is converted to IOP in millimeters of mercury using a conversion chart. The examiner records the scale reading, weight, converted IOP, time of day, ocular medications, and time since last instillation of ocular medication, as well as the conversion chart used.

9. The instrument is calibrated before each use by placing it on a polished metal sphere and checking to be sure that the scale reading is zero. If the reading is not zero, the instrument must be repaired.

10. After each use, the tonometer plunger and footplate should be rinsed with water, followed by alcohol, and then wiped dry with lint-free material. It is important to prevent foreign material from drying within the footplate because this affects the movement of the plunger. The most common "foreign material" that finds its way onto the plunger tip is fluid from the patient's tear film. The instrument can be sterilized with ultraviolet radiation, steam, ethylene oxide, or a variety of solutions that have been indicated for the Goldmann prism.

11. If the tonometer is not going to be used for a while, it is best to disassemble the unit, clean it, and store it in its case. Disassembly allows for better cleaning of the barrel and plunger apparatus, and case storage protects the instrument from becoming bent or otherwise damaged and thrown out of calibration.

The Schiøtz tonometer is portable, sturdy, relatively inexpensive, and easy to operate. The instrument is accurate over a wide range of IOPs, although pressures may vary from those obtained with Goldmann applanation tonometry, particularly when relatively untrained examiners are administering the test.[57-59] An important concern is that placing the heavy tonometer (total weight at least 16.5 g) on the eye raises IOP. The rise in pressure reflects the dispensability of the ocular coats, a property termed ocular rigidity. All of the tables that relate the change in volume to the IOP assume a normal ocular rigidity, and this introduces a substantial error for some measurements. Eyes with high ocular rigidity (e.g., high hyperopia[60] or long-standing glaucoma[53]) give falsely high Schiøtz IOP readings, whereas eyes with low ocular rigidity (e.g., myopia,[60] strong miotic therapy,[60] retinal detachment surgery,[61,62] or compressible gas[63]) give falsely low Schiøtz IOP readings. It is possible to estimate ocular rigidity by comparing applanation and Schiøtz measurements[4] or by repeating the Schiøtz measurements with two or more weights using the Friedenwald nomogram.[53]

The Schiøtz tonometer may also affect the IOP estimation by altering the outflow facility, rate of aqueous humor formation, episcleral venous pressure, and blood volume of the eye.[64] Although none of these alterations is as important during tonometry as it is during tonography (see Chapter 4), they add to the uncertainty of the measurement. The Schiøtz pressure reading is also influenced by the size of the footplate hole and the thickness and curvature of the cornea.[65]

Electronic Schiøtz Tonometer

The electronic Schiøtz tonometer has a continuous recording of IOP that is used for tonography. The scale is also magnified, which makes it easier to detect small changes in IOP.

Continuous Monitoring of Intraocular Pressure

There have been a few attempts to monitor IOP continuously in animal and human eyes. The devices described consist of applanation instruments inside contact lenses or suction cups[66,67] or strain gauges in encircling bands that resemble scleral buckling elements.[68] None of these instruments has achieved widespread use. The development of such a device would greatly aid our understanding of aqueous humor dynamics and glaucoma.

DISTRIBUTION OF INTRAOCULAR PRESSURE IN THE GENERAL POPULATION

There have been a number of studies on the distribution of IOP in the normal population (Table 5-1). In a classic study Leydhecker and co-workers[69] performed Schiøtz tonometry on more than 10,000 normal individuals. They found the mean (±SD) IOP to be 15.8 ± 2.6 mm Hg. At first glance the pressure readings appeared to be distributed in a normal fashion (also referred to as a gaussian or bell-shaped distribution). However, closer inspection of the data revealed that the distribution was not gaussian, but rather skewed to the right.[70,71] This distinction is important because it means we cannot define an upper limit for IOP by adding 2 or 3 standard deviations to the mean. This conclusion is supported by a number of studies, all of which have found a much higher prevalence of elevated IOP (e.g., > 20 or 21 mm Hg) than would be predicted by gaussian statistics (Table 5-2). Unfortunately, the skewed distribution also means that an abnormal IOP must be defined empirically—that is, an abnormal pressure is one that causes optic nerve damage in a particular eye. Because eyes differ markedly in their susceptibility to the effects of pressure, it is difficult to know *a*

Table 5-1

Mean Intraocular Pressure Measurements in the General Population

Author	Technique	Individuals (n)	Mean	Standard Deviation
Leydhecker and others[69]	Schiøtz	10,000	15.5	2.6
Linner[186]	Schiøtz	78	16.7	2.4
Becker[187]	Schiøtz	909	16.1	2.8
Johnson[188]	Schiøtz	7577	15.4	2.6
	Applanation	70	13.7	2.5
Soeteren[189]	Schiøtz	95	15.5	2.4
	Applanation	123	13.2	2.4
Goldmann[3]	Applanation	50	15.6	2.9
Goldmann[4]	Applanation	400	15.4	2.5
Draeger	Applanation	178	14.5	2.8
Armaly[70]	Applanation	2316	15.9	3.1
Loewen and others[190]	Applanation	4661	16.2	3.8
Ruprecht and others[191]	Applanation	8899	16.2	3.4

Table 5-2

Prevalence of Elevated Intraocular Pressure in the General Population

Location	Age (Years)	Individuals or Eyes	Cut-off Intraocular Pressure (mm Hg)	Prevalence of High Pressure (%)
Skovde, Sweden[192]	> 40	7275	> 21	4.5
Ferndale, Wales[193]	40-74	4231	> 20	9.4
Framingham, Mass[194]	52-85	5223 (eyes)	> 21	7.6
Dalby, Sweden[195]	55-70	1511	> 20.5	7.3

Modified from Leske MC: *Am J Epidemiol* 118:166, 1983.

priori what level of IOP will be harmful to a given patient. Some individuals develop glaucomatous damage at IOPs near the population mean, whereas others maintain normal optic nerves and visual function for many years despite IOPs of 30 or even 40 mm Hg.

Similar mean IOPs are found using applanation and Schiøtz tonometry (see Table 5-1). Given the theoretic and practical shortcomings of Schiøtz tonometry, this suggests some combination of compensating errors for the indentation technique.

As a general rule, IOPs are similar in the right and left eyes of normal individuals. Although differences of 4 mm Hg or more between the eyes are seen in less than 4% of normal individuals,[72,73] such differences are common in patients with glaucoma. Davanger[72] reported that 10% of patients with glaucoma had pressure differences greater than 6 mm Hg.

FACTORS THAT INFLUENCE INTRAOCULAR PRESSURE

Many different factors affect IOP (Table 5-3). A few of the more important factors are discussed here.

Table 5-3

Factors Influencing Intraocular Pressure (IOP)

Factors	Association	Comments
Demographic		
Age	Mean IOP increases with increasing age	May be mediated partially through cardiovascular factors
Sex	Higher IOP in women	Effect more marked after age 40 years
Race	Higher IOP among blacks	
Heredity	IOP inherited	Polygenic effect
Systemic		
Diurnal variation	Most people have a diurnal pattern of IOP	Quite variable in some individuals
Seasonal variation	Higher IOP in winter months	
Blood pressure	IOP increases with increasing blood pressure	
Obesity	Higher IOP in obese people	
Posture	IOP increases from sitting to inverted position	Greater effect below horizontal
Exercise	Strenuous exercise lowers IOP transiently	Long-term training has a lesser effect
Neural	Cholinergic and adrenergic input alters IOP	
Hormones	Corticosteroids raise IOP; diabetes associated with increased IOP	
Drugs	Multiple drugs alter IOP	
Ocular		
Refractive error	Myopic individuals have higher IOP	IOP correlates with axial length
Eye movements	IOP increases if eye moves against resistance	
Eyelid closure	IOP increases with forcible closure	
Inflammation	IOP decreases unless aqueous humor outflow affected more than inflow	
Surgery	IOP generally decreases unless aqueous humor outflow affected more than inflow	

Age

Most studies[70,74-76] find a positive correlation between IOP and age. The effect of increasing age on IOP is the result, at least in part, of increased blood pressure, increased pulse rate, and obesity.[77,78] It is unclear whether the rise in IOP with age represents an increase for all individuals or a greater skewness of the data—that is, a greater minority of the people having higher pressure while the majority show no change. It should be pointed out that a number of studies find little correlation between IOP and age.[78] In addition, one investigative team found that IOP declined with age in a group of Japanese workers.[79,80]

Sex

It has been reported that women have higher IOPs than men, especially after age 40.[70] However, this finding was not confirmed in another study.[81]

Race

In the United States blacks have higher IOPs than whites.[75,82,83] In part, this difference appears to be racial or genetic. There is one report that the Zuni Indians of New Mexico have relatively low IOPs.[84] It is unclear whether this phenomenon is caused by genetic or environmental factors. Because the definitions of, and differences between, various racial and ethnic groups are increasingly indistinct, it is difficult to predict the ultimate clinical utility of these observations.

Heredity

There appears to be a hereditary influence on IOP,[70,85,86] which is polygenic in nature.[85,87] A number of studies have indicated that first-degree relatives of patients with open-angle glaucoma have higher IOPs than the general population.[70,88] In contrast, one study found that spouses have similar levels of IOP, which suggests that there are important environmental influences as well.[89]

Diurnal Variation

Over the course of the day, IOP varies an average of 3 to 6 mm Hg in normal individuals.[90-97] Patients with glaucoma have much wider swings of IOP that can reach 30 mm Hg or even 50 mm Hg in rare cases.[90,92,95,98] In many people the diurnal variation of IOP follows a reproducible pattern, with the maximum pressure in the midmorning hours and the minimum pressure late at night or early in the morning. However, some individuals peak in the afternoon or evening, and others follow no consistent pattern.[95,98-102]

Most of the diurnal pressure variation is caused by fluctuations in the rate of aqueous humor formation. There has been controversy about whether there are also diurnal variations in the facility of aqueous humor outflow, but recent studies indicate that this effect is small at most.[98,103-108] The rate of aqueous formation falls to low levels during sleep and increases during the day, most likely in response to circulating catecholamines.[109,110] The decrease in aqueous flow during sleep is not as pronounced in untreated primary open-angle glaucoma patients as in normal controls, but the magnitude of the difference is so small that clinical relevance is unlikely.[111] A few investigators have postulated that the diurnal IOP variation follows the diurnal glucocorticoid cycle, with IOP peaking about 3 to 4 hours after plasma cortisol.[112]

The diurnal variation in IOP has extremely important clinical implications for glaucoma patients. The fact that the pressure can vary dramatically during a given day makes it unreasonable to assume that a single pressure taken at a specific time is representative of the average pressure the patient experiences over time. It is quite possible that this single pressure represents a high- or low-point, and that the patient's average pressures are substantially different.[97,113] This is of particular concern in patients with normal-tension glaucoma, in whom it may be important to know whether the pressures are always in the low/normal range, or if they sail into the 20s every evening.[114,115] A full 24-hour diurnal curve measurement is often prohibitively difficult to arrange in today's climate of cost containment. A modified diurnal curve is much more practical, while still providing useful information. It is often fairly easy to measure an "office diurnal curve," which generally means checking the pressure every 1 or 2 hours from about 8 AM to 6 PM. Pressure swings of 6 or 8 mm Hg are not uncommon.[96] Knowing the patient's daily pressure excursions allows the physician to tailor therapy toward blunting peaks in pressure, as well as controlling the average pressure during a certain time of day. In addition to measuring a modified diurnal curve, the patient's follow-up visits can be scheduled at differing times of the day. Home tonometry has been suggested as a method of following patients' pressures away from the office. It is unclear whether this method is practical in large populations, although it has been a successful adjunct in certain circumstances.[116]

Seasonal Variation

A seasonal variation of IOP has been reported, with higher IOPs in the winter months.[77,102,117,118] This phenomenon has been attributed to changes in the number of hours of light and to alterations of atmospheric pressure.[118]

Cardiovascular Factors

A number of studies* have shown a correlation between IOP and systemic blood pressure. The relationship is such that large changes in blood pressure are accompanied by small changes in IOP. For example, Bulpitt and co-workers[81] have estimated that systemic blood pressure must rise by 100 mm Hg to increase IOP by 2 mm Hg. Normally, IOP fluctuates 1 to 3 mm Hg as arterial pressure varies with each cardiac cycle.[121] The magnitude of this IOP fluctuation is related to the height of the ocular pressure[121,122] and to the variation of arterial pressure. Systemic hypertension and glaucoma show only a modest association, and the bulk of the effect is attributable to perfusion pressure or other vascular effects, rather than increased IOP.[123] Slower changes in IOP are seen with the Traube-Hering waves. A few researchers believe that IOP also correlates with pulse rate and hemoglobin concentration.[78]

Elevations of episcleral venous pressure, whether from local or systemic conditions, are associated with increased IOP. The rise in IOP is usually in the same range as the rise in episcleral venous pressure.

Alterations in serum osmolality produce changes in IOP. This is best exemplified by the marked changes in IOP that occur during hemodialysis.[124-126] Hyperosmotic drugs such as glycerine, urea, and mannitol are administered systemically to reduce IOP during acute episodes of glaucoma.

Exercise

Strenuous exercise produces a transient reduction of IOP.[127-132] This phenomenon is at least in part caused by acidosis and alterations in serum osmolality.[128,132] In one study a program of conditioning reduced baseline IOP in normal volunteers.[133]

Postural Changes

When normal individuals go from the sitting to the supine position, IOP rises by as much as 6 mm Hg.[134-141] An even greater response is seen in patients with open-angle glaucoma or normal-tension glaucoma.[134,137-139,142,143] When normal volunteers are placed in an inverted position, IOP increases markedly—that is, from an average of 16.8 mm Hg to 32.9 mm Hg in one study.[144] Once again, the rise is greater in glaucomatous eyes.[145] The increase in IOP occurs very rapidly and probably reflects changes in arterial and venous pressure.[135] It is unlikely that such brief elevations of IOP are dangerous in normal individuals, but they may be harmful in patients with advanced glaucoma.[141]

Neural Factors

A number of investigators have postulated that IOP is under neural control. As of yet there is no proof for this hypothesis, although some interesting observations have been made. Sympathectomy produces a transient reduction in IOP and an increase in outflow facility from a release of cate-

*Refs: 75, 77, 78, 81, 88, 119, 120.

cholamines.[146,147] In a similar fashion, adrenergic agonists and cyclic adenosine monophosphate are capable of reducing IOP.[148-150]

Other investigators have explored neural control of IOP by the parasympathetic system. Stimulation of the third cranial nerve reduces IOP.[151] Cholinergic drugs lower IOP by increasing outflow facility. Conversely, ganglionic blocking drugs increase IOP.[152]

Finally, other investigators have sought central nervous system centers that might control IOP. Some researchers have found that stimulation of specific diencephalic areas in experimental animals alters IOP, whereas other researchers[153,154] believed these effects were nonspecific in nature. The third ventricle is close to the hypothalamus and other diencephalic centers. Infusion of a number of substances—including calcium, prostaglandins, arachidonic acid, cyclic nucleotides, hyperosmotic solutions, and hypoosmotic solutions—alters IOP.[155-157]

Psychiatric Disorders

Ocular self-mutilation is a rare finding in psychotic and other severely disturbed patients.[158-162] The authors have seen one young man who pressed and rubbed his fists against his eyes continually unless he was heavily medicated or physically restrained. At the time of our examination his vision was 20/200 in his better eye, with no light perception in the worse eye. Both eyes showed extensive cupping typical of glaucomatous damage, although his pressures were entirely normal and he exhibited no other risk factors for glaucoma.

Hormonal Factors

As mentioned previously, the diurnal intraocular fluctuation may follow the glucocorticoid cycle.[112] Administration of corticosteroids topically, periocularly, and systemically raises IOP.

Some researchers have questioned whether sex hormones have an influence on IOP. It has been noted that IOP varies with the menstrual cycle[163-165] and is low in the third trimester of pregnancy.[163,165,166] However, other studies have not found good correlations between IOP and serum levels of progesterone and estrogen.[167,168] Pharmacologic doses of progesterones and estrogens reduced IOP in experimental animals and man.[165]

Diabetic individuals have higher IOPs than the general population. The reason for this association is unclear. A careful population-based study found that diabetic patients did not have an increased prevalence of glaucoma when selection bias was ruled out.[169]

Other hormones, including growth hormone, thyroxine, aldosterone, vasopressin, and melanocyte-stimulating hormone, may influence IOP physiologically or when administered in pharmacologic doses.[170]

Refractive Error

A number of studies have reported higher IOPs in myopic individuals.[88,171,172] IOP also correlates with axial length.[173] This has been reported in several studies involving pediatric patients, with some investigators suggesting that the increased pressure leads to the increase in axial length.[174-176]

Foods and Drugs

A variety of foods and drugs can alter IOP transiently (Table 5-4).

Eye Movements

If the eye moves against mechanical resistance, IOP can rise substantially.[177-180]

Eyelid Closure

Forcible eyelid closure raises IOP by 10 to 90 mm Hg.[181] Repeated eyelid squeezing reduces IOP.[182] Widening of the lid fissure increases IOP by approximately 2 mm Hg.[183] Conversely, with Bell's palsy IOP is slightly reduced.[184,185]

Table 5-4

Food and Drugs Influencing Intraocular Pressure (IOP)

Agent	Association	Comments
General anesthesia[196]	IOP is reduced in proportion to depth of anesthesia	Exceptions are ketamine and trichlorethylene[197-199]
Alcohol[200,201]	Reduces IOP	Acts through inhibition of antidiuretic hormone and reduction of aqueous formation[200]
Marijuana	Reduces IOP	Acts through local, vascular, and central effects
Corticosteroids	Raise IOP	
Topical cycloplegic agents[202,203]	Raise IOP	Effect greater on glaucomatous eyes
Water	Raises IOP	Large volumes of fluid (> 500 ml) can raise IOP

Inflammation

IOP is usually reduced when the eye is inflamed because aqueous humor formation is reduced. However, if the outflow channels are more affected than the ciliary body, IOP can be elevated.

Surgery

In most cases IOP is reduced after ocular surgery. However, if the outflow channels are affected by inflammation or by the surgery itself (e.g., by viscoelastic substances or by an incision that reduces support for the trabecular meshwork), IOP can be elevated.

REFERENCES

1. Davson H: *The intraocular pressure.* In Davson H, editor: *The eye, vol 1-a, Vegetative physiology and biochemistry,* ed 3, London, 1984, Academic Press.
2. Baum J, and others: Assessment of intraocular pressure by palpation, *Am J Ophthalmol* 119:650, 1995.
3. Goldmann H: Un nouveau tonometre a applanation, *Bull Soc Ophthalmol Fr* 67:474, 1954.
4. Goldmann H, Schmidt TH: Uber applanationstonometrie, *Ophthalmologica* 134: 221, 1957.
5. Phelps CD, Phelps GK: Measurement of intraocular pressure: a study of its reproducibility, *Graefes Arch Clin Exp Ophthalmol* 198:39, 1976.
6. Moltolko MA, and others: Sources of variability in the results of applanation tonometry, *Can J Ophthalmol* 17:93, 1982.
7. Craven ER, and others: Applanation tonometer tip sterilization for adenovirus type 8, *Ophthalmology* 94:1538, 1987.
8. Machesney W, Salz JJ: A simple, convenient tonometer tip disinfection technique, *Ophthalmic Surg* 19:748, 1998.
9. Pepose JS, and others: Disinfection of Goldmann tonometers against human immunodeficiency virus type 1, *Arch Ophthalmol* 107:983, 1989.

10. Threlkeld AB, and others: Efficacy of a disinfectant wipe method for the removal of adenovirus 8 from tonometer tips, *Ophthalmology* 100:1841, 1993.
11. Maldonado MJ, and others: Goldmann applanation tonometry using sterile disposable silicone tonometer shields, *Ophthalmology* 103:815, 1996.
12. Moses RA: The Goldmann applanation tonometer, *Am J Ophthalmol* 46:865, 1958.
13. Holladay JT, Allison ME, Prager TC: Goldmann applanation tonometry in patients with regular corneal astigmatism, *Am J Ophthalmol* 96:90, 1983.
14. Koester CJ, Campbell CJ, Donn A: Ophthalmic optical instruments: two recent developments, *Jpn J Ophthalmol* 24:1, 1980.
15. Currie ZI, and others: Dysthyroid eye disease masquerading as glaucoma, *Ophthalmic Physiol Opt* 11:176, 1991.
16. Spierer A, Eisenstein Z: The role of increased intraocular pressure on upgaze in the assessment of Graves ophthalmopathy, *Ophthalmology* 98:1491, 1991.
17. Moniz E, and others: Removal of hepatitis B surface antigen from a contaminated applanation tonometer, *Am J Ophthalmol* 91:522, 1981.

18. Chronister CL, Russo P: Effects of disinfecting solutions on tonometer tips, *Optom Vis Sci* 67:818, 1990.
19. Centers for Disease Control: Recommendations for preventing possible transmission of human T-lymphotropic virus type III/lymphadenopathy-associated virus in tears, *MMWR Morb Mortal Wkly Rep* 34:533, 1985.
20. Birch-Hirschfeld A: *Die Krankeiten der Orbita.* In Axenfeldt T, Elschnig A, editors: *Handbuch der gesamten Augenheilkunde,* vol 9, part 1, Berlin, 1930, Springer-Verlag.
21. Krakau CET, Wilke K: On repeated tonometry, *Acta Ophthalmol Scand Suppl* 49:611, 1971.
22. Moses RA: Repeated applanation tonometry, *Ophthalmologica* 142:663, 1961.
23. Ehlers N, Bramsen T, Sperling S: Applanation tonometry and central corneal thickness, *Acta Ophthalmol Scand Suppl* 53:34, 1975.
24. Johnson M, and others: Increased corneal thickness simulating elevated intraocular pressure, *Arch Ophthalmol* 96:664, 1978.
25. Olson PF, and others: Measurement of intraocular pressure after epikeratophakia, *Arch Ophthalmol* 101:1111, 1983.

150. Neufeld AH, Jampol LM, Sears ML: Cyclic AMP in the aqueous humor: the effects of adrenergic agents, *Exp Eye Res* 14:242, 1972.

151. Armaly MF: Studies on intraocular effects of orbital parasympathetics. II. Effect on intraocular pressure, *Arch Ophthalmol* 62:117, 1959.

152. Barany EH: Relative importance of autonomic nervous tone and structure as determinants of outflow resistance in normal monkey eyes (*Ceropithecus ethiops* and *Macaca irus*). In Rohen JW, editor: *The structure of the eye,* Stuttgart, 1965, Schattauer.

153. Gloster J, Greaves DP: Effect of diencephalic stimulation upon intraocular pressure, *Br J Ophthalmol* 41:513, 1957.

154. von Sallmann L, Lowenstein O: Responses of intraocular pressure, blood pressure and cutaneous vessels to electric stimulation of the diencephalon, *Am J Ophthalmol* 39:11, 1955.

155. Krupin T, and others: Increased intraocular pressure and hypothermia following injections of calcium into the rabbit third ventricle, *Exp Eye Res* 27:129, 1978.

156. Krupin T, and others: Increased intraocular pressure after third ventricle injections of prostaglandin E1 and arachidonic acid, *Am J Ophthalmol* 81:346, 1976.

157. Krupin T, Podos SM, Becker B: Alterations of intraocular pressure after third ventricle injections of osmotic agents, *Am J Ophthalmol* 76:948, 1973.

158. Slamovits T: Popping eyes, *Surv Ophthalmol* 33:273, 1989.

159. Witherspoon CD, and others: Ocular self-mutilation, *Ann Ophthalmol* 21:255, 1989.

160. Jones NP: Self-enucleation and psychosis, *Br J Ophthalmol* 74:571, 1990.

161. Kennedy BL, Feldmann TB: Self-inflicted eye injuries: case presentations and a literature review, *Hosp Community Psychiatry* 45:470, 1994.

162. Yucel B, Ozkan S: A rare case of self-mutilation: self-enucleation of both eyes, *Gen Hosp Psychiatry* 17:310, 1995.

163. Becker B, Friedenwald JS: Clinical aqueous outflow, *Arch Ophthalmol* 50:557, 1952.

164. Dalton K: Influence of menstruation on glaucoma, *Br J Ophthalmol* 51:692, 1967.

165. Paterson GD, Miller SJH: Hormonal influences in simple glaucoma, *Br J Ophthalmol* 47:129, 1963.

166. Phillips CI, Gore SM: Ocular hypotensive effect of late pregnancy with and without high blood pressure, *Br J Ophthalmol* 69:117, 1985.

167. Feldman F, Bain J, Matuk AR: Daily assessment of ocular and hormonal variables throughout the menstrual cycle, *Arch Ophthalmol* 96:1835, 1978.

168. Green K, Cullen PM, Phillips CI: Aqueous humor turnover and intraocular pressure during menstruation, *Br J Ophthalmol* 68:736, 1984.

169. Tielsch JM, and others: Diabetes, intraocular pressure, and primary open-angle glaucoma in the Baltimore Eye Survey, *Ophthalmology* 102:48, 1995.

170. Kass MA, Sears ML: Hormonal regulation of intraocular pressure, *Surv Ophthalmol* 22:153, 1977.

171. Daubs JG, Pitts-Crick R: Effect of refractive error on the risk of ocular hypertension and open-angle glaucoma, *Trans Ophthalmol Soc UK* 101:121, 1981.

172. Perkins ES, Phelps CD: Open-angle glaucoma, ocular hypertension, low-tension glaucoma, and refraction, *Arch Ophthalmol* 100:1464, 1982.

173. Tomlinson A, Phillips CI: Applanation tension and axial length of the eyeball, *Br J Ophthalmol* 54:548, 1970.

174. Parssinen O: Intraocular pressure in school myopia, *Acta Ophthalmol Scand Suppl* 68:559, 1990.

175. Edwards MH, Brown B: Intraocular pressure in a selected sample of myopic and nonmyopic Chinese children, *Optom Vis Sci* 70:15, 1993.

176. Quinn GE, and others: Association of intraocular pressure and myopia in children, *Ophthalmology* 102:180, 1995.

177. Moses RA, Lurie P, Wette R: Horizontal gaze position effect on intraocular pressure, *Invest Ophthalmol Vis Sci* 22:551, 1982.

178. Pohjanpelto P: The thyroid gland and intraocular pressure, *Acta Ophthalmol Scand Suppl* 97:1, 1968.

179. Saunders RA, Helveston EM, Ellis FD: Differential intraocular pressure in strabismus diagnosis, *Ophthalmology* 87:59, 1981.

180. Zappia RJ, Winkelman JZ, Gay AJ: Intraocular pressure changes in normal subjects and the adhesive muscle syndrome, *Am J Ophthalmol* 71:880, 1971.

181. Coleman DJ, Trokel S: Direct-recorded intraocular pressure variations in a human subject, *Arch Ophthalmol* 82:637, 1969.

182. Green K, Luxenberg MN: Consequences of eyelid squeezing on intraocular pressure, *Am J Ophthalmol* 88:1072, 1979.

183. Moses RA, and others: Proptosis and increase of intraocular pressure in voluntary lid fissure widening, *Invest Ophthalmol Vis Sci* 25:989, 1984.

184. Losada F, Wolintz AH: Bell's palsy: a new ophthalmologic sign, *Ann Ophthalmol* 5:1093, 1973.

185. Starrels ME, Krupin T, Burde RM: Bell's palsy and intraocular pressure, *Ann Ophthalmol* 7:1067, 1975.

186. Linner E: Adrenocortical steroids and aqueous humor dynamics, *Doc Ophthalmol* 13:210, 1959.

187. Becker B: The decline in aqueous secretion and outflow facility with age, *Am J Ophthalmol* 46:731, 1958.

188. Johnson LV: Tonographic survey, *Am J Ophthalmol* 61:680, 1966.

189. Soeteren T: Scleral rigidity in normal human eyes, *Acta Ophthalmol (Copenh)* 38:303, 1960.

190. Loewen U, Handrup B, Redeker A: Results of a glaucoma mass screening program, *Klin Mbl Augenheilk* 169:754, 1976.

191. Ruprecht KW, Wulle KG, Christl HL: Applanation tonometry within medical diagnostic "check-up" programs, *Klin Mbl Augenheilk* 172:332, 1978.

192. Stromberg U: Ocular hypertension, *Acta Ophthalmologica (Suppl) (Copenh)* 69:7, 1962.

193. Hollows FC, Graham PA: Intraocular pressure, glaucoma and glaucoma suspects in a defined population, *Br J Ophthalmol* 50:570, 1966.

194. Leibowitz HM, and others: The Framingham eye study monograph, *Surv Ophthalmol* 24:336, 1980 (Suppl).

195. Bengtsson B: The prevalence of glaucoma, *Br J Ophthalmol* 65:46, 1981.

196. Duncalf D: Anesthesia and intraocular pressure, *Trans Am Acad Ophthalmol Otolaryngol* 79:562, 1975.

197. Maddox TS Jr, Kielar RA: Comparison of the influence of ketamine and halothane anesthesia on intraocular tensions of nonglaucomatous children, *J Pediatr Ophthalmol* 11:90, 1974.

198. Schreuder M, Linssen GH: Intra-ocular pressure and anesthesia: direct measurements by needling the anterior chamber in the monkey, *Anesthesia* 27:165, 1972.

199. Schutten WH, Van Horn DL: The effects of ketamine sedation and ketamine-pentobarbital anesthesia upon the intraocular pressure of the rabbit, *Invest Ophthalmol* 16:531, 1977.

200. Houle RE, Grant WM: Alcohol, vasopressin and intraocular pressure, *Invest Ophthalmol* 6:145, 1967.

201. Peczon JD, Grant WM: Glaucoma, alcohol, and intraocular pressure, *Arch Ophthalmol* 73:495, 1965.

202. Lazenby GW, Reed JW, Grant WM: Short-term tests of anticholinergic medication in open-angle glaucoma, *Arch Ophthalmol* 80:443, 1968.

203. Valle O: Effect of cyclopentolate on the aqueous dynamics in incipient or suspected open-angle glaucoma, *Acta Ophthalmologica (Copenh)* 80:52, 1973.

PART III

Clinical Examination of the Eye

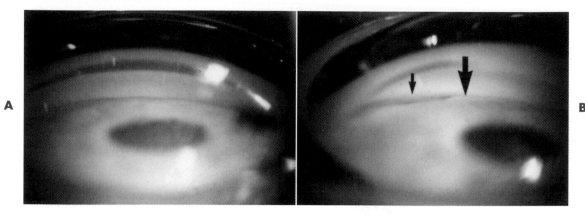

Figure 6-10   **A,** An eye with appositional angle closure. No trabecular meshwork is visible. **B,** With indentation gonioscopy, parts of the trabecular meshwork are visualized *(small arrow)* but there is a broad peripheral anterior synechia *(large arrow),* which precludes visualization of the remainder of the trabecular meshwork. (From Alward WLM: *Color atlas of gonioscopy,* St Louis, 1994, Mosby.)

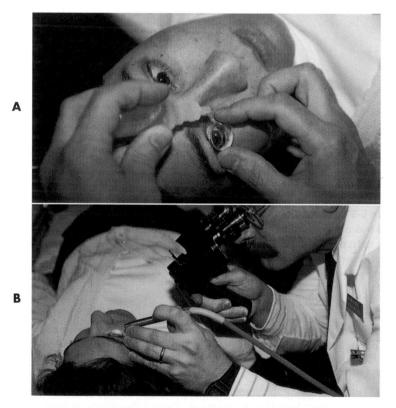

Figure 6-11   **A,** Saline is used to bridge the gap between the Koeppe lens and the cornea in a supine patient. **B,** Examination of supine patient with Koeppe lens using counterbalanced biomicroscope and Barkan illuminator. (Courtesy of Paul R. Lichter, M.D. and A. Tim Johnson, M.D., Ph.D., University of Michigan. From Alward WLM: *Color atlas of gonioscopy,* St Louis, 1994, Mosby.)

right-hand thumb and index finger for the right eye and between the left-hand thumb and index finger for the left eye and inserts the lens between the lids. After the space beneath the lens is filled with isotonic sodium chloride solution, an assistant can steady it with a muscle hook or an applicator. If the patient is less cooperative, then more viscous 1% methylcellulose is used instead of isotonic sodium chloride solution.

REFERENCES

1. Alward W: *Color atlas of gonioscopy,* Barcelona, 1994, Mosby-Wolfe.
2. Fisch B: *Gonioscopy and the glaucomas,* Boston, 1993, Butterworth-Heinemann.
3. Grant WM, Schuman JS: *The angle of the anterior chamber.* In Epstein DL, Allingham RR, Schuman JS, editors: *Chandler & Grant's glaucoma,* ed 4, Baltimore, 1996, Williams & Wilkins.
4. Palmberg P: *Gonioscopy.* In Ritch R, Shields MB, Krupin T, editors: *The glaucomas,* St Louis, 1996, Mosby.
5. Forbes M: Gonioscopy with corneal indentation: a method for distinguishing between appositional closure and synechial closure, *Arch Ophthalmol* 76:488, 1966.
6. Shaffer RN: *Stereoscopic manual of gonioscopy,* St Louis, 1962, Mosby.

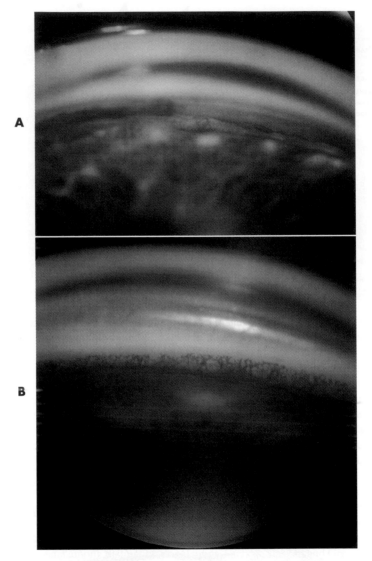

Figure 7-3   **A,** Blood in the angle following traumatic angle recession. Jugular compression resulted in discharge of blood from Schlemm's canal into the anterior chamber in this patient who had suffered angle recession some months previously. The patient had experienced periodic blurring of vision with pressure elevation as a result of this blood in the anterior chamber. It was resolved with laser applied to the bleeding point. **B,** Iris processes covering angle. This 33-year-old female had iris sweeping up over the trabecular meshwork in a dense syncytium. This is similar to the concave iris insertion in trabeculodysgenesis (see Chapter 21). Such patients often present with glaucoma before the age of 30.

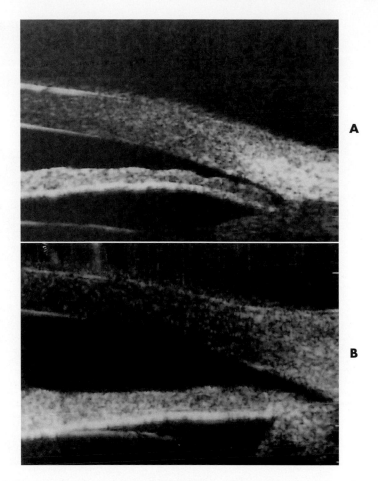

Figure 7-4   **A,** Bowing of iris into angle during attack of pupillary-block angle-closure glaucoma. **B,** Following laser iridectomy the contour of the iris has become flat, falling away from the angle. (From Pavlin CJ, Foster FS: *Ultrasound in biomicroscopy in glaucoma.* In Ritch R, Shields MB, Krupin T, editors: *The glaucomas,* ed 2, St Louis, 1996, Mosby.)

Anatomic Features of Narrow-Angled Eyes

In contrast, the lens of the shallow-chambered, narrow-angled eye is well anterior to the ciliary body ring, and the iris is held more snugly against a much larger area of the posterior iris surface (Fig. 7-3). Therein results a physiologic or relative pupillary block. In such an eye a somewhat higher pressure is required in the posterior chamber to push aqueous humor through this tight iris-lens apposition than is necessary for the looser apposition of the wide-angled eye.[19] An exaggeration of this pupillary block is the chief cause of angle-closure glaucoma. The slight excess pressure in the posterior chamber lifts the iris root forward and may be adequate to push the iris against the trabecular meshwork in some eyes (see Fig. 8-1, *C* and *D*). If the angle is sufficiently narrow, and the iris base sufficiently distensible, the iris is forced against the surface of the trabecular meshwork, blocking aqueous flow into Schlemm's canal, and an attack of angle-closure glaucoma ensues. The alternative route for aqueous egress provided by a patent iridotomy can completely reverse this propensity for angle occlusion by the iris base, as demonstrated dramatically with ultrasonic biomicroscopy (Fig. 7-4).

An important exception to the usual narrow-angle configuration is the anatomic abnormality associated with plateau iris. In this condition the peripheral iris is displaced anteriorly into the angle by anomalously positioned and rotated ciliary processes behind the iris root.[20] This has been demonstrated both by ultrasonic biomicroscopy[21] and by histology.[22] Pupillary dilation may bunch up the peripheral iris and occlude the angle. Pupillary block plays only a small role in the mechanism;

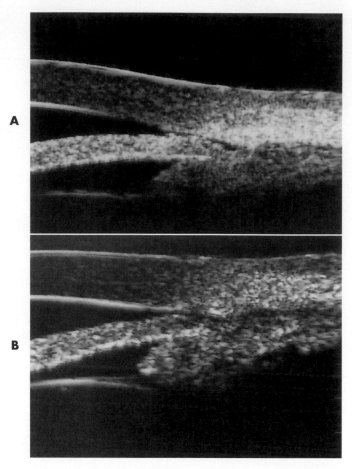

Figure 7-5 **A,** Plateau iris syndrome with anteriorly rotated ciliary process pressing peripheral iris forward toward the angle. **B,** Following laser iridotomy there is virtually no change in either iris or angle configuration. (From Pavlin CJ, Foster FS: *Ultrasound in biomicroscopy in glaucoma.* In Ritch R, Shields MB, Krupin T, editors: *The glaucomas,* ed 2, St Louis, 1996, Mosby.)

neither iridotomy nor lens removal favorably affects this configuration (Fig. 7-5). Gonioscopically, there may be a marked V-shaped recess between the peripheral iris and the trabecular meshwork with miosis.

GONIOSCOPIC ANATOMY AND MICROSCOPIC INTERPRETATION
Pupil and Iris

It is best to start gonioscopy by looking at the pupil for rapid orientation. The anterior lens surface can be observed for focal opacifications *(glaukomflecken)* of the anterior lens and for posterior synechiae. This position is also excellent for viewing the white dandrufflike flecks of exfoliation on the pigment at the posterior edge of the pupil, which is typical of exfoliative syndrome.[23,24] Iridodonesis is present to a small degree in some deep-chambered normal eyes and is easily observed if of a pathologic degree.

The first of the three major iris features the examiner should carefully evaluate is the *contour* of the iris, noting its flatness when the anterior chamber is deep, its convexity (or even bowing) in eyes with a shallow anterior chamber, or its peripheral concavity in eyes with high myopia or signs of pigment dispersion.[25,26] After assessing the configuration of the peripheral iris, attention should be paid to the *site of iris insertion*—both its apparent and actual juncture in the angle. Indentation gonioscopy is particularly helpful in distinguishing iris-trabecular touch (apposition) from genuine adhesion. The level of iris insertion can be described in reference to structures within the angle re-

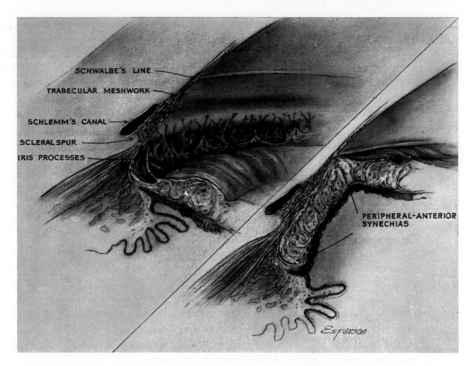

SCHWALBE'S LINE

TRABECULAR MESHWORK

SCHLEMM'S CANAL

SCLERAL SPUR

IRIS PROCESSES

PERIPHERAL-ANTERIOR SYNECHIAS

Esperson

Figure 7-6   Difference between iris processes and peripheral anterior synechiae.

cess—at the level of the upper trabecular meshwork and Schwalbe's line; at the level of the filtering trabecular meshwork; just below the scleral spur; below the spur in the ciliary body; or deep posteriorly in the ciliary band. Anteriorly inserting irides, at the level of the spur or lower trabecular meshwork, have been described among Asians[7,8] and in patients with hyperopia. Third, the examiner should estimate the *angulation* between the iris insertion and the slope of the inner cornea in the angle, in approximate steps of 10°. As discussed in the next chapter, this assessment of angle width is the basis of many gonioscopic grading systems. Last, abnormalities such as neovascularization, hypoplasia, atrophy, and polycoria should be noted.

Ciliary Body, Iris Processes, and Synechiae

Beyond the final iris roll is the angle recess. At birth this recess is incompletely developed. By the age of 1 year the recess has formed a concavity into the anterior surface of the ciliary body. The ciliary body appears as a densely pigmented band deep to the trabecular surface. Its anterior extension merges into the scleral spur, which appears as a white line between the ciliary body and the more anterior pigmented trabecular band. If there is no pigment in the trabecular meshwork, the ciliary body will be the only pigmented structure in the angle wall. In angle recession (Fig. 7-3, *A*) the ciliary body may be broadly exposed. Irregular, threadlike fibers of the anterior iris stroma sometimes arborize across the angle recess and are called iris processes (Fig. 7-3, *B*). Gonioscopically, the processes usually seem to terminate near the spur, but some may extend in front of Schlemm's canal, occasionally running as high as Schwalbe's line. Larger processes represent an incomplete embryologic separation of the iris from the angle wall, which is seen in exaggerated form in the pathologic congenital syndrome of Axenfeld. Most of the fibers lose their pigment at the scleral spur and then merge with the innermost layer of the trabecular meshwork called the uveal meshwork.

In blue eyes the iris processes are light gray and difficult to see, but in brown eyes the pigmented processes stand out prominently against the light background of the scleral spur. The neophyte gonioscopist may misinterpret these processes as peripheral anterior synechiae. They do not interfere in any way with outflow of aqueous humor (Fig. 7-6).

True synechiae are formed when the peripheral iris becomes attached to the trabecular wall. There are several clues for distinguishing iris processes from peripheral anterior synechiae. Iris processes are fibers or syncytial sheets that closely follow or bridge the concavity of the angle recess and that usually allow a view of the angle recess behind them unless they are extraordinarily dense. Peripheral anterior synechiae are actual adhesions of iris tissue that cover and occlude variable amounts of the angle. They can insert low at the level of the scleral spur (such as after laser trabeculoplasty) to as high as Schwalbe's line and beyond (as with the irido-corneo-endothelial syndromes). Often normal angle structures can be seen in one area but are concealed by the synechiae in other areas. Synechiae can form only when the iris is pushed against the trabecular meshwork, as in angle-closure glaucoma, or when the iris is pulled up onto the meshwork as the result of the shrinkage of inflammatory products or fibrovascular membranes attached to both iris and meshwork. In the area of a synechia, peripheral iris tissue butts flat against the trabecular surface; it does not wrap around the angle recess as does an iris process—a distinction well appreciated during indentation gonioscopy.

Scleral Spur

The most anterior projection of the sclera internally is the scleral spur. In wide-angled eyes it is seen gonioscopically as a gray-white line of varying width at the outer end of the angle recess, and it is the point of attachment of the ciliary body and the point of termination of most of the iris processes. If blood is in Schlemm's canal, it lies just anterior to the spur.

The spur forms the posterior concavity of the scleral sulcus. Schlemm's canal is held in the sulcus by the corneoscleral trabecular sheets that form an inner wall to the sulcus. Most of these sheets insert at the spur. The spur is also the insertion point for most of the longitudinal muscle fibers of the ciliary body, whose action alters the facility of aqueous outflow (see Fig. 7-1). The spur's crisp white appearance is the most helpful landmark in orienting the gonioscopist. It is also prominent in ultrasonic biomicroscopy because unlike other angle structures such as the posterior trabecular meshwork, it can be readily identified and thus used as an important landmark in quantifying angle measurements.[27]

Schwalbe's Line

Another important gonioscopic landmark, Schwalbe's line, marks the most anterior extension of the meshwork and the termination of Descemet's membrane of the cornea. By slit-lamp examination of normal eyes it often can be seen somewhere in the limbal circumference as a hazy zone of the inner corneal surface. With an indirect contact lens the corneal parallelepiped of the slit-lamp beam comes together at this point (Fig. 7-7). With the use of the Koeppe contact lens, Schwalbe's

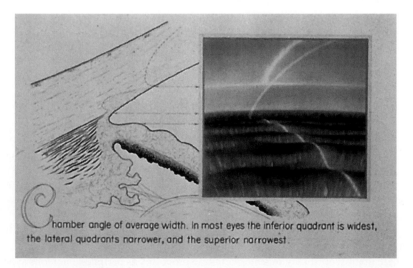

chamber angle of average width. In most eyes the inferior quadrant is widest, the lateral quadrants narrower, and the superior narrowest.

Figure 7-7   Parallelepiped method of identifying the boundary between cornea (thick light beam) and anterior trabecular meshwork (thin strip of light). (From Palmberg P: *Gonioscopy.* In Ritch R, Shields MB, Krupin T: *The glaucomas,* ed 2, St Louis, 1996, Mosby.)

line is seen as a translucent or white ledge that projects slightly into the anterior chamber,[28] or it may be a vague line of demarcation between the smooth surface of Descemet's membrane that covers the inner cornea and the less transparent rough texture of the uveal meshwork.

The line itself is composed of a bundle of collagenous connective tissue fibers running circumferentially around the eye at the end of Descemet's membrane. Here the corneal radius of curvature changes to the larger radius of the sclera. This change in curvature and the beginning roughness of the trabecular surface provide a lodging place for the pigment granules that may be carried into the inferior angle by the aqueous convection currents (Sampaolesi's line). Such pigmentation is rare in healthy young eyes but becomes increasingly common in older or diseased eyes.

Trabecular Meshwork and Trabecular Pigment Band

Between Schwalbe's line and the scleral spur lies the trabecular meshwork, through which aqueous humor flows to Schlemm's canal. The internal layer of the trabecular meshwork is a syncytium of fibers called the uveal meshwork. The outer portion of the trabecular meshwork is composed of corneoscleral trabecular sheets that insert into the scleral sulcus and the spur. These sheets are not visible gonioscopically.

GONIOSCOPIC APPEARANCE

Gonioscopically, the trabecular meshwork has an irregularly roughened surface, which in childhood appears as a glistening, translucent-like semitransparent gelatin with a stippled surface. With increasing age its transparency decreases. The roughness of its surface is caused by the large openings of the uveal meshwork. It should be stressed that the examiner's gaze should parallel the iris as near as possible when looking at the trabecular surface. With indirect gonioscopy, such as with the Zeiss lens, having the patient look away from the viewing mirror gives an optimal view of the meshwork in wide-angle eyes. In the narrow-angled eye the convex plane of the iris forces a more oblique visualization (optimized with the patient looking toward the viewing mirror), which allows the angle recess to be seen, but which may give a somewhat foreshortened and distorted appearance to the meshwork.

Just anterior to the scleral spur is the effective filtering portion of the meshwork, lying in front of Schlemm's canal. In aging and disease processes the aqueous flow carries pigment from the iris and deposits it in varying amounts and depths in the meshwork, giving rise to the trabecular pigment band, which tends to be denser in the lower angle. Such pigmentation can be homogenous in appearance (as in the pigment dispersion syndrome) or variegated (as seen after anterior segment trauma). The presence and extent of trabecular pigmentation may provide valuable clinical information, such as suggesting an occult case of pseudoexfoliative syndrome or being indicative of a favorable response to laser trabeculoplasty.

REFERENCES

1. Hogan MJ, Alvarado JA, Weddell J: *Histology of the human eye,* Philadelphia, 1971, WB Saunders (atlas and textbook).
2. Lütjen-Dricoll E, Rohen JW: *Morphology of aqueous outflow pathways in normal and glaucomatous eyes.* In Ritch R, Shields MB, Krupin T, editors: *The glaucomas,* ed 2, St Louis, 1996, Mosby.
3. Allen L, Burian HM, Braley AE: A new concept of the anterior chamber angle, *Arch Ophthalmol* 62:966, 1959.
4. Barkan O, Boyle SF, Maisler S: On the genesis of glaucoma: an improved method based on slitlamp microscopy of the angle of the anterior chamber, *Am J Ophthalmol* 19:209, 1936.
5. Spaeth GL: Gonioscopy: uses old and new. The inheritance of occludable angles, *Ophthalmology* 85:222, 1978.
6. Spaeth GL: The normal development of the human anterior chamber angle: a new system of descriptive grading, *Trans Ophthalmol Soc UK* 91:709, 1971.
7. Oh YG, and others: The anterior chamber angle is different in different racial groups: a gonioscopic study, *Eye* 8:104, 1994.
8. Nguyen N, and others: A high prevalence of occludable angles in a Vietnamese population, *Ophthalmology* 103:1426, 1996.
9. Arkell SM, and others: The prevalence of glaucoma among Eskimos of northwest Alaska, *Arch Ophthalmol* 105:482, 1987.
10. Alsbirk PH: Early detection of primary angle-closure glaucoma: limbal and axial chamber depth screening in a high risk population (Greenland Eskimos), *Acta Ophthalmol Scand Suppl* 66:556, 1988.
11. Van Rens GH, and others: Primary angle-closure glaucoma among Alaskan Eskimos, *Doc Ophthalmol* 70:265, 1988.
12. Loh RCK: The problem of glaucoma in Singapore, *Singapore Med J* 9:76, 1968.
13. Hu Z: An epidemiologic investigation of glaucoma in Beijing and Shun-yi county, *Chin J Ophthalmol* 25:115, 1989.
14. Hung PT: Aetiology and mechanism of primary angle-closure glaucoma, *Asia-Pac J Ophthalmol* 2:82, 1990.
15. Kitazawa Y: Epidemiology of primary angle-closure glaucoma, *Asia-Pac J Ophthalmol* 2:78, 1990.
16. Shiose Y, and others: Epidemiology of glaucoma in Japan: a nationwide glaucoma survey, *Jpn J Ophthalmol* 35:133, 1991.
17. Salmon JF, Martell R: The role of ethnicity in primary angle-closure glaucoma, *S Afr Med J* 84:623, 1994.

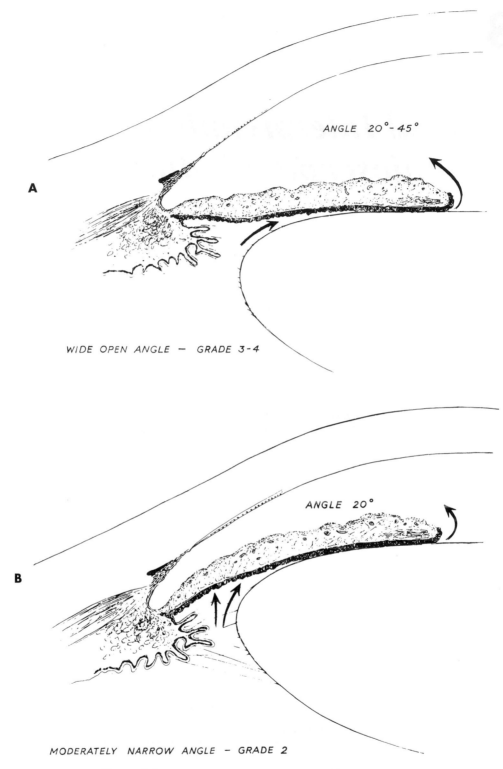

ANGLE 20°- 45°

A

WIDE OPEN ANGLE — GRADE 3-4

ANGLE 20°

B

MODERATELY NARROW ANGLE — GRADE 2

Figure 8-1   **A** through **D,** Grading of angles by estimated angulation.

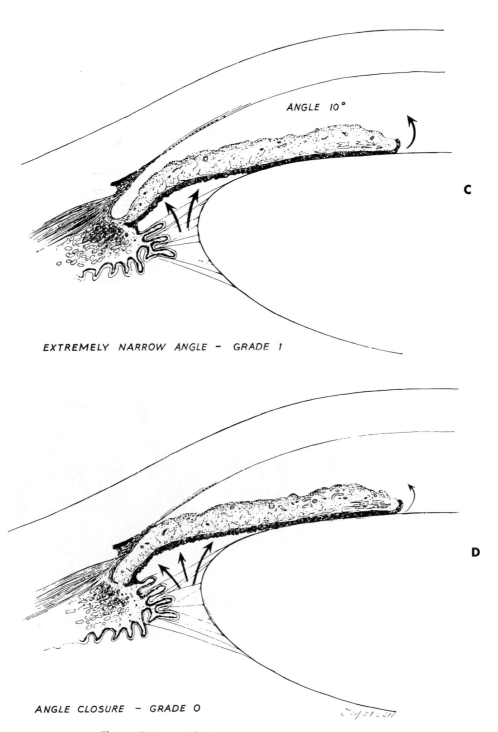

ANGLE 10°

C

EXTREMELY NARROW ANGLE - GRADE 1

D

ANGLE CLOSURE - GRADE 0

Figure 8-1, cont'd   For legend see opposite page.

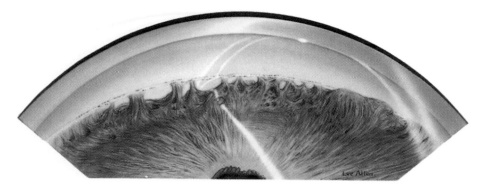

Figure 8A-12   Axenfeld's anomaly with dense iris adhesions that almost completely cover the trabecular meshwork. Particles of pigment are deposited along a very prominent Schwalbe's ring. (From Burian HM: *Arch Ophthalmol* 53:767, 1955. Copyright 1955 by the American Medical Association.)

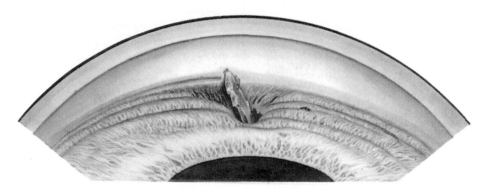

Figure 8A-13   Glass in the inferior angle after trauma. The patient had broken his glasses while working in a sawmill. A fragment of glass was removed earlier. The patient presented with discomfort and injection. The chip of glass is wedged between the trabecular meshwork and the iris, distorting both structures. There is a small tear in the iris and clotted blood under the fragment. Some blood is present in Schlemm's canal. (Copyright by Abbott Laboratories, North Chicago, Ill.)

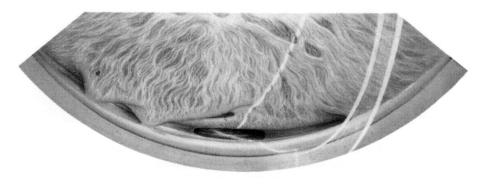

Figure 8A-14   Aphakic glaucoma status after surgical cyclodialysis showing an open cleft with surrounding synechiae. (From Alward WLM: *Color atlas of gonioscopy,* London, 1994, Mosby. Illustration by Lee Allen.)

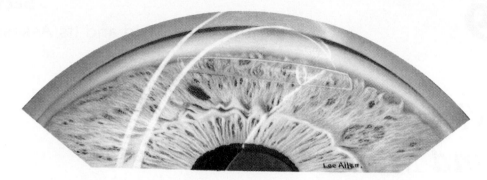

Figure 8A-15 Inferior scroll of Descemet's membrane after surgery. (From Alward WLM: *Color atlas of gonioscopy,* London, 1994, Mosby. Illustration by Lee Allen.)

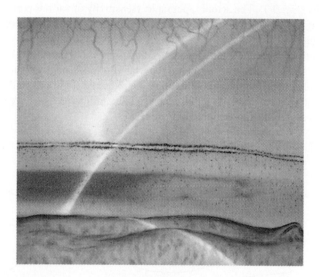

Figure 8A-16 Gonioscopic view of an angle showing blood in Schlemm's canal. There is, incidentally, a prominent Schwalbe's line. (From Alward WLM: *Color atlas of gonioscopy,* London, 1994, Mosby. Illustration by Lee Allen.)

9

Visual Field Theory and Methods

THE NORMAL VISUAL FIELD

The normal visual field has been described as an island of vision in a sea of darkness.[1] This island has a sharp central peak, corresponding to the fovea, with sloping sides. The sides are slightly steeper superiorly and nasally.[2] The island of vision extends 60° superiorly and nasally, 75° inferiorly, and 100° temporally (Fig. 9-1). The actual topography (sensitivity of various parts) of the island depends on the level of light adaptation of the retina.[3] The peak has its greatest sensitivity when the retina is completely light adapted and therefore can see the weakest stimulus. The edges of the island have poor light sensitivity, so stimuli must be up to 3500 times more intense to be perceived.[4,5] If the retina is fully dark adapted, the fovea (center of the island) is less sensitive than the periphery.

Visual field testing is usually done in the photopic (light-adapted) or mesopic (partially light-adapted) state. Thus in the normal visual field examination, the fovea is the most sensitive point tested and represents the peak.

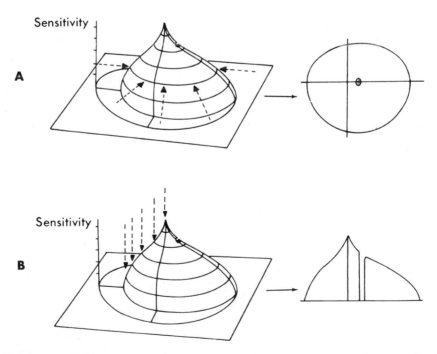

Figure 9-1 **A,** Isopter (kinetic) perimetry. Test object of fixed intensity is moved along several meridians toward fixation. Points where the object is first perceived are plotted in a circle. **B,** Static perimetry. Stationary test object is increased in intensity from below threshold until perceived by the patient. Threshold values yield a graphic profile section. (Modified from Aulhorn E, Harms H. In Leydhecker W, editor: *Glaucoma, Tutzing symposium,* Basel, 1967, S Karger.)

Visual Acuity Versus Visual Field

Visual acuity measurement tests the resolving power of the retina for objects of distinct form. Visual field measurement tests a more primitive retinal function—*differential light sensitivity*. Differential light sensitivity is the measure of the ability of the retina to distinguish a stimulus that is some degree brighter than the background illumination.

Terminology and Definitions

Fixation. That part of the visual field corresponding to the fovea centralis. Also, the inability of patients to keep their eyes directed at the center of the visual field apparatus. Patients with poor fixation move their eyes repeatedly and produce an unreliable visual field test result.

Central field. That portion of the visual field within 30° of fixation.

Bjerrum's area (arcuate area). That portion of the central field extending from the blind spot and arcing above or below fixation in a broadening path to end at the horizontal raphe nasal to fixation. Bjerrum's area usually is considered to be within the central 25° of the visual field. This part of the visual field is quite susceptible to glaucomatous damage (see Fig. 11-9). Bjerrum's area does not include nonspecific peripheral depression that is commonly seen along the uppermost border of automated visual field charts. These defects may appear to arc because of the placement of test points, but they do not constitute a classic arcuate scotoma (Fig. 9-2; see also Fig. 11-2).

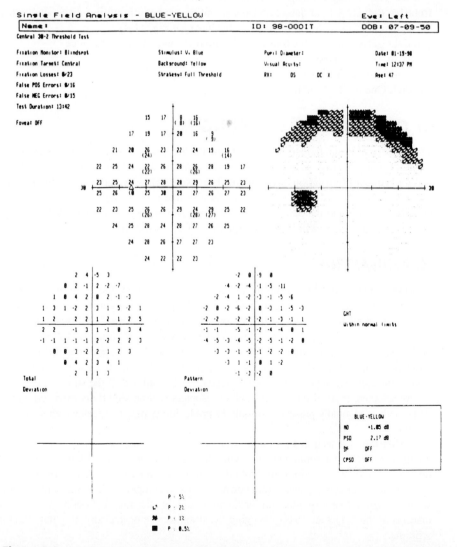

Figure 9-2 The dark areas at the top of this printout are artifacts. The patient has a normal field.

Peripheral field. That portion of the visual field from 30° to the far periphery. The shape of the normal peripheral field is governed by the shape and structures of the face.

Static perimetry. Visual field test wherein the position of the stimulus is held constant while the stimulus intensity is varied.

Kinetic perimetry. Visual field test wherein the intensity and size of the stimulus are held constant while the stimulus location is moved.

Isopter. The outline of a contiguous area of the visual field capable of perceiving a given stimulus. The isopter is most often used to define an area outlined by a given stimulus in kinetic perimetry.

Threshold. At a given retinal point, the intensity of a stimulus that is perceived 50% of the times it is presented.

Fluctuation. The variability in visual field measurement.

Short-term fluctuation. The variability within a field at the time of its measurement.

Long-term fluctuation. The variability between two visual fields performed at different times on the same eye that cannot be attributed to pathologic change.

Short wavelength automated perimetry. Visual field test in which short wavelength-sensitive (blue) cones are isolated by using blue light stimuli projected on a yellow background. Also called *blue on yellow* perimetry.

Depression. A reduction in sensitivity greater than the expected normal reduction.

Scotoma. A localized defect or depression in the visual field.

Absolute defect. A field defect that persists when the maximum stimulus of the testing apparatus is used. The normal blind spot is an absolute scotoma.

Relative defect. A field defect that is present to weaker stimuli but disappears when tested with brighter stimuli. A defect that is not absolute (see Fig. 11-4).

Candela per square meter (cd/m²). The international unit of luminance.

Apostilb. 0.1 millilambert = 3.183 cd/m².

Log unit. Logarithm base 10 of the luminance in apostilbs.

Decibel. One tenth of the log unit.

THEORY OF VISUAL FIELD TESTING

The purpose of visual field testing is to define the topography of the island of vision to recognize any variation from normal. It is used to detect abnormalities and to follow abnormalities while the patient is under observation or treatment. The visual field is tested by adapting the eye to the background luminance and then presenting a stimulus that is some degree brighter than the background at a given position in the field. The ability of the patient to perceive the stimulus may be tested kinetically, statically, or with some combination of the two techniques.

KINETIC PERIMETRY

In kinetic perimetry the stimulus usually is presented in the periphery and moved at approximately 2° per second toward fixation until the patient first perceives it. The stimulus is moved to another meridian in the periphery out of view and advanced toward fixation again until the patient sees it. By repeating these maneuvers at approximately 15° intervals around 360° of the visual field, the examiner defines a series of points that can be connected to describe an isopter corresponding to the stimulus used (see Fig. 9-1). By decreasing or increasing the size or brightness of the stimulus, a smaller or larger isopter will be outlined. If the stimulus is presented into randomly selected areas of the visual field, the isopters will be slightly constricted and irregular compared with sequentially presented stimuli. Reproducibility may be greater with sequentially presented stimuli.[6]

After initial detection a scotoma can be defined more precisely with kinetic perimetry by placing the stimulus in the scotoma and moving the stimulus outward until it is perceived. This process is repeated in various directions until all edges of the scotoma have been defined. If the edges of the scotoma are sloping (the change from normal to abnormal regions within the field is gradual), a brighter stimulus will define a smaller scotoma, and a dimmer stimulus will define a larger scotoma. If the margins of the defect are steep, changing the stimulus size or intensity may not affect the size of the scotoma.

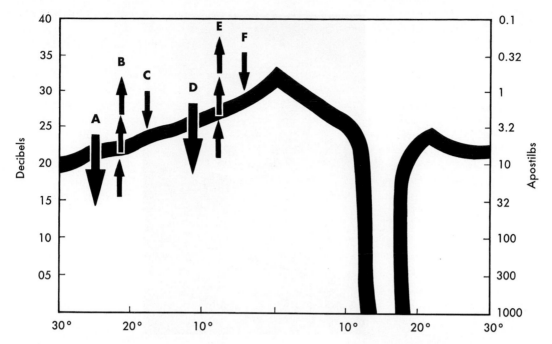

Figure 9-3   Static testing for threshold sensitivity. **A,** A bright stimulus is presented that the patient can see. **B,** The stimulus intensity is decreased until the patient can no longer see it. **C,** The stimulus intensity is then increased again until the patient just sees it. This establishes the threshold sensitivity for that spot in the retina. **D** through **F,** A similar maneuver then is carried out in an adjacent part of the retina. The increment of change in stimulus intensity governs the sensitivity of the test.

STATIC PERIMETRY

In static perimetry the test stimulus size usually remains constant throughout the test. For full-threshold testing, each point in the visual field is evaluated by positioning the stimulus at that point and varying the intensity until the threshold for that particular retinal location is defined for those testing conditions (Fig. 9-3). This process is repeated until all of the positions of the retina to be measured have been tested.

The more retinal positions tested, the more defects will be found and quantified. There is, however, a point of diminishing returns, at approximately 80 locations, wherein patient fatigue seriously reduces the accuracy and consistency of responses.[7,8] If a 6° separation of retinal locations is chosen, about 75 to 80 positions are required to test the central 30° of vision. Most computerized perimeters (Figs. 9-4 and 9-5) use static visual field testing techniques for their standard tests.

Alternatives to standard full-threshold testing of each retinal position have been devised to reduce the number of patient responses required without reducing the amount of information obtained at each testing session.[9-12] Such alternatives include threshold-related testing and zone testing, as well as algorithms that use less precise bracketing to estimate the threshold. These methods generally produce results that are similar to, but somewhat more variable than, standard threshold determining strategies.[13-16]

Threshold-Related Testing

The "normal" state of the visual field is a statistically determined figure obtained from the testing of many normal individuals of different ages. It is clear that each retinal location has a statistically determined normal sensitivity that can be expressed in decibels of stimulus intensity related to stimulus size, background intensity, and patient age.[17] It is also clear that this sensitivity is not

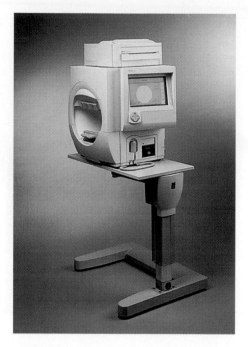

Figure 9-4 Humphrey 700 series perimeter.

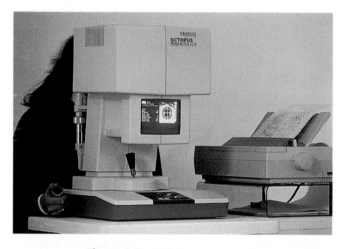

Figure 9-5 Octopus 123 perimeter.

constant from patient to patient or even within the same patient from test to test. Therefore for a particular retinal location to have a strong possibility of being abnormal, its sensitivity should be reduced from normal by about 2 standard deviations of the mean of normal, or approximately 4 or 5 dB. This is not to say that defects cannot occur with a smaller variance from normal than 4 or 5 dB. Rather, it may be impossible to know whether such smaller differences are abnormal or not.

In threshold-related testing (Fig. 9-6) if the patient is presented with a stimulus that is roughly 4 dB brighter than the expected normal level for that retinal position and the patient sees it, the location is considered normal, and the stimulus is moved to the next position without measuring the threshold of the location precisely.

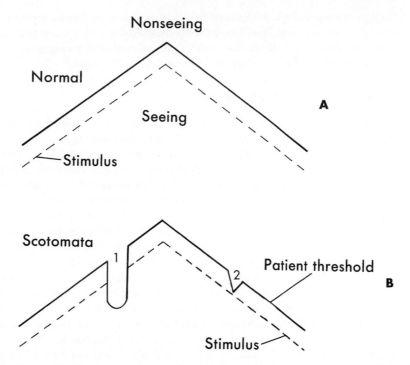

Figure 9-6   Threshold-related testing. **A,** A single stimulus usually 4 or 5 dB brighter than the anticipated threshold is exposed across the visual field. If the patient sees it, that part of the field is considered normal. **B,** Defect 1 will be detected by the technique, but defect 2 will be missed.

The disadvantage of this technique is that it only finds defects equal to or greater in depth than the suprathreshold stimulus used. This technique also provides no information regarding subtle variation in the contour of the field, which is important in recognizing early changes from normal.[18] The rapidity of testing normal areas using the technique, however, allows a larger area of the retina to be examined. If defects are detected, they can be quantified with the full-thresholding strategy.

Zone Testing

Zone testing uses three levels, or zones, of stimulus intensity to locate and then quantify defects. The first zone is a suprathreshold stimulus 4 or 5 dB brighter than the anticipated normal threshold as described in the section on threshold-related testing. If the patient sees this stimulus, the response is recorded as normal. If the patient fails to see the initial stimulus, a maximally bright stimulus is shown. If the patient sees this stimulus (but failed to see the initial, relatively dim, stimulus), the machine indicates a relative defect. If the patient fails to see either stimulus, the machine records an absolute defect. Responses can thus be grouped in three zones—normal, relative defect, or absolute defect. There are multiple variations on this theme that allow a greater number of zones to be defined, or for zones to be defined at different levels. The obvious disadvantage of this technique is that subsequent testing can only recognize major change because the difference between the test stimuli is great. The advantage is that it is fast.

Screening Tests

Screening tests for visual field defects are available by manual perimetry and with most computerized perimeters. Unfortunately, they only detect rather large changes in the visual field.[19-21] Most screening programs use a technique that recognizes defects that are greater than 4 or 5 dB below an expected level. As such, they may not detect early glaucomatous defects. Also, if a defect is found, the patient must undergo a full visual field examination to establish a baseline against which future change can be measured. Therefore in persons suspected of having visual field defects, screening programs and other fast strategies that reduce examination time at the expense of evaluating the critical sensitivity area within 5 dB of threshold are of questionable value.[17]

Other Static Testing Techniques

Single-stimulus level static testing was used commonly in some of the early computerized perimeters. Because the visual threshold slopes from the center to the periphery of vision, a single-stimulus intensity cannot be effective in testing a large area of the retina. This technique is useful only as a relatively crude screening method. A variety of innovative screening techniques has been developed to aid clinicians in obtaining the maximum amount of useful information in the minimum amount of time. A few of these bear mention for illustrative purposes.

Snowfield, or noisefield, perimetry is performed by having the patient observe a computer screen (Fig. 9-7) or home television set.[22-24] The screen projects a "noise" pattern of small (roughly 1 to 4 mm), irregularly shaped dark and bright spots oscillating at 50 Hz. Patients with localized defects notice the defective region as a smudge or blank area on the screen. In simple terms, they detect the noise pattern in normal regions of the field, and its absence in the abnormal areas is perceivable. Detection takes only seconds in alert patients, but not all patients can cooperate fully with the test requirements. The information gained is useful mainly for screening.[25,26] Optokinetic perimetry is a novel approach to visual field screening in which the patient is presented a series of cards with static stimuli arranged in a set pattern. While maintaining steady fixation, the patient is asked how many spots she sees.[27-29] Stimuli in defective areas of the field are not detected, and by evaluating the points missed during the test, the examiner can gain a fairly clear idea of the nature and extent of the field loss.[30-33] This method is very fast, taking perhaps only 30% to 50% of the total time needed for screening fields conventionally.

The Future of Visual Field Testing

The current generation of computerized perimeters allows placement of stimuli of varying sizes, intensities, and colors into backgrounds of varying intensities, and they accurately chart the patient's responses. This flexibility facilitates design of an almost infinite number of testing protocols. Recent improvements have involved both hardware and software. A wide variety of test and interpretation protocols are in use, and more are being developed continually. Most commercially available protocols have been standardized against groups of normal patients, and a few disease-specific protocols have been standardized against groups of patients with the target condition.[4,34-38] Although

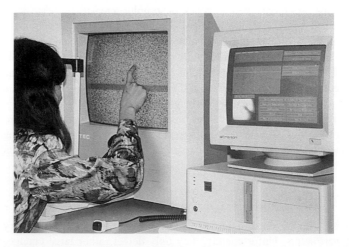

Figure 9-7   Patient viewing "snowfield" on computer monitor. Defects are noticed by the patient as smudges or fuzzy areas on screen.

these programs do not fully replace careful interpretation by a trained observer, they certainly help to guide us toward more consistent evaluation of visual field information. Some programs, such as the Swedish Interactive Testing Algorithm from Humphrey Systems, allow the machine to adjust the testing algorithm in real time to shorten the test.

Differential light sensitivity is a rather primitive retinal function. Quigley and Green found that up to 50% of retinal nerve fibers may be lost before a diagnostic glaucomatous visual field defect is detected by manual kinetic measurement.[39] Computerized static perimetry with statistical analysis of the results is more sensitive,[40] but some amount of nerve fiber loss precedes even computerized field loss in most cases.[41] These lost nerve fibers assist in other visual functions that may be more sophisticated than simple differential light sensitivity. One of the more intriguing ways that this has been investigated recently is with *blue-on-yellow,* or *short wavelength, automated perimetry* (SWAP). A series of studies have indicated that the short wavelength-sensitive (blue) system may be more sensitive to early glaucoma.[42-44] The test is similar to conventional perimetry except blue stimuli are projected on a yellow background to isolate the short wavelength-sensitive system. The results of these studies have been quite interesting. In one study, Johnson and co-workers[45] tested 38 ocular hypertensive patients and 62 normal controls with conventional white-on-white (w/w) perimetry and subsequently with SWAP (see also p. 173). All 38 ocular hypertensive patients had normal w/w perimetry at the time the study began. Nine of these eyes had a defect detected by SWAP at the beginning of the study. Five years later, 5 of the 9 eyes that initially showed a SWAP defect but were normal by w/w perimetry had developed w/w visual field loss. The w/w defects were in the same locations of the visual field as the SWAP defects, but the SWAP defects were larger. No eye that was initially normal on SWAP testing developed w/w field loss during the period of study. Thus SWAP perimetry was very sensitive (100%) for early glaucoma; its specificity (using w/w defects as the standard) was 55% (5/9) at 5 years, but this may rise with longer follow-up.

Other studies have generated similar findings. The general pattern is that SWAP defects, although similar in location and shape, appear earlier and are larger than subsequent W/W defects.[46-49] This method is not entirely without cost, however. SWAP perimetry takes longer than equivalent W/W perimetry, and increased patient fatigue and decreased dynamic range may contribute to significantly higher fluctuation values. The increased testing time and fluctuation have limited the use of SWAP in routine clinical settings.

In addition to perimetric techniques, there are a host of other psychophysical methods of detecting and following glaucomatous damage. Some of these are discussed in Chapter 12.

COMBINED STATIC AND KINETIC PERIMETRY

Combined static and kinetic perimetry uses the speed of kinetic perimetry and the sensitivity of static testing. It is used routinely in manual perimetry, and rarely with automated perimeters. Generally, the peripheral field and scotomata are defined by kinetic methods, and the central field is examined by static perimetry. With manual perimetry, a threshold stimulus is chosen for testing the central field. This stimulus is chosen by a variety of methods, but commonly it is the weakest stimulus visible at the point either 15° above or 15° below the horizontal meridian 25° temporal to fixation.

Aulhorn and Harms,[3] Armaly,[50-52] Drance and Anderson,[18] and Rock and co-workers[53] have suggested methods using this approach to rapidly detect and define scotomata. The threshold stimulus is used to kinetically define the central field and any scotomata demonstrated by the static presentations. Static stimuli are presented at various locations for no more than 1 second. Hesitant or absent patient response indicates a potential defect, which then can be more completely analyzed by kinetic perimetry using varying stimulus sizes and intensities (Fig. 9-8).

With automated perimetry the central field is examined in the standard static fashion, and one or two peripheral isopters are examined to avoid missing defects that do not involve the central field.[54-56] The peripheral field can be examined by static threshold perimetry, but this is a time-consuming and tedious process. Full-threshold testing of the periphery costs a great deal in terms of patient fatigue and satisfaction for relatively little gain, and is therefore performed rarely. Static two- or three-zone screening tests are a reasonable compromise that allow the examiner to deemphasize but not ignore the periphery.

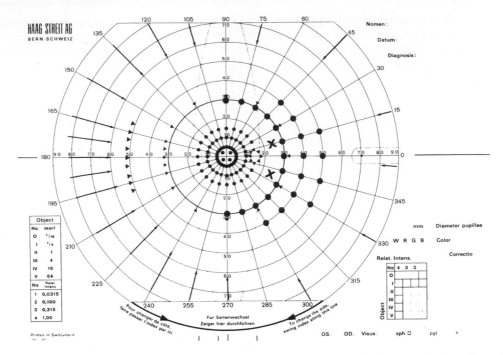

Figure 9-8   Goldmann visual field chart illustrating both static *(dots)* and kinetic *(arrows)* points of examination. Note that 72 points are tested statically with a threshold target in the central field. This is considered a reliable search for early glaucomatous field defects. The I-4-e target is used to check for nasal step in the peripheral field. Testing of the peripheral temporal field for a step will identify the occasional patient in whom this is the earliest evidence of glaucomatous damage. Tangent screen can be tested in a similar manner within the central 30° by exposing and hiding the stimulus to stimulate static perimetry.

REFERENCES

1. Harrington DO, Drake MV: *The visual fields: a textbook and atlas of clinical perimetry,* ed 6, St Louis, 1990, Mosby.
2. Hoskins HD Jr, Migliazzo C: Development of a visual field screening test using a Humphrey visual field analyzer, *Doc Ophthalmol Proc Series* 42:85, 1985.
3. Aulhorn E, Harms H: *Visual perimetry.* In Jameson D, Hurvich LM, editors: *Handbook of sensory physiology,* vol 7, New York, 1972, Springer-Verlag.
4. Zulauf M: Normal visual fields measured with Octopus program G1. I. Differential light sensitivity at individual test locations, *Graefes Arch Clin Exp Ophthalmol* 232:509, 1994.
5. Zulauf M, and others: Normal visual fields measured with Octopus program G1. II. Global visual field indices, *Graefes Arch Clin Exp Ophthalmol* 232:516, 1994.
6. Gandolfo E, and others: Effects of random presentation on kinetic threshold, *Doc Ophthalmol Proc Series* 42:539, 1985.
7. Hudson C, and others: Fatigue effects during a single session of automated static threshold perimetry, *Invest Ophthalmol Vis Sci* 35:268, 1994.
8. Wild JM, and others: Long-term follow-up of baseline learning and fatigue effects in the automated perimetry of glaucoma and ocular hypertensive patients, *Acta Ophthalmol Scand Suppl* 69:210, 1991.

9. Araujo ML, and others: Evaluation of baseline-related suprathreshold testing for quick determination of visual field non-progression, *Arch Ophthalmol* 111:365, 1993.
10. Flanagan JG, and others: Evaluation of FASTPAC, a new strategy for threshold estimation with the Humphrey Field Analyzer, in a glaucomatous population, *Ophthalmology* 100:949, 1991.
11. Vivell PM, and others: [Comparative study of various perimetry strategies], *Fortschr Ophthalmol* 88:819, 1991.
12. Zeyen TG, and others: Priority of test locations for automated perimetry in glaucoma, *Ophthalmology* 100:518, 1993.
13. Fingeret M: Clinical alternative for reducing the time needed to perform automated threshold perimetry, *J Am Optom Assoc* 66:699, 1995.
14. Nordmann JP, and others: Static threshold visual field in glaucoma with the Fastpac algorithm of the Humphrey Field Analyzer: is the gain in examination time offset by any loss of information? *Eur J Ophthalmol* 4:105, 1994.
15. Schaumberger M, and others: Glaucomatous visual fields: FASTPAC versus full threshold strategy of the Humphrey Field Analyzer, *Invest Ophthalmol Vis Sci* 36:1390, 1995.

16. Young IM, and others: Comparison between Fastpac and conventional Humphrey perimetry, *Aust N Z J Ophthalmol* 22:95, 1994.
17. Gloor BP, Simitrakos SA, Rabineau PA: *Long-term follow-up of glaucomatous fields by computerized (Octopus) perimetry.* In Krieglstein GK, editor: *Glaucoma update III,* Berlin, 1987, Springer-Verlag.
18. Drance SM, Anderson DR: *Automatic perimetry in glaucoma: a practical guide,* New York, 1985, Grune & Stratton.
19. Hong C, and others: Detection of glaucomatous visual field defect using a screening program of Humphrey Field Analyzer, *Korean J Ophthalmol* 4:23, 1990.
20. Marraffa M, and others: Comparison of different screening methods for the detection of visual field defect in early glaucoma, *Int Ophthalmol* 13:43, 1989.
21. Sponsel WE, and others: Prevent Blindness America visual field screening study. The Prevent Blindness America Glaucoma Advisory Committee, *Am J Ophthalmol* 120:699, 1995.
22. Aulhorn E, Kost G: [White noise field campimetry: a new form of perimetric examination], *Klin Mbl Augenheilk* 192:284, 1988.
23. Shirato S, and others: Subjective detection of visual field defects using home TV set, *Jpn J Ophthalmol* 35:273, 1991.

24. Schiefer U, Stercken-Sorrenti G: [A new white-noise campimeter], *Klin Mbl Augenheilk* 202:60, 1993.

25. Adachi M, Shirato S: The usefulness of the noise-field test as a screening method for visual field defects, *Jpn J Ophthalmol* 38:392, 1994.

26. Kolb M, and others: Scotoma perception in white-noise-field campimetry and post-chiasmal visual pathway lesions, *Ger J Ophthalmol* 4:228, 1995.

27. Clark BJ, and others: Oculokinetic perimetry for the assessment of visual fields, *Arch Dis Child* 65:432, 1990.

28. Damato BE, and others: The detection of glaucomatous visual field defects by oculo-kinetic perimetry: which points are best for screening, *Eye* 3:727, 1989.

29. Damato BE, and others: A hand-held OKP chart for the screening of glaucoma: preliminary evaluation, *Eye* 4:632, 1990.

30. Felius J, and others: Oculokinetic perimetry compared with standard perimetric threshold testing, *Int Ophthalmol* 16:221, 1992.

31. Greve M, Chisholm IA: Comparison of the oculokinetic perimetry glaucoma screener with two types of visual field analyzer, *Can J Ophthalmol* 28:201, 1993.

32. Vernon SA, Quigley HA: Improving the sensitivity of the OKP visual field screening test with the use of neutral density filters, *Eye* 8:406, 1994.

33. Wishart PK: Oculokinetic perimetry compared with Humphrey visual field analysis in the detection of glaucomatous visual field loss, *Eye* 7:113, 1993.

34. Asman P, Heijl A: Glaucoma hemifield test: automated visual field evaluation, *Arch Ophthalmol* 110:812, 1992.

35. Funkhouser A, and others: A comparison of five methods for estimating general glaucomatous visual field depression, *Graefes Arch Clin Exp Ophthalmol* 230:101, 1992.

36. Kaufmann H, and others: Evaluation of visual fields by ophthalmologists and by OCTOSMART program, *Ophthalmologica* 201:104, 1990.

37. Morgan RK, and others: Statpac 2 glaucoma change probability, *Arch Ophthalmol* 109:1690, 1991.

38. Smith SD, and others: Analysis of progressive change in automated visual fields in glaucoma, *Invest Ophthalmol Vis Sci* 37:1419, 1996.

39. Quigley HA, Green WR: The histology of human glaucoma cupping and nerve damage: clinicopathologic correlation in 21 eyes, *Ophthalmology* 10:1803, 1979.

40. Katz J, and others: Automated perimetry detects visual field loss before manual Goldmann perimetry, *Ophthalmology* 102:21, 1995.

41. Sommer A, and others: Clinically detectable nerve fiber atrophy precedes the onset of glaucomatous field loss, *Arch Ophthalmol* 109:77, 1991.

42. Bielik M, and others: PERG and spectral sensitivity in ocular hypertensive and chronic open-angle glaucoma patients, *Graefes Arch Clin Exp Ophthalmol* 229:401, 1991.

43. Heron G, and others: Foveal and non-foveal measures of short wavelength sensitive pathways in glaucoma and ocular hypertension, *Ophthalmic Physiol Opt* 7:403, 1987.

44. Heron G, and others: Central visual fields for short wavelength sensitive pathways in glaucoma and ocular hypertension, *Invest Ophthalmol Vis Sci* 29:64, 1988.

45. Johnson CA, and others: Progression of early glaucomatous visual field loss as detected by blue-on-yellow and standard white-on-white automated perimetry, *Arch Ophthalmol* 111:651, 1993.

46. Felius J, and others: Functional characteristics of blue-on-yellow perimetric thresholds in glaucoma, *Invest Ophthalmol Vis Sci* 36:1665, 1995.

47. Johnson CA, and others: Blue-on-yellow perimetry can predict the development of glaucomatous visual field loss, *Arch Ophthalmol* 111:645, 1993.

48. Johnson CA, and others: Short-wavelength automated perimetry in low-, medium-, and high-risk ocular hypertensive eyes: initial baseline results, *Arch Ophthalmol* 113:70, 1995.

49. Sample PA, and others: Color perimetry for assessment of primary open-angle glaucoma, *Invest Ophthalmol Vis Sci* 31:1869, 1990.

50. Armaly MF: Ocular pressure and visual fields: a ten-year follow-up study, *Arch Ophthalmol* 81:25, 1969.

51. Armaly MF: Selective perimetry for glaucomatous defects in ocular hypertension, *Arch Ophthalmol* 87:518, 1972.

52. Armaly MF: Visual field defects in early open-angle glaucoma, *Trans Am Ophthalmol Soc* 69:147, 1971.

53. Rock WJ, Drance SM, Morgan RW: Visual field screening in glaucoma: an evaluation of the Armaly technique for screening glaucomatous visual fields, *Arch Ophthalmol* 89:218, 1973.

54. Ballon BJ, and others: Peripheral visual field testing in glaucoma by automated kinetic perimetry with the Humphrey Field Analyzer, *Arch Ophthalmol* 110:1730, 1992.

55. Miller KN, and others: Automated kinetic perimetry with two peripheral isopters in glaucoma, *Arch Ophthalmol* 107:1316, 1989.

56. Stewart WC, and others: Peripheral visual field testing by automated kinetic perimetry in glaucoma, *Arch Ophthalmol* 106:202, 1988.

10

Techniques and Variables in Visual Field Testing

A number of factors can affect a visual field test[1-16] other than the disease being studied. It is important to minimize the influence of these variables as completely as possible in order to accurately assess and precisely document the abnormalities present so that deviations from normal and future changes can be recognized easily. Fluctuation, the combination of normal physiologic variability and measurement error, complicates the recognition of pathologic change. If all other possible variables are eliminated, then change in the disease must be responsible for any alteration in the visual field. Unfortunately it is impossible to eliminate all other variables. Awareness of factors influencing the visual field, however, can help minimize these variables and improve interpretation (Box 10-1).

PATIENT VARIABLES

Age

With age, the visual field has a linear decrease in sensitivity and the slope steepens.[13,17,18] The increase in fluctuation that occurs as the test moves toward the periphery is also greater with age. The combined effect of these variables is a field with an increasingly steep slope as one moves away from fixation. The effect of age on the central field is gradual and can usually be ignored in the evaluation of individual patients. Mean sensitivity of the visual field decreases approximately 0.58 to 1.0 dB per decade.[9] Increased age may be associated with increased variability in repeated test results over time. The standard deviation of the mean sensitivity of points tested ranges from about 1.0 to 2.0 dB in the normal central field of a young patient. Patients older than 60 years of age may have standard deviations up to twice that amount centrally and up to 10 dB per point at 30° eccentricity.*

Fixation

Most patients maintain acceptable fixation on the central target of the perimeter.[20-22] Patients with poor fixation can be encouraged to stabilize their fixation, but this does not always prevent them from looking around.[23] Technicians and computerized systems usually monitor or grade patient fixation in some way. Machines that monitor fixation continuously, generally by some form of eye movement or pupillary reflex assessment, often have algorithms that disregard responses generated during fixation losses. These machines return to the same test location later during the examination and present the stimulus again. The intention of this programming is to ensure that all responses recorded by the machine occur during periods of steady fixation. Other machines use a monitoring system with a blind spot fixation in which stimuli are projected on the physiologic blind spot at intervals throughout the test. If fixation is steady these stimuli will continue to land on the blind spot and will not be detected. If fixation has shifted the stimuli will land on photoreceptors and be detected. The machine records and/or alerts the operator that a fixation loss has occurred. If the patient

*Refs: 2, 4, 5, 13, 14, 16, 18, 19.

Box 10-1
Some Artifacts That Affect Visual Field Results

Examination Artifacts

Technician: results vary with different technicians
Equipment: results vary with different equipment
Test: results vary with different types of tests
Software: results vary with different testing or interpretation algorithms

Eye Artifacts

Refraction: should have distance prescription with proper addition for near vision
Pupil size: should be 3 mm or more; must be consistent
Fixation: results vary with quality of fixation control
Media opacity: visual acuity should be recorded

Patient Artifacts

Misunderstanding the test
Fatigue
Inattentiveness
Physiologic/pathologic/psychologic/mental status
Systemic illness, hangover, anxiety, and so on

Analysis Artifacts

Is the visual field normal? Requires standards for normal
Has the visual field changed? Requires knowledge of fluctuation
Misinterpretation

---

generates fixation losses more than 20% to 30% of the time the test can be considered only an approximation of the true visual field.[24,25]

Reliability

In addition to monitoring fixation, patient reliability should be graded as good or poor by the technician. Computerized machines can provide some index of reliability based on false-positive or false-negative responses and fixation losses.[26] Fatigue, drugs, age, and illness can all affect patient reliability and must be considered when assessing the accuracy of a given test.

Patient variability is usually reduced with repeated testing (learning curve).[27,28] Thus the first visual field may be the least accurate. Patients with experience on manual perimeters may have less of a learning curve effect.[29] We tend to repeat the initial test if the results are abnormal in any way. Although computerized machines are automated, they are not automatic. Patient/technician interaction can have a substantial impact on the reliability of the examination and may also aid in patient satisfaction.

OCULAR VARIABLES
Pupil Size

A pupillary diameter of less than 3 mm can cause generalized depression of the visual field.[30] It is usually best to test the field with a pupil that is at least 3 mm in diameter. If it is not possible to dilate the pupil to 3 mm the test should be performed with a pupil that is no smaller than that which existed during previous tests.[31,32]

Media Clarity

Any opacity of the ocular media can cause a localized or generalized depression in the visual field. This is particularly problematic when following a glaucoma patient who is developing cataracts. As

RIGHT   C30-2

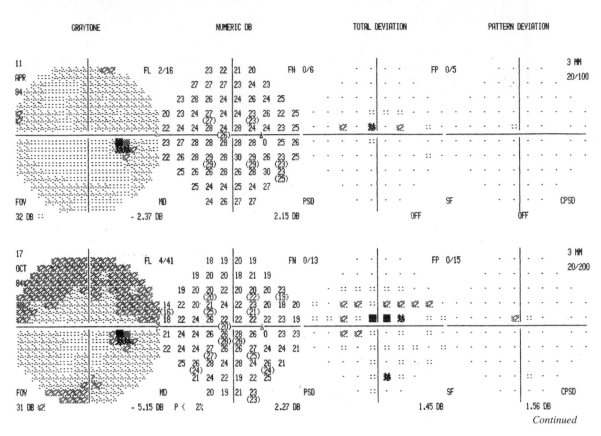

Figure 10-1   Developing cataract in a glaucoma patient. Note the increasing depression of the visual field in the left grey-scale printout and in the total deviation graphic presentation *(third from the left)*. The pattern deviation that is presented in the *far right column* shows little change over time. Cataract extraction with intraocular lens implantation was performed prior to the last field test. Note that the generalized depression and the total deviation have reversed while the pattern deviation remains similar. This methodology allows improved ability to follow glaucoma patients in the presence of developing cataracts.

the lens opacity become denser, field defects may appear to enlarge or become denser because of the reduced amount of light reaching the retina or because of image distortion or light scattering.[33,34] Patterns of localized loss tend to remain consistent before and after cataract extraction, however.[35] Visual acuity, refraction, and the appearance of the lens can help in determining the influence of cataract on the field. If acuity has dropped by more than one line on the Snellen chart, the examiner should suspect that the cataract is accentuating the appearance of visual field defects. Some analysis programs compensate for this reduction by removing generalized depression from the visual field so that scotomata are exposed (Fig. 10-1).

Refractive Correction

Proper refraction with appropriate correction for presbyopia and patient age are required for accurate testing. In one series of experiments overcorrection of +1.00 D in the sphere reduced mean sensitivity 3.6 + 0.8 dB, and overcorrection of +2.00 D caused a reduction of 5.3 + 0.9 dB.[36,37] Another study found a decrease in threshold sensitivity as high as 7.6 dB with +6.00 D overcorrection.[38]

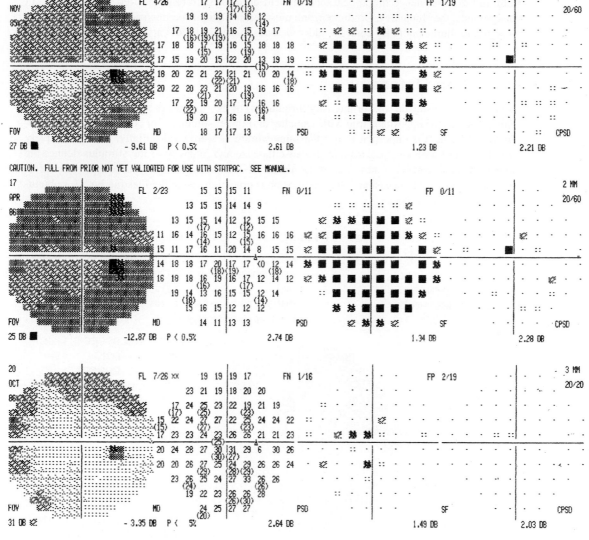

Figure 10-1, cont'd For legend see opposite page.

TESTING VARIABLES

Technician

It is virtually impossible for two technicians to administer a manual visual field examination in precisely the same manner. Even the same technician varies his or her technique from one examination to another. Thus to accurately interpret visual fields the interpreter must be familiar with the skills and variations of the technician performing the tests. The technician can improve patient performance by monitoring it consistently during the examination, but this has few advantages over intermittent monitoring following a brief introductory orientation.[39] Computerized perimetry has a great advantage over manual perimetry because it allows repeated performance of a standardized test.

Background Illumination

The level of background illumination affects the contour of the hill of vision and thus the appearance of the visual field. Brighter background illumination increases the slope of the central field and may influence the appearance of field defects. Different perimeters have different backgrounds; the Humphrey, Goldmann, and most recent Octopus perimeters use 31.5 apostilbs of background illumination. By contrast, older Octopus machines used 4 apostilbs of background illumination.

Stimulus Size and Intensity

Obviously, increasing the size or intensity (brightness) of the stimulus projects more light onto the retina, whereas the opposite is true with a smaller or dimmer stimulus. For comparison with previous visual fields it is important to use the same stimuli as were used initially. This is relatively straightforward with kinetic perimetry because the size and intensity of the stimulus defines the isopter. Mistakes can occur, however, if the technician uses the same color ink to represent different isopters on various occasions. Standardization is crucial in visual field testing both for obtaining and recording results.

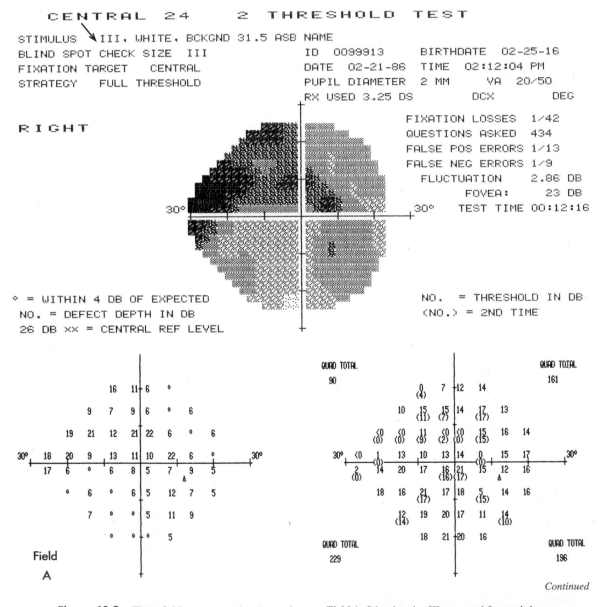

Field A

Continued

Figure 10-2   These field tests were taken 1 month apart. **Field A,** Stimulus size III was used first and shows a dense arcuate defect superonasally. **Field B,** Stimulus size V shows a subtle field defect superonasally in the grey scale. Care must be taken not to be misled by the change in stimulus size when interpreting a field change.

Static automated perimetry produces reports that resemble each other superficially regardless of the stimulus size used during the test. A change in stimulus size can produce a different test result, however. The authors use a Goldmann size III stimulus for virtually all conventional automated perimetric testing. The small benefit gained by using nonstandard testing parameters is rarely worth the risk of forgetting to reset the machine to standard parameters before administering the next test. If an apparent large change occurs between tests, however, the examiner should check the stimulus used in order to ensure that identical parameters were employed (Fig. 10-2).

Stimulus Exposure Time

Temporal summation, the ability of the visual apparatus to accumulate information over time, can influence visual field testing for stimulus exposure times less than 0.5 seconds (Fig. 10-3). Most manual perimetry is performed with exposure times of approximately 1 second, so temporal summation has little influence. The computerized Octopus perimeter has a stimulus exposure time of 0.1

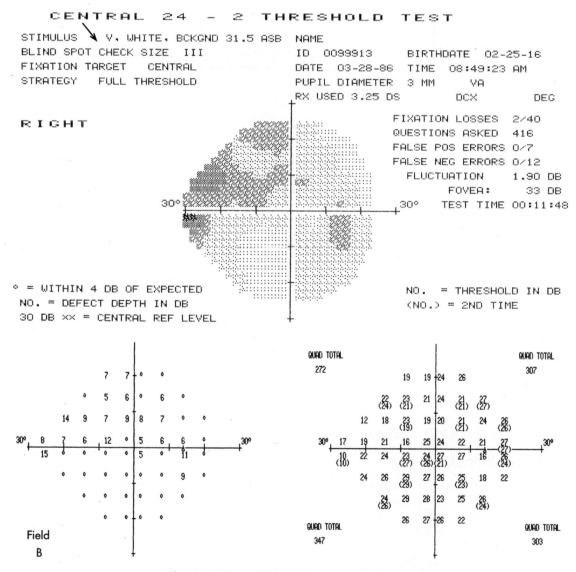

Figure 10-2, cont'd For legend see opposite page.

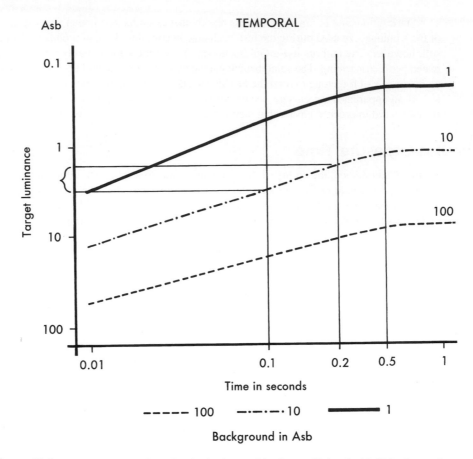

Figure 10-3 Temporal summation related to background luminance. Using the 10-dB background curve, approximately a 3-dB increase ({) can be anticipated by increasing stimulus exposure time from 0.1 to 0.2 seconds. (Modified from Aulhorn E, Harms H: In Jameson D, Hurvich LM: editors: *Handbook of sensory physiology,* vol 7, New York, 1972, Springer-Verlag.)

second, whereas the Humphrey Field Analyzer uses twice that time. This may contribute to the fact that patients see slightly dimmer stimuli with the Humphrey machine.[10,40]

Area Tested

To compare visual field charts, the same region of the visual field must be tested during serial examinations (Fig. 10-4). For most purposes tests that examine alongside vertical and horizontal meridians are more useful than are tests that examine on the meridian (the latter are rarely used today).

EQUIPMENT AND TECHNIQUES

General Principles

Regardless of the equipment used, there are certain fundamental requirements for accurate visual field testing. Accurate distance refraction, with the appropriate addition for the distance from patient to stimulus, should be used. Because accommodative capacity varies with age, the amount of addition should be adjusted for the patient's age and the instrument used (Table 10-1).

In kinetic perimetry the rate of motion of the test object should be constant within a given test and for subsequent field examinations. Two degrees per second is conventional. The test object should be moved from the nonseeing area of the visual field to the seeing area. Most important, however, is that the same technique be used each time.

Constant fixation is necessary to obtain reliable visual fields. The visual field is mapped accu-

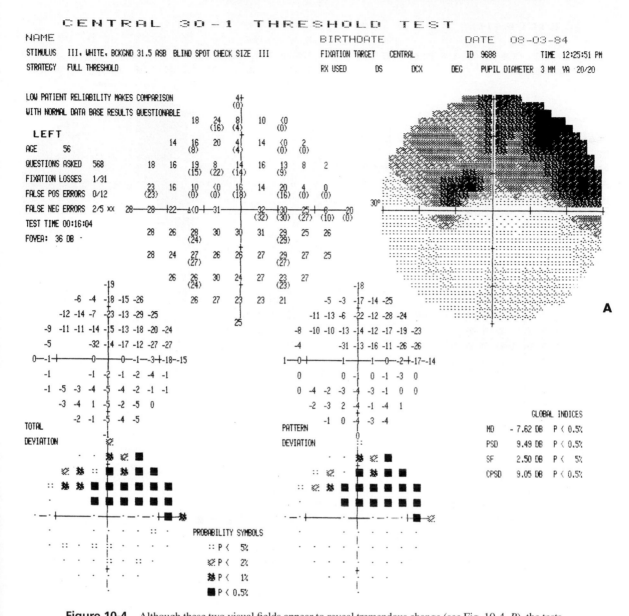

Figure 10-4   Although these two visual fields appear to reveal tremendous change (see Fig. 10-4, *B*), the tests were performed on the same day. **A,** The 30-1 visual field positions the spot on the horizontal and vertical midlines and then positions subsequent spots 6° off these midlines. *Continued*

Table 10-1

Addition for Near, Bowl Perimetry

Age	Octopus, Model 500	Octopus, Model 201	Humphrey Analyzers	Goldmann Perimeter
30-39	Plano	Plano	+1.00	+0.50
40-44	+1.00	+0.50	+1.50	+1.00
45-49	+1.25	+1.00	+2.00	+1.50
50-54	+1.75	+2.00	+2.50	+2.25
55-59	+2.00	+2.00	+3.00	+3.00
>59	+2.00	+2.00	+3.00	+3.50

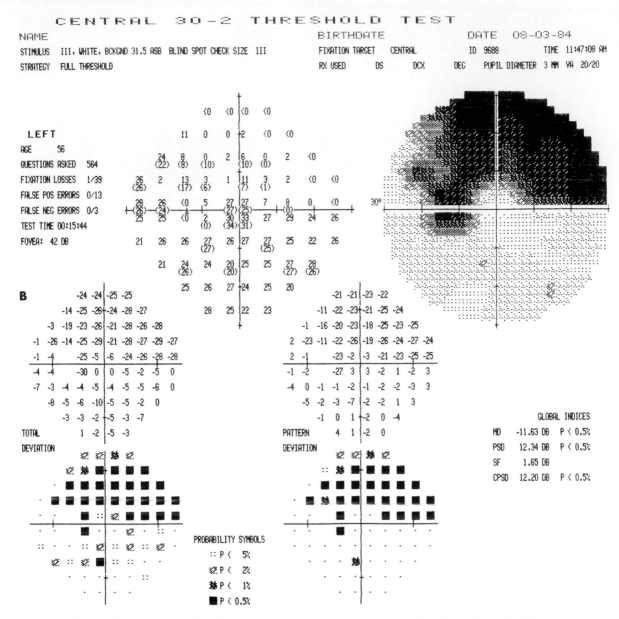

Figure 10-4, cont'd   **B,** The 30-2 program positions the spots 3° to either side of the midlines. The 30-2 program is better for recognizing change along midlines such as those that occur in patients with glaucoma and neurologic deficits.

rately only if the patient looks steadily at the central fixation target. Some assessment of the patient's fixation should be recorded on the field chart, and the patient should be gently encouraged throughout the test to look at the fixation target.

For valid comparison of visual fields, follow-up field examinations should use the same stimulus sizes and intensities for kinetic perimetry; the stimulus size and testing strategy should be duplicated for sequential static examinations. Other variables such as pupil size, technician, visual acuity, and testing equipment should be standardized as much as possible to reduce artifactual field fluctuations and to facilitate recognition of true pathologic change.

Tangent Screen

The tangent screen may be used at 1 or 2 meters.[41] It should be large enough to allow testing of the full 30° of the central field at whichever distance is chosen and should have a uniform illumination of 7 foot-candles. Examiners can use the tangent screen for either kinetic or static testing. For sta-

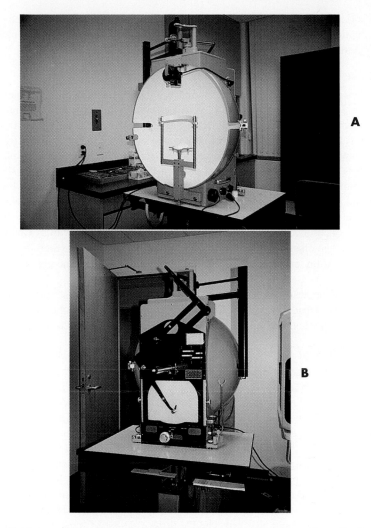

Figure 10-5 Goldmann perimeter for visual field examination as viewed from the patient's side (**A**) and the examiner's side (**B**).

tic testing the test object is placed on the side of the test wand so that it can be obscured by being rotated out of view. The wand should be covered by black felt material similar in composition to the tangent screen so that the wand itself is largely unseen during the test.[42] While the patient maintains steady fixation the wand is moved to the area of interest and the target is quickly rotated in and out of view. The patient responds to the on/off presentation.

The smallest test object the patient can see consistently just temporal to the blind spot is used for testing the central field. For a 1-meter test distance this is usually a white test object that is 1 mm in diameter.

Fixation can be tested repeatedly by concealing and exposing the test object in the blind spot area. If the patient sees it, fixation has shifted. The test strategy is the same as that used for the central 30° of the visual field during Goldmann perimetry.

Bowl Perimetry

Goldmann developed the first bowl perimeter that provided standardized background and stimulus intensity. He improved fixation monitoring by allowing the technician to see the patient's eye through a telescope. He also provided a system for simplified test recording and facilitated reproducible test object positioning and movement. The perimeter that bears his name is the standard for manual bowl perimetry (Fig. 10-5). Many of its features have been incorporated into computerized visual field machines.

Using the light meter provided, the machine should be calibrated each day before the initial examination. The maximum stimulus, V4e, should be 1000 apostilbs; the background, or bowl, illumination should match the V1e stimulus, equivalent to 31.5 apostilbs.

Preparing the Patient

Patient preparation for the examination is similar whether the bowl perimeter is to be used for manual or computerized testing. Refractive correction with the appropriate addition should be inserted into the lens holder for examination of the central portion of the visual field.

The patient should be comfortably seated so that his or her chin and forehead are firmly against the supports and the eye is centered in the observer's telescope or display screen. After the patient is positioned, the lens holder should be placed as close as possible to the patient's eye without touching the lashes. The eye should be centered in the lens holder. Corrective lenses should be "full-field" type with thin rims so that they do not interfere with peripheral vision. For manual machines the patient should be instructed to push the button on the patient response indicator if one is available. If not, the patient should tap the table with a coin to indicate when he or she sees the test object. Verbal responses are discouraged because they move the head and adversely affect fixation and concentration. For automated machines the patient uses the patient response button.

It is important to encourage the patient throughout the test, even if the computer is doing the testing. Most patients prefer to interact with another person rather than with a machine; reliability is increased when a technician is present during computerized perimetry.[9]

Technique of Manual Bowl (Goldmann) Perimetry (See Fig. 9-8)

Aulhorn and Harms,[40] Armaly,[43,44] Drance and co-workers,[45] and others[46] have contributed concepts that provide the basis for techniques in glaucomatous visual field testing and analysis. For the central field a test object that is just detectable at the temporal horizontal meridian at 25° eccentricity, 15° above and 15° below this point, is most useful. This threshold target is used to define the limits of the central isopter and blind spot by kinetic perimetry. Particular attention is given to the nasal and temporal meridians in looking for a step. Careful investigation of the 5°, 10°, and 15° isopters is necessary to reveal the isolated scotomata that are characteristic of early glaucoma. These three central isopters are examined by static and, if necessary, by kinetic perimetry (from nonseeing to seeing). Any paracentral field defects found with the threshold target should be checked at least twice because artifacts are possible in any subjective test. Hesitant responses (especially in the Bjerrum area) should be noted. The I2e is the established standard test stimulus for the central visual field and provides a comparison for other patients and eyes. Selected higher-intensity objects will determine the density of a defect. An I4e test object is used to test the far periphery, and a V4e stimulus will outline the maximum area of the visual field.

Technique of Computerized Bowl Perimetry

The Octopus was the first computerized visual field machine that provided enough flexibility to allow accurate detection and quantification of visual field defects. This machine uses only static testing strategies. The Humphrey and some other computerized perimeters offer a kinetic option,[47,48] but the overwhelming majority of clinical tests are performed using static techniques.

Each of these machines provides a variety of testing programs for different situations. The physician should designate the program to be used for each patient. In most practices it is appropriate to have a standard program that is used for all patients by default. If a particular patient has special needs or circumstances the physician can order a test that addresses that patient's needs. If a wide variety of tests are used routinely it is difficult to gain sufficient experience with any one test to interpret the results optimally. We have found it much better to be comfortable with a few tests we know well than to try to master the entire menu offered by the manufacturer.

In addition to perhaps dozens of standard options, computerized machines offer custom programs that allow the examiner to tailor the area tested as well as the testing algorithm. This sounds like a good feature, but using custom programs is a risky practice. Remember that the hallmark of successful serial perimetry is consistency. For a custom test to be useful in the future it must be duplicated exactly on subsequent examinations. It is not practical in most busy clinics and practices to take the time to reprogram the machine before each test. It is also difficult to remember to do this for the occasional patient.

For glaucoma testing, most visual field defects are located in the central 30° of the visual field (Fig. 10-6). The Octopus G-1 and Humphrey 30-2 or 24-2 are the most popular current glaucoma programs on these respective machines. These and similar programs on the Dicon and other machines test the central 24° to 30° with test points that are 3° to 6° apart. The number of points tested varies but is roughly 60 to 70 depending on the program. In each case the test grid is chosen to gather sufficient information without tiring the patient excessively. For the most part there is a direct relationship between the amount of time spent testing and the amount of information obtained. Patient fatigue leads to errors that may be clinically significant, however, and there is a point of diminishing returns with automated perimetric tests.[49,51] Several programs allow the machine or the examiner to shorten the test if certain parameters are met (indicating that further testing is unlikely to improve the quality of the result or change the ultimate interpretation). For example, the patient may be a young adult with no obvious pathology and a previously normal baseline examination. Rechecking a representative sample of the previous test points may be enough to reassure the examiner that no change has occurred. The most sophisticated programs, like the Humphrey Swedish Interactive Thresholding Algorithm program, spend more time testing suspicious areas of the field and less time on normal or clearly defective areas.

Defects that approach fixation are especially worrisome and can be plotted within 1.0° or 1.5° accuracy using macular programs. Central fields can also be plotted using the Goldmann or tangent screen perimeter in glaucoma patients who have only one central island remaining. Full-field automated tests are very time-consuming and discouraging for these patients, and they do not provide enough information to warrant the time and aggravation they cause.

Glaucomatous defects may occur solely in the peripheral visual field. This is rare, however, and probably occurs in 0% to 8% of cases depending on the examination technique.[52-59] Many of the computerized perimeters supply a separate program that carefully examines the nasal area to detect most isolated peripheral defects. Other machines have screening programs that test the periphery. If the periphery is tested, the lens holder and lens should be removed from in front of the eye.

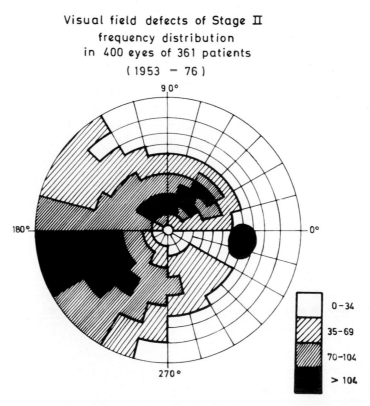

Figure 10-6 Frequency distribution of the location of early glaucomatous visual field defects found in 400 eyes of 361 patients. (From Aulhorn E: In Krieglstein GK, Leydecker W, editors: *Glaucoma update,* Berlin, 1979, Springer-Verlag.)

The constant dilemma facing physicians with computerized perimeters is matching a patient's ability with the program(s) to be used.[60] Younger, more vigorous patients can tolerate longer tests. Most people are fatigued after 20 minutes of consecutive testing and need a rest. The machine never gets tired and is capable of testing the visual field in minute detail. Patient reliability decreases, however, with increasing fatigue. The physician must select the appropriate tests to obtain the most accurate information for each patient. Most patients can tolerate a full-threshold visual field that measures the central 30° visual field (Fig. 10-7); subsequent testing can be used to recognize change. Depending on the results of the initial test, follow-up visual field tests may be performed with a program that tests only the central 24°. This allows speedier testing, although the ability to recognize early change may be reduced in rare cases.[61] In addition to employing time-saving steps such as faster pacing when appropriate, software programs that allow the machine to interact with the patient and modify the test based on a real-time evaluation of the patient's responses allow faster testing without sacrificing sensitivity or accuracy.

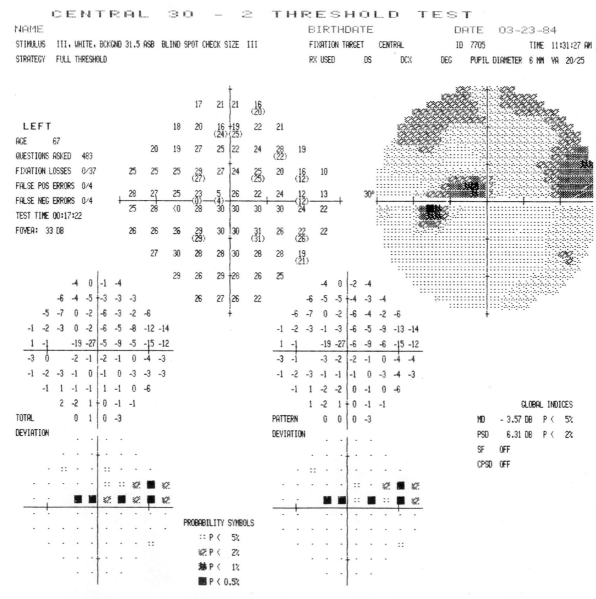

Figure 10-7 The grey scale *(upper right)* indicates depression superiorly, just above the macula, and in the upper nasal aspect of the field. The total deviation plot *(lower left)* shows the significance of this deviation compared with a normal population of this patient's age. The pattern deviation *(lower right)* subtracts generalized depression, of which there is very little in this patient, leaving the scotomatous defect obvious.

REFERENCES

1. Anderson DR: *Testing the field of vision,* St Louis, 1982, Mosby.
2. Bebie H, Fankhauser F, Spahr J: Static perimetry: accuracy and fluctuations, *Acta Ophthalmol* 54:339, 1976.
3. Flammer J, and others: JO and STATJO: programs for investigating the visual field with the Octopus automatic perimeter, *Can J Ophthalmol* 18:115, 1983.
4. Flammer J, Drance SM, Schulzer M: The estimation and testing of the components of long-term fluctuation of the differential light threshold, *Doc Ophthalmol* 35:383, 1983.
5. Flammer J, and others: Differential light threshold in automated static perimetry: factors influencing short-term fluctuation, *Arch Ophthalmol* 102:876, 1984.
6. Flammer J, and others: Differential light threshold: short- and long-term fluctuation in patients with glaucoma, normal controls, and patients with suspected glaucoma, *Arch Ophthalmol* 102:704, 1984.
7. Flammer J, and others: Quantification of glaucomatous visual field defects with automated perimetry, *Invest Ophthalmol Vis Sci* 26:176, 1985.
8. Flammer J, and others: The Octopus glaucoma G-1 program, *Glaucoma* 9:67, 1987.
9. Greve EL, Bakker D, van den Berg TJTP: Physiological factors in computer-assisted perimetry: automatic and semi-automatic perimetry, *Doc Ophthalmol* 42:137, 1985.
10. Hoskins HD Jr, Migliazzo D: Development of a visual field screening test using a Humphrey visual field analyzer, *Doc Ophthalmol* 42:85, 1985.
11. Jaffee GJ, Alvarado JA, Juster RP: Age-related changes of the normal visual field, *Arch Ophthalmol* 104:1021, 1986.
12. Katz J, Sommer A: Asymmetry and variation in the normal hill of vision, *Arch Ophthalmol* 104:65, 1986.
13. Katz J, Sommer A: A longitudinal study of the age-adjusted variability of automated visual fields, *Arch Ophthalmol* 105:1083, 1987.
14. Parrish RK, Schiffman J, Anderson DR: Static and kinetic visual field testing: reproducibility in normal volunteers, *Arch Ophthalmol* 102:1497, 1984.
15. Sommer A, Quigley HA, Robin AL; Evaluation of nerve-fiber layer assessment, *Arch Ophthalmol* 102:1766, 1984.
16. Wilensky JT, Joondeph BC: Variation in visual field measurements with an automated perimeter, *Am J Ophthalmol* 97:328, 1984.
17. Haas A, Flammer J, Schneider U: Influence of age on the visual field of normal subjects, *Am J Ophthalmol* 101:199, 1986.
18. Heijl A, Bengtsson B: The effect of perimetric experience in patients with glaucoma, *Arch Ophthalmol* 114:19, 1996.
19. Lewis RA, and others: Variability of quantitative automated perimetry in normal observers, *Ophthalmology* 93:878, 1986.
20. Eizenman M, and others: Stability of fixation in healthy subjects during automated perimetry, *Can J Ophthalmol* 27:336, 1992.
21. Johnson CA, Nelson-Quigg JM: A prospective three-year study of response properties of normal subjects and patients during automated perimetry, *Ophthalmology* 100:269, 1993.

22. Rohrschneider K, and others: Stability of fixation: results of fundus-controlled examination using the scanning laser ophthalmoscope, *Ger J Ophthalmol* 4:197, 1995.
23. Sanabria O, and others: Pseudo-loss of fixation in automated perimetry, *Ophthalmology* 98:76, 1991.
24. Katz J, Sommer A: Reliability indexes of automated perimetric tests, *Arch Ophthalmol* 106:1252, 1988.
25. Bickler-Bluth, and others: Assessing the utility of reliability indices for automated visual fields: testing ocular hypertensives, *Ophthalmology* 96:616, 1989.
26. Lee M, and others: The influence of patient reliability on visual field outcome, *Am J Ophthalmol* 117: 756, 1994.
27. Werner EB, and others: Effect of patient experience on the results of automated perimetry in glaucoma suspect patients, *Ophthalmology* 97:44, 1990.
28. Heijl A, Bengtsson B: The effect of perimetric experience in patients with glaucoma, *Arch Ophthalmol* 114:19, 1996.
29. Werner EB, and others: Effect of patient experience on the results of automated perimetry in clinically stable glaucoma patients, *Ophthalmology* 95:764, 1988.
30. McCluskey DJ, and others: The effect of pilocarpine on the visual field in normals, *Ophthalmology* 93:843, 1986.
31. Lindenmuth KA, and others: Effects of pupillary constriction on automated perimetry in normal eyes, *Ophthalmology* 96:1298, 1989.
32. Kudrna GR, and others: Pupillary dilation and its effects on automated perimetry results, *J Am Optom Assoc* 66:675, 1995.
33. Lam GL, and others: Effect of cataract on automated perimetry, *Ophthalmology* 98:1066, 1991.
34. Klein BE, and others: Visual sensitivity and age-related eye diseases: the Beaver Dam Study, *Ophthalmic Epidemiol* 3:47, 1996.
35. Budenz DL, and others: The effect of simulated cataract on the glaucomatous visual field, *Ophthalmology* 100:511, 1993.
36. Goldstick BJ, Weinreb RN: The effect of refractive error on automated global analysis program G-1, *Am J Ophthalmol* 104:229, 1987.
37. Weinreb RN, Perlman JP: The effect of refractive correction on automated perimetric thresholds, *Am J Ophthalmol* 101:706, 1986.
38. Heuer DK, and others: The influence of refraction accuracy on automated perimetric threshold measurements, *Ophthalmology* 94:1550, 1987.
39. Johnson LN, and others: Effect of intermittent versus continuous patient monitoring on reliability indices during automated perimetry, *Ophthalmology* 100:76, 1993.
40. Aulhorn E, Harms H: *Visual perimetry.* In Jameson D, Hurvich LM, editors: *Handbook of sensory physiology,* vol 7, New York, 1972, Springer-Verlag.
41. Garber N: Tangent screen perimetry (continuing education credit), *J Ophthalmic Nurs Technol* 13:69, 1995.

42. West RW: Standardization of the tangent screen examination: some neglected parameters, *Am J Optom Physiol Opt* 65:580, 1988.
43. Armaly MF: Ocular pressure and visual fields: a 10-year follow-up study, *Arch Ophthalmol* 81:25, 1969.
44. Armaly MF: Selective perimetry for glaucomatous defects in ocular hypertension, *Arch Ophthalmol* 87:518, 1972.
45. Drance SM, and others: A screening method for temporal visual defects in chronic simple glaucoma, *Can J Ophthalmol* 7:428, 1972.
46. Rock WJ, Drance SM, Morgan RW: Visual field screening in glaucoma: an evaluation of the Armaly technique for screening glaucomatous visual fields, *Arch Ophthalmol* 89:287, 1973.
47. Ballon BJ, and others: Peripheral visual field testing in glaucoma by automated kinetic perimetry with the Humphrey Field Analyzer, *Arch Ophthalmol* 110:1730, 1992.
48. Stewart WC: Static versus kinetic testing in the nasal peripheral field in patients with glaucoma, *Acta Ophthalmol (Copenh)* 70:79, 1992.
49. Marra G, Flammer J: The learning and fatigue effect in automated perimetry, *Graefes Arch Clin Exp Ophthalmol* 229:501, 1991.
50. Wild JM, and others: Long-term follow-up of baseline learning and fatigue effects in the automated perimetry of glaucoma and ocular hypertensive patients, *Acta Ophthalmol (Copenh)* 69:210, 1991.
51. Hudson C, and others: Fatigue effects during a single session of automated static threshold perimetry, *Invest Ophthalmol Vis Sci* 35:268, 1994.
52. Coughlan M, Freidmann AI: The frequency distribution of early field defects in glaucoma, *Doc Ophthalmol* 26:345, 1981.
53. Feruno F, Matsuo H: Early stage progression in glaucomatous visual field changes, *Doc Ophthalmol* 19:247, 1979.
54. Gloor BP, Vokt BA: Long-term fluctuations versus actual field loss in glaucoma patients, *Dev Ophthalmol* 12:48, 1985.
55. Heijl A, Lundqvist L: The location of earliest glaucomatous visual field defects documented by automatic perimetry, *Doc Ophthalmol* 85:153, 1983.
56. LeBlanc RP: Peripheral nasal field defects, *Doc Ophthalmol* 14:131, 1977.
57. LeBlanc RP, Lee A, Baxter M: Peripheral nasal field defects, *Doc Ophthalmol* 42:377, 1985.
58. Werner EB, Beraskow J: Peripheral nasal field defects in glaucoma, *Ophthalmology* 86:1875, 1979.
59. Werner EB, Drance SM: Early visual field disturbances in glaucoma, *Arch Ophthalmol* 95:1173, 1977.
60. Aulhorn E, Durst W, Gauger E: A new quick-test for visual field examination in glaucoma, *Doc Ophthalmol* 14:75, 1979.
61. Fingeret M: Clinical alternative for reducing the time needed to perform automated threshold perimetry, *J Am Optom Assoc* 66:699, 1995.

11

Visual Field Interpretation

GLAUCOMATOUS CHANGES IN THE VISUAL FIELD
Anatomy of Visual Field Defects

Visual field defects reflect visual pathway abnormalities, so their appearance should correlate well with the anatomic arrangement of neurons in that pathway (Fig. 11-1). Glaucomatous field damage results from damage to the intraocular portion of the optic nerve extending from the retinal ganglion cells to just posterior to the lamina cribrosa.

Types of Visual Field Loss

Generalized Loss

Generalized, or diffuse, visual field loss is thought to be caused by a diffuse loss of axons, whereas localized defects result from loss or damage to a contiguous group of axons. The early visual field investigators recognized that generalized constriction, enlargement of the blind spot, and diminished night vision were all seen in early glaucoma. Unfortunately, these same findings occur with age and with other nonspecific forms of visual field loss. Previously it was impossible to quantify these changes precisely enough to define normal limits and recognize variations from those limits. This was because isopter plotting with manual Goldmann kinetic perimetry has inherent variability that makes it difficult to distinguish or quantitate mild generalized loss. The quantitative measurements made by static automated perimetry, however, are ideally suited to comparisons between a patient and his or her age-matched normal. Thus we are better able to recognize and quantify diffuse visual field loss (Fig. 11-2).

Localized Defects (Scotomata)

Scotomata, or localized depressions of the visual field, are more easily recognized than are generalized depressions because the normal neighboring field makes the defect stand out. The margins or walls of the defect may be steep or sloping. Scotomata are also described as *absolute* or *relative*.[1] In an absolute scotoma the brightest stimulus of the machine is not perceived. In a relative scotoma the brightest stimulus is visible, but dimmer stimuli are not.

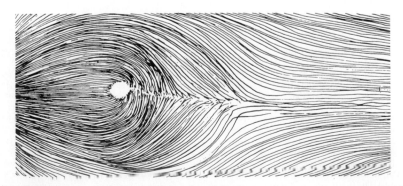

Figure 11 1 Pattern of the nerve fiber layer shown in a drawing of the region of the temporal raphe that has been reconstructed from low-power photographs. (From Vrabee F: *Am J Ophthalmol* 62:926, 1966.)

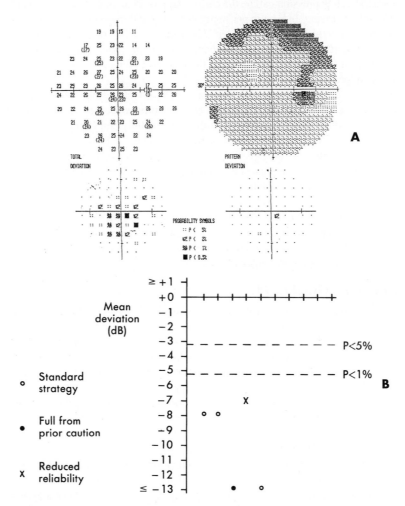

Figure 11-2 **A,** Computerized perimeters have their greatest value in having a normal database against which individual patients' results can be compared. In this figure the grey scale indicates a superior visual field loss. The total deviation plot *(lower left),* however, indicates central visual field depression as compared with normal eyes. The pattern deviation *(lower right)* indicates only a single spot adjacent to fixation that is reduced below normal. The pattern deviation has subtracted the general depression that is present to expose any scotomatous defect that may be deeper than the general depression. This patient actually does not have glaucoma but rather a cataract is causing this central depression. The superior field slopes more precipitously than does the inferior field, causing the grey scale to appear more depressed in that area. This does not necessarily represent pathology. The deviation plots indicate decreasing probability that a spot may be normal by increasing the density of the symbol. A totally black square has a probability of being normal of less than 0.5%. **B,** This graph, taken from a Humphrey STATPAC printout, indicates how a patient's visual fields compare with normal data. The horizontal line at the zero point represents a normal mean sensitivity level. Negative numbers extending down from that point indicate a mean decibel shift below normal. As can be seen, a mean deficit of slightly more than 3 dB occurs in less than 5% of normal eyes, whereas a mean deficit of slightly more than 5 dB occurs in less than 1% of normal eyes. This patient has had five visual fields. The first two were done with standard strategy. The third was full from prior strategy, which is not calibrated for STATPAC. The fourth had reduced reliability. The fifth was done with standard strategy. It appears that the patient started with a mean deviation of -8 dB, which is distinctly pathologic, and the field has worsened over time. (From the Humphrey STATPAC program.)

Glaucomatous Visual Field Defects

Generalized Depression

Generalized depression can be the earliest sign of glaucoma, but it can also occur with aging, miosis, or hazy media. In kinetic perimetry generalized depression is seen as a generalized constriction of the peripheral and central isopters. Unfortunately, this too is a rather nonspecific finding. Kinetic perimetry, at least by manual methods, lacks the precision necessary to differentiate generalized depression from normal aging unless there is an obvious difference between the patient's two eyes or the depression is substantial.

Generalized depression can increase the physician's suspicion that glaucomatous damage has occurred, especially if it is unilateral or more pronounced in the eye with the higher pressure or larger cup:disc ratio. Interestingly, both the Humphrey and Octopus field machines use *MD* to represent the amount of generalized loss found in the field (Figs. 11-3 and 11-4). On the Octopus machine this stands for "mean defect." If the patient has loss (i.e., a defect), then the MD has a positive sign indicating the presence of a defect. If the patient sees better than expected, the MD has a negative sign; a negative defect indicates above-normal sensitivity. On the Humphrey machine MD stands for "mean deviation" and measures the difference between the patient's response and normal. If the patient has field loss the MD has a negative sign; if the patient sees better than expected the MD is positive—just the reverse of the Octopus nomenclature. Luckily it is easy to tell which system is being used clinically, and in common parlance an abnormal MD means that the patient has some component of generalized loss.

Irregularity of the Visual Field

There may be a lack of uniformity in the visual field. With computerized perimetry, this "roughness" appears as a variation of decibel level among contiguous points that is greater than that anticipated in normal patients of the same age. These areas of loss appear nonuniformly throughout the field. This variation is expressed statistically as the standard deviation of the deviations found in the field (Humphrey) or the variance (square of standard deviation) of the mean of all points tested (Octopus). Humphrey uses the term *pattern standard deviation,* whereas Octopus uses the term *loss variance.* These functions are sensitive to localized loss but are relatively unaffected by generalized loss (see Figs. 11-3 and 11-4).

Nasal Step or Depression

The nasal portion of the visual field is often affected early in glaucoma, and defects may persist until the last stages of the disease.[2] The nasal area is the most important region of the midperipheral and peripheral field to test.[3] Depression may be evidenced by hesitancy in patient response when

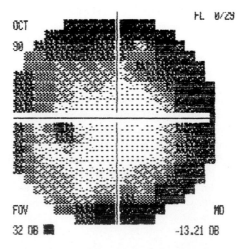

Figure 11-3   Humphrey field showing moderate to severe generalized depression. The mean deviation (MD; *lower right*) is −13.21.

testing this area, as an inward turning of the isopter in manual perimetry, or by reduced sensitivity on static testing. If a true step that respects the horizontal raphe develops, a defect is present. Such defects may occur centrally (Fig. 11-5), peripherally, or both (Fig. 11-6) and may be isolated or associated with other Bjerrum area defects.

Temporal Step or Depression

A temporal depression or step may develop as an isolated finding or in conjunction with other glaucomatous defects. They may be detected at any stage of glaucoma but are more commonly found as a component of late-stage disease.[4] Drance and co-workers[5] suggest careful testing of the tem-

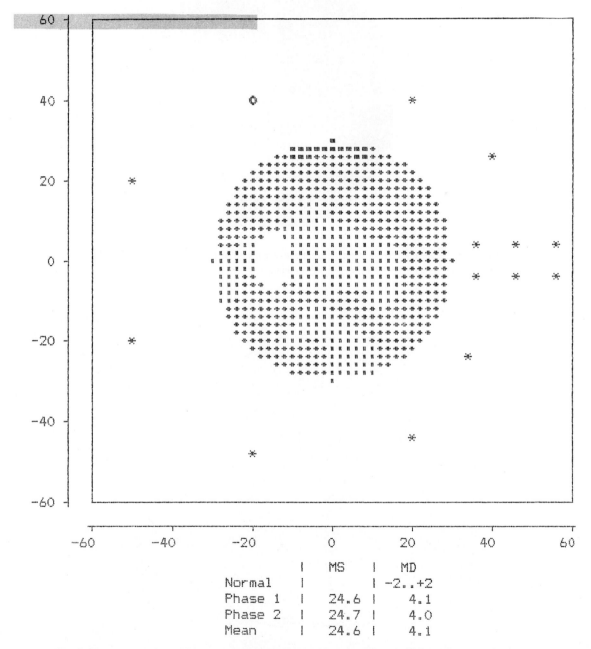

Figure 11-4 Octopus field showing slight generalized depression. The mean defect (MD) is +4.1. *MS,* mean sensitivity; *MS + MD,* normal sensitivity for the patient's age.

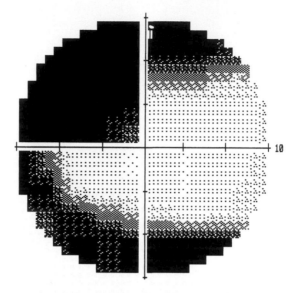

Figure 11-5 Central 10° field from the right eye of a patient with advanced glaucoma. The nasal horizontal step (*left side in this figure*) runs all the way to fixation.

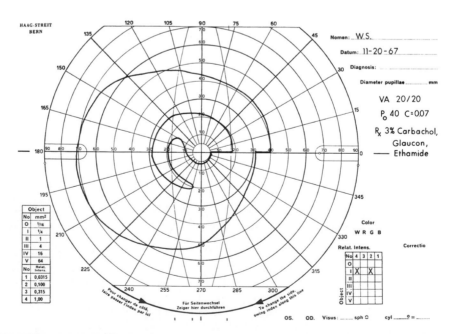

Figure 11-6 Note the inferior nasal step present on the peripheral and central isopters in this patient. There is an inferior arcuate scotoma present also.

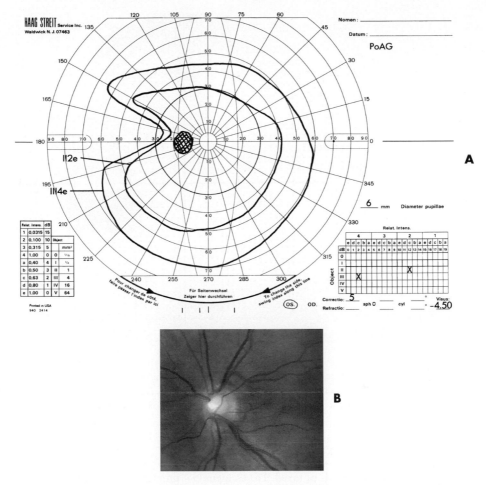

Figure 11-7   Visual field temporal defect. **A** and **B,** Note the temporal wedge that occurred in this patient with erosion of the nasal aspect of the optic nerve.

poral area to recognize the occasional patients who may develop this condition as their only defect (Fig. 11-7).

Enlargement of the Blind Spot

Enlargement and baring of the blind spot are considered nonspecific changes that can occur in normal patients (Fig. 11-8). If the blind spot enlarges in an arcuate manner, it is called a *Seidel's scotoma* and may be seen in early glaucoma (Fig. 11-9).

Isolated Paracentral Scotomata

Careful manual perimetry using combined static and kinetic techniques may demonstrate small paracentral scotomata. In a classic study, Aulhorn and Harms[6] found similar small defects that did not connect to the blind spot in 20% of glaucomatous visual fields. Early glaucomatous defects may have a small dense center. If the glaucoma is progressive, these defects enlarge, deepen, and coalesce over time to form arcuate scotomata. Inconsistency of responses in the paracentral area may be an early sign of glaucomatous change.[5,7,8]

Static testing through these scotomata may confirm that they are true defects. Because many computerized perimeters provide programs with a 6° separation of test sites, a scotoma smaller than 6° may be missed. Consequently some investigators advocate using spots separated by 3° in glaucoma testing. This can be done with most computerized machines by using two programs (e.g., 30-1 and 30-2 in the Humphrey machine). This testing will take up to an hour per eye, and the

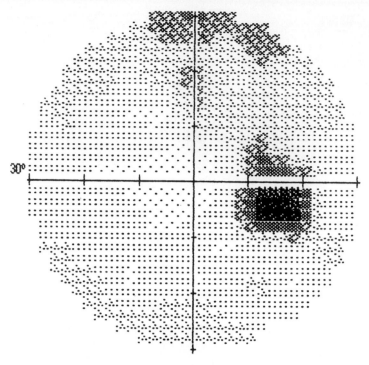

Figure 11-8   Visual field chart from the right eye of a 56-year-old woman with early glaucoma. Generalized blind spot enlargement is not necessarily a glaucomatous defect. This blind spot is roughly 14° × 14°, with sloping margins. The normal blind spot is about 7° vertically and 5.5° horizontally, with sharp borders.

patient's endurance will be taxed. The Octopus G-1 program has test points packed more tightly in the central and Bjerrum regions to avoid missing small but significant paracentral scotomata (Fig. 11-10). Computerized static perimetry is sensitive enough in the majority of clinical situations to detect most defects with a single test using a 6° spot separation. Newer approaches, such as Humphrey's Swedish Interactive Thresholding Algorithm program, focus testing attention on pathologic areas of the field.

Arcuate Defects (Nerve Fiber Bundle Defects)

The arcuate scotoma represents a complete nerve fiber bundle defect. It begins at the blind spot, arcs around fixation, and ends at the horizontal nasal raphe. The defect may break through into the periphery nasally and then expand further to ultimately become an altitudinal defect (Fig. 11-11).

End-Stage Defects

Central and Temporal Islands

In the later stages of glaucoma most of the axons at the superior and inferior poles of the disc are destroyed, leaving only the papillomacular bundle and some nasal fibers. This destruction produces the characteristic end-stage field, with a small central island and a larger temporal crescent remaining. The central island may split fixation so that only fibers from half of the papillomacular bundle remain (Fig. 11-12). Kolker[9] found that patients with split fixation are more susceptible to central vision loss at surgery, although this still is a very rare outcome.[10] These patients may need to have their pressures controlled in the mid teens to avoid further progression.

Reversal of Visual Field Defects

Fluctuation and increasing familiarity with the test or random chance may cause subsequent visual field examinations to appear improved.[11,12] Nevertheless, reversibility of visual field defects seems to be a real phenomenon in some patients following therapy for glaucoma.[13-16]

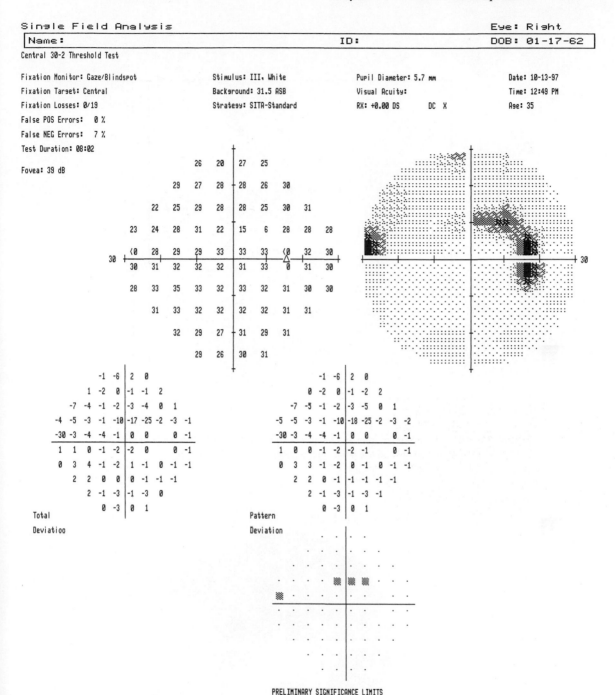

Single Field Analysis   Eye: Right

Name: ID: DOB: 01-17-62

Central 30-2 Threshold Test

Fixation Monitor: Gaze/Blindspot   Stimulus: III, White   Pupil Diameter: 5.7 mm   Date: 10-13-97
Fixation Target: Central   Background: 31.5 ASB   Visual Acuity: Time: 12:49 PM
Fixation Losses: 0/19   Strategy: SITA-Standard   RX: +0.00 DS   DC X   Age: 35
False POS Errors: 0 %
False NEG Errors: 7 %
Test Duration: 08:02

Fovea: 39 dB

PRELIMINARY SIGNIFICANCE LIMITS

Total Deviation Probability Plot, GHT, and Global Indices will be in a future software rev.

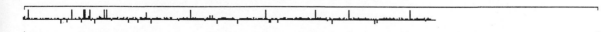

Figure 11-9 Chart from the right eye of a patient with normal-tension glaucoma showing a Seidel's scotoma extending from the blind spot. There is also a small peripheral superior nasal step defect.

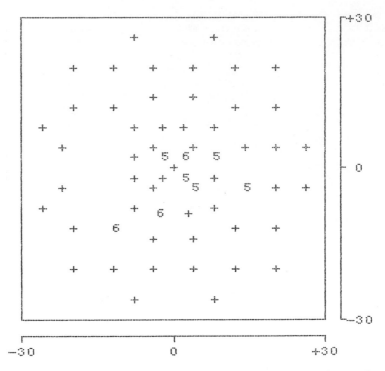

Figure 11-10   Test grid pattern from the Octopus G-1 program. Twenty-one test points are placed in the central 12° × 12° rather than only 16 test points in the Octopus 31 or 32 program.

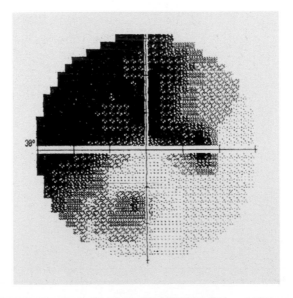

Figure 11-11   Field from the right eye of patient with advanced glaucoma. The superior arcuate defect has expanded to include the entire superonasal quadrant and includes half of the superotemporal quadrant as well. The inferior half of the field is much less severely affected.

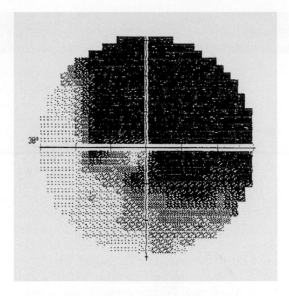

Figure 11-12 Central island of a patient's left eye with field defects encroaching on fixation. The temporal field is partially spared.

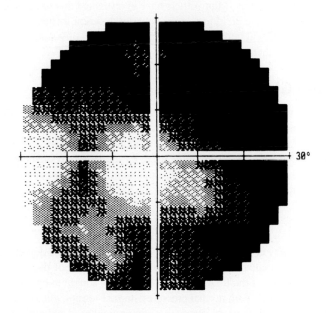

Figure 11-13 The superior field (left eye) exhibits similar but more advanced loss compared with the inferior field. If the disease is unchecked, both fields will continue to progress.

ANALYSIS OF VISUAL FIELD LOSS

Chronic Open-Angle Glaucoma

Any of the preceding types of visual field loss may be seen in chronic open-angle glaucoma.[17] In the early stages there may be a generalized depression that progresses gradually or sometimes in steps from paracentral scotomata to arcuate to altitudinal to end-stage defects. Defects usually become denser and then increase in area in one hemifield before progressing to the next hemifield (Fig. 11-13). Scotomata may show episodic (stepwise), linear, or curvilinear progression.[18-20]

Many recent investigations have suggested that the two forms of glaucomatous visual field loss, diffuse and localized, may have different pathogenic origins.[21] It has been speculated that in-

> **Box 11-1**
> **Some Causes of Nerve Fiber Bundle–Associated Visual Field Defects**
>
> | | |
> |---|---|
> | Chorioretinitis | Optic nerve ischemia |
> | Myopic retinal degeneration | Optic nerve compressive lesions |
> | Refractive scotomata | Optic neuritis |
> | Trauma | Drusen of optic nerve head |
> | Retinal laser damage glaucoma | |

creased intraocular pressure (IOP) may cause diffuse loss[22] but have less influence on the development of localized defects.[23] Observer bias may have some influence on these findings, however, because patients with mild diffuse loss and normal pressure are often not identified as abnormal. Conversely, patients with elevated IOPs are examined closely because of the pressure , and because suspicion is high mild diffuse defects are recognized. Patients with dense localized defects tend to have localized optic nerve changes and may have visual field studies based on the appearance of the optic nerve. If the IOP is normal a diagnosis of glaucoma is more likely when the field defect is local and dense rather than diffuse or nonspecific. Drance,[24] however, found that patients with increased IOP with localized defects in one hemifield had nearly double the amount of generalized reduction in sensitivity in the other hemifield compared with a similar group of patients with normal-tension glaucoma. Many others have investigated this issue, and there is general agreement that early glaucomatous field loss may appear in different forms.

Future studies will help clarify the types and causes of visual field loss in glaucoma. Currently the only effective therapy is lowering elevated IOP.

Angle-Closure Glaucoma

During the acute phase of angle-closure glaucoma in patients with high IOP, corneal edema and retinal ischemia can produce bizarre field defects that have little clinical value for following disease progression. After the pressure has been normalized, field defects may remain and may sometimes be extensive if ischemic atrophy of the nerve has occurred. In such cases pallor of the nerve may be more severe than cupping. This is one situation in which glaucomatous field defects may not correspond well to the amount of cupping of the nerve head.[25-27]

Other Causes

Other diseases may cause arcuate nerve fiber bundle visual field defects (Box 11-1) that may be confused with glaucomatous damage. Generally, if excavation of the optic nerve does not correspond with the appearance of the field, other causes must be sought to explain the defect. If visual field defects occur or progress with normal pressures, normal-tension glaucoma may be the cause (see Chapter 17), but the examiner must be sure that other retinal or visual pathway lesions are not present, *especially if the process is occurring unilaterally.* Glaucoma is a jigsaw puzzle in which all the "pieces" of the disease should fit. If a piece does not fit properly, the physician should be suspicious that it may belong to some other puzzle (disease). Generally, the configuration of the optic nerve and the appearance of the visual field correspond. Superior visual field defects are accompanied by erosion of the inferior portion of the optic disc and vice versa. The nerve in a patient with a temporal visual field defect should have a thinned nasal rim. Although normal-tension glaucoma may account for 10% or more of glaucoma patients, depending on definitions and the patient population being studied, IOP is elevated at some time in most glaucoma patients. If these factors do not occur in appropriate patterns, the possibility of glaucoma is not excluded, but the physician's suspicions should be heightened and a thorough evaluation should be undertaken to exclude other possible diseases.

Esterman Disability Rating

Assessment of disability resulting from visual field loss is often needed, although it can be difficult to quantitate. The American Medical Association (AMA) recently adopted the Esterman disability rating.[1,28,29] This binocular assessment used by government and industry is described more fully in *AMA Guidelines to Impairment* and *Physicians Desk Reference for Ophthalmology.*

ANALYSIS OF COMPUTERIZED STATIC PERIMETRY

Computerized static perimetry provides numbers that represent the patient's responses to stimuli in various areas of the retina. These numbers can be manipulated mathematically and statistically to provide information about the reliability of patient responses and test results. Although not identical, Goldmann visual field plots and computer-generated grey-scale visual field patterns usually are similar (Fig. 11-14).

Reliability Indexes

False-Positive and False-Negative Responses

Reliability indexes usually include false-positive and false-negative responses and some analysis of fixation. *False-positive responses* occur when the patient indicates that he or she has seen a stimulus when one was not presented. This is usually a reaction to random noise generated by the perimeter. *False-negative responses* occur when the patient fails to respond to a stimulus that is at least as bright or brighter than one that he or she had previously recognized in that position. This indicates that the response was erroneous at least one of the two times that the position was tested. The lower the percentage of false-positive or false-negative responses, the more reliable is the test. False-positive or false-negative scores in excess of 20% to 30% indicate a test of questionable reliability.

Fixation Reliability

Fixation reliability can be monitored in a number of ways. The technician can offer a subjective assessment of the patient's fixation reliability; the computer may stop the test if a video or infrared fixation monitor indicates that the eye has shifted; or the blind spot may be stimulated periodically (Heijl-Krakau technique) with a bright stimulus, anticipating that the properly fixing patient will not see it.

All of these techniques have flaws. It is difficult for technicians to see tiny fixation shifts, and only with considerable experience are they able to judge the shifts' effects on the test. In addition, it is practically impossible for a technician in a darkened room to maintain concentration on patients' eye movements all day long. Automatic fixation monitors that interrupt the test can be quite precise; however, most patients cannot fixate "perfectly."[30] Even the most attentive patient will have minor head and eye movements associated with breathing, heartbeat, etc. If the monitor is set to be very sensitive, the test will be prolonged by frequent interruptions. If the monitor is too insensitive, it has little value. Although constant monitoring is desirable, it is probably not necessary in most patients.[31]

The blind spot is not constant. Only one of eight to ten presentations is directed at the blind spot, so the computer has no way of knowing about the patient's fixation between those checks. If the computer incorrectly located the blind spot at the beginning of the test, subsequent checks might fall outside the real blind spot and give a false impression of bad fixation. If there is a large scotoma adjacent to the blind spot or a hemianopic field defect, fixation may be poor but the blind spot check will fall into the scotoma and falsely indicate good fixation.

Most patients either fixate well or poorly. Fixation behavior can be improved by encouragement from the technician, but the improvement may be small and inconsistent from test to test. Generally, the clinician needs to know the quality of fixation to help judge the accuracy of the field, and this can be provided by any of the preceding methods. Fixation losses exceeding 20% are considered poor in most circumstances, although the exact effect of such losses on the usefulness of the test is unclear and may vary substantially from patient to patient.

Global Indexes

Global indexes, which reflect the results of the visual field examination, are mathematic summaries of the actual sensitivity data produced by the examination (Figs. 11-15 and 11-16).

Fluctuation

Short-Term Fluctuation

Short-term fluctuation (SF) is measured by most computerized perimeters. This statistical analysis is the result of checking several loci in the visual field twice. The Octopus G-1 program tests each

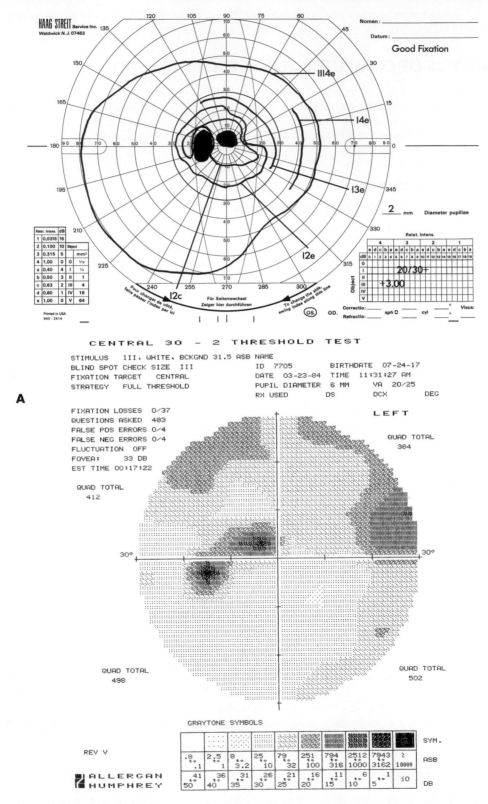

Figure 11-14 Comparison of Goldmann perimetry with automated threshold perimetry. **A,** Shortly following the Goldmann test *(top),* this patient had full-threshold 30-2 Humphrey perimetry. Computerized perimetry *(bottom)* depicts the paracentral scotoma and nasal step that were demonstrated by Goldmann perimetry.

Continued

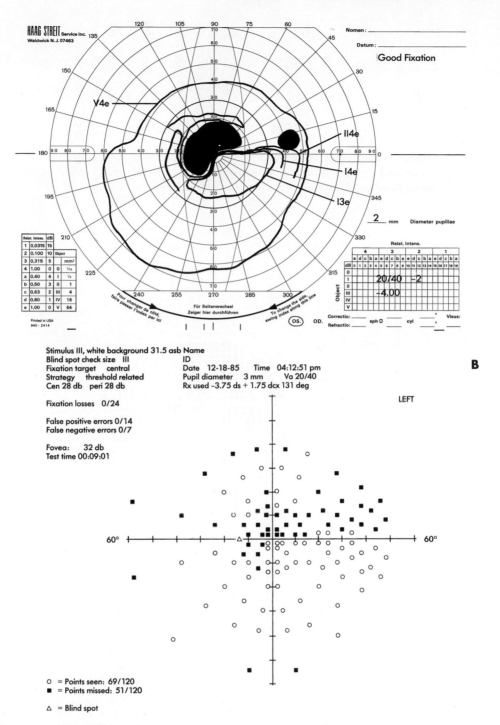

Figure 11-14, cont'd B, Goldmann perimetry *(top)* demonstrates an altitudinal type of defect with a large arcuate scotoma. A similar pattern is seen on the full-field suprathreshold screening test performed by the Humphrey perimeter *(bottom)*. The *black squares* indicate areas of deficit.

MD: -23.20 dB   P < 0.5 %

PSD: 11.08 dB   P < 0.5 %

SF: 5.90 dB   P < 0.5 %

CPSD: 8.85 dB   P < 0.5 %

Figure 11-15 Detail of visual field indexes from Humphrey field analyses. *MD*, mean deviation; *PSD*, pattern standard deviation; *SF*, short-term fluctuation; *CPSD*, corrected pattern standard deviation. *P* values indicate the likelihood that values are normal. These values are severely disturbed.

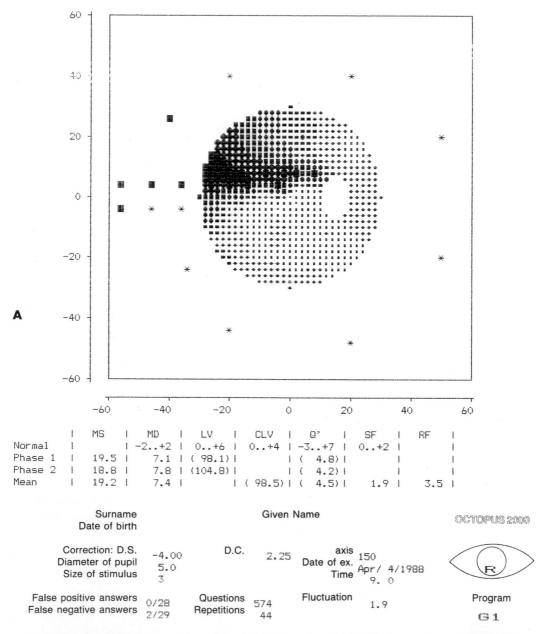

A

	MS	MD	LV	CLV	Q'	SF	RF
Normal		-2..+2	0..+6	0..+4	-3..+7	0..+2	
Phase 1	19.5	7.1	(98.1)		(4.8)		
Phase 2	18.8	7.8	(104.8)		(4.2)		
Mean	19.2	7.4		(98.5)	(4.5)	1.9	3.5

Surname   Given Name   OCTOPUS 2000
Date of birth

Correction: D.S. -4.00   D.C.   2.25   axis 150
Diameter of pupil 5.0   Date of ex. Apr/ 4/1988
Size of stimulus   3   Time   9. 0

False positive answers 0/28   Questions   574   Fluctuation   1.9   Program
False negative answers 2/29   Repetitions 44   G 1

Figure 11-16 **A,** Grey-scale printout of the Octopus G-1 program indicating an upper arcuate defect in the right eye. Global indexes are printed below the grey-scale plot.   *Continued*

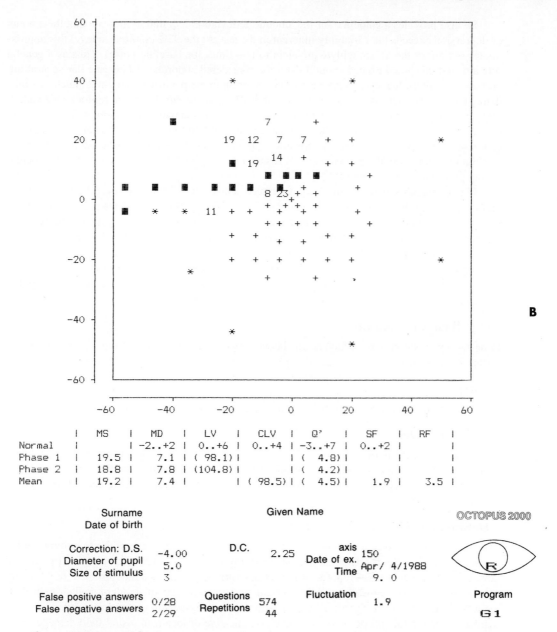

	MS		MD		LV		CLV		Q'		SF		RF	
Normal			-2..+2		0..+6		0..+4		-3..+7		0..+2			
Phase 1		19.5		7.1		(98.1)			(4.8)					
Phase 2		18.8		7.8		(104.8)			(4.2)					
Mean		19.2		7.4			(98.5)	(4.5)			1.9		3.5	

Surname	Given Name	OCTOPUS 2000
Date of birth		

Correction: D.S. −4.00   D.C. 2.25   axis 150
Diameter of pupil 5.0   Date of ex. Apr/ 4/1988
Size of stimulus 3   Time 9. 0

False positive answers 0/28   Questions 574   Fluctuation 1.9   Program
False negative answers 2/29   Repetitions 44   G 1

Figure 11-16, cont'd B, Raw data provided by the G-1 program. The *crosses* indicate normal spots, the *black squares* indicate absolute defects, and the *numbers* represent depth of defect in decibels. *MS,* mean sensitivity, *MD,* mean defect; *LV,* loss variance; *CLV,* corrected loss variance; *SF,* short-term fluctuation; *RF,* reliability factor (the ratio of false-positives and false-negatives expressed as a percentage).

point in the central field twice. The variability that is noted between each of the double tests is reported as its root mean square and defined as SF. For most normal young subjects, overall SF is between 1.5 and 2.5 dB.[32,33] SF is affected by age and eccentricity from fixation. Although the overall SF printed on the field chart may be as high as 2.5 dB in normals, a fluctuation of 2.5 dB a few degrees from fixation in a young patient with clear media is unusual whereas fluctuation at 30° eccentricity in a normal 70-year-old individual may be 8 or 10 dB.[34-36]

SF is increased in glaucoma suspects,[37-40] patients who cannot cooperate well for the test, and patients who have decreased sensitivity in areas of the visual field.[41,42] It is also increased in cooperative patients with significant localized field loss. In these patients the first test point may be in a fairly normal area of retina and the subsequent retest in an adjacent scotoma (or vice versa) because of a minor shift in fixation.

SF also provides a guideline for the amount of deviation required to indicate that the amount of depression exceeds the variability inherent in the test. At the 95% confidence level this approximates two times the SF (roughly equivalent to two times the baseline noise). Thus as a general rule a deviation should exceed about 5 dB to be considered abnormal.[43] This rule has several important exceptions, however. Because normal variation in the parafoveal region is much less than that in the midperiphery, deviations smaller than 5 dB can represent significant reproducible pathology when they occur near fixation. Conversely, as mentioned above, a deviation of 10 dB or more may occur at 30° in a normal middle-aged patient. In addition to the age of the patient and the location of the test point, the status of surrounding points can help determine whether a small deviation is significant. A mildly depressed point has a greater likelihood of being pathologic if its neighboring points are also depressed.[35,36]

Fluctuation also increases in areas of reduced sensitivity.[12] There are several possible explanations for this. It is well known that an area of inconsistency often precedes a permanent depression with Goldmann perimetry. Inconsistent responses on Goldmann perimetry appear as increased fluctuation on computerized automated perimetry. Another explanation is that the nature of the test for fluctuation—repeating the test twice during the examination—means that different areas of the field may be tested because of a small fixation shift. In an area of pathology the second test can examine a slightly different area that legitimately has different sensitivity. The machine compares the first and second tests and indicates the difference between them as SF.

Long-Term Fluctuation

Long-term fluctuation is that which occurs between two separate visual field tests. This is discussed further in the section on recognition of change.

Mean Sensitivity

Mean sensitivity is the average of the patient's responses for all of the points tested.

Mean Deviation or Defect

MD is the measurement of how the mean of the patient's responses varies from the mean of the responses of a series of normal patients of similar age under similar testing conditions. It is a statement of the generalized depression of the visual field and is useful in recognizing early diffuse visual field loss in glaucoma.

Standard Deviation or Variance

The standard deviation of the mean of the patient's responses is the same as the square root of the variance. The Humphrey perimeter analysis program reports standard deviation (pattern standard deviation), whereas Octopus reports variance (loss variance). Each is a measurement of the variation in responses across the visual field. Normal patients have a small standard deviation, indicating a "smooth" surface to the hill of vision. A high standard deviation or variance indicates an irregular surface to the hill of vision and may be indicative of localized visual field damage.[32,39,41] These indexes can be corrected by SF and then are labeled as *corrected* (i.e., *corrected* pattern standard deviation or *corrected* loss variance). When the indexes have been corrected, they become more sensitive to recognizing true localized defects in the visual field because the variability caused by SF is removed.

Graphic Plots

One of the greatest values of computerized perimetry lies in the ability of the computer to analyze the numeric data and present them graphically for easier comprehension. The grey-scale printout of the Octopus was the first of these. Printouts that show variation from normal are widely available today (Fig. 11-17). The Humphrey STATPAC analysis printout includes probability maps that allow quick assessment of the likelihood that a response is disturbed. Patterns of disturbed points are easily detected. These printouts can also be adjusted for generalized depression so that scotomata are more obvious. This latter function is especially useful for follow-up of patients with glaucoma and other causes of generalized depression such as constricted pupils or cataracts (Figs. 11-18 and 11-19).

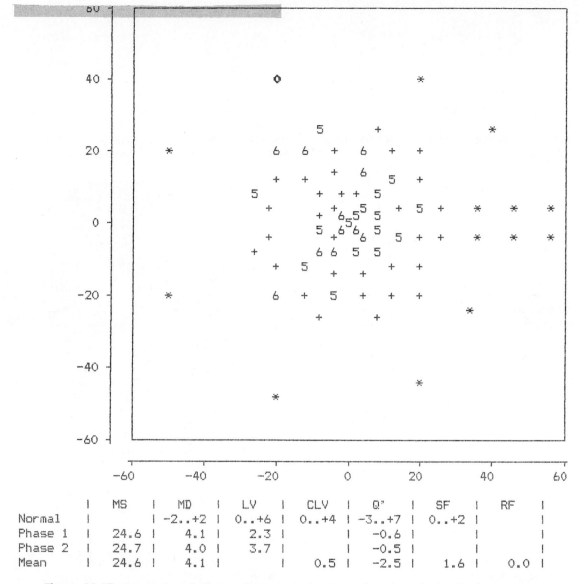

	MS	MD	LV	CLV	Q"	SF	RF
Normal		-2..+2	0..+6	0..+4	-3..+7	0..+2	
Phase 1	24.6	4.1	2.3		-0.6		
Phase 2	24.7	4.0	3.7		-0.5		
Mean	24.6	4.1		0.5	-2.5	1.6	0.0

Figure 11-17 Printout from the Octopus G-1 program showing a subtraction scale plot. *Numbers* represent depth of the defect at the corresponding point.

Area of the Visual Field to be Tested

Most computerized perimeters measure the threshold sensitivity of 56 to 72 locations in the central 25° to 30°. Flammer and co-workers[44] and Jenni and co-workers[43] developed the G-1 program to focus more attention on the areas of particular interest in glaucoma (see Fig. 11-10).

Long-Term Analysis

By selecting a series of similar tests, computerized perimeters can analyze the results over time to evaluate whether the visual field is changing. This may be accomplished by linear regression or *t*-test techniques.[45] Even with these methods, however, several visual fields of good reliability from the same eye are needed to analyze change well. Trying to recognize change from fewer fields is fraught with hazard and requires a large amount of change.[46,47] This is discussed further in the section on recognition of change.

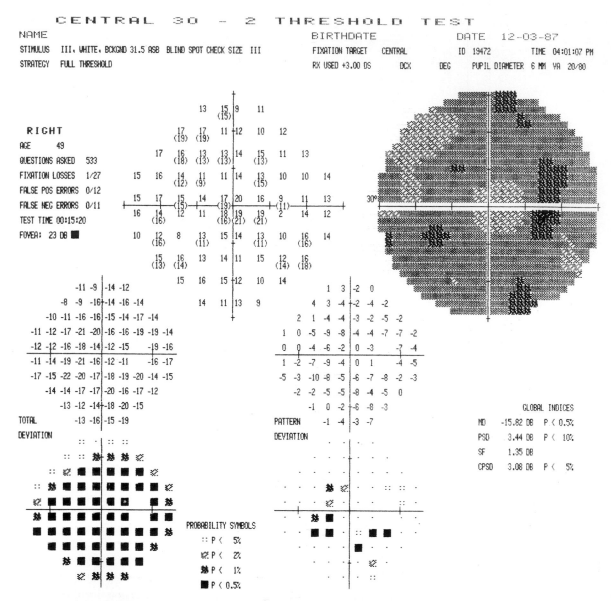

Figure 11-18 This patient has aphakia, glaucoma, and vitreous debris. His refractive correction was incorrectly chosen as a +3 sphere, which failed to fully correct his aphakia. There is marked depression of the grey scale *(upper right)* and generalized depression noted on the total deviation plot *(lower left)*. The pattern deviation plot *(lower right)* recognizes this general depression, eliminates it, and prints out a defect in the inferior and superior arcuate areas. These defects are consistent with glaucoma.

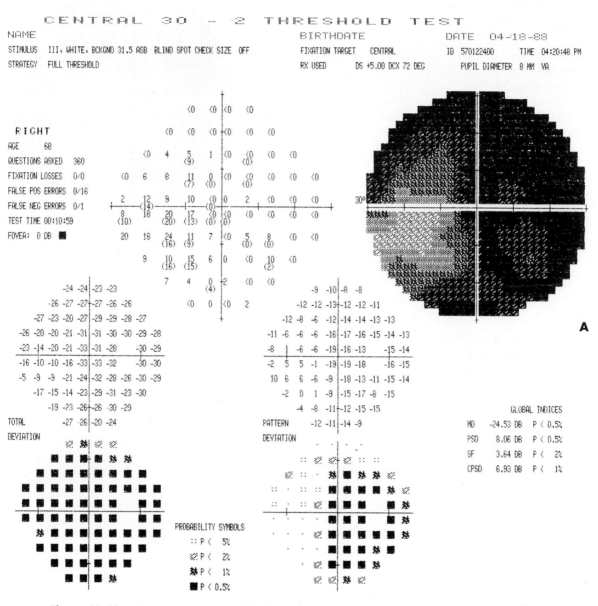

Figure 11-19 Bitemporal hemiopia. **A,** Right eye.

Continued

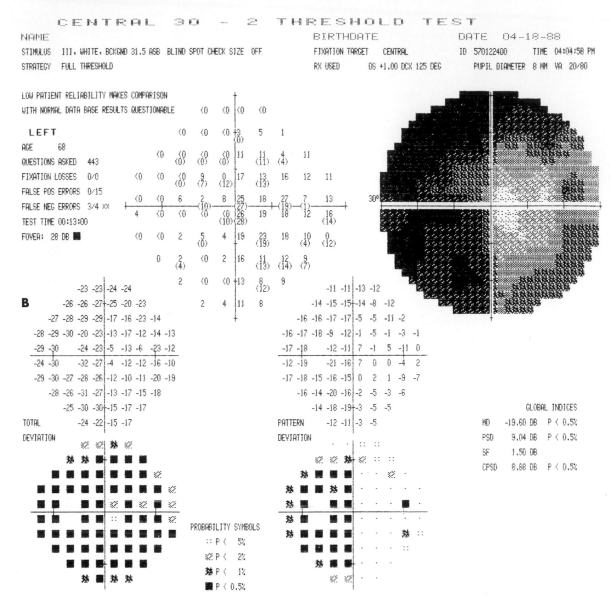

Figure 11-19, cont'd **B,** Left eye. The grey-scale image *(upper right)* could be misinterpreted as advanced glaucomatous visual field loss. The total deviation pattern *(lower left)* indicates marked generalized depression. The pattern deviation *(lower right),* however, demonstrates a hemiopic defect. The right eye has such poor vision that the patient's fixation shifted slightly to the left, which explains the overlapping of the vertical meridian.

DETERMINATION OF NORMAL VISUAL FIELD

Evaluation of the visual field in glaucoma patients or glaucoma suspects attempts to answer two important questions: Is the visual field abnormal? (detection) and has it worsened? (progression).

There are three basic ways by which the physician can determine whether the field is abnormal: (1) by recognizing deviation from normal values, (2) by recognizing variation between two eyes of the same patient, and (3) by establishing significant variation within the given field. Several of the computerized machines have analysis programs that will indicate abnormalities by graphic plots or by a written phase.[35,36,48,49]

Deviation From Normal Values

There are no published normal values for Goldmann perimetry. This is probably because results vary widely from technician to technician and from technique to technique. Certain guidelines,

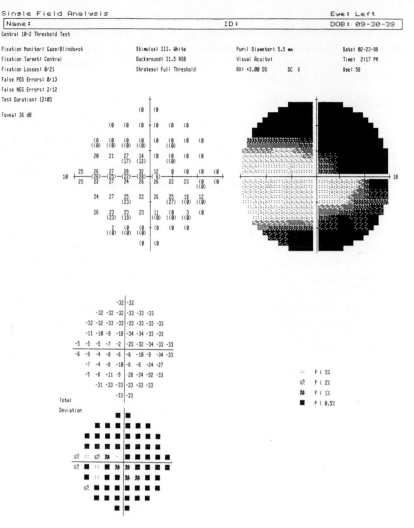

Figure 11-20 Humphrey STATPAC with probability map. The *upper numerical printout* represents sensitivity measured during the test. The *lower numerical printout* represents deviation from normal. *Symbols* represent the likelihood that measured points are within normal limits, according to the key at the *lower right.*

however, are helpful. Generally, the I2e isopter falls between 25° and 30°. The I4e isopter usually falls between 40° and 50° nasally. In the absence of lens opacity in patients older than 75 years of age, these isopters may contract 5° or so. Contraction may be greater in the presence of cataracts.

Graphic Plot of Points Varying From Normal

The Humphrey and Octopus perimeters have age-matched normal values stored in their computer memories for each point tested. The Humphrey perimeter provides the deviation from normal in a graphic printout through its STATPAC program.[50] For each point tested, STATPAC provides the statistical probability that the patient's threshold would be found in the normal population (Fig. 11-20). The Octopus program provides a printout of how many decibels a point deviates from the norm for that age (see Fig. 11-17). Regardless of the technique used, it is unwise to depend on one or two deviant points within a field to indicate abnormality unless they are severely depressed or contiguous.

Global Indexes

Measurements of single points are more likely to contain error than are averages of measurements of all points within the visual field. Therefore global indexes are helpful in recognizing deviation from normal. The Octopus MD may be statistically abnormal with less deviation from normal than that required for a single point. For the Octopus, 95% of the population will fall within 2 dB of the normal mean sensitivity provided on the Octopus printout.[37] By contrast, an individual point may need to be depressed two to three times this amount to be even mildly suspicious. The Humphrey printout provides a table indicating the lower 5% probability of normal for each of the global indexes. Deviations greater than these may be abnormal. The greater the deviation, the greater the likelihood will be of abnormality.

Comparison With the Other Eye

Published data[51] indicate that the mean sensitivities of the two eyes fall within 1 dB 95% of the time and within 1.4 dB 99% of the time. Therefore unexplained variation of mean sensitivity between the two eyes greater than 1 dB would be suspicious and greater than 2 dB may be abnormal. If the lower sensitivity occurs in the eye with higher IOP or greater excavation of the optic nerve head, it would be highly suspicious of glaucomatous visual field loss.[52]

Localized Variation Within the Visual Field

Localized depression within the field may not be enough to cause a statistically significant reduction of mean sensitivity or be deep enough to be recognized by the computers as an increased MD. However, one of the most important types of early change in glaucoma is mild inconsistent depression in the paracentral area.[8,53,54] Careful examination of the raw data may show a small cluster of points that vary from their neighbors by no more than 2 or 3 dB. These may be early visual field defects. The Humphrey corrected pattern standard deviation and the Octopus corrected loss variance are designed to highlight these defects statistically (Fig. 11-21). Occasionally such deviations may be so subtle as to fail to reach statistical significance. Katz and Sommer[55] suggest comparing the upper and lower hemifields for earlier recognition of glaucomatous change based on evidence that change in one hemifield precedes change in the other.

It is often difficult to be certain that minor changes in the visual field represent true deviations from normal. Minor change in an eye with other suspicious findings, such as increased IOP or optic nerve cupping, lends them credibility. Persistence on repeated examinations often confirms them.

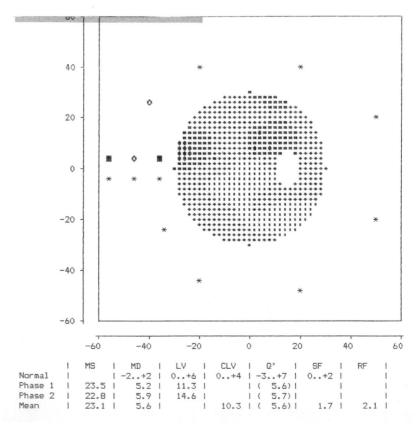

	MS	MD	LV	CLV	Q'	SF	RF
Normal		-2..+2	0..+6	0..+4	-3..+7	0..+2	
Phase 1	23.5	5.2	11.3		(5.6)		
Phase 2	22.8	5.9	14.6		(5.7)		
Mean	23.1	5.6		10.3	(5.6)	1.7	2.1

Figure 11-21   Subtle superior peripheral nasal step and a subtle superior Seidel's scotoma in the right eye of a patient with normal-tension glaucoma. Note the slightly elevated mean defect (*MD*) and moderately elevated corrected loss variance (*CLV*), which help alert the physician to the presence of an abnormality.

RECOGNITION OF CHANGE

Change from one field to another is difficult to determine because of the fluctuation that occurs within and between tests. With Goldmann perimetry, areas of isopters within the central 30° were found to fluctuate by as much as 30% between tests in patients whose glaucoma was apparently controlled.[56] As described previously, computerized perimetry suffers from the same problem (Fig. 11-22), but the amount of intertest variation is reduced by the administration of a more standardized test. Also, the amount of fluctuation can be measured easily and analyzed both for populations and for individual patients.

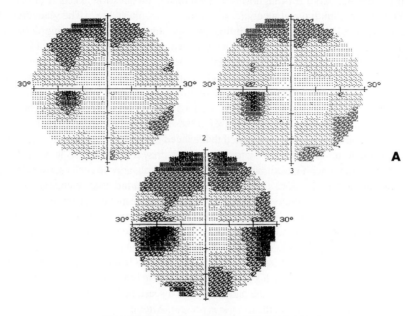

A

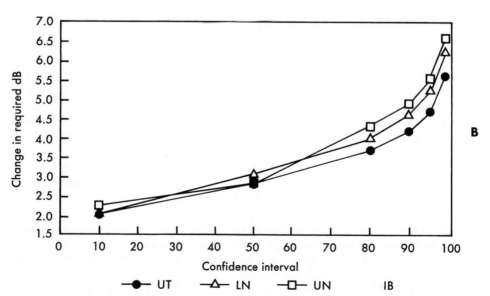

**CHANGE IN MS FROM FIELD 1 TO FIELD 2
VS CONFIRMED LOSS FOR MINIMUM DAMAGE**

B

Figure 11-22 **A,** These three visual fields were performed approximately 4 months apart. The second field (*bottom*) shows apparent worsening compared with the first and third fields, which appear quite similar. This amount of fluctuation is not uncommon in glaucoma patients. **B,** Confidence level of change between the two fields. To obtain 95% confidence levels, the change in the portion of the field under study must be at least 5 to 7 dB when comparing two fields. *UT,* upper temporal; *LN,* lower nasal; *UN,* upper nasal; *IB,* interior Bjerrum. (From Hoskins HD Jr, Magee SD: A system for the analysis of automated visual fields. Paper presented at the Seventh International Visual Field Symposium of the International Perimetric Society, Amsterdam, September 7-10, 1986.)

To address this problem investigators have assembled large databases of normal and glaucomatous patients to aid the examiner, by way of the statistical analysis program on the computer, in determining whether or not a field is normal or has worsened. The glaucoma hemifield test, available with the Humphrey STATPAC, compares the patient's upper and lower fields and then compares the patient's results with results from a large group of glaucoma patients.[35,36] If the patient's hemifields differ in ways consistent with defects observed in the group of known glaucoma patients, the field chart indicates an abnormal test (Fig. 11-23). When the deviation is less certain the machine may indicate a "borderline" result. If the patient's hemifields are normal or do not differ in ways seen in the glaucoma population the machine reports the glaucoma hemifield test (GHT) result as normal. After the diagnosis has been made, the question asked of the visual field shifts from "Does the patient have glaucoma?" to "Is the glaucoma stable?" The glaucoma change probability test was developed to help answer this question. In this statistical manipulation a series of three or more of the patient's fields are compared with a similar series of fields from a large database of stable glaucoma patients.[57] If changes in the patient's field exceed those found in the stable glaucoma population the machine indicates that glaucomatous change may have taken place.

In all cases the examiner is attempting to distinguish physiologic fluctuation from pathologic progression. SF, the intratest variation, ranges from 1.5 to 2.5 dB in the central field of normal patients. Approximately 95% of responses in these patients fall within two times the SF. Therefore deviations within the given visual field that exceed two times that amount may be abnormal.

Long-term fluctuation, the intertest variation, may reach 1 to 2 dB in normal patients and possibly more in patients with glaucomatous damage.[37] Thus changes in mean sensitivity must exceed this by some amount to be considered true change. We found that a change in mean sensitivity of 6 dB or more in the entire central field was required between the first and second visual fields to be 95% confident that the third field would confirm a downward trend.[43] This is a great amount of change, and the ophthalmologist would hope to recognize smaller amounts with some certainty. There are several techniques to help do this. The important axiom to repeat the field before initiating or changing therapy certainly applies here. Visual field data, like the data from any medical test, are accumulated to assist the physician in refining his or her diagnosis. There is a certain chance that a patient has the disease in question. The chance that the patient has the disease before the test results are known corresponds to the prior probability that the disease is present. After the test results are known the posterior probability that the disease exists may be higher or lower than the prior probability. With an accurate and appropriate test the disease may be ruled in or out by the results. A patient with a very large cup:disc ratio and high pressures who shows a Bjerrum scotoma on visual field testing is easy to diagnose. This occurs when the prior probability of the disease is high and the test results are pathognomonic.

As the prior probability becomes lower and the test results less definitive, small irregularities in the test results become more worrisome. It is under circumstances like these that visual field examinations may have to be repeated several times to improve accuracy and reduce fluctuation. One of the potential techniques is to establish a baseline from the averaged results of three visual field tests performed approximately a few weeks apart. If subsequent fields, as compared by *t*-test, vary from this baseline, two additional fields are performed and averaged with the follow-up field. The average of the baseline visual fields is then compared with the average of the follow-up fields by *t*-test, and smaller deviations can be recognized as statistically significant because there are more observations (see Fig. 11-3).[52] This works well in experimental situations or for long-term patients for whom there is already a wealth of data, but it is impractical in a busy or managed care clinic where the luxury of testing a patient half a dozen times or more within several weeks may not exist.

A second technique is to perform linear regression analysis of the visual fields over time. This technique incorporates fluctuation into the analysis and recognizes a series of visual fields whose means produce a slope that is significantly different from zero. If the slope is negative, the field may be deteriorating. At least five observations (visual field examinations) are needed for such analysis, and more observations are better.

There are a host of other techniques to manipulate and display the data from the patient's test to help the examiner reach a conclusion. One of the more popular of these is the probability map and pattern deviation printout on the Humphrey machine (see Fig. 11-20). The probability maps compare the patient's response at each point to a large age-matched control group. If the patient's response falls within a range that encompasses 95% of normals, a small dot is printed on the field chart at the test point. If less than 5% but more than 2% of normals generated a response as low as the patient, a different, more dense, symbol is printed. The darkest symbol is used if less than 1 in 200 nor-

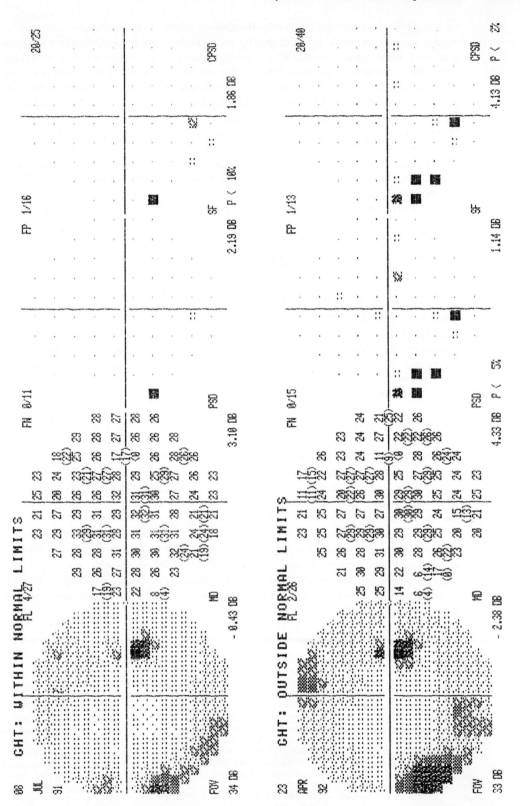

Figure 11-23 The upper field shows a slight disturbance along the border of the inferior nasal quadrant and falls within normal limits on the glaucoma hemifield test (GHT). The lower field, taken 9 months later, shows an intensified defect, which has deepened to form an inferior peripheral nasal step. It now falls outside the acceptable limits of normal on the GHT. Also note the probability maps, which show only one or two disturbed points on the first test but more than half a dozen on the subsequent examination.

mals had a value as low as the patient's. Because the points are tested in pseudorandom order, contiguous points with similar levels of depression are highly significant. Sometimes it is important to separate generalized loss, such as that caused by cataract, from localized loss, which is more often seen with moderate glaucomatous damage. The pattern deviation (not to be confused with the pattern *standard* deviation) of the Humphrey is a method to assist with this interpretation. The pattern deviation essentially subtracts generalized depression from the field to compensate for developing media opacities (see Fig. 10-1). The physician must judge whether this depression is due to glaucoma or has some other cause. The precise manipulation performed by the computer to produce the pattern deviation plot is quite complicated, but the resultant printout is very easy to read.

An additional widely used method of comparing serial visual data is to compare visual field indexes over time. A patient who has a steadily increasing corrected loss variance (CLV) on the Octopus (or CPSD on the Humphrey) may have a subtle deepening of his or her scotoma. The field should be repeated, perhaps several times depending on the level of pathology and the degree of glaucoma control indicated by the remainder of the history and physical examination.

THE FUTURE OF COMPUTERIZED PERIMETRY

Although in its present form computerized perimetry may not always offer a diagnostic advantage over meticulously performed combined kinetic and static manual perimetry,[58] the consistency of computerized perimetry provides less variation in technique over time than does manual perimetry. In addition, only the very best technicians can hope to equal or surpass the current generation of computerized machines. The average human is really no match for the computer in this realm. Computers also offer rapid statistical data analysis, graphic presentation of results, and simplified storage and retrieval of data. All of these factors make computerized perimetry the standard method for assessing the visual field.

As more and more patients are followed up over a longer time, ophthalmologists are gaining a better understanding of what represents true glaucomatous change in the visual field.[34,47] By increasing the frequency of field examinations, more data points will be available and the time needed to recognize incremental change will be reduced. This will help physicians initiate and change therapy sooner and should reduce the number of patients who progress to blindness from glaucoma.[45,59] In patients whose glaucoma is poorly controlled or who have central fixation threatened, three or four well-standardized visual field examinations per year will demonstrate progression of the disease earlier than any other currently available technique.

Perimetric software such as the Swedish Interactive Thresholding Algorithm program offered by Humphrey promises to make perimetry faster and more acceptable to patients. Artificial intelligence or pseudoartificial intelligence will allow the machines to refine the information they gather from the patient and to make more accurate diagnostic suggestions.[60] The hope is that we can improve the predictive or confirmatory value of visual field testing and thus improve our ability to diagnose and follow glaucoma.

REFERENCES

1. American Medical Association: *Guides to the evaluation of permanent impairment,* ed 2, Chicago, 1984, The Association.
2. Weber JT, and others: The visual field in advanced glaucoma, *Int Ophthalmol* 13:47, 1989.
3. Stewart WC, Shields MB: The peripheral visual field in glaucoma: re-evaluation in the age of automated perimetry, *Surv Ophthalmol* 36:59, 1991.
4. Pennebaker GE, Stewart WC: Temporal visual field in glaucoma: a re-evaluation in the automated perimetry era, *Graefes Arch Clin Exp Ophthalmol* 230:111, 1992.
5. Drance SM, and others: A screening method for temporal visual defects, *Am J Ophthalmol* 104:577, 1987.
6. Aulhorn E, Harms H: *Early visual field defects in glaucoma.* In Leydhecker W, editor: *Glaucoma: Tutzing Symposium,* 1966, Basel, 1967, Karger.
7. Hart WM Jr, Becker B: The onset and evolution of glaucomatous visual field defects, *Ophthalmology* 89:268, 1982.
8. Werner EB, Drance SM: Early visual field disturbances in glaucoma, *Arch Ophthalmol* 95:1173, 1977.
9. Kolker AE: Visual prognosis in advanced glaucoma: a comparison of medical and surgical therapy for retention of vision in 101 eyes with advanced glaucoma, *Trans Am Ophthalmol Soc* 75:539, 1977.
10. Martinez A, and others: Risk of postoperative visual loss in advanced glaucoma, *Am J Ophthalmol* 115:332, 1993.
11. Krakau CE: Hazards in evaluation of visual field decay, *Doc Ophthalmol* 63:239, 1986.
12. Krakau CET, Holmin C: *The effect of argon laser trabeculoplasty (ALT) on the visual field decay.* In Krieglstein GK, editor: *Glaucoma update III, Glaucoma Society of the International Congress of Ophthalmology, Amsterdam, September 1986,* New York, 1987, Springer-Verlag.
13. Heijl A, Bengtsson B: *The short-term effect of laser trabeculoplasty on the glaucomatous visual field.* In Heijl A, Greve EL, editors: *Sixth International Visual Field Symposium, Santa Margherita Ligure, 1984,* Dordrecht, 1985, Dr W Junk Publishers.

14. Holmin C, Krakau CET: *The visual field before and after argon laser trabeculoplasty: regression analysis based on computerized perimetry.* In Heijl A, Greve EL, editors: *Sixth International Visual Field Symposium, Santa Margherita Ligure, 1984,* Dordrecht, 1985, Dr W Junk Publishers.

15. Traverso CE, and others: *The effect of argon laser trabeculoplasty on the visual field of patients with glaucoma.* In Heijl A, Greve EL, editors: *Sixth International Visual Field Symposium, Santa Margherita Ligure, 1984,* Dordrecht, 1985, Dr W Junk Publishers.

16. Katz LJ, and others: Reversible optic disk cupping and visual field improvement in adults with glaucoma, *Am J Ophthalmol* 107:485, 1989.

17. Asman P: Computer-assisted interpretation of visual fields in glaucoma, *Acta Ophthalmol Scand Suppl* 206:1, 1992.

18. Holmin C, Krakau CET: Visual field decay in normal subjects and in cases of chronic glaucoma, *Graefes Arch Clin Exp Ophthalmol* 213:291, 1980.

19. Mikelberg FS, Drance SM: The mode of progression of visual field defects in glaucoma, *Am J Ophthalmol* 98:443, 1984.

20. Mikelberg FS, and others: The rate of progression of scotomas in glaucoma, *Am J Ophthalmol* 101:1, 1986.

21. Drance SM: Diffuse visual field loss in open-angle glaucoma, *Ophthalmology* 98:1533, 1991.

22. Flammer J: *Psychophysics in glaucoma: a modified concept of the disease.* In Greve EL, Leydhecker W, Raitta C, editors: *The Second European Glaucoma Symposium,* The Hague, 1985, Dr W Junk Publishers.

23. Lachenmayr BJ, and others: Diffuse and localized glaucomatous field loss in light-sense, flicker and resolution perimetry, *Graefes Arch Clin Exp Ophthalmol* 229:267, 1991.

24. Drance SM, and others: Diffuse visual field loss in chronic open-angle and low-tension glaucoma, *Am J Ophthalmol* 104:577, 1987.

25. Reference deleted in pages.

26. Reference deleted in pages.

27. Reference deleted in pages.

28. Esterman B: Functional scoring of the binocular field, *Ophthalmology* 89:1226, 1982.

29. Mills RP, Drance SM: Esterman disability rating in severe glaucoma, *Ophthalmology* 93:371, 1986.

30. Eizenman M, and others: Stability of fixation in healthy subjects during automated perimetry, *Can J Ophthalmol* 27:336, 1992.

31. Johnson LN, and others: Effect of intermittent versus continuous patient monitoring on reliability indices during automated perimetry, *Ophthalmology* 100:76, 1993.

32. Flammer J, and others: Quantification of glaucomatous visual field defects with automated perimetry, *Invest Ophthalmol Vis Sci* 26:176, 1985.

33. Heijl A: *The implications of the results of computerized perimetry in normals for the statistical evaluation of glaucomatous visual fields.* In Krieglstein GK, editor: *Glaucoma update III,* Berlin, 1987, Springer-Verlag.

34. Heijl A, and others: Test-retest variability in glaucomatous visual fields, *Am J Ophthalmol* 108:130, 1989.

35. Asman P, Heijl A: Glaucoma hemifield test: automated visual field evaluation, *Arch Ophthalmol* 110:812, 1992.

36. Asman P, Heijl A: Weighting according to location in computer-assisted glaucoma visual field analysis, *Acta Ophthalmol (Copenh)* 70:671, 1992.

37. Bebie H: *Computerized techniques of visual field analysis.* In Drance SM, Anderson DR, editors: *Automatic perimetry in glaucoma: a practical guide,* Orlando, 1985, Grune & Stratton.

38. Brenton RS, Argus WA: Fluctuations on the Humphrey and Octopus perimeters, *Invest Ophthalmol Vis Sci* 28:767, 1987.

39. Flammer J, and others: Differential light threshold: short and long-term fluctuation in patients with glaucoma, normal controls, and patients with suspected glaucoma, *Arch Ophthalmol* 102:704, 1984.

40. Werner EB, Saheb N, Thomas D: Variability of static visual field threshold responses in patients with elevated IOPs, *Arch Ophthalmol* 100:1627, 1984.

41. Flammer J, and others: Differential light threshold in automated static perimetry: factors influencing short-term fluctuation, *Arch Ophthalmol* 102:876, 1984.

42. Magee SD, Hoskins HD, Kidd MN: Long-term fluctuation in glaucomatous visual field. Paper presented at the annual meeting of the Association for Research in Vision and Ophthalmology, Sarasota, Fla, May 1987.

43. Jenni A, and others: Special Octopus software for clinical investigations, *Doc Ophthalmol* 35:351, 1983.

44. Flammer J, and others: JO and STATJO: programs for investigating the visual field with the Octopus automatic perimeter, *Can J Ophthalmol* 18:115, 1983.

45. Smith SD, and others: Analysis of progressive change in automated visual fields in glaucoma, *Invest Ophthalmol Vis Sci* 37:1419, 1996.

46. Schulzer M: Errors in the diagnosis of visual field progression in normal-tension glaucoma, *Ophthalmology* 101:1589, 1994.

47. Fitzke FW, and others: Analysis of visual field progression in glaucoma, *Br J Ophthalmol* 80:40, 1996.

48. Hirsbrunner HP, and others: Evaluating a perimetric expert system: experience with Octosmart, *Graefes Arch Clin Exp Ophthalmol* 228:237, 1990.

49. Kaufmann H, and others: Evaluation of visual fields by ophthalmologists and by OCTOSMART program, *Ophthalmologica* 201:104, 1990.

50. Heijl A, Asman P: A clinical study of perimetric probability maps, *Arch Ophthalmol* 107:199, 1989.

51. Brenton RS, and others: Interocular differences of the visual field in normal subjects, *Invest Ophthalmol Vis Sci* 27:799, 1986.

52. Anderson DR, Knighton RW: Perimetry and acuity perimetry. Paper presented at the meeting of the American Glaucoma Society, Iowa City, June 1987.

53. Reference deleted in pages.

54. Werner EB, Drance SM: Increased scatter of responses as a precursor of visual field changes in glaucoma, *Can J Ophthalmol* 12:140, 1977.

55. Katz J, Sommer A: Similarities between the visual fields of ocular hypertensive and normal eyes, *Arch Ophthalmol* 104:1468, 1986.

56. Hoskins HD, Simmons S, unpublished data, 1984.

57. Morgan RK, and others: Statpac 2 glaucoma change probability, *Arch Ophthalmol* 109:1690, 1991.

58. Kidd MN, Hokins HD, Magee SD: Confidence intervals for change in automated visual fields, *Br J Ophthalmol* 591, 1988.

59. Quigley HA, and others: Rate of progression in open-angle glaucoma estimated from cross-sectional prevalence of visual field damage, *Am J Ophthalmol* 122:355, 1996.

60. Blondeau P, Phelps CD: *Peripheral acuity in normal subjects.* In Heijl A, Greve EL, editors: *Sixth International Visual Field Symposium, Santa Margherita Ligure, 1984,* Dordrecht, 1985, Dr W Junk Publishers.

12

Other Psychophysical Tests

Psychophysics examines how the mind interprets physical stimuli. Examination of the visual field, which requires patients to respond to a physical light stimulus, is a psychophysical test. The current method of visual field testing measures differential light sensitivity, which is the ability to recognize a difference in light intensity between a stimulus and its background. This is most commonly accomplished by projecting a white light on a dimly illuminated white background and asking the patient to respond if he or she sees the stimulus. This is referred to as *conventional perimetry*. Although conventional perimetry has served the ophthalmic community well over the past century, it has limitations.

Studies have indicated that as many as 50% of optic nerve fibers may be lost before a field defect is detected with Goldmann kinetic perimetry.[1] Although computerized static perimetry is more sensitive,[2] it is still far from ideal. In addition to suboptimal sensitivity, conventional perimetric methods are time-consuming and relatively imprecise. The tests can take 30 to 60 minutes per patient, and many patients find the tests boring, tedious, or even demoralizing. Differential light sensitivity is a relatively primitive function. It seems reasonable to suspect that more sophisticated visual functions may be impaired early in the disease process and that testing them would provide earlier recognition of the disease state. A variety of other psychophysical tests have been investigated in the hope that they would provide a faster, more reproducible, more sensitive, and reasonably reliable test.[3-9]

There are two basic directions that new research in glaucoma testing has taken. The first is improved detection of early glaucoma. The second is better methods of glaucoma follow-up, particularly with regard to visual field interpretation and assessment of visual field progression.[10-14] Many tests currently being investigated seek to isolate one or another part of the visual system in an effort to detect early abnormalities. Conventional perimetry stimulates a broad spectrum of retinal ganglion cells. Redundancy within the visual system may mask functional loss due to early glaucoma.[15] An ideal test would either isolate the subset of retinal ganglion cells first damaged by glaucoma or stress the visual system to the point that redundancy would no longer effectively obscure functional loss.

COLOR PERCEPTION

Color perception is primarily a foveal and macular function.[16-19] Several investigators have found color vision defects in glaucoma patients.[19a-19c] Patients with advanced glaucoma had the greatest defects in color vision and non-glaucomatous controls had the least. Patients with either ocular hypertension or early glaucoma exhibited intermediate color vision loss. These results paved the way for further investigations into the effectiveness of color-specific perimetry in glaucoma detection. The most promising of these methods concentrates on the short wavelength region of the spectrum. The blue-yellow (short wavelength) system is affected more frequently and earlier in glaucoma patients and glaucoma suspects than in normals. In the late 1980s Johnson and co-workers[20] performed perimetry using a blue test stimulus on a yellow background and a standard white-on-white test in patients with early glaucomatous field loss, patients with ocular hypertension (OHT), and normal control subjects. The blue-on-yellow (b/y) test detected up to 10% more abnormalities in the patients with OHT than did the standard white-on-white (w/w) test. In patients with early glaucomatous field loss, the blue-on-yellow test detected up to 15% more abnormalities. These preliminary results have been followed by a series of studies in several sites[7,9] that verify the sensitivity of b/y or short-wavelength automated perimetry (SWAP) in glaucoma detection.

One of the seminal studies was a prospective 5-year investigation in which Johnson and co-workers[21] studied 38 patients with OHT and 62 normal controls. At the beginning of the study all of the eyes in the OHT group ($n = 76$) had normal w/w fields by conventional Humphrey perimetry. Nine of these 76 eyes had abnormal SWAP tests. After 5 years of follow-up, five of nine eyes with abnormal SWAP tests had developed w/w field defects. None of the 67 eyes with initially normal SWAP tests developed w/w field defects. The w/w field defects that developed during the follow-up period all occurred in areas that had previously been abnormal on SWAP testing. The authors concluded that SWAP testing appeared to detect glaucomatous visual field loss earlier than did standard w/w perimetry.[21]

In a later study of 232 patients with OHT, Johnson and co-workers found that the presence of SWAP defects correlated with the appearance of the vertical cup:disc ratio, patient age, family history of glaucoma, and intraocular pressure.[22] Thirty-three percent of patients at highest risk of developing glaucoma had SWAP defects, whereas only 10% of patients in the low-risk category had SWAP defects. The authors concluded that their findings supported the theory that SWAP defects precede conventional perimetric defects in patients with primary open-angle glaucoma. Their findings were very similar to those of Sample and co-workers.[23]

SWAP is not without drawbacks, however. Although most investigators agree that SWAP is more sensitive than conventional perimetry in detecting early glaucoma, its clinical utility remains unclear.

SWAP fields are more difficult to perform and interpret than are conventional fields. Wild and co-workers[9] found that the corrected interindividual variability in SWAP fields is roughly twice that found in conventional fields. This means that it may be more difficult to distinguish a pathologic change from normal fluctuation. Additionally, SWAP field testing requires about 15% more time per eye. For patients with normal or slightly abnormal fields this can add 1 to 3 minutes to a test that many already find trying. One of the authors (MVD) recently performed a test field on himself with this technology. The conventional 30-2 field took an average of 11 minutes, 58 seconds per eye; the SWAP field test took 13 minutes, 49 seconds. The SWAP targets were harder to see, making the test seem more difficult. The ultimate clinical utility of this technology will depend on the relationship between its increased sensitivity and the increased variability, time, and difficulty encountered in routine patient examinations.

CONTRAST SENSITIVITY

Contrast sensitivity is a measure of a subject's ability to recognize a simple grating pattern of bars or stripes varying from lighter to darker in a sinusoidal pattern (Fig. 12-1). As the bars become narrower, increasing contrast is required for the pattern to become visible to the normal observer. The width of the bars is defined as spatial frequency, which expresses the number of pairs of dark and light bars subtended in 1° of angle at the eye. A high spatial frequency implies narrow bars, whereas a low spatial frequency indicates wide bars. In addition to spatial frequency, the temporal frequency can be varied.

The Arden Contrast Sensitivity Plates are standard photographs of increasing contrast bars presented in six spatial frequencies: 0.2, 0.4, 0.8, 1.6, 3.2, and 6.4 cycles per degree at a viewing distance of 50 cm. These plates are useful in screening for deficits in optic nerve function that occur in various forms of optic neuritis and may be more sensitive than Snellen visual acuity tests or visual evoked potentials.[24-27] Their usefulness in glaucoma is disputed.[28-32] Although high-frequency loss is correlated with glaucomatous visual field damage, many studies find a large overlap with normal eyes; hence the diagnostic usefulness of the tests is limited.

Temporal frequency defines the rate at which the dark and light bars are reversed or modulated (usually on a video monitor). Long temporal frequencies (1 Hz) improve the visibility of high spatial frequency patterns, whereas shorter temporal frequencies enhance visibility of low spatial frequency patterns. This suggests that there may be separate neuronal pathways for the detection of high- and low-frequency patterns.

High spatial frequency contrast sensitivity deficits result from many factors, including aging and poor accommodation. The most common deficit in glaucoma is recognition of low spatial frequency patterns modulated at 8 Hz or more. Such defects have been found in the perifoveal visual field of OHT patients with no demonstrable visual field loss and in glaucoma patients with definite field defects.[33-38]

Flicker fusion is similar to temporal frequency contrast sensitivity but uses a diffuse target in-

Figure 12-1 Examples of Arden gratings. Note that the pattern is less visible toward the top of each picture. The *upper picture* shows a low-frequency pattern; the *lower picture* shows a high-frequency pattern.

stead of phase reversal (counterphase) measurement. A number of studies have investigated temporal frequency sensitivity using both diffuse and counterphase targets. Glaucoma patients have generally demonstrated deficits at modulation rates between 8 and 30 Hz.[33-38]

The overriding difficulty with contrast sensitivity as a testing modality is the difficulty in separating normal from abnormal. Simply stated, these techniques are quite good at separating normal patients from patients with moderately advanced glaucoma, but so are many other methods. Contrast sensitivity tests are also good at separating populations of patients with early glaucoma from populations of normal patients. The overlap in test results between normal, OHT, and early glaucoma patients is so great, however, that it is not practical at this time to use contrast sensitivity testing to diagnose glaucoma in individual patients. These techniques often produce consistent or confirmatory results, but they rarely produce diagnostic results in the absence of other easily obtainable information.

Interesting recent work has indicated a tendency toward reversal of early contrast sensitivity defects in glaucoma patients following treatment.[39,40] If these preliminary results prove generalizable, this may be an area in which contrast sensitivity testing has clinical utility. Although color vision and contrast sensitivity testing currently lack the specificity to be of good diagnostic or prognostic value in glaucoma, they do indicate that loss of visual function occurs early in glaucoma in the macular area. The redundancy of the nervous system is exemplified by the macular region of the eye, where it has been estimated that loss of 80% of macular nerve fibers could occur and still allow 20/20 visual acuity.[41] This redundancy prevents us from recognizing early functional change by measuring the rather crude function of differential light sensitivity that is the basis of standard perimetry. By attempting to measure more sophisticated visual functions, recognition of functional damage before major loss of neurons occurs may be possible. Such testing may also allow measurement of smaller increments of change and therefore recognition of inadequate therapy earlier in the course of the disease.

Frequency doubling contrast sensitivity tests are effective as screening examinations for early glaucoma.[41a] They produce very good sensitivity and specificity compared to conventional automated perimetry tests and require only a few minutes' test time per eye. These tests may find greater clinical use when a faster thresholding strategy is offered and an expanded normative database is available.

In addition to color and contrast sensitivity testing, visual fields measured with high-pass perimetry have been investigated.[41b-41h] High-pass perimetry uses ring-shaped targets of different sizes but constant contrast. The result is that targets are either resolvable or completely invisible. The test apparatus is a personal computer and monitor, which tend to require less dedicated space than most conventional automated perimeters. This method correlates well with conventional perimetry under most testing conditions, with the added benefit of significant time savings in many patients.

ELECTROPHYSIOLOGIC TESTING

Visual evoked potentials represent an objective way of measuring the response of the occipital cortex to stimulation of the retina with light or a pattern.[42-44] Visual evoked potential data seem to confirm contrast sensitivity data that glaucoma damage reduces sensitivity to low spatial frequency patterns presented at rather high temporal frequency rates, but the results are nonspecific.[45-48]

Measurement of pattern electroretinographic response in glaucoma patients has revealed similar findings that low spatial frequency patterns presented at high temporal frequencies elicit the greatest number of defects in OHT and glaucoma patients.[42,49-55] There is the same problem of lack of specificity for glaucomatous damage as exists with color and contrast testing.

REFERENCES

1. Quigley HA, Addicks EM, Green WR: Quantitative nerve damage in human glaucomas. III. Quantitative correlation of nerve fiber loss and visual field defect in glaucoma, ischemic neuropathy, papilledema, and toxic neuropathy, *Ophthalmology* 100:135, 1982.
2. Sommer A, and others: Clinically detectable nerve fiber atrophy precedes the onset of glaucomatous field loss, *Arch Opthhalmol* 109:77, 1991.
3. Fristrom B: Peripheral colour contrast thresholds in ocular hypertension and glaucoma, *Acta Ophthalmol Scand* 75:376, 1997.

4. Marraffa M, and others: Does nerve fiber layer thickness correlate with visual field defects in glaucoma? A study with the nerve fiber analyzer, *Ophthalmologica* 211:338, 1997.
5. Parisi V, and others: Electrophysiological assessment of visual pathways in glaucoma, *Eur J Ophthalmol* 7:229, 1997.
6. Roy M, and others: Pattern electroretinogram and spatial contrast sensitivity in primary congenital glaucoma, *Ophthalmology* 104:2136, 1997.
7. Teesalu P, and others: Correlation of blue-on-yellow visual fields with scanning confocal laser optic disc measurements, *Invest Ophthalmol Vis Sci* 38:2452, 1997.

8. Yoshiyama KK, Johnson CA: Which method of flicker perimetry is most effective for detection of glaucomatous visual field loss? *Invest Ophthalmol Vis Sci* 38:2270, 1997.
9. Wild JM, and others: Statistical aspects of the normal visual field in short-wavelength automated perimetry, *Invest Ophthalmol Vis Sci* 39:54, 1998.
10. Stamper RL, Hsu-Winges C, Sopher M: Arden contrast sensitivity testing in glaucoma, *Arch Ophthalmol* 100:947, 1982.
11. Hitchings RA, and others: Contrast sensitivity gradings in glaucoma family screening, *Br J Ophthalmol* 65:518, 1981.

12. Arden GB, Jacobson JJ: A simple grading test for contrast sensitivity: preliminary results indicate value for screening in glaucoma, *Invest Ophthalmol Vis Sci* 17:23, 1978.

13. Sample PA, Weinreb RN, Bornton RM: Acquired dyschromatopsia in glaucoma, *Surv Ophthalmol* 31:54, 1986.

14. Drance SM, and others: Acquired color vision changes in glaucoma, *Arch Ophthalmol* 99:829, 1981.

15. Johnson CA: Early loss of visual function in glaucoma, *Optom Vis Sci* 72:359, 1995.

16. Davson H: *Physiology of the eye,* New York, 1980, Academic Press.

17. Gouras P, Zrenner E: Color coding in the primate retina, *Vision Res* 21:1591, 1981.

18. Pokorny J, and others, editors: *Congenital and acquired color vision defects,* New York, 1979, Grune & Stratton.

19. Sample PA, Weinreb RN, Boynton RM: Acquired dyschromatopsia in glaucoma, *Surv Ophthalmol* 31:54, 1986.

19a. Drance SM, and others: Acquired color vision changes in glaucoma, *Arch Ophthalmol* 99:829, 1981.

19b. Adams AJ, and others: Spectrosensitivity in color discrimination changes in glaucoma and glaucoma suspect patients, *Invest Ophthalmol Vis Sci* 23:516, 1982.

20. Johnson CA, Adams AJ, Lewis RA: *Automated perimetry of short wavelength-sensitive mechanisms in glaucoma and other hypertension: preliminary findings.* In Heijl A, editor: *Perimetry update 1988/89,* Amsterdam, 1989, Kugler & Ghedini.

21. Johnson CA, and others: Blue on yellow perimetry can predict the development of glaucomatous visual field loss, *Arch Ophthalmol* 111:645, 1993.

22. Reference deleted in pages.

23. Sample PA, Weinreb RN: Color perimetry for assessment of primary open-angle glaucoma, *Invest Ophthalmol Vis Sci* 31:1869, 1990.

24. Arden GB, Gucukoglu AG: Grating test of contrast sensitivity in patients with retrobulbar neuritis, *Arch Ophthalmol* 96:1626, 1978.

25. Minassian DC, Jones BR, Zargarizadeh A: The Arden grating test of visual function: a preliminary study of its practicability and application in a rural community in north-west Iran, *Br J Ophthalmol* 62:210, 1978.

26. Skalka HW: Comparison of Snellen acuity, VER acuity, and Arden grating scores in macular and optic nerve diseases, *Br J Ophthalmol* 64:24, 1980.

27. Weatherhead RG: Use of the Arden grating test for screening, *Br J Ophthalmol* 64:591, 1980.

28. Arden GB, Jacobson JJ: A simple grating test for contrast sensitivity: preliminary results indicate value in screening for glaucoma, *Invest Ophthalmol Vis Sci* 17:23, 1978.

29. Lundh BL: Central contrast sensitivity tests in the detection of early glaucoma, *Acta Ophthalmol (Copenh)* 63:481, 1985.

30. Regan D, Neima D: Low-contrast letter charts in early diagetic retinopathy, ocular hypertension, glaucoma and Parkinson's disease, *Br J Ophthalmol* 68:885, 1984.

31. Vaegan: The clinical value of printed contrast sensitivity tests, *J Physiol (Lond)* 300:76, 1979.

32. Stamper RL, Hsu-Winges C, Sopher M: Arden contrast sensitivity testing in glaucoma, *Arch Ophthalmol* 100:947, 1982.

33. Atkin A, and others: Abnormalities of central contrast sensitivity in glaucoma, *Am J Ophthalmol* 88:205, 1979.

34. Atkin A, and others: Flicker threshold and pattern VEP latency in ocular hypertension and glaucoma, *Invest Ophthalmol Vis Sci* 24:1524, 1983.

35. Bodis-Wollner I: Pathophysiology of the visual system, The Hague, 1981, Dr. W. Junk, Publisher.

36. Brussell EM, and others: Multiflash campimetry as an indicator of visual field loss in glaucoma, *Am J Optom Physiol Opt* 63:32, 1986.

37. Neima D, Le Blanc R, Regan D: Visual field defects in ocular hypertension and glaucoma, *Arch Ophthalmol* 102:1042, 1984.

38. Regan D, Neima D: Balance between pattern and flicker sensitivities in the visual field of ophthalmological patients, *Br J Ophthalmol* 68:310, 1984.

39. Pomerance GN, Evans DW: Test-retest reliability of the CSV-1000 contrast test and its relationship to glaucoma therapy, *Invest Ophthalmol Vis Sci* 35:3357, 1994.

40. Bose SJ, and others: Nimodipine, a centrally active calcium antagonist, exerts a beneficial effect on contrast sensitivity in patients with normal-tension glaucoma and in control subjects, *Ophthalmology* 102:1236, 1995.

41. Frisen L: The neurology of visual acuity, *Brain* 103:639, 1980.

41a. Johnson CA, Samuels SJ: Screening for glaucomatous field loss with frequency doubling perimetry, *Invest Ophthalmol Vis Sci* 38:413, 1997.

41b. Chauhan BC, House PH: Inratest variability in conventional and high-pass resolution perimetry, *Ophthalmology* 98:79, 1991.

41c. Lachenmayr B, and others: Light-sense, flicker and resolution perimetry in glaucoma: a comparative study, *Graefes Arch Clin Exp Ophthalmol* 229:246, 1991.

41d. Sample PA, and others: High-pass resolution perimetry in eyes with ocular hypertension and primary open-angle glaucoma, *Am J Ophthalmol* 113:309, 1992.

41e. Chauhan BC, and others: Comparison of reliability indices in conventional and high-pass resolution perimetry, *Ophthalmology* 100:1089, 1993.

41f. Frisen L: High-pass resolution perimetry: a clinical review, *Doc Ophthalmol* 83:1, 1993.

41g. Frisen L, Nikolajeff F: Properties of high-pass resolution perimetry targets, *Acta Ophthalmol (Copenh)* 71:320, 1993.

41h. Martinez GA, and others: Comparison of high-pass resolution perimetry and standard automated perimetry in glaucoma, *Am J Ophthalmol* 119:195, 1995.

42. Marx MS, and others: Signs of early damage in glaucomatous monkey eyes: low spatial frequency losses in the pattern ERG and VEP, *Exp Eye Res* 46:173, 1988.

43. Johnson MA, and others: Pattern-evoked potentials and optic nerve fiber loss in monocular laser-induced glaucoma, *Invest Ophthalmol Vis Sci* 30:897, 1989.

44. Boschi A, and others: Contribution of pattern electroretinogram and pattern visual evoked potential in early diagnosis of primary open angle glaucoma, *Bull Soc Belge Ophthalmol* 244:85, 1992.

45. Schmeisser ET, Smith TJ: Flicker visual evoked potential differentiation of glaucoma, *Optom Vis Sci* 69:458, 1992.

46. Follman P, and others: Assessment of optic nerve function by visual evoked potential recordings in the diagnosis of glaucoma, *Doc Ophthalmol* 40:265, 1984.

47. Howe JW, Mitchell KW: Visual evoked potential changes in chronic glaucoma and ocular hypertension, *Trans Ophthalmol Soc UK* 105:457, 1986.

48. Towle V, and others: The visual evoked potential in glaucoma and ocular hypertension: effects of check size, field size and stimulation rate, *Invest Ophthalmol Vis Sci* 24:175, 1983.

49. Bobak P, and others: Pattern electroretinograms and visual evoked potentials in glaucoma and multiple sclerosis, *Am J Ophthalmol* 96:72, 1983.

50. Bodis-Wollner I, and others: Methodological aspects of signal-to-noise evaluation of simultaneous pattern electroretinogram and visual evoked potential recordings, *Doc Ophthalmol* 40:39, 1984.

51. Trick GL: Retinal potentials in patients with primary open-angle glaucoma: physiological evidence for temporal frequency tuning defects, *Invest Ophthalmol Vis Sci* 26:1750, 1985.

52. Trick GL: PRRP abnormalities in glaucoma and ocular hypertension, *Invest Ophthalmol Vis Sci* 27:1730, 1986.

53. Wanger P, Persson HE: Pattern-reversal electroretinograms in unilateral glaucoma, *Invest Ophthalmol Vis Sci* 24:749, 1983.

54. Wanger P, Persson HE: Pattern-reversal electroretinograms in ocular hypertension, *Doc Ophthalmol* 61:27, 1985.

55. Vaegan SL, and others: Flash and pattern electroretinogram changes with optic atrophy and glaucoma, *Exp Eye Res* 60:697, 1995.

13

Optic Nerve Anatomy and Pathophysiology

In the past decade two significant changes have evolved in articulating the underlying pathogenic mechanisms of chronic open-angle glaucoma. The first has been the elimination of intraocular pressure (IOP) from the essential definition of the disease.[1-3] In other words, glaucomatous optic neuropathy is thought of as an optic nerve disorder in which IOP is one important causative, dose-related risk factor among several others. The other important shift has been in the conceptual framework for pathogenesis. At one time theories of glaucomatous pathophysiology were considered either "mechanical" or "vasogenic." However, such a dichotomy has proven useless clinically and of marginal rhetorical value. Instead a multifactorial spectrum of tantalizing observations is proving most useful in underpinning theoretic and experimental advances.

All glaucomatous atrophy shares the following features:[4] (1) progressive death of retinal ganglion cells, manifesting as (2) characteristic histopathologic alteration of the optic nerve—known as excavation—which is functionally apparent as (3) sequential visual field deterioration in characteristic patterns. Detailed understanding of the microanatomy of the optic nerve is intimately entwined with the current concepts of glaucomatous pathophysiology.

ANATOMY OF THE OPTIC NERVE HEAD

The optic nerve head (ONH) can be divided into four anatomic parts: the surface layer and the prelaminar, laminar, and retrolaminar portions. Each portion of the ONH is made up of axons (nerve fibers) grouped into bundles, blood vessels, and supporting glial tissue.

The superficial nerve fiber layer (SNFL) of the ONH has its most anterior limit at the point where the nerve contacts the vitreous. For histopathologic and clinical purposes, the peripheral edge of the nerve is defined by the anterior limits of the scleral ring. The posterior limit of the SNFL is recognized histologically as the point at which the axon bundles have completed their 90° turn from the plane of the retina and have reached the level of the choroid. The prelaminar portion of the ONH is the indistinct segment of the axons surrounded by the outer retina, choriocapillaris, and choroid; structurally the astroglial component here is considerably increased compared with the SNFL. The laminar portion of the nerve is contained within the lamina cribrosa; here the glial-wrapped axon bundles are confined in the relatively rigid pores of the specialized laminar scleral plates. Posterior to this is the retrolaminar portion of the optic nerve, where its thickness is doubled by the presence of myelinating oligodendrocytes. These and other eponymic details are illustrated in Figure 13-1.

In the human eye the distribution of the nerve fibers from the peripheral retina toward the optic nerve is such that axons from peripheral ganglion cells are progressively overlayered by axons derived from cell bodies closer to the optic nerve (Fig. 13-2).[5] These peripheral fibers remain peripheral as they enter the disc; central fibers enter centrally, adjacent to the physiologic cup. This topographic arrangement correlates with the clinical progression of the glaucomatous visual field: paracentral scotomas appear early in the disease as the cup enlarges, and the peripheral field remains until the peripheral axons in the nerve are affected.[6]

The arterial blood supply to the ONH varies among individuals,[7-11] but there is general agreement about its fundamental components (Fig. 13-3).[12] The central retinal artery (CRA) and the short

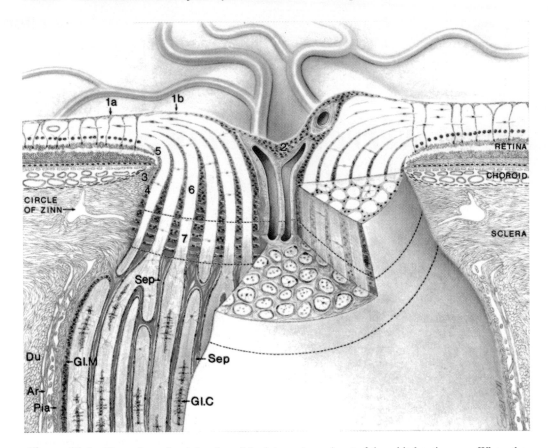

Figure 13-1 Three-dimensional drawing of the intraocular and part of the orbital optic nerve. Where the retina terminates at the optic disc edge, the Müller cells *(1a)* are in continuity with the astrocytes, forming the internal limiting membrane of Elschnig, *(1b)*. In some specimens Elschnig's membrane is thickened in the central portion of the disc to form the central meniscus of Kuhnt, *(2)*. At the posterior termination of the choroid on the temporal side, the border tissue of Elschnig *(3)* lies between the astrocytes surrounding the optic nerve canal *(4)*, and the stroma of the choroid. On the nasal side, the choroidal stroma is directly adjacent to the astrocytes surrounding the nerve. This collection of astrocytes *(4)*, surrounding the canal is know as the *border tissue of Jacoby*. This is continuous with a similar glial lining called the *intermediary tissue of Kuhnt (5)*, at the termination of the retina. The nerve fibers of the retina are segregated into approximately 1000 bundles, or fascicles, by astrocytes *(6)*. On reaching the lamina cribrosa *(upper dotted line)*, the nerve fascicles, *(7)* and their surrounding astrocytes are separated from each other by connective tissue *(blue)*. This connective tissue is the cribriform plate, which is an extension of scleral collagen and elastic fibers through the nerve. The external choroid also sends some connective tissue to the anterior part of the lamina. At the external part of the lamina cribrosa *(lower dotted line)*, the nerve fibers become myelinated and columns of oligodendrocytes *(black and white cells)* and a few astrocytes *(red-colored cells)* are present within the nerve fascicles. The astrocytes surrounding the fascicles form a thinner layer here than in the laminar and prelaminar portion. The bundles continue to be separated by connective tissue all the way to the chiasm *(Sep)*. This connective tissue is derived from the pia mater *(Pia)* and is know as the *septal tissue*. A mantle of astrocytes *(GLM)*, continuous anteriorly with the border tissue of Jacoby, surrounds the nerve along it orbital course. The dura *(Du)*, arachnoid *(Ar)*, and pia matter are shown. The central retinal vessels are surrounded by a perivascular connective tissue throughout their course in the nerve; this connective tissue blends with the connective tissue of the cribriform plate in the lamina cribrosa; it is called the central supporting connective tissue strand here. (From Anderson D: *Arch Ophthalmol* 82:506-530, 1969. Copyright 1969. American Medical Association.)

posterior ciliary arteries (SPCAs) all contribute directly or indirectly to a capillary plexus that supplies the ONH. The venous drainage of the ONH is almost entirely through branches of the central retinal vein, although important choroidal collaterals exist; these collaterals may appear as retinociliary shunts in instances of disturbed retinal circulation.

The branches of the CRA supply the SNFL. This is the network responsible for the flame-

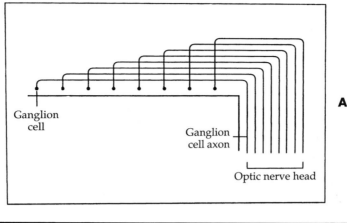

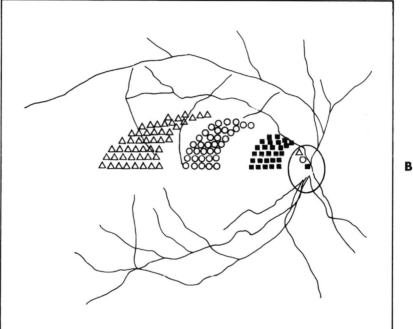

Figure 13-2 **A,** Schematic diagram of the axonal arrangement in humans shows that the closer the ganglion cell is to the optic nerve, the more superficial its axon is in the nerve fiber layer. Thus axons from cells in the periphery occupy the periphery of the optic nerve, and axons from cells closer to the disc occupy the center of the nerve head. (From Airaksinen PJ, Alanko HI: *Graefes Arch Clin Ophthalmol* 220:193, 1983.) **B,** Schematic diagram of the horizontal topography of axonal bundles from arcuate areas of the retina as they project into the anterior part of the optic nerve viewed ophthalmoscopically. Bjerrum areas of disc correspond to approximately the central 30° of the superior and inferior temporal quadrants. Peripherally located ganglion cells project to the peripheral optic nerve *(triangles),* centrally located ganglion cells to intermediate portions of the nerve *(circles),* and peripapillary ganglion cells to the central portion of the nerve *(squares).* (From Minckler DS: *Arch Opthalmol* 98:1635, 1980.)

(splinter-) disc hemorrhages seen clinically, and it is also the vascular bed that appears in fluorescein angiograms of the ONH. The prelaminar ONH is supplied by branches of the SPCAs, which enter the disc substance through the adjacent sclera and posterior to the choroidal bed (see Figs. 13-1 and 13-3). With one prolific exception,[7-10,13,14] most investigators maintain that vessels derived from the peripapillary choroid make only a minor contribution to the blood supply of the anterior ONH.[11,12,15-21]

The laminar portion is vascularized primarily by centripetal SPCAs, although an axial longitudinal anastomotic capillary bed has been described.[11] The ability of that network to provide col-

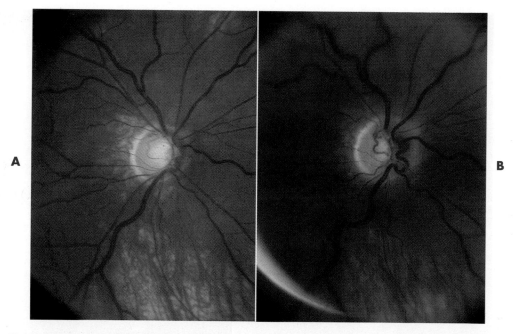

Figure 14-6 This 5-year-old child underwent two goniotomies. **A,** The optic nerve before the first goniotomy. **B,** The optic nerve before the second goniotomy. Note an increasing thickness of the rim with an increasing pinkness of the nerve head as pressure is lowered after each goniotomy.

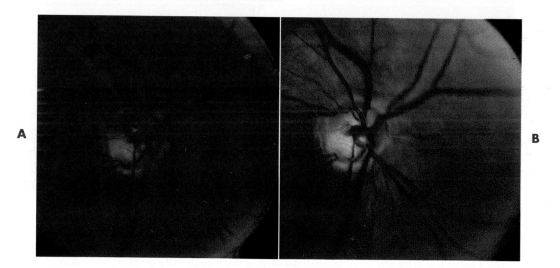

Figure 14-7 **A,** Extension of the cup (notching) inferotemporally. **B,** 7 years later, note thinning of the neural rim and shifts of the positions of blood vessels. (From Campbell DG, Netland PA: *Stereo atlas of glaucoma,* St Louis, 1998, Mosby.)

cause profound visual field loss that may recover dramatically when the compression is relieved.[72] In glaucoma this phenomenon exists to a small degree, in that apparent recovery of visual field loss has occurred following treatment of the glaucoma. Spaeth and co-workers[12,73] suggest this as one way of recognizing the adequacy of treatment. In our experience, however, this recovery is never great and is certainly not manifest when defects in the nerve fiber layer have already appeared. As the axons die, they occupy less space in the scleral canal, and the cup enlarges. Quigley[74] found up to 40% of some nerves could be lost without having any recognizable field defect on Goldmann perimetry. Thus nerve damage can occur and progress with little or no field defect. Despite advances in computerized perimetry and other psychophysical tests for early glaucoma, progressive optic disc cupping without visual field loss remains an early indicator of glaucoma, assuming no other disease process is occurring.[3-6]

Position of Central Retinal Vessels and Branches

It has been observed that there is local susceptibility to NRR loss in the rim sector farthest from the major trunk of the central retinal vessels.[25] This specific relationship of glaucomatous loss can be useful to monitor in circumstances with an unusually shaped NRR.

As the cup enlarges, the retinal vessels, which usually pass perpendicularly through the disc tissue to reach the retina, are displaced externally following the receding nasal wall of the cup. Where the vessels shift from a more vertical orientation along the cup wall to a horizontal orientation on the retinal surface, there is a bend in the vessel. Change in the shape or position of that bend, as may be seen when comparing serial photographs, is a sensitive indicator of disc change and can be monitored with computer analysis (Fig. 14-7).[75]

Vessels that pass circumferentially across the temporal aspect of the cup have been called circumlinear vessels. If they pass the exposed depths of the cup, they are "bared."[76] Baring of circumlinear vessels is seen because as the cup recedes, it exposes the vessels. Baring of circumlinear vessels is seen commonly in glaucomatous cups, but it may be seen in normal cups as well.[77]

PERIPAPILLARY DISC CHANGES

By paying attention to alterations in the area immediately surrounding the optic disc, valuable information can be determined about the glaucoma status of the ONH. Four phenomena should be evaluated—optic disc splinter hemorrhages; changes in the RNFL; variations in the diameter of retinal arterioles; and patterns of peripapillary choroidal atrophy (PPCA).

Optic Disc Hemorrhages

Nearly 30 years ago Drance and co-workers[78] revived interest in splinter hemorrhages on the ONH in glaucoma patients. These are either flame-shaped or blot hemorrhages that can occur at any location around the disc rim (Fig. 14-8). They usually are located within the nerve fiber layer extending across the disc rim into the retina, but they may occur deep in the disc tissue. They last for a variable interval between 2 and 35 weeks.[79] Because they appear in areas of preserved NRR, they are not usually seen in advanced cases of cupping in which little rim remains.[34]

The literature on optic disc hemorrhage has been dominated by case series and case-controlled studies in eyes under surveillance for glaucoma.[80] As a result, many assertions about the association of disc hemorrhage with one type of glaucoma (e.g., "low-tension glaucoma"[79,81-83]) or about the specificity of this finding for predicting glaucomatous loss[84-86] reflect this selection bias. A comprehensive Australian population-based study, using subjects rather than eyes, provides a more broad-based context for assigning meaning to disc hemorrhages.[87]

This epidemiologic survey of mostly whites in the Blue Mountains near Sydney used a thorough glaucoma assessment including computerized fields and disc photographs on all participants. An overall prevalence rate of optic disc hemorrhage of 1.4% was found; this was slightly higher than the rates of 0.8%[84] and 0.9%[88] reported in the only two other population-based studies in the literature. Positive correlation was seen with increasing age and among women; no correlation was identified with a history of vascular events, smoking, aspirin use, or myopia.[87] Most remarkable was that 70% of all disc hemorrhages were seen in subjects *without* any definite signs of glaucoma. Only 1 out of 4 patients over 50 years old with a disc hemorrhage demonstrated other disc and visual field signs of glaucoma. Thus the specificity of this sign as a screening tool does not seem particularly good, as reported elsewhere.[89]

Nevertheless, among patients known to have glaucoma, disc hemorrhages were decidedly more common (13.8%); for every high-pressure glaucoma eye there were three eyes with "low pressure" disease. And when compared with normals, patients with ocular hypertension had twice the frequency of disc hemorrhage.[87] Others have demonstrated a strong association between disc hemorrhages in glaucomatous eyes with RNFL loss (especially inferotemporally), NRR notching, and discrete visual field loss.[80,90,91] Such hemorrhages may precede progression of the disease,[80,90,92-97] with subsequent disc and field changes manifesting between 1 and 7 years later.[95,97] Others report

126. Papastathopoulos KI, Jonas JB: Focal narrowing of retinal arterioles in optic nerve atrophy, *Ophthalmology* 102:1706, 1995.

127. Rankin SJ, Drance SM: Peripapillary focal retinal arteriolar narrowing in open angle glaucoma, *J Glaucoma* 5:22, 1996.

128. Primrose J: The incidence of the peripapillary halo glaucomatosus, *Trans Ophthalmol Soc UK* 89:585, 1969.

129. Wilensky JT, Kolker AE: Peripapillary changes in glaucoma, *Am J Ophthalmol* 81:341, 1976.

130. Anderson DR: *Correlation of the peripapillary anatomy with the disc damage and field abnormalities in glaucoma.* In Greve EL, Heijl A, editors: *Fifth International Visual Field Symposium,* Dordrecht, Netherlands, 1983, Dr W Junk.

131. Anderson DR: *Relationship of peripapillary halos and crescents to glaucomatous cupping.* In Krieglstein GK, editor: *Glaucoma update III,* Berlin/Heidelberg, 1987, Springer-Verlag.

132. Buus DR, Anderson DR: Peripapillary crescents and halos in normal-tension glaucoma and ocular hypertension, *Ophthalmology* 96:16, 1989.

133. Kasner O, Feuer WJ, Anderson DR: Possibly reduced prevalence of peripapillary crescents in ocular hypertension, *Can J Ophthalmol* 24:211, 1989.

134. Nevarez J, Rockwood EJ, Anderson DR: The configuration of peripapillary tissue in unilateral glaucoma, *Arch Ophthalmol* 106:901, 1988.

135. Rockwood EJ, Anderson DR: Acquired peripapillary changes and progression in glaucoma, *Graefes Arch Clin Exp Ophthalmol* 226:510, 1988.

136. Tezel G, and others: Parapapillary chorioretinal atrophy in patients with ocular hypertension: I. An evaluation as a predictive factor for the development of glaucomatous damage, *Arch Ophthalmol* 115:1503, 1997.

137. Heijl A, Samander C: Peripapillary atrophy and glaucomatous field defects, *Doc Ophthalmol Proc Series* 35:1, 1985.

138. Park KH, and others: Correlation between peripapillary atrophy and optic nerve damage in normal-tension glaucoma, *Ophthalmology* 103:1899, 1996.

139. Tezel G, and others: Comparative optic disc analysis in normal pressure glaucoma, primary open-angle glaucoma, and ocular hypertension, *Ophthalmology* 103:2105, 1996.

140. Tezel G, and others: Parapapillary chorioretinal atrophy in patients with ocular hypertension: II. An evaluation of progressive changes, *Arch Ophthalmol* 115:1509, 1997.

141. Derick RJ, and others: A clinical study of peripapillary crescents of the optic disc in chronic experimental glaucoma in monkey eyes, *Arch Ophthalmol* 112:846, 1994.

142. Airaksinen PJ, and others: *Change of peripapillary atrophy in glaucoma.* In Krieglstein GK, editor: *Glaucoma update III,* Berlin/Heidelberg, 1987, Springer-Verlag.

143. Jonas JB, Naumann GO: Parapapillary chorioretinal atrophy in normal and glaucoma eyes. II. Correlations, *Invest Ophthalmol Vis Sci* 30:919, 1989.

144. Jonas JB, and others: Parapapillary chorioretinal atrophy in normal and glaucoma eyes. I. Morphometric data, *Invest Ophthalmol Vis Sci* 30:908, 1989.

145. Kubota T, Jonas JB, Naumann GO: Direct clinico-histological correlation of parapapillary chorioretinal atrophy, *Br J Ophthalmol* 77:103, 1993.

146. Sugiyama K, and others: The association of optic disc hemorrhage with retinal nerve fiber layer defect and peripapillary atrophy in normal-tension glaucoma, *Ophthalmology* 104:1926, 1997.

147. Jonas JB, Schiro D: Localised wedge shaped defects of the retinal nerve fibre layer in glaucoma, *Br J Ophthalmol* 78:285, 1994.

148. Jonas JB, Xu L: Parapapillary chorioretinal atrophy in normal-pressure glaucoma, *Am J Ophthalmol* 115:501, 1993.

149. Nicolela MT, and others: Various glaucomatous optic nerve appearances: a color Doppler imaging study of retrobulbar circulation, *Ophthalmology* 103:1670, 1996.

150. Goldmann H: *Problems in present-day glaucoma research.* In Streiff EB, Babel F, editors: *Modern problems in ophthalmology,* Basel, 1957, S Karger.

151. Alvarado JA, Hogan MJ, Weddell JE: *Histology of the human eye,* Philadelphia, 1971, WB Saunders.

152. Jonas JB, and others: Optic disc size and optic nerve damage in normal pressure glaucoma, *Br J Ophthalmol* 79:1102, 1995.

153. Caprioli J: *Quantitative measurements of the optic nerve head.* In Ritch R, Shields MB, Krupin T, editors: *The glaucomas,* ed 2, St Louis, 1996, Mosby.

154. Zangwill L, de Souza-Lima M, Weinreb RN: *Confocal scanning laser ophthalmoscopy to detect glaucomatous optic neuropathy.* In Schuman JS, editor: *Imaging in glaucoma,* Thorofare, NJ, 1997, SLACK.

155. de Souza-Lima M: *Scanning laser polarimetry to assess the nerve fiber layer.* In Schuman JS, editor: *Imaging in glaucoma,* Thorofare, NJ, 1997, SLACK.

156. Schuman JS: *Optical coherence tomography for imaging and quantitation of nerve fiber layer thickness.* In Schuman JS, editor: *Imaging in glaucoma,* Thorofare, NJ, 1997, SLACK.

157. Schuman JS: *Imaging of the optic nerve head and nerve fiber layer in glaucoma.* In Epstein DL, Allingham RR, Schuman JS, editors: *Chandler and Grant's glaucoma,* ed 4, Baltimore, 1996, Williams & Wilkins.

158. Shields MB: The future of computerized image analysis in the management of glaucoma, *Am J Ophthalmol* 108:319, 1989.

159. Chauhan BC, and others: Test-retest variability of topographic measurements with confocal scanning laser tomography in patients with glaucoma and control subjects, *Am J Ophthalmol* 118:9, 1994.

160. Cioffi GA, and others: Confocal laser scanning ophthalmoscope: reproducibility of optic nerve head topographic measurements with the confocal laser scanning ophthalmoscope, *Ophthalmology* 100:57, 1993.

161. Brigatti L, Caprioli J: Correlation of visual field with scanning confocal optic disc measurements in glaucoma, *Arch Ophthalmol* 113:1191, 1995.

162. Cucevic V, and others: Use of a confocal laser scanning ophthalmoscope to detect glaucomatous cupping of the optic disc, *Aust N Z J Ophthalmol* 25:217, 1997.

163. Uchida H, Brigatti L, Caprioli J: Detection of structural damage from glaucoma with confocal laser image analysis, *Invest Ophthalmol Vis Sci* 37:2393, 1996.

164. Tjon-Fo-Sang MJ, de Vries MJ, Lemij HG: Measurement by nerve fiber analyzer of retinal nerve fiber layer thickness in normal subjects and patients with ocular hypertension, *Am J Ophthalmol* 122:220, 1996.

165. Tjon-Fo-Sang MJ, Lemij HG: The sensitivity and specificity of nerve fiber layer measurements in glaucoma as determined with scanning laser polarimetry, *Am J Ophthalmol* 123:62, 1997.

166. Tjon-Fo-Sang MJ, and others: Improved reproducibility of measurements with the nerve fiber analyzer, *J Glaucoma* 6:203, 1997.

167. Anton A, and others: Nerve fiber layer measurements with scanning laser polarimetry in ocular hypertension, *Arch Ophthalmol* 115:331, 1997.

168. Poinoosawmy D, and others: Variation of nerve fibre layer thickness measurements with age and ethnicity by scanning laser polarimetry, *Br J Ophthalmol* 81:350, 1997.

169. Niessen AG, and others: Retinal nerve fiber layer assessment by scanning laser polarimetry and standardized photography, *Am J Ophthalmol* 121:484, 1996.

PART IV

Clinical Entities

15

Angle-Closure Glaucoma With Pupillary Block

PRIMARY ANGLE-CLOSURE GLAUCOMA WITH PUPILLARY BLOCK

Historical Review

The Hippocratic aphorisms include two mentions of blindness, one of which may refer to glaucoma: "When headache develops in cases of ophthalmia and accompanies it for a long time there is a risk of blindness."[1] Gradually the different causes of blindness were separated, with the most important distinction between cataract (which was treatable by couching) and glaucoma (which was not). Thirteenth century Syrian Salah-ad-din-ibin Yusuf al-kahal bi Hamah described a condition that he called "migraine of the eye" or "headache of the pupil," which resembles acute angle-closure glaucoma in that it consists of pain, hemicrania, and dilation of the pupil.[1]

Itinerant British oculist Richard Banister published a clear description of end-stage or absolute glaucoma in which he observed that the eye was hard to palpation.[2] Further descriptions of congestive glaucoma and the firmness of the eye were published by Platner, Guthrie, Beer, and Demours.[2] Demours also reported halo vision in glaucoma.[2]

In 1853, von Arlt ascribed the cause of glaucoma to the struggle for a livelihood, grief, weeping, vexation, eyestrain, and a damp dwelling.[3] Most other scientists in the 18th and 19th centuries viewed glaucoma as a disease of the vitreous humor that was associated with iritis and arthritis. Following the development of the ophthalmoscope in 1851 by von Helmholtz, Jacobson, Jaeger, von Graefe, and Weber disproved this theory by noting glaucomatous cupping in eyes with clear vitreous bodies.[2] The lack of vitreous involvement in glaucomatous eyes was confirmed histopathologically by Mackenzie and Muller.[2]

Another important step in our understanding of glaucoma came from studies by Leber, Weber, and Knies of the aqueous humor circulation in animal and human eyes.[2] The association between shallow anterior chambers and acute attacks of angle-closure glaucoma became clear in the late 19th century.[4,5] It was during this time that von Graefe,[5] in one of the landmark papers of ophthalmology, proposed iridectomy as a treatment for glaucoma. In the 1920s Curran,[6] Banziger,[7] and Raeder[8] independently put forth theories regarding the mechanism of pupillary block and further proposed that peripheral iridectomy cured angle-closure glaucoma by relieving this block. The efficacy of peripheral iridectomy as a treatment for glaucoma was confirmed by many physicians, including Gifford,[9] O'Connor,[10] Elschnig,[11] Barkan,[12] and Chandler.[13] With the development of gonioscopy by Trantas, Salzmann, Koeppe, and Troncoso, the mechanism of angle closure was confirmed; and glaucoma was classified in modern terms by Barkan according to the state of the angle.[14] This classification system was elaborated by Sugar[15] and later adopted by a variety of organizations, including the American Academy of Ophthalmology.[16]

Our understanding of angle-closure glaucoma was greatly enhanced by ultrasonic biometry and the ultrasonic biomicroscope. These modalities showed that eyes with pupillary block angle-closure glaucoma tend to be shorter; more hyperopic; and have a steeper corneal curvature, a shallower anterior chamber, and a thicker and more anteriorly placed lens than that in eyes with normal or open-angle glaucoma.[17,18]

Today glaucoma is classified into open-angle and angle-closure forms (see Chapter 1). In open-angle glaucoma there is increased resistance to aqueous humor outflow through the trabecular meshwork–Schlemm's canal–episcleral venous system by a variety of mechanisms that do not involve obstruction by the iris. In the angle-closure glaucomas there is increased resistance to outflow because the peripheral iris covers the trabecular meshwork, preventing the aqueous humor from reaching the outflow channels.

The angle-closure glaucomas are classified according to the presence or absence of pupillary block. When pupillary block is present, aqueous humor is restricted in its passage from the posterior chamber to the anterior chamber. This creates a pressure differential that is adequate to push or balloon the peripheral iris forward into contact with the trabecular meshwork. Nonpupillary block angle-closure glaucoma refers to conditions in which the iris is pushed or pulled against the trabecular meshwork by mechanisms other than pupillary block. The pupillary block angle-closure glaucomas are further divided into primary and secondary forms, depending on whether there is a known additional ocular or systemic disorder that accounts for the increased resistance to aqueous humor flow from the posterior to the anterior chamber. However, the distinction between primary pupillary block glaucoma and that caused by swelling of the crystalline lens as a result of aging is quite blurred.

Angle-closure glaucoma has often been described by the adjective pairs *congestive/noncongestive and compensated/uncompensated*. These terms have been abandoned because they neither specify the pathophysiology of the condition nor indicate the correct treatment. Furthermore, congestion and corneal edema are not invariably a part of angle-closure glaucoma and may occur in some forms of open-angle glaucoma such as that associated with iridocyclitis or pigmentary glaucoma. The congestion and corneal decompensation are more a function of the rapidity with which the pressure rises and its ultimate severity rather than the cause. Today the terms *acute, subacute,* and *chronic* are often used to reflect the time course and/or presence of symptoms. These descriptions can apply to any form of angle-closure glaucoma—pupillary block or nonpupillary block, primary or secondary.

Pathophysiology

The pathophysiology of primary pupillary block angle-closure glaucoma involves the following fundamental factors: (1) lens–iris apposition with resultant bowing forward of the peripheral iris; and (2) an anatomically predisposed eye that allows the anterior displaced peripheral iris to occlude the trabecular meshwork. Because the posterior iris surface is in contact with the anterior surface of the lens, aqueous humor passes from the posterior to the anterior chamber against the resistance caused by this lens–iris contact. The iris sphincter muscle can be thought of as having a posterior vector of force that causes the central iris to "hug" the anterior lens surface.[19] The dilator muscle may also contribute to some of this posterior force vector. The resistance to flow, referred to as *relative pupillary block,* causes a slight pressure differential so that the pressure in the posterior chamber is slightly higher than that in the anterior chamber (Fig. 15-1). Under normal circumstances, this pressure differential is of little significance; however, if the pupillary block were to increase, the pressure posterior to the iris would increase—forcing the peripheral iris to billow forward like a sail in the wind. As the iris becomes more elastic with age, the amount of forward billowing would increase.

If the peripheral iris bows forward slightly or if the anterior chamber is relatively large, the effect on intraocular pressure (IOP) and anterior chamber dynamics would be inconsequential. However, if the peripheral iris bows forward enough to cover the trabecular meshwork, the normal outflow of aqueous humor from the anterior chamber would be blocked and the IOP would increase[20] (Fig. 15-2). Angle-closure glaucoma typically occurs in eyes with small anterior segments in which even a relatively small forward bow of the peripheral iris may contact the trabecular meshwork. The tight junctions of the posterior pigment epithelium prevent fluid flow through the iris.

IOP and outflow facility are normal in eyes with shallow but open angles no matter how narrow the angle appears. In contrast, when the iris is in contact with the trabecular meshwork, IOP rises and outflow facility falls in proportion to the extent of the angle closed; the resultant IOP would depend on the function (outflow facility) of the remaining unobstructed angle. As noted previously, increased pupillary block and angle-closure glaucoma typically occur in eyes with small anterior segments. This anatomic configuration is inherited under polygenic influence[21] and includes the following features:

1. Shallow anterior chamber both centrally[22-24] and peripherally.[23,25,26] Both Lowe[21] and Alsbirk[27] found angle-closure glaucoma to be uncommon in eyes with central anterior cham-

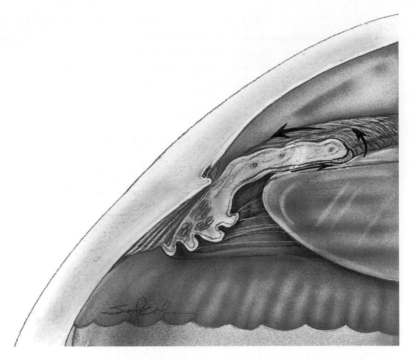

Figure 15-1 Relative pupillary block.

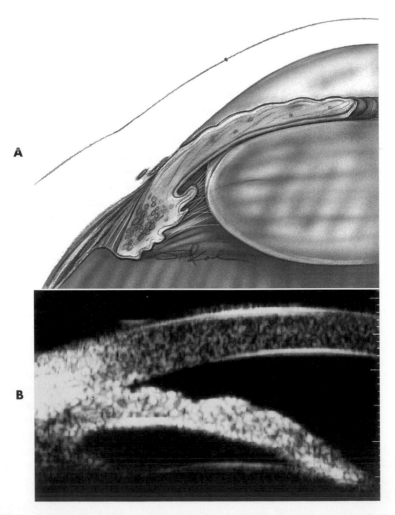

Figure 15-2 **A,** Pupillary block leading to angle closure. **B,** Ultrasound biomicroscopic photograph illustrating central posterior iris apposition causing the iris to bow forward and occlude the anterior chamber angle. (Courtesy of Robert Ritch, M.D.)

ber depths of 2.5 mm or greater (Table 15-1). Although one authority has reported that primary angle-closure glaucoma with pupillary block can occur in eyes with deep anterior chambers (≥2.6 mm), this has to be a rare phenomenon and may have other explanations.[28]

2. Decreased anterior chamber volume. Using photogrammetric images, Lee and co-workers[18] computed that anterior chamber volume was approximately 50% lower in eyes with angle-closure glaucoma than in normal eyes (Table 15-2).

3. Short axial length of the globe.[17,23]

4. Small corneal diameter.[25,29]

5. Increased posterior corneal curvature (i.e., decreased radius of posterior corneal curvature).[30-32]

6. Decreased corneal height.[24]

7. Anterior position of the lens with respect to the ciliary body.[24]

8. Increased curvature of the anterior lens surface.[33]

9. Increased thickness of the lens.[17,24,33,34]

10. More anterior insertion of the iris into the ciliary body, giving a narrower approach to the angle recess.

Each of these factors acts to increase the contact between the iris and lens, to add to the resistance to flow from posterior to anterior chamber, and to accentuate relative pupillary block. A strong correlation was recently found between an increase in the lens thickness: ocular axial length ratio and the need for peripheral iridotomy.[35] However, none of the biometric factors considered alone or together allow the ophthalmologist to diagnose or predict angle-closure glaucoma; such diagnosis and prediction require the synthesis of clinical data, including history, slit-lamp findings, IOP, and gonioscopic examination.

The biometric peculiarities of eyes predisposed to angle-closure glaucoma are accentuated by three trends associated with aging. First, the lens grows in thickness throughout life.[36,37] Second, the

Table 15-1

Central Anterior Chamber Depth and Angle-Closure Glaucoma in a Group of Eskimos

Anterior Chamber Depth (mm)	Prevalence of Angle-Closure Glaucoma (%)
>2.5	0
2.0–2.49	1
1.5–1.99	20
<1.5	85

Modified from Alsbirk PH: *Acta Ophthalmol (Copenh)* 53:89, 1975.

Table 15-2

Anterior Chamber Diameter and Volume In Eyes With Various Forms of Angle-Closure Glaucoma

	Anterior Chamber Diameter (mm)*	Anterior Chamber Volume (μl)*
Normal eyes (first series)	12.3 ± 0.5	149.5 ± 25.1
Normal eyes (second series)	12.5 ± 0.4	167.9 ± 31.5
Eyes with acute angle-closure glaucoma	11.4 ± 0.8	81.4 ± 14.1
Fellow eyes	11.3 ± 0.7	76.0 ± 25.1
Subacute angle-closure glaucoma	11.5 ± 0.6	94.3 ± 24.3
Chronic angle-closure glaucoma	10.9 ± 0.7	91.2 ± 26.0
Narrow angles without glaucoma	11.3 ± 0.7	91.3 ± 24.4
Plateau iris	11.6 ± 0.6	112.6 ± 26.4

Modified from Lee DA, Brubaker RF, Ilstrup DM: *Arch Ophthalmol* 102:46, 1984, American Medical Association.
*Values are mean ± SD.

lens assumes a more anterior position with age.[36] Third, the pupil becomes increasingly miotic with age. All of these age-associated changes increase the contact between the iris and lens, potentiate pupillary block, and reduce anterior chamber depth and volume. It is estimated that central anterior chamber depth decreases 0.01 mm/year.[37]

The mechanisms described above are sufficient to explain the development of a gradual closure of the angle (chronic or "creeping" angle closure). Many cases of acute or subacute angle-closure glaucoma are precipitated by a specific event that accentuates the pupillary block (Box 15-1). Moderate pupillary dilation is the most immediate cause of increased pupillary block; pupil dilation itself may be precipitated by an event such as pharmacologic dilation or a prone position. It is thought that the posterior vector of force of the iris sphincter muscle reaches its maximum when the pupil is moderately dilated to a diameter of 3.0 to 4.5 mm.[19,38] Furthermore, when the pupil is moderately dilated, the peripheral iris is under less tension and is more easily pushed forward into contact with the trabecular meshwork. Finally, dilation may also thicken and bunch the peripheral iris in the angle. In contrast, when the pupil is *widely* dilated, there is little or no contact between the lens and the iris and minimum pupillary block. This fact explains why acute angle-closure glaucoma rarely occurs while the pupil is in the process of dilating due to a topical agent; the dilation occurs rapidly enough that pupillary block does not have time to develop. Rather, pupillary block tends to occur as the pupil slowly recovers because the pupil will have a longer time at middilation. Pupillary block can also be increased by marked pupillary miosis.

It is common for acute angle-closure glaucoma to be precipitated in predisposed individuals by an emotional upset (e.g., bad news, pain, fear, illness, an accident) or dim illumination (e.g., in a restaurant or theater). Emotional upset dilates the pupil through increased sympathetic tone to the iris dilator muscle, whereas dim illumination dilates the pupil through decreased cholinergic tone to the iris sphincter muscle. Acute angle-closure glaucoma can also be triggered in predisposed individuals by a variety of medications applied topically, systemically, or transdermally. These medications include tranquilizers, bronchodilators, vasoconstrictors, appetite suppressants, antiParkinsonian agents, cold preparations, antinausea agents, and antispasmodics (Box 15-2).[39-41] These drugs dilate the pupil through an anticholinergic effect on the iris sphincter muscle or a sympathomimetic effect on the iris dilator muscle.

Other drugs that cause extreme pupillary miosis (e.g., cholinesterase inhibitors) can also trigger angle-closure glaucoma. Intranasal use of cocaine has reportedly induced an attack of angle-closure glaucoma.[42] An additional precipitating factor may be forward lens movement, which occurs in a variety of situations such as reading, changes in body position, and miotic therapy. Mapstone and Clark[43] proposed that anterior chamber depth fluctuates in a diurnal fashion, reaching its shallowest state during the evening. They postulated that this phenomenon may play a role in precipitating attacks of angle-closure glaucoma. This theory requires further study. It is of some interest that subacute attacks of angle closure may spontaneously resolve in the evening or during the night because aqueous secretion decreases during those hours.[44]

Mapstone and Clark[45] believe that parasympathetic dysfunction may play a role in precipitating closed angles. They found reduced systemic parasympathetic tone and postulate that reduced parasympathetic tone in the eye could lead to middilation of the pupil, increasing relative pupillary block.

Box 15-1
Precipitating Factors for Angle Closure

Mydriasis
  Emotional upset
  Dim illumination
  Medications (see Box 15-2)
  Evening hours
  Systemic parasympathetic dysfunction
Extreme miosis
Prone position

In summary the pathophysiology of primary angle-closure glaucoma with pupillary block involves at least three factors: (1) a small anterior segment that provides the anatomic predisposition for increased pupillary block; (2) aging changes, such as lens thickening or forward lens position, which accentuate pupillary block: and, in some cases; (3) a precipitating factor, such as midpupillary dilation, extreme miosis, or forward lens movement, to trigger an acute attack.

Epidemiology

The incidence and prevalence of primary angle-closure glaucoma with pupillary block in a population are influenced by a number of factors, including age distribution, gender, racial makeup, range of refraction, and heredity. In one study in Olmsted County, Minnesota, the incidence of angle-closure glaucoma was 8.3 per 100,000 population 40 years of age and older.[46] In this same study, 14% of participants were blind in at least one eye at the time of diagnosis and a further 4% became monocularly blind over a 5-year follow-up. In Taiwan, the prevalence of angle-closure glaucoma in a rural population was about 3%, with an additional 2% angle-closure suspects.[47]

Age

Most studies have noted that primary angle-closure glaucoma with pupillary block occurs with greatest frequency in the sixth and seventh decades of life.[48-50] Several age-associated changes increase relative pupillary block, including increased lens thickness, a more anterior position of the lens, and pupillary miosis. It should be emphasized, however, that primary angle-closure glaucoma with pupillary block can occur in patients of any age, including children.[51,52]

Gender

Most studies have reported that primary angle-closure glaucoma with pupillary block occurs two to three times more commonly in women than in men.[53-57] The increased prevalence of angle closure in women probably reflects the fact that women have shallower anterior chambers.[37,58] The one exception to this observation may be in those of black African ancestry, in whom the occurrence of angle-closure glaucoma is equal in men and women.[59]

Box 15-2
Classes of Drugs Capable of Precipitating
Angle-Closure Glaucoma In Susceptible Eyes

Sympathomimetic agents
Cocaine
Epinephrine
Dipivefrin
Ephedrine
Pseudoephedrine
Hydroxyamphetamine
Norepinephrine
Dopamine
Naphazoline
Tetrahydrozoline
Methoxamine
Clonidine
Stimulants
   Amphetamines
   Caffeine
   Methylphenidate

Strong parasympathomimetic agents
   (e.g., echothiophate, pilocarpine > 2%)
Parasympatholytic agents
Cyclopentolate
Tropicamide
Atropine
Homatropine
Scopolamine
Antiparkinson agents
Phenothiazines
Antihistamines and H_1 antagonists
Vasodilators

Modified from Mandelkorn RM, Zimmerman TJ: In Ritch, R, Shields MB, editors: *The secondary glaucomas,* St Louis, 1982, Mosby.

Race

Primary angle-closure glaucoma with pupillary block occurs one fourth to one tenth as frequently as does primary open-angle glaucoma in white individuals living in the United States and western Europe.[48,60-63] One study states that primary angle-closure glaucoma occurs in 0.1% of whites older than 40 years of age and comprises about 6% of the total glaucoma cases.[64] Within this group angle-closure glaucoma affects fewer individuals of Mediterranean origin than of northern European origin.[56] Primary acute angle-closure glaucoma with pupillary block seems to occur less frequently in individuals of black African ancestry,[59,65] and those blacks who are affected generally have a chronic asymptomatic form of the disease.[59,66-69] Some investigators postulate that black patients are less likely to develop primary acute angle-closure glaucoma because they have thinner lenses or weaker iris sphincter muscles that generate less pupillary block.[23]

Primary acute angle-closure glaucoma with pupillary block occurs infrequently in some mongoloid populations, including Pacific islanders, American Indians, and Tibetans,[70-72] and often in other populations, including Eskimos (Inuit) in such diverse places as Greenland, Alaska, and northern Canada.[73-75] Alsbirk[76] reported that 10% of Eskimo women and 2.1% of Eskimo men over 40 years of age are affected by angle-closure glaucoma. The prevalence of angle-closure glaucoma is equal to that of open-angle glaucoma in such south Asian countries as India and Sri Lanka.[77,78] Primary angle-closure glaucoma appears to be relatively more common among most eastern and southeast Asian peoples, including the Chinese, Malaysian, Burmese, Filipino, and Vietnamese.[72,79,80] Some of these cases may be the chronic or creeping angle-closure type.[81] Conversely, Japanese patients seem to have primary angle-closure glaucoma less frequently than do other Asians.[82,83]

Heredity

Most cases of primary angle-closure glaucoma with pupillary block are sporadic in nature—that is, there is no family history of glaucoma. However, several pedigrees are reported to have a high prevalence of primary angle-closure glaucoma,[84,85] some with autosomal-dominant and some with autosomal-recessive patterns of inheritance. Tornquist[32,86] has suggested that the configuration of the anterior chamber is inherited under polygenic influence, and this explains the familial occurrence of primary angle-closure glaucoma rather than a specific gene linked to the disease. Shallow anterior chambers and narrow angles are more common in relatives of patients with primary angle-closure glaucoma than in individuals whose relatives do not have the disorder.[86-88]

Refractive Error

The prevalence of primary angle-closure glaucoma with pupillary block is much higher in individuals with hyperopic eyes, which typically have shallow anterior chambers.[37] Although rare, angle-closure glaucoma can occur in myopic eyes.[89]

Seasonal Incidence

Many reports have indicated that primary angle-closure glaucoma with pupillary block occurs more commonly in the winter months.[90-92] This has been variously attributed to low levels of illumination, increased cloudiness, changeable weather, and low sunspot activity.[93]

CLINICAL PRESENTATIONS: PRIMARY ANGLE-CLOSURE GLAUCOMA WITH PUPILLARY BLOCK

As noted previously, when the angle closes suddenly and completely the pressure rises rapidly to high levels, causing symptoms and damage to the optic nerve at a fairly rapid pace. This form of glaucoma is called *acute angle-closure glaucoma*. If the attack is spontaneously aborted, such as may occur from a bright light that constricts the pupil or during sleep, and if the sequence—attack and spontaneous resolution—occurs more than once, then the patient is said to have *subacute angle-closure glaucoma*. If the angle closes slowly over a long period of time without symptoms, this is called *chronic* (or creeping) *angle-closure glaucoma*. Both subacute and chronic angle-closure types ultimately may result in an attack that does not resolve spontaneously. One can often elicit a history of one or more subacute attacks in patients with both acute angle-closure attacks and chronic angle-closure glaucoma. Thus these may be different phases of the same disease process. These same temporal relationships may be seen in other forms of angle closure glaucoma as well.

Acute Primary Angle-Closure Glaucoma With Pupillary Block

Symptoms

The typical patient with an acute attack of primary angle-closure glaucoma due to pupillary block will have a sudden onset of pain or aching on the side of the affected eye. This pain is accompanied by blurred vision, colored haloes around lights, redness, and sometimes nausea, vomiting, and sweating. The pain occurs in the trigeminal distribution and may be localized by the patient to the eye, orbit, head, ear, sinuses, or teeth. The discomfort may be mild to severe—so severe in fact that the glaucoma attack may masquerade as an acute intracranial process such as an aneurysm. The pain appears to be related more to the rapid rise in IOP than to the absolute level of the pressure itself. The blurred vision occurs at first as a result of distortion of the corneal lamellae and later as a result of corneal epithelial edema. The corneal edema acts as a diffraction grating that breaks white light into its component colors, causing patients to note colored haloes or rainbows around incandescent lights. During these episodes, the blue-green colors are central and the yellow-red colors are peripheral. In a recent study of over 5000 Taiwanese patients with angle-closure glaucoma, symptoms of angle closure were present in only 35% of patients.[47]

Autonomic stimulation during an acute attack can result in nausea, vomiting, sweating, and bradycardia. These symptoms are sometimes confused with those caused by a flulike illness or to an acute abdomen. Occasionally systemic symptoms such as abdominal or chest pain are predominant and may make diagnosis difficult.[94] Angle closure can be associated with or precipitated by pituitary apoplexy[95] and childbirth.[96]

Most attacks of angle-closure glaucoma are unilateral. However, 5% to 10% of the attacks may affect both eyes simultaneously.[50] Patients who develop acute attacks of angle-closure glaucoma may relate that they have had similar but less severe episodes in the past. They may recall mild episodes of discomfort or blurring that were relieved by sleep or by exposure to bright light.

Findings

Acute attacks of primary angle-closure glaucoma with pupillary block are usually accompanied by a variety of physical findings (Boxes 15-3 and 15-4), including the following:

1. Diminished visual acuity.
2. Conjunctival hyperemia that is more marked near the limbus (i.e., ciliary flush).
3. Corneal edema, which at times involves only the epithelium, whereas at other times the stroma is also thickened and thrown into striae.
4. A shallow anterior chamber both centrally and peripherally.
5. Minimal to moderate anterior chamber reaction caused by increased aqueous humor protein concentration.[97] Severe or prolonged attacks may produce heavy anterior chamber cell and flare, but keratic precipitates are rarely seen.

Box 15-3
Physical Findings In Acute Angle-Closure Glaucoma With Pupillary Block

Findings During An Acute Attack of Angle-Closure Glaucoma	Findings Suggesting Previous Episodes of Acute Angle-Closure Glaucoma
Diminished vision	Posterior synechiae
Ciliary flush	Peripheral anterior synechiae
Corneal edema	Diminished outflow facility
Shallow anterior chamber	Glaukomflecken
Anterior chamber cell and flare	Sector or generalized iris atrophy
Moderately dilated and sluggishly reactive pupil	Optic nerve cupping and/or pallor
Markedly elevated intraocular pressure	Visual field loss
Closed angle on gonioscopy	
Diminished outflow facility	
Hyperemic and swollen optic disc	
Constricted visual field	

Box 15-4
Differential Diagnosis of Acute Angle-Closure Glaucoma

Acute primary angle-closure glaucoma
Sudden total angle closure in chronic angle-closure glaucoma
Aqueous misdirection glaucoma
Neovascular glaucoma
Iridocorneal endothelial syndrome
Plateau iris syndrome with angle closure
Secondary angle closure with pupillary block
Uveitis associated with increased intraocular pressure
   Glaucomatocyclitic crisis
   Herpes simplex keratouveitis
   Herpes zoster uveitis
   Sarcoid uveitis
Pigmentary glaucoma
Exfoliative glaucoma (may have associated angle closure)
Posttraumatic glaucoma
Phacolytic glaucoma

---

6. A moderately dilated, vertically oval, sluggish, or nonreactive pupil. The high IOP causes ischemia and paresis of the pupillary sphincter.[98-100]

7. Markedly elevated IOP, usually in the range of 45 to 75 mm Hg.

8. A closed angle on gonioscopy, which is the critical test for diagnosing angle-closure glaucoma. It is sometimes difficult to evaluate the angle during an acute attack because of corneal edema and hazy media. In this situation gonioscopy should be repeated after the IOP is reduced by medical treatment, allowing the cornea to clear. One or two drops of anhydrous glycerin can also be administered to the anesthetized eye to clear the cornea and improve the gonioscopic examination. If the view remains hazy, gonioscopy of the fellow eye can confirm the presence of narrow angles. Furthermore, the peripheral anterior chamber depth appears shallow in both eyes by the van Herick test.[101]

9. A hyperemic, swollen optic disc. The optic disc is swollen during an attack of angle-closure glaucoma from hydropic degeneration and impaired axoplasmic flow. The optic disc may be swollen when hypotony follows an acute attack of angle-closure glaucoma. The disc does not appear pale or cupped during the acute attack unless there have been previous episodes of angle closure or concomitant glaucoma from another cause.[102] When IOP was raised to high levels in experimental studies in monkey eyes, the optic discs appeared swollen for 4 to 5 days and then became pale and cupped.[103] The appearance of the optic disc is altered if there is a concomitant central or branch vein occlusion.[104-106] It is also possible for a central retinal vein occlusion to cause a transient shallowing of the anterior chamber (see Chapter 16).[107,108]

10. A normal or constricted visual field. Visual field examinations are generally not performed during acute attacks of angle-closure glaucoma. Following an attack visual fields often demonstrate superior constriction or nerve fiber bundle defects.[102,109]

11. Diminished tonographic outflow facility. The resistance to outflow is directly related to the extent of the angle closure. The resistance also depends on whether the open portions of the angle have been damaged by previous attacks of angle closure.

A patient examined during an acute attack of primary angle-closure glaucoma with pupillary block may demonstrate signs that are actually the sequelae of previous attacks, including posterior synechiae, peripheral anterior synechiae, impaired outflow facility, anterior subcapsular lens opacities (Glaukomflecken of Vogt), sector or generalized atrophy of the iris, pallor and cupping of the optic disc, and visual field loss (see Boxes 15-3 and 15-4). The iris atrophy is probably ischemic in origin and is more often located superiorly than inferiorly. This process releases a considerable amount of pigment, which is then deposited on the iris surface, corneal endothelium, and trabecular meshwork. The ischemia may contribute to the severe pain during the acute attack.

Many of the above signs and symptoms could occur as a result of an abrupt and profound rise in IOP regardless of cause. The ophthalmologist must distinguish primary acute angle-closure glaucoma with pupillary block from other forms of angle-closure glaucoma as well as open-angle glaucoma with sudden markedly high levels of IOP. The differential diagnosis includes neovascular glaucoma, plateau iris syndrome, hypertensive iridocyclitis, aqueous misdirection, posttraumatic recessed angle, exfoliative glaucoma, pigmentary glaucoma, and glaucomatocyclitic crisis (see Box 15-4). A special situation exists with exfoliative syndrome, which can produce very high IOPs in the presence of an open angle. However, exfoliative syndrome is also associated with an increased prevalence of narrow angles and an increased risk of pupillary block narrow-angle glaucoma.[110]

These entities are usually diagnosed readily by a careful history of the temporal course of events, a slit-lamp examination, and gonioscopy of the involved and the fellow eyes. The examination also serves to detect secondary forms of angle closure that are associated with aqueous misdirection, ciliary body swelling, posterior segment tumor, central retinal vein occlusion, and nanophthalmos. It is crucial that both eyes be examined in order to determine whether the condition is bilateral and to assess the potential for the second eye to become involved. Indentation gonioscopy (with a Zeiss, Sussman, or similar gonioscopy lens) should also be performed to differentiate appositional from synechial closure (see Chapters 6 and 8).

Treatment

The treatment of acute primary angle-closure glaucoma with pupillary block can be divided into four stages:
1. Immediate medical therapy to stop the acute attack, thereby minimizing damage to the optic nerve, trabecular meshwork, and lens and reducing the formation of posterior and peripheral anterior synechiae.
2. Protection of the fellow eye, initially with medical treatment. In most cases the fellow eye is subject to the same hereditary and aging influences as is the involved eye and is predisposed to develop acute angle-closure glaucoma because of a shallow anterior chamber and increased pupillary block. Furthermore, a patient who develops acute angle-closure glaucoma in one eye is often frightened and in pain, both of which serve to increase sympathetic stimulation to the fellow eye. The resulting mydriasis may precipitate acute angle-closure glaucoma in the predisposed fellow eye.
3. Definitive treatment of iridotomy in both the involved and fellow eyes. This will prevent further encroachment of the iris on the angle as well as future attacks of angle-closure glaucoma, at least those cases caused by pupillary block.
4. Management of the long-term sequelae of the angle-closure attack.

The crucial step in the medical treatment of acute primary angle-closure glaucoma with pupillary block is to pull the iris away from the trabecular meshwork; this is accomplished most effectively by producing moderate pupillary miosis with cholinergic agents. Miosis tightens and thins the peripheral iris, pulling it away from the trabecular meshwork, and thereby allows aqueous humor to leave the eye (Fig. 15-3). Unfortunately, in most acute attacks of angle-closure glaucoma with pupillary block the IOP is so high that the pupillary sphincter muscle is ischemic and unresponsive to topical miotic agents.[98-100] In such cases IOP must be reduced by other medical means before pilocarpine can produce pupillary miosis.

The physician should immediately administer some combination of a topical β-adrenergic antagonist,[111] a topical α-adrenergic agent such as apraclonidine, an oral or parenteral carbonic anhydrase inhibitor (CAI)[112] and, if necessary, a hyperosmotic agent (Table 15-3). These agents will begin lowering the IOP, helping to alleviate pain, allowing the cornea to be cleared with a topical hyperosmotic agent for further diagnostic evaluation, and allowing a miotic to pull the iris away from the trabecular meshwork and middilation.

Assuming there are no contraindications, any of the commonly used topical β-adrenergic antagonists can be administered to the affected eye to reduce aqueous humor formation and IOP. Timolol or levobunalol will begin to take effect within about 20 minutes of administration. Apraclonidine 0.5%, which also reduces aqueous formation, is often helpful in reducing IOP rapidly.[113] Similarly, the CAI acetazolamide can be given orally in a dose of 500 mg. If the patient is nauseous or vomiting, acetazolamide (500) mg may be administered intravenously.

Hyperosmotic agents dehydrate the vitreous and allow the lens–iris diaphragm to move posteriorly; they are often the most effective means of lowering IOP during acute episodes of angle-

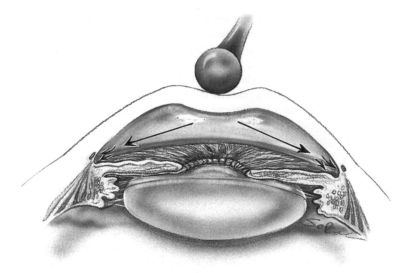

Figure 15-4 Depressing the central cornea with a blunt instrument forces aqueous humor into the periphery of the anterior chamber where it may open the angle.

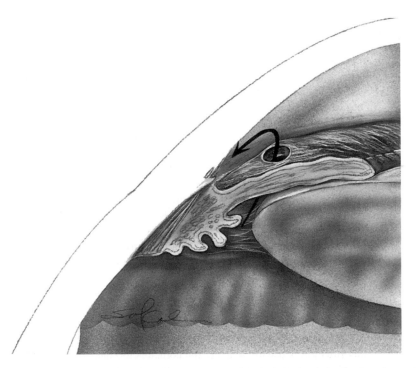

Figure 15-5 Patent iridectomy reduces pupillary block and equilibrates pressure in posterior and anterior chambers.

anterior chambers there is an insufficient pressure differential to push the peripheral iris forward against the trabecular meshwork (Fig. 15-5). The peripheral anterior chamber depth increases after iridectomy or iridotomy, whereas the central depth is unchanged.[22,25,123] If iridectomy is not performed, repeated attacks of angle closure damage the optic nerve and lead to the formation of peripheral anterior synechiae. If extensive peripheral anterior synechiae develop, an iridectomy may no longer be adequate to control the glaucoma and filtering surgery may be required.

Argon and Nd.YAG LPI have largely replaced surgical iridectomy as the preferred technique for performing iridectomy.[124,125] (See Chapter 30 for details of this technique.) The term *iridotomy* is used to indicate laser-induced openings in the iris, whereas *iridectomy* indicates surgical removal of iris tissue. The terms are often used interchangeably, however. Although surgical iridectomy is a relatively safe and simple procedure, it is invasive and presents a small but still present risk of intraocular complications such as cataract, bleeding, and endophthalmitis. Surgical iridectomy is now reserved for situations in which the laser fails to produce a patent iridectomy; laser iridectomies close repeatedly; the laser is not available or not functioning properly; opacities of the media interfere with laser treatment; or the patient is uncooperative or unable to sit at the slit lamp. In some eyes with very shallow anterior chambers, posterior pressure with the Abraham or similar lens deepens the chambers sufficiently to allow laser treatment without significant damage to the cornea.

LPIs, especially those performed with the argon as opposed to the Nd:YAG laser, may close at a later date and subject the eye to redevelopment of angle closure.[126] Fleck[126] has calculated that a 15-μm opening is theoretically large enough to prevent pupillary block; however, localized iris edema, pigment epithelial proliferation, and changes in iridotomy size after pupil dilation may obstruct a small opening. Therefore he recommends (and experience confirms) that an iridotomy of at least 200 μm should be created. For most patients, an iridotomy of 150 μm is sufficient.

If an acute attack can be terminated by medical means, the physician can proceed directly to laser iridectomy or wait 1 or 2 days for the cornea to clear and intraocular inflammation to subside. If the latter option is chosen, the eye is treated with topical pilocarpine and a topical corticosteroid preparation until surgery. The physician must observe the patient carefully to ensure that a repeat attack does not occur.

Some eyes that develop acute primary angle-closure glaucoma with pupillary block eventually require filtering surgery for IOP control.[127-129] This has stirred considerable controversy with regard to whether some cases of acute angle-closure glaucoma should be treated primarily by drainage operations rather than progressing through the sequence of iridectomy, medical treatment, and then filtering surgery. Considerable literature suggests that it is difficult, if not impossible, to predict which patients will require subsequent filtration.[127-131] Iridectomy combined with medical treatment gave results equal to those obtained by primary filtering surgery, with fewer surgical complications.[129-131] Many eyes were well controlled after iridectomy despite extensive damage from acute attacks of glaucoma.

The development of laser surgery has done much to settle this dispute. The current recommendation is for all eyes to receive an LPI first.[132] Residual glaucoma is then treated in a stepwise fashion with medical therapy, laser trabeculoplasty, and filtering surgery as needed.

Fellow eyes (i.e., contralateral eyes that did not develop angle-closure glaucoma) should also receive LPI. A number of studies indicate that 40% to 80% of fellow eyes develop angle-closure glaucoma over a 5- to 10-year period. Fellow eyes have occasionally developed angle closure after 25 or 30 years.[133-137] The incidence of angle-closure glaucoma in fellow eyes is reduced somewhat by the prophylactic long-term administration of miotic agents. However, this approach is not recommended because miotic agents do not provide total protection against acute attacks, and their chronic administration may favor the development of peripheral anterior synechiae and chronic angle-closure glaucoma.

A few physicians disagree with the management proposed above for fellow eyes. They instead select the fellow eyes for iridectomy on the basis of provocative tests.[138,139] Most authorities reject this approach, however, because of lack of prospective data on the sensitivity and specificity of provocative tests. One prospective study demonstrated that no clinical test, including a provocative one, is helpful in predicting future angle-closure attacks.[140] Furthermore, the availability of the laser markedly alters the risk:benefit ratio for prophylactic iridotomy. Finally, physicians must consider that some patients wait for days before seeking medical care for acute attacks of angle-closure glaucoma.[50,141] Surprisingly, some may delay despite the fact that they sustained severe damage when their first eye developed angle-closure glaucoma. Except in unusual circumstances, current opinion holds that it is safer to perform prophylactic laser iridotomies in fellow eyes than to observe them for the development of angle closure or treat them with chronic miotic therapy. The exceptions to this rule include fellow eyes that have little pupillary block because of anisometropia, recessed angles, or peaked pupils.

Complications and Sequelae of Acute Angle-Closure Glaucoma

In the early postiridotomy period, elevated IOP may occur as a result of incomplete or sealed iridotomy, unrecognized plateau iris syndrome, inflammation, extensive peripheral anterior synechiae,

Table 15-4

Occurrence of Elevated Intraocular Pressure and Cataract After Surgical Iridectomy For Angle-Closure Glaucoma

Study	Postoperative or Late Intraocular Pressure Elevation (%)	Surgery for Residual Glaucoma (%)	Visually Significant Cataract (%)	Patients Requiring Cataract Surgery (%)
Williams and co-workers[144]	31	8	19	6
Lowe[147]	29	0	54	0
Floman and co-workers[146]	70	NA	57	NA
Krupin and co-workers[129]	24	2	55	10
Playfair and Watson[127]	28	16	NA	21
Burris[148]	72	32	44	40
Saraux and Offre[148]	39	0	NA	NA
Bobrow and Drews[148]	52	4	41	19

Modified from Bobrow JC, Drews RC: *Glaucoma* 3:319, 1981.
NA, Not available.

or corticosteroid administration.[142,143] Elevated IOP can also occur months to years later and has been reported in 24% to 72% of eyes following iridectomy for angle-closure glaucoma (Table 15-4).[127,129,144-148] Patients must be warned of the need for lifelong care even when iridectomy has apparently "cured" their glaucoma. Elevated IOP is seen more commonly in eyes with extensive peripheral anterior synechiae. However, increased IOP is also found in eyes without synechiae, causing some authorities to propose that even transient apposition between the iris and trabecular meshwork damages the outflow channels. Elevated IOP also occurs in some fellow eyes that never had an acute attack of angle-closure glaucoma (see Box 15-3).* This suggests two alternative hypotheses—either intermittent, subclinical apposition between the iris and the trabecular meshwork damages the outflow channels, or anatomically narrow angles are associated with an underlying defect of the outflow channels.

The treatment of the residual glaucoma after iridotomy is similar to that for open-angle glaucoma, with a stepwise escalation of medical therapy, laser trabeculoplasty, and filtering surgery as needed. Laser trabeculoplasty can be effective unless there are extensive peripheral anterior synechiae.[150] Some researchers have reported that synechial closure may be alleviated by argon laser gonioplasty.[151-153] Laser gonioplasty reportedly lowers IOP in cases not only of recent origin but even in cases in which synechial closure has been present for years.[153] There is no question that laser gonioplasty can be useful to allow better visualization of the trabecular meshwork when performing laser trabeculoplasty in patients with narrow angles. It is also possible to anatomically pull some synechiae from the trabecular meshwork with this technique. However, the long-term effectiveness of laser goniosynechialysis has not yet been proven. The synechiae often reappear over time.

There are a few reports that peripheral anterior synechiae can be lysed surgically if glaucoma is uncontrolled after an iridectomy.[154] Goniosynechialysis using viscoelastic dissection has also been proposed.[155] Medical therapy is often still required after synechialysis. Surgical goniosynechialysis is a less complicated procedure that is less likely to result in long-term complications than is filtration surgery, but its long-term effectiveness has not been confirmed.

The development of visually significant cataract is a relatively common occurrence following surgical iridectomy (Tables 15-4 and 15-5).† Cataract formation is not surprising in eyes that have had an acute angle-closure attack given the extreme disturbance of ocular physiology during the attack. Furthermore, early cataract formation is often a precursor to pupillary block, so many patients

*Refs. 127, 129, 144, 146, 148, 149.
†Refs: 129, 131, 144, 146-148, 156, 157.

Table 15-5

Occurrence of Elevated Intraocular Pressure and Cataract After Prophylactic Surgical Iridectomy

Study	Postoperative or Late Intraocular Pressure Elevation (%)	Surgery for Residual Glaucoma (%)	Visually Significant Cataract (%)	Patients Requiring Cataract Surgery (%)
Williams and co-workers[144]	0	0	2	0
Sugar[156]	0	0	31	NA
Kirsch[149]	NA	NA	Same as	Control group
Lowe[147]	12	NA	40	0
Godel and Regenbogen[157]	0	0	40	NA
Floman and co-workers[146]	35	NA	42	NA
Krupin and co-workers[129]	12	0	37	2
Playfair and Watson[127]	2	0	NA	4
Bobrow and Drews[148]	54	5	45	25

Modified from Bobrow JC, Drews RC: *Glaucoma* 3:319, 1981.
NA, Not available.

already have some lens opacity when the attack occurs. Whether surgical iridectomy plays an additional role in cataract formation has been debated. Most investigators today believe that surgical iridectomy plays a major role in the initiation and development of lens changes. Other important factors in the development of cataract include the age of the patient, the preexisting state of the lens, the occurrence of an acute attack, and the need for filtering surgery. Although argon laser can produce localized lens changes, no data exist to implicate LPI as a cause of generalized lens opacity. A review of patients treated with argon laser peripheral iridotomy showed no statistically significant differences from age- and sex-matched controls in the development or severity of cataract development.[158] Aqueous misdirection syndrome has been reported following LPI.[159]

A decrease in central corneal endothelial cell density has been reported following acute attacks of angle-closure glaucoma.[160-162] The decrease in cell density correlates with the duration of the attack; in fact, longer attacks may cause as much as 77% endothelial cell loss.[27,162] The loss of endothelial cells also correlates with other indicators of ocular damage, including visual field loss and optic disc cupping.[163] Occasionally corneal decompensation requiring penetrating keratoplasty occurs after an acute attack. Patients with Fuchs' endothelial dystrophy have shallower anterior chambers depths, shorter axial lengths, and a greater propensity for increased IOP after penetrating keratoplasty.[164]

The argon laser can cause a superficial corneal burn, especially if a contact lens is not used during LPI. These burns usually disappear after a few days. The Nd:YAG laser can cause a localized area of denuded corneal endothelial cells, especially if a contact lens is not used[165] or if the treated iris is very close to the corneal endothelium.[166,167] However, there is usually no generalized decrease in endothelial cell density following LPI.[168-172] Patients with preexisting endothelial dystrophy who suffer an acute angle-closure attack may be more susceptible to the effects of LPI and develop corneal decompensation after treatment.[167,169]

Subacute Primary Angle-Closure Glaucoma With Pupillary Block

Subacute primary angle-closure glaucoma with pupillary block is also referred to by the terms *prodomal, intermittent,* and *subclinical glaucoma.*[128,173] This is a milder form of angle closure in which symptoms may be modest or absent. Patients often report that they have experienced mild episodes of discomfort, blurred vision, and halo vision that were relieved by sleep or exposure to bright light. The symptoms occur more often at night or with dim illumination. It is possible to confuse subacute angle closure with transient ischemic attacks or other neurologic causes of intermittent visual loss.[143,174]

It is postulated that the milder course of subacute episodes reflects a variation in angle width that prevents total angle closure. It is also possible that moderate IOP elevations during subacute attacks decrease aqueous humor formation or reduce pupillary block by causing mydriasis. Between episodes of subacute angle closure, IOP and outflow facility are generally normal and no peripheral anterior synechiae are present. On rare occasions subacute angle-closure glaucoma is seen as intermittent ocular hypertension.[175] Patients with subacute angle-closure glaucoma may progress to either an acute attack or chronic angle-closure glaucoma. Subacute primary angle-closure glaucoma with pupillary block is treated with LPI.

Chronic Primary Angle-Closure Glaucoma With Pupillary Block

Chronic primary angle-closure glaucoma with pupillary block is also referred to as *creeping angle closure*.[176-178] This entity is often misdiagnosed because it closely resembles primary open-angle glaucoma in that patients are asymptomatic and have quiet eyes, cupping and atrophy of the optic discs, and visual field loss. IOP is moderately elevated and often poorly responsive to medical treatment.[178] Gonioscopy is the key to the diagnosis of chronic angle-closure glaucoma and should be performed on all patients suspected of glaucoma. In contrast to the open angle of open-angle glaucoma, gonioscopy in chronic angle-closure glaucoma reveals a very narrow angle with apposition between the iris and the trabecular meshwork over most of the circumference of the angle. The apposition usually begins in the superior angle and progresses in both directions toward the 6 o'clock position.[14,179,180] When approximately two thirds of the angle is occluded, IOP rises substantially. The height of the IOP is directly related to the extent of angle closure and the competency of the remaining open angle.

Peripheral anterior synechiae may be present but are usually far less extensive than are the areas of apposition. As noted previously, apposition and synechiae may be distinguished by indentation gonioscopy.[181] When synechiae are present, they are continuous rather than scattered as would be seen after acute angle-closure glaucoma. It is thought that the absence of vascular congestion explains the relative paucity of peripheral anterior synechiae despite long-term apposition between the iris and the trabecular meshwork. Chronic angle-closure glaucoma is usually seen as described above but may also occur after subacute or acute angle closure, which produces extensive peripheral anterior synechiae and damaged outflow channels. Chronic angle-closure glaucoma is the most common form of angle closure seen in black patients in the United States and Africa,[182-184] although open-angle glaucoma is much more common than is angle closure in people of black African descent.

The treatment for primary chronic angle-closure glaucoma with pupillary block is LPI. Whether filtering surgery should be employed primarily in some of these cases has been debated.[144] Once again this question has largely been settled by the availability of the laser. Following LPI, residual glaucoma is treated in the usual fashion by medical therapy, laser trabeculoplasty, and filtering surgery as indicated.

Primary Angle-Closure Glaucoma Suspect

Ophthalmologists commonly examine asymptomatic patients and find shallow anterior chambers and anatomically narrow angles. An estimated 2% to 6% of eyes have suspiciously narrow angles (grade II or less), and 0.6% to 1.1% have critically narrow angles (grade I or less).[101,185] Narrow angles are found more frequently in older, hyperopic patients and in certain ethnic groups such as the Chinese, the Vietnamese, and Inuit Eskimos (Table 15-6).

With practice, shallow anterior chambers can be detected with the naked eye or with a hand-held illuminator directed from the temporal side along the plane of the iris (Fig. 15-6). However, most anatomically narrow angles are identified on slit-lamp examination by noting shallow central[186,187] and peripheral[188] anterior chamber depths. In young patients central anterior chamber depths may be normal even though the peripheral chambers are shallow. This discrepancy may be related to the relatively small size of the lens in young individuals. These young patients are at risk for developing angle closure if their pupils are dilated. One useful technique for detecting narrow angles is to compare the peripheral anterior chamber depth with the thickness of the cornea. If the peripheral anterior chamber depth is less than one fourth the thickness of the cornea, the angles are

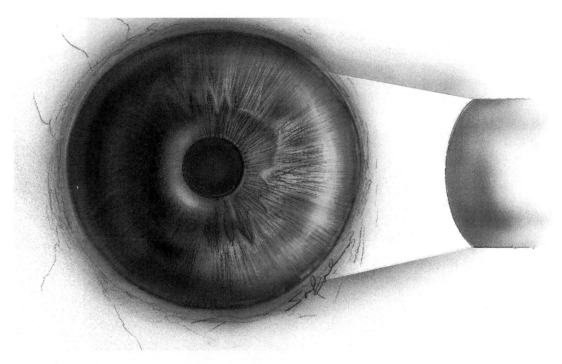

Figure 15-6   Illumination from the temporal side casts shadow on iris if there is considerable bombé.

Table 15-6

Frequency of Narrow Angles by Age and Refractive Error as Estimated by Slit-Lamp Examination

Age (yr)	Hyperopia > 1 Di		Intermediate Refractive Error − 1 to + 1 Di		Myopia > 1 Di	
	Grade I and II Angles (%)	Grade III and IV Angles (%)	Grade I and II Angles (%)	Grade III and IV Angles (%)	Grade I and II Angles (%)	Grade III and IV Angles (%)
0–19	0	100	0	100.0	0	100
20–39	0	100	0.7	99.3	0.2	99.8
40–59	2	98	1.0	99.0	0.3	99.7
>60	3.5	96.5	2.0	98.0	0	100

Modified from van Herick W, Shaffer RN, Schwartz A: *Am J Opthalmol* 68:626, 1969. Published with permission from *The American Journal of Ophthalmology*. Copyright by the Ophthalmic Publishing Company.

very likely to be shallow (Fig. 15-7).[101] It should be emphasized that the techniques described here are used to indicate the need for careful gonioscopy rather than to replace gonioscopy.

A few authorities prefer the Koeppe gonioscopy system for distinguishing narrow but open angles from closed angles because they believe the Koeppe system offers greater flexibility in the angles of viewing and illumination, making it easier to observe the trabecular meshwork over a convex iris.[189] However, the Koeppe system is awkward to set up and is time consuming. Most physicians prefer the Zeiss (or similar) four-mirror prism because it is rapid, relatively atraumatic, and useful for indenting the central cornea to distinguish appositional closure from peripheral anterior synechiae.[181] It is important to emphasize, however, that the key feature of any gonioscopy system is the skill and experience of the examiner.

An ectopic lens can cause severe pupillary block if it comes forward into the pupil or anterior chamber (Fig. 15-11).[226,227] Dislocation of the lens may also allow the vitreous face to come forward and obstruct the pupil. Other possible causes of glaucoma associated with ectopic lenses include uveitis, trauma, and phacolytic reaction. In most cases of ectopia lentis and pupillary block the patient is given a systemic hyperosmotic agent, a topical β-adrenergic antagonist, an α-adrenergic agonist and, if necessary, an oral CAI to reduce IOP. The hyperosmotic agent also shrinks the vitreous, allowing the lens to move posteriorly. If the lens is caught in the pupil or anterior chamber, weak mydriatic agents are administered. If the zonules are known to be intact, a cycloplegic drug may be used to pull the lens posteriorly. Once the lens is in the posterior chamber, the pupil is constricted by miotic agents and an LPI is performed. The iridotomy should be placed in such a position that the lens will not occlude the opening. The patient is then treated long-term with miotic agents to prevent forward migration of the dislocated or subluxated lens. There are a few situations in which a dislocated or subluxated lens should be removed, including the inability to reposit it in the posterior chamber, severe diplopia, reduction of visual acuity related to cataract or high astigmatism, phacolytic glaucoma, and intractable uveitis. The choice between anterior cataract extraction and lensectomy through the pars plana depends on the position and condition of the lens. Intraocular surgery in these situations is associated with a high rate of complications, in part caused by the condition of the eyes and in part caused by the associated systemic diseases (e.g., homocystinuria).

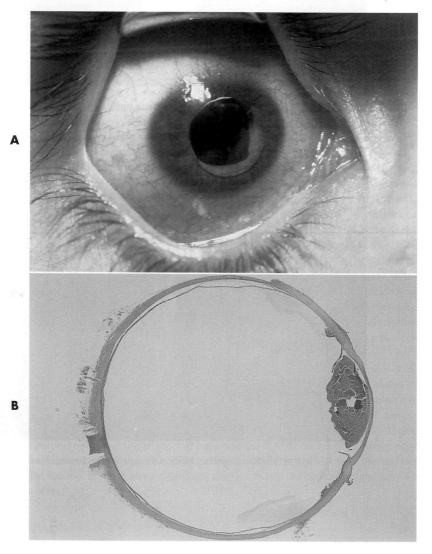

Figure 15-11 **A,** Lens prolapsed into pupil and anterior chamber. **B,** Light micrograph of crystalline lens dislocated into the anterior chamber. (Courtesy of William H. Spencer, M.D.)

Microspherophakia

Microspherophakia (i.e., a small round lens), ectopia lentis, and glaucoma may occur as an isolated familial condition[228] or may be associated with a variety of diseases, including Marfan syndrome, homocystinuria,[229] Klinefelter's syndrome,[230] mandibulofacial dysostosis,[231] and Alport's syndrome.[232] Most commonly, however, microspherophakia is associated with the Weill-Marchesani syndrome, which is characterized by short, stocky habitus, short fingers and toes, brachycephaly, and limited finger and wrist mobility. In microspherophakia, the equatorial diameter of the lens is decreased while the thickness is increased, giving it a spheric or globular shape (Fig. 15-12, *A*).[233-236]

When the pupil is dilated, the entire circumference of the lens is visible at the slit lamp (Fig. 15-12, *B*). Dislocation of the lens is common and often occurs at a relatively young age. Pupillary block and glaucoma occur through one of two mechanisms; either the lens dislocates into the pupil and anterior chamber or long zonules allow the lens to come forward into the pupil. The physician should be suspicious of microspherophakia when angle-closure glaucoma occurs in young myopic individuals or when a myopic individual has a shallow anterior chamber.

When an acute episode of glaucoma occurs in an individual with Weill-Marchesani syndrome, the status of the zonules is usually unknown. If the physician knows that the zonules are intact, a cycloplegic agent should be administered to pull the lens posteriorly. If the zonules are not intact, however, dilating the pupil allows the lens to come forward into the anterior chamber. Furthermore, miotic agents often aggravate pupillary block in spherophakia.[237] Thus the safest approach is to avoid both miotics and cycloplegics and to administer hyperosmotic agents, CAIs, and topical β-adrenergic antagonists and then to place the patient in the supine position. The hyperosmotic drugs shrink the vitreous and allow the lens to move posteriorly, thereby reducing pupillary block. An argon or Nd:YAG LPI is then performed in both eyes. LPI is preferable to surgical iridectomy because the latter is associated with a high rate of complications. Ritch and Wand[238] have suggested that prophylactic LPI be performed in all individuals with the Weill-Marchesani syndrome.

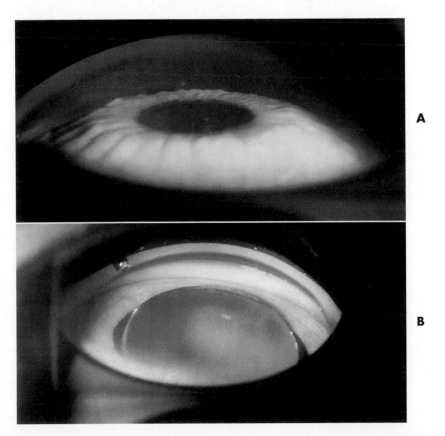

A

B

Figure 15-12 **A,** Gonioscopic view of a spherophakic lens displacing the iris and shallowing the anterior chamber. **B,** Gonioscopic view after pupillary dilation showing the entire circumference of the lens in the pupil.

Cystinosis

Pupillary block and angle-closure glaucoma have been reported in young women with cystinosis. The iris thickens and becomes rigid from deposited cystine crystals.[239]

Retinopathy of Prematurity

Angle-closure glaucoma can occur in patients with retinopathy of prematurity. The mechanisms are varied and include neovascularization, pupillary block, and pushing forward of the lens–iris diaphragm.[240,241] In known cases of retinopathy of prematurity, periodic gonioscopy is indicated and the pupil should be dilated with care. If pupillary block appears to be part of the mechanism, a peripheral LPI should be performed. If a narrow angle is encountered in a young individual, retinopathy of prematurity as well as ectopia lentis and microspherophakia should be considered.

Blackball Hyphema

Parrish and Bernardino[242] reported that pupillary block may be a part of the syndrome of elevated IOP associated with a blackball hyphema. The clot appears to block the pupil via a collar-button effect, preventing aqueous from getting from the posterior to the anterior chamber. In these cases, surgical iridectomy may be of value, although once the eye is open it may be reasonable to remove some or most of the clot.

REFERENCES

1. Lowe RF: Primary angle-closure glaucoma: a short history, *Trans Ophthalmol Soc Aust* 24:80, 1965.
2. Duke Elder S: *System of ophthalmology, vol 11, Diseases of the lens and vitreous: glaucoma and hypotony,* St Louis, 1969, Mosby.
3. Ritch R, Liebmann JM, Lowe RF: *The history of angle-closure glaucomas: from congestive to multiple mechanisms.* In Van Buskirk EM, Shields MB, editors: *100 Years of progress in glaucoma,* Philadelphia, 1997, Lippincott-Raven.
4. Smith P: On the shallow anterior chamber of primary glaucoma, *Ophthalmol Rev* 6:181, 1887.
5. von Graefe A: Uber die iridectomie bei glaukom und uber den glaucomatosen process, *Graefes Arch Clin Exp Ophthalmol* 3:456, 1857.
6. Curran EJ: New operation for glaucoma involving a new principle in the etiology and treatment of chronic primary glaucoma, *Arch Ophthalmol* 49:131, 1920.
7. Banziger T: Die Mechanik des Acute glaukom und die deutung der iridektomie wirkung bei demselben, *Dutsch Ophth Gesellsch* 43:43, 1922.
8. Raeder JG: Untersuchungen uber die lage und deche der linse in Menschlichen Auge bei physiologischen und pathogischen zustanden, nach einer neuen methode gemessen. II. Die lage der linse bei glaukomatosen zustanden, *Graefes Arch Clin Exp Ophthalmol* 112:1, 1923.
9. Gifford N: Peripheral iridotomy (Curran) as the treatment of glaucoma, *Am J Ophthalmol* 4:889, 1921.
10. O'Connor R: Peripheral iridotomy (Curran) in glaucoma, *Am J Ophthalmol* 18:146, 1935.
11. Elschnig A: Curran's irodotomie gengen glaukom, *Klin Monatsbl Augenheilkd* 70.657, 1923.

12. Barkan O: Iridectomy in narrow angle glaucoma, *Am J Ophthalmol* 37:504, 1954.
13. Chandler PA: Narrow-angle glaucoma, *Arch Ophthalmol* 47:695, 1952.
14. Barkan O: Glaucoma: classification, causes and surgical control. Results of microgonioscopic research, *Am J Ophthalmol* 21:1099, 1938.
15. Sugar HS: Newer conceptions in the classification of the glaucomas, *Am J Ophthalmol* 32:425, 1949.
16. Friedenwald JS: Symposium on primary glaucoma. I. Terminology, pathology and physiological mechanisms, *Trans Am Acad Ophthalmol Otolaryngol* 53:169, 1949.
17. Lowe RF: The causes of shallow anterior chambers in primary angle-closure glaucoma: ultrasonic giometry of normal and angle-closure eyes, *Am J Ophthalmol* 67:87, 1969.
18. Lee DA, Brubaker RF, Illstrup DM: Anterior chamber dimensions in patients with narrow angles and angle-closure glaucoma, *Arch Ophthalmol* 102:46, 1984.
19. Mapstone R: Mechanics of pupil block, *Br J Ophthalmol* 52:19, 1968.
20. Mapstone R: The mechanism and clinical significance of angle-closure, *Glaucoma* 2:249, 1980.
21. Lowe RF: Primary angle-closure glaucoma: inheritance and environment, *Br J Ophthalmol* 56:13, 1972.
22. Weekers R, Grieten J: La measure de la profondeur de la chambre anterieure en clinique, *Bull Soc Belge Ophtalmol* 129:361, 1961.
23. Clemmesen V, Luntz MH: Lens thickness and angle-closure glaucoma: a comparative oculometric study in South African negroes and Danes, *Acta Ophthalmol (Copenh)* 54:193, 1976.

24. Tomlinson A, Leighton DA: Ocular dimensions in the heredity of angle-closure glaucoma, *Br J Ophthalmol* 57:475, 1973.
25. Tornquist R: Peripheral chamber depth in shallow anterior chamber, *Br J Ophthalmol* 43:169, 1959.
26. Aizawa K: Studies on the depth of the anterior chamber, *Jpn J Ophthalmol* 4:272, 1960.
27. Alsbirk PH: Anterior chamber depth and primary angle-closure glaucoma. I. An epidemiologic study in Greenland Eskimos, *Acta Ophthalmol (Copenh)* 53:89, 1975.
28. Mapstone R: Closed-angle glaucoma in eyes with non-shallow anterior chambers, *Trans Ophthalmol Soc UK* 101:218, 1981.
29. Alsbirk PH: Corneal diameter in Greenland Eskimos: anthropometric and genetic studies with special reference to primary angle-closure glaucoma, *Acta Ophthalmol (Copenh)* 53:635, 1975.
30. Grieten J, Weekers R: Etude des dimensions de la chambre anterieure de l'oeil humain: 3e partic. Dans le glaucome a angle ferme et dans le glaucome a angle ouvert, *Opthalmologica* 143:409, 1962.
31. Lowe RF, Clark BAJ: Posterior corneal curvature correlations in normal eyes and in eyes involved with primary angle-closure glaucoma, *Br J Ophthalmol* 57:464, 1973.
32. Tornquist R: Chamber depth in primary acute glaucoma, *Br J Ophthalmol* 40:421, 1956.
33. Lowe RF, Clark BAJ: Radius of curvature of the anterior lens surface, *Br J Ophthalmol* 57:471, 1973.
34. Gernet H, Jurgens V: Echographische Befunde beim primar-chronischen Glaukom, *Graefes Arch Clin Exp* 168:419, 1965.
35. Banals WC, and others: Biometric variables in patients with occludable anterior chamber angles, *Am J Ophthalmol* 110:186, 1990.

36. Lowe RF: Anterior lens displacement with age, *Br J Ophthalmol* 54:117, 1970.

37. Fontana ST, Brubaker RF: Volume and depth of the anterior chamber in the normal aging human eye, *Arch Ophthalmol* 98:1803, 1980.

38. Lowe RF: Aetiology of the anatomical base for primary angle-closure glaucoma, *Br J Ophthalmol* 54:161, 1970.

39. Grant WM: Ocular complications of drugs: glaucoma, *JAMA* 207:2089, 1969.

40. Grant WM: *Toxicology of the eye,* ed 2, Springfield, Ill, 1974, Charles C Thomas.

41. Mandelkorn RM, Zimmerman TJ: *Effects of nonsteroidal drugs on glaucoma.* In Ritch R, Shields MB, editors: *The secondary glaucomas,* St Louis, 1982, Mosby.

42. Mitchell JD, Schwartz AL: Acute angle-closure glaucoma associated with intranasal cocaine abuse, *Am J Ophthalmol* 122:425, 1996.

43. Mapstone R, Clark CV: Diurnal variation in the dimensions of the anterior chamber, *Arch Ophthalmol* 103:1485, 1985.

44. Reiss GR, and others: Aqueous humor flow during sleep, *Invest Ophthalmol Vis Sci* 25:75, 1984.

45. Mapstone R, Clark CV: The prevalence of autonomic neuropathy in glaucoma, *Trans Ophthalmol Soc UK* 194:265, 1985.

46. Erie JC, Hodge DO, Gray DT: The incidence of primary angle-closure glaucoma in Olmsted County, Minnesota, *Arch Ophthalmol* 115:177, 1997.

47. Congdon NG, and others: Screening techniques for angle-closure glaucoma in rural Taiwan, *Acta Ophthalmol Scand* 74:113, 1996.

48. Lehrfeld L, Reber J: Glaucoma at the Wills Hospital, *Arch Ophthalmol* 18:712, 1937.

49. Lowe RF: Angle-closure glaucoma: acute and subacute attacks: clinical types, *Trans Ophthalmol Soc Aust* 21:65, 1961.

50. Hillman JS: Acute closed-angle glaucoma: An investigation into the effect of delay in treatment, *Br J Ophthalmol* 63:817, 1979.

51. Appleby RS Jr, Kinder RSL: Bilateral angle-closure glaucoma in a 14-year old boy, *Arch Ophthalmol* 86:449, 1971.

52. Fivgas GD, Beck AD: Angle-closure glaucoma in a 10-year-old girl, *Am J Ophthalmol* 124:251, 1997.

53. Host JC: A statistical study of glaucoma, *Am J Ophthalmol* 30:1267, 1947.

54. Posner A, Schlossman A: The clinical course of glaucoma, *Am J Ophthalmol* 31:915, 1948.

55. Lemoine AN: Glaucoma, *Am J Ophthalmol* 33:1353, 1950.

56. Lowe RF: Comparative incidence of angle-closure glaucoma among different national groups in Victoria, Australia, *Br J Ophthalmol* 47:721, 1963.

57. Smith R: The incidence of the primary glaucomas, *Trans Ophthalmol Soc UK* 78:215, 1958.

58. Olurin O: Anterior chamber depths of Nigerians, *Ann Ophthalmol* 9:315, 1977.

59. Alper MG, Laubach JL: Primary angle-closure glaucoma in the American negro, *Arch Ophthalmol* 79:663, 1968.

60. Barkan O: Primary glaucoma: pathogenesis and classification, *Am J Ophthalmol* 37:724, 1954.

61. Hollows FC, Graham PA: *The Ferndale glaucoma survey.* In Hunt LB, editor: *Glaucoma symposium,* London, 1966, Churchill Livingstone.

62. Bankes JLK, and others: Bedford glaucoma survey, *BMJ* 1:791, 1968.

63. Norskov K: Primary glaucoma as a cause of blindness, *Acta Ophthalmol (Copenh)* 46:853, 1968.

64. Hollows FC, Graham PA: Intraocular pressure, glaucoma and glaucoma suspects in a defined population, *Br J Ophthalmol* 50:570, 1966.

65. Luntz MH: Primary angle-closure glaucoma in urbanized South African Caucasoid and Negroid communities, *Br J Ophthalmol* 57:445, 1973.

66. Venable HP: Glaucoma in the Negro, *J Natl Med Assoc* 44:7, 1952.

67. Sarkies JWR: Primary glaucoma amongst Gold Coast Africans, *Br J Ophthalmol* 37:615, 1953.

68. Roger FC: Eye diseases in the African continent, *Am J Ophthalmol* 45:343, 1958.

69. Neumann E, Zauberman H: Glaucoma survey in Liberia, *Am J Ophthalmol* 59:8, 1965.

70. Elliott R: Ophthalmic disease in Western Samoa, *Trans Ophthalmol Soc NZ* 12:87, 1959.

71. Holmes WJ: Glaucoma in the Central and South Pacific, *Am J Ophthalmol* 51:253, 1961.

72. Congdon N, Wang F, Tielsch JM: Issues in the epidemiology and population-based screening of primary angle-closure glaucoma, *Surv Ophthalmol* 36:411, 1992.

73. Lloyd JPF: A preliminary survey of 44 consecutive cases of congestive glaucoma, *Trans Ophthalmol Soc UK* 68:89, 1948.

74. Alsbirk PH: Angle-closure glaucoma surveys in Greenland Eskimos: A preliminary report, *Can J Ophthalmol* 8:260, 1973.

75. Drance SM: Angle-closure among Canadian Eskimos, *Can J Ophthalmol* 8:252, 1973.

76. Alsbirk PH: Early detection of primary angle-closure glaucoma: limbal and axial chamber depth screening in a high risk population (Greenland Eskimos), *Acta Ophthalmol (Copenh)* 66:556, 1988.

77. Linner E: Assessment of glaucoma as a cause of blindness, India, *WHO SE Asia Regiona/Ophthalmol* 55:2, 1982.

78. Pararajasegaram R: Glaucoma pattern in Ceylon, *Trans Asia Pac Acad Ophthalmol* 3:23, 1979.

79. Lim ASM: Primary angle-closure glaucoma in Singapore, *Aust J Ophthalmol* 7:23, 1979.

80. Nguyen N, and others: A high prevalence of occludable angles in a Vietnamese population, *Ophthalmology* 103:1426, 1996.

81. Lowe RF: Clinical types of primary angle closure glaucoma, *Aust NZ J Ophthalmol* 16:245, 1988.

82. Kitazawa Y: Epidemiology of primary angle-closure glaucoma, *Asia Pac J Ophthalmol* 2:78, 1990.

83. Shiose Y, and others: Epidemiology of glaucoma in Japan: a nationwide glaucoma survey, *Jpn J Ophthalmol* 35:133, 1991.

84. Probert LA: A survey of hereditary glaucoma, *Can Med Assoc J* 66:563, 1952.

85. Biro I: Notes upon the question of hereditary glaucoma, *Ophthalmologica* 122:228, 1951.

86. Tornquist R: Shallow anterior chamber in acute glaucoma: a clinical and genetic study, *Acta Ophthalmol Scand Suppl* 39:1, 1953.

87. Kellerman L, Posner A: The value of heredity in the detection and study of glaucoma, *Am J Ophthalmol* 40:681, 1955.

88. Patterson G: Studies on siblings of patients with both angle-closure and chronic simple glaucoma, *Trans Ophthalmol Soc UK* 81:561, 1961.

89. Hagen JC III, Lederer CM Jr: Primary angle closure glaucoma in a myopic kinship, *Arch Ophthalmol* 103:363, 1985.

90. Pillat G: Statistisches zum primarren Glaukom in China, *Graefes Arch Clin* 129:299, 1933.

91. Weinstein P: Ueber das Vorkommen des Glaukoms, *Klin Monatsbl Augenheilkd* 93:794, 1934.

92. Sautter VH, Daubert K: Meterologische Studie uber das akute Glaukom, *Ophthalmologica* 129:381, 1955.

93. Hillman JS, Turner JDC: Association between acute glaucoma and the weather and sunspot activity, *Br J Ophthalmol* 61:512, 1977.

94. Watson N, Kirkby GR: Acute glaucoma presenting with abdominal symptoms, *BMJ* 299:254, 1989.

95. Goldey SH, and others: Pituitary apoplexy precipitating acute angle closure, *Arch Ophthalmol* 110:1687, 1992 (letter).

96. Kearns P, Dhillon B: Angle-closure glaucoma precipitated by labour, *Acta Ophthalmol* 68:225, 1990.

97. Bessiere E, and others: Pre- and postoperative study of the aqueous humor production in the primary glaucomas, *D'Ophtalmologie* 34:67, 1974.

98. Charles ST, Hamasaki DI: The effect of intraocular pressure on the pupil size, *Arch Ophthalmol* 83:729, 1970.

99. Ruthowski PC, Thompson HS: Mydriasis and increased intraocular pressure. I. Pupillographic studies, *Arch Ophthalmol* 87:121, 1972.

100. Anderson DR, Davis EB: Sensitivities of ocular tissues to acute pressure-induced ischemia, *Arch Ophthalmol* 93:267, 1975.

101. van Herick W, Shaffer RN, Schwartz A: Estimation of width of angle of anterior chamber: incidence and significance of the narrow angle, *Am J Ophthalmol* 68:626, 1969.

102. Douglas GR, Drance SM, Schulzer M: The visual field and nerve head in angle-closure glaucoma: a comparison of the effects of acute and chronic angle closure, *Arch Ophthalmol* 93:409, 1975.

103. Zimmerman LE, de Venecia G, Hamasaki DI: Pathology of the optic nerve in experimental acute glaucoma, *Invest Ophthalmol Vis Sci* 6:109, 1967.

104. Verhoeff FH: The effect of chronic glaucoma on the central retinal vessels, *Arch Ophthalmol* 42:145, 1913.

105. Vannas S, Tarkkanen A: Retinal vein occlusion and glaucoma: a tonographic study of the influence of glaucoma and of its prognostic significance, *Br J Ophthalmol* 44:583, 1960.

106. Hitchings RA, Spaeth GL: Chronic retinal vein occlusion and glaucoma, *Br J Ophthalmol* 60:694, 1976.

107. Hyams SW, Neumann E: Transient angle-closure glaucoma after retinal vein occlusion: report of two cases, *Br J Ophthalmol* 56:353, 1972.

108. Grant WM: Shallowing of the anterior chamber following occlusion of the central retinal vein, *Am J Ophthalmol* 75:384, 1973.

109. McNaught EI, and others: Pattern of visual damage after acute angle-closure glaucoma, *Trans Ophthalmol Soc UK* 94:406, 1974.

110. Gross FJ, Tingey D, Epstein DL: Increased prevalence of occludable angles and angle-closure glaucoma in patients with pseudoexfoliation, *Am J Ophthalmol* 117:333, 1994.

111. Airaksinen PJ, and others: Management of acute closed-angle glaucoma with miotics and timolol, *Br J Ophthalmol* 63:822, 1979.

112. Ganias F, Mapstone R: Miotics in closed-angle glaucoma, *Br J Ophthalmol* 59:205, 1975.

113. Kravitz PL, Podos SM: Use of apraclonidine in the treatment of acute angle-closure glaucoma, *Arch Ophthalmol* 108:1208, 1990.

114. Wollensak J: Prophylaxis and treatment of narrow-angle glaucoma, *Glaucoma* 1:91, 1979.

115. Halasa AH, Rutkowski PC: Thymoxamine therapy for angle-closure glaucoma, *Arch Ophthalmol* 90:177, 1973.

116. Rutkowski PC, and others: Alpha-adrenergic receptor blockade in the treatment of angle-closure glaucoma, *Trans Am Acad Ophthalmol Otolaryngol* 77:137, 1973.

117. Wand M, Grant WM: Thymoxamine hydrochloride: an alpha-adrenergic blocker, *Surv Ophthalmol* 25:75, 1980.

118. Allinson RW, and others: Reversal of mydriasis by dapiprazole, *Ann Ophthalmol* 22:131, 1990.

119. Hogan TS, and others: Dose-response study of dapiprazole HCl in the reversal of mydriasis induced by 2.5% phenylephrine, *J Ocul Pharmacol Ther* 13:297, 1997.

120. Anderson DR: Corneal indentation to relieve acute angle-closure glaucoma, *Am J Ophthalmol* 88:1091, 1979.

121. Ritch R: Argon laser treatment for medically unresponsive attacks of angle-closure glaucoma, *Am J Ophthalmol* 94:197, 1982.

122. Shin DH: Argon laser treatment for relief of medically unresponsive angle-closure glaucoma attacks, *Am J Ophthalmol* 94:821, 1982.

123. Jacobs IH, Krohn DL: Central anterior chamber depth after laser iridectomy, *Am J Ophthalmol* 89:865, 1980.

124. Abraham RK, Miller GL: Outpatient argon laser iridotomy for angle-closure glaucoma: a two-year study, *Trans Am Acad Ophthalmol Otolaryngol* 79:529, 1975.

125. Rivera AH, Brown RH, Anderson DR: Laser iridotomy vs. surgical iridectomy: have the indications changed? *Arch Ophthalmol* 103:1350, 1985.

126. Fleck BW: How large must an iridotomy be? *Br J Ophthalmol* 74:583, 1990.

127. Playfair TJ, Watson PG: Management of acute primary angle-closure glaucoma: a long-term follow-up of the results of peripheral iridectomy used as an initial procedure, *Br J Ophthalmol* 63:17, 1979.

128. Playfair TJ, Watson PG: Management of chronic or intermittent primary angle-closure glaucoma: a long-term follow-up of the results of peripheral iridectomy used as an initial procedure, *Br J Ophthalmol* 63:23, 1979.

129. Krupin T, and others: The long-term effects of iridectomy for primary acute angle-closure glaucoma, *Am J Ophthalmol* 86:506, 1978.

130. Forbes M, Becker B: Iridectomy in advanced angle-closure glaucoma, *Am J Ophthalmol* 57:57, 1962.

131. Murphy MB, Spaeth GL: Iridectomy in primary angle-closure glaucoma: classification and differential diagnosis of glaucoma associated with narrowness of the angle, *Arch Ophthalmol* 91:114, 1974.

132. Quigley HA: Long-term follow-up of laser iridotomy, *Ophthalmology* 88:218, 1981.

133. Winter FC: The second eye in acute, primary, shallow-chamber angle glaucoma, *Am J Ophthalmol* 40:557, 1955.

134. Bain WES: The fellow eye in acute closed-angle glaucoma, *Br J Ophthalmol* 41:193, 1957.

135. Lowe RF: Acute angle-closure glaucoma. The second eye: an analysis of 200 cases, *Br J Ophthalmol* 46:641, 1962.

136. Ritzinger I, Benedikt O, Dirisamer F: Surgical or conservative prophylaxis of the partner eye after primary acute angle block glaucoma, *Klin Monatsbl Augenheilkd* 164:645, 1974.

137. Snow TI: Value of prophylactic peripheral iridectomy on the second eye in angle-closure glaucoma, *Trans Ophthalmol Soc UK* 97:189, 1977.

138. Hyams SW, Friedman Z, Keroub C: Fellow eye in angle-closure glaucoma, *Br J Ophthalmol* 59:207, 1975.

139. Mapstone R: The fellow eye, *Br J Ophthalmol* 65:410, 1981.

140. Wilensky JT, and others: Follow-up of angle-closure suspects, *Am J Ophthalmol* 115:338, 1993.

141. Lloyd JPF: A preliminary survey of 44 consecutive cases of congestive glaucoma, *Trans Ophthalmol Soc UK* 68:89, 1948.

142. Akingbehin AO: Corticosteroid-induced ocular hypertension. I. Prevalence in closed-angle glaucoma, *Br J Ophthalmol* 66:536, 1982.

143. Akingbehin AO: Corticosteroid-induced ocular hypertension. II. An acquired form, *Br J Ophthalmol* 66:541, 1982.

144. Williams DJ, Gillis JP Jr, Hall GA: Results of 233 peripheral iridectomies for narrow-angle glaucoma, *Am J Ophthalmol* 65:548, 1968.

145. Galin MA, Obstbaum SA, Hung PT: Glaucoma report: rethinking prophylactic iridectomy, *Ann Ophthalmol* 8:1333, 1976.

146. Floman N, Berson P, Landau L: Peripheral iridectomy in closed angle glaucoma: late complications, *Br J Ophthalmol* 61:101, 1977.

147. Lowe RF: Primary angle-closure glaucoma: a review 5 years after bilateral surgery, *Br J Ophthalmol* 57:457, 1973.

148. Bobrow JC, Drews RC: Long-term results of peripheral iridectomy, *Glaucoma* 3:319, 1981.

148a. Saraux H, Offre H: Long-term study of patients with iridectomy for angle-closure glaucoma, *Glaucoma* 1:149, 1979.

149. Kirsch RE: A study of provocative tests for angle closure glaucoma, *Arch Ophthalmol* 74:770, 1965.

150. Shirakashi M, Iwata K, Nakayama T: Argon laser trabeculoplasty for chronic angle-closure glaucoma uncontrolled by iridotomy, *Acta Ophthalmol (Copenh)* 67:265, 1989.

151. Fu YA, Liaw ZC: Argon laser gonioplasty with trabeculoplasty for chronic angle-closure glaucoma before and after peripheral iridectomy, *Ann Ophthalmol* 19:419, 1987.

152. Weiss HS, and others: Argon laser gonioplasty in the treatment of angle closure glaucoma, *Am J Ophthalmol* 114:14, 1992.

153. Wand M: Argon laser gonioplasty for synechial angle closure, *Arch Ophthalmol* 110:363, 1992.

154. Campbell DG, Vella A: Modern goniosynechialysis for the treatment of synechial angle-closure glaucoma, *Ophthalmology* 97:551, 1990.

155. Shingleton BJ, and others: Surgical goniosynechialysis for angle closure glaucoma, *Ophthalmology* 97:551, 1990.

156. Sugar HS: Cataract formation and refractive changes after surgery for angle-closure glaucoma, *Am J Ophthalmol* 69:747, 1970.

157. Godel V, Regenbogen L: Cataractogenic factors in patients with primary angle-closure glaucoma after peripheral iridectomy, *Am J Ophthalmol* 83:180, 1977.

158. Maltzman BA, Agin M: Argon peripheral iridotomy and cataract formation, *Ann Ophthalmol* 20:28, 1988.

159. Cashwell LF, Martin TJ: Malignant glaucoma after laser iridotomy, *Ophthalmology* 99:651, 1992.

160. Setala K: Corneal endothelial cell density after an attack of acute glaucoma, *Acta Ophthalmol (Copenh)* 57:1004, 1979.

161. Olsen T: The endothelial cell damage in acute glaucoma: on the corneal thickness response to intraocular pressure, *Acta Ophthalmol (Copenh)* 58:257, 1980.

162. Bigar F, Witmer R: Corneal endothelial changes in primary acute angle-closure glaucoma, *Ophthalmology* 89:596, 1982.

163. Markowitz SN, Morin JD: The endothelium in primary angle-closure glaucoma, *Am J Ophthalmol* 98:103, 1984.

164. Pitts JF, Jay JL: The association of Fuchs corneal endothelial dystrophy with axial hypermetropia, shallow anterior chamber and angle closure glaucoma, *Br J Ophthalmol* 74:601, 1990.

165. Power WJ, Collum LM: Electron microscopic appearance of human corneal endothelium following Nd:YAG laser iridotomy, *Ophthalmol Surg* 23:347, 1992.

166. Martin NF, and others: Endothelium damage thresholds for retrocorneal Q-switched neodymium:YAG laser pulses in monkeys, *Ophthalmology* 92:1382, 1985.

167. Schwartz AL, Martin NF, Weber PA: Corneal decompensation after argon laser iridectomy, *Arch Ophthalmol* 106:1572, 1988.

168. Hirst LW, and others: Corneal endothelial changes after argon laser iridotomy and panretinal photocoagulation, *Am J Ophthalmol* 93:473, 1982.

169. Smith J, Whitted P: Corneal endothelial changes after argon laser iridotomy, *Am J Ophthalmol* 98:153, 1984.

170. Thoming C, Van Buskirk EM, Samples JR: The corneal endothelium after laser therapy for glaucoma, *Am J Ophthalmol* 103:518, 1987.

171. Panek WC, Lee DA, Christensen RE: Effects of argon laser iridotomy on the corneal endothelium, *Arch Ophthalmol* 105:395, 1988.

172. Panek WC, Lee DA, Christensen RE: The effects of Nd:YAG laser iridotomy on the corneal endothelium, *Am J Ophthalmol* 111:505, 1991.

173. Chandler PA, Trotter RR: Angle-closure glaucoma, subacute types, *Arch Ophthalmol* 53:305, 1955.

174. Ravits J, Seybold ME: Transient monocular visual loss from narrow-angle glaucoma, *Arch Neurol* 41:991, 1984.

175. Mapstone R: Mechanisms in ocular hypertension, *Br J Ophthalmol* 63:325, 1979.

176. Gorin G: Shortening of the angle of the anterior chamber in angle-closure glaucoma, *Am J Ophthalmol* 49:141, 1960.

177. Lowe RF: Primary angle-closure of provocative tests, *Br J Ophthalmol* 51:727, 1967.

178. Pollack IP: Chronic angle-closure glaucoma: diagnosis and treatment in patients with angles that appear open, *Arch Ophthalmol* 85:676, 1971.

179. Phillips CI: Closed-angle glaucoma: significance of sectoral variations in angle depth, *Br J Ophthalmol* 40:136, 1956.

180. Bhargava SK, Leighton DA, Phillips CI: Early angle-closure glaucoma, *Arch Ophthalmol* 89:369, 1973.

181. Forbes M: Gonioscopy with corneal indentation: a method for distinguishing between appositional closure and synechial closure, *Arch Ophthalmol* 76:488, 1966.

182. Venable HP: Glaucoma in the Negro, *J Natl Med Assoc* 44:7, 1952.

183. Neumann E, Zauberman H: Glaucoma survey in Liberia, *Am J Ophthalmol* 59:8, 1965.

184. Avshalom A, and others: Israeli ophthalmologists in Africa, *J Israel Med Assoc* 70:254, 1966.

185. Spaeth GL: The normal development of the human anterior chamber angle: a new system of descriptive grading, *Trans Ophthalmol Soc UK* 91:709, 1971.

186. Smith RJH: A new method of estimating the depth of the anterior chamber, *Br J Ophthalmol* 63:215, 1979.

187. Jacobs IH: Anterior chamber depth measurement using the slit-lamp microscope, *Am J Ophthalmol* 88:236, 1979.

188. Chan RY, Smith JA, Richardson KT: Anterior segment configuration correlated with Shaffer's grading of anterior chamber angle, *Arch Ophthalmol* 99:104, 1981.

189. Campbell DG: A comparison of diagnostic techniques in angle-closure glaucoma, *Am J Ophthalmol* 88:197, 1979.

190. Patel KH, and others: Incidence of acute angle-closure glaucoma after pharmacologic mydriasis, *Am J Ophthalmol* 120:709, 1995.

191. Wilensky JT, Ritch R, Kolker AE: Should patients with anatomically narrow angles have prophylactic iridectomy? *Surv Ophthalmol* 41:31, 1996.

192. Harris LS, Galin MA: Pprone provocative testing for narrow angle glaucoma, *Arch Ophthalmol* 87:493, 1972.

193. Becker B, Thompson HE: Tonography and angle-closure glaucoma: diagnosis and therapy, *Am J Ophthalmol* 46:305, 1958.

194. Gloster J, Poinoosawmy D: Changes in intraocular pressure during and after the dark room test, *Br J Ophthalmol* 57:170, 1973.

195. Friedman Z, Neumann E: Comparison of prone-position, dark-room, and mydriatic test for angle-closure glaucoma before and after peripheral iridectomy, *Am J Ophthalmol* 74:24, 1972.

196. Hyams SW, Friedman Z, Neumann E: Elevated intraocular pressure in the prone position: a new provocative test for angle-closure glaucoma, *Am J Ophthalmol* 66:661, 1968.

197. Neumann E, Hyams SW: Gonioscopy and anterior chamber depth in the prone-position provocative test for angle-closure glaucoma, *Ophthalmologica* 167:9, 1973.

198. Mapstone R: Provocative tests in closed-angle glaucoma, *Br J Ophthalmol* 60:115, 1976.

199. Drance SM: Angle closure glaucoma among Canadian Eskimos, *Can J Ophthalmol* 8:252, 1973.

200. Hung PT, Chow LH: Provocation and mechanism of angle-closure glaucoma after iridectomy, *Arch Ophthalmol* 97:1862, 1979.

201. Ritch R: *Glaucoma secondary to lens intumescence and dislocation.* In Ritch R, Shields MB, editors: *The secondary glaucomas,* St Louis, 1982, Mosby.

202. Tomey KF, al Rajhi-AA: Neodymium:YAG laser iridotomy in the initial management of phacomorphic glaucoma, *Ophthalmology* 99:660, 1992.

203. Neuschler R: Myopia transitoria in corso di terapie con dichlorfenamide, *Bull Ocul* 43:507, 1964.

204. Muirhead JF, Scheie HS: Transient myopia after acetazolamide, *Arch Ophthalmol* 63:315, 1960.

205. Fan JT, Johnson DH, Burk RR: Transient myopia, angle-closure glaucoma, and choroidal detachment after oral acetazolamide, *Am J Ophthalmol* 115:813, 1993 (letter).

206. Beasley FJ: Transient myopia during trichlormethazide therapy, *Ann Ophthalmol* 12:705, 1980.

207. Edwards TS: Transient myopia due to tetracycline, *JAMA* 186:69, 1963.

208. Yasuna E: Acute myopia associated with prochloroperazine (Compazine) therapy, *Am J Ophthalmol* 54:793, 1962.

209. Belci C: Miopia transitori in corso di terapia con diuretici, *Bull Ocul* 47:24, 1968.

210. Sanford-Smith JH: Transient myopia after aspirin, *Br J Ophthalmol* 58:698, 1974.

211. Maddalena MA: Transient myopia associated with acute glaucoma and retinal edema following vaginal administration of sulfanilamide, *Arch Ophthalmol* 80:186, 1968.

212. Schroeder W, Schwarzer J: Transitorische myopie mit Winkelblockglaucoma, *Klin Montasbl Augenheilkd* 172:762, 1978.

213. Epstein DL: *Chandler and Grants glaucoma,* Philadelphia, 1986, Lea & Febiger.

214. Sugar HS: Pupil block in aphakic eyes, *Am J Ophthalmol* 46:831, 1958.

215. Chandler PA: Glaucoma from pupillary block in aphakia, *Arch Ophthalmol* 67:44, 1962.

216. Francois J: Aphakic glaucoma, *Ann Ophthalmol* 6:429, 1974.

217. Ferayonri JJ: Intraocular lenses and secondary glaucoma: a retrospective study, *Ann Ophthalmol* 10:1447, 1978.

218. Layden WE: Pseudophakia and glaucoma, *Ophthalmology* 89:875, 1982.

219. Cohen JS, and others: Complications of extracapsular cataract surgery: the indications and risks of peripheral iridectomy, *Ophthalmology* 91:826, 1984.

220. Van Buskirk EM: Pupillary block after intraocular lens implantation, *Am J Ophthalmol* 95:55, 1983.

221. Obstbaum SA, and others: Laser photomydriasis in pseudophakic pupillary block, *J Am Intraocul Implant Soc* 7:28, 1981.

222. Mandelcorn MS: Laser iridotomy in post-traumatic and postsurgical pupillary block: a report of five cases, *Can J Ophthalmol* 13:163, 1978.

223. Kokoris N, Macy JI: Laser iridectomy treatment of acute pseudophakic pupillary block glaucoma, *J Am Intraocul Implant Soc* 8:33, 1982.

224. Murphy GE: Long-term gonioscopy follow-up of eyes with posterior chamber lens implants and no iridectomy, *Ophthalmic Surg* 17:227, 1986.

225. Weinreb RN, and others: Pseudophakic pupillary block with angle-closure glaucoma in diabetic patients, *Am J Ophthalmol* 102:325, 1986.

226. Hein HF, Muttzman B: Long-standing anterior dislocation of the crystalline lens, *Ann Ophthalmol* 7:66, 1975.

227. Nelson LP, Maumenee IH: Ectopia lentis, *Surv Ophthalmol* 27:143, 1982.

228. Johnson VP, Grayson M, Christain JC: Dominant microspherophakia, *Arch Ophthalmol* 85:534, 1971.

229. Cross HE, Jensen AD: Ocular manifestations in the Marfan syndrome and homocysteinuria, *Am J Ophthalmol* 75:405, 1973.

230. Bessiere E, Riviere J, Leuret JP: An association of Klinefelter's disease and congenital anomalies, captodactyly and microphakia, *Bull Soc Ophtalmol Fr* 62:197, 1962.

231. Magnasco A: Unusual malformation association: mandibulofacial dysostosis and bilateral microspherophakia, *Ann Ophthalmol* 91:489, 1965.

232. Sohar E: Renal disease, inner ear deafness and ocular changes: a new heredofamilial syndrome, *Arch Intern Med* 97:627, 1956.
233. Meyer SJ, Holstein T: Spherophakia with glaucoma and brachydactyly, *Am J Ophthalmol* 24:247, 1941.
234. Probert LA: Spherophakia with brachydactyly: comparison with Marfan's syndrome, *Am J Ophthalmol* 36:1571, 1953.
235. McGavic JS: Weill-Marchesani syndrome, *Am J Ophthalmol* 62:820, 1966.

236. Feiler-Ofrey V, Stein R, Godel V: Marchesani's syndrome and chamber angle anomalies, *Am J Ophthalmol* 65:862, 1968.
237. Urbanek J: Glaucoma juvenile inversum, *Z Augenheilk* 77:171, 1930.
238. Ritch R, Wand M: Treatment for the Weill-Marchesani syndrome, *Ann Ophthalmol* 13:665, 1981.
239. Wan WL, Minckler DS, Rao NA: Pupillary block glaucoma associated with childhood cystinosis, *Am J Ophthalmol* 101:700, 1986.

240. Michael AJ, and others: Management of late-onset angle-closure glaucoma associated with retinopathy of prematurity, *Ophthalmology* 98:1093, 1991.
241. Ueda N, Ogino N: Angle-closure glaucoma with pupillary block mechanism in cicatricial retinopathy of prematurity, *Ophthalmologica* 196:15, 1988.
242. Parrish R, Bernardino V Jr: Iridectomy in the surgical management of eight-ball hyphema, *Arch Ophthalmol* 100:435, 1982.

16

Angle-Closure Glaucoma Without Pupillary Block

PATHOPHYSIOLOGY

There are many diseases and conditions that produce angle-closure glaucoma without pupillary block. It is important for clinicians to understand these diseases and conditions—not because they are common causes of glaucoma, but rather because they are capable of producing severe elevations of intraocular pressure (IOP) and marked loss of vision. The term *without pupillary block* is actually an oversimplification. Unless the patient has previously undergone an iridectomy or has developed iris atrophy, in many eyes there can be some degree of pupillary block. However, in the diseases discussed in this chapter, pupillary block contributes little to the development of angle closure (i.e., angle closure would develop even if a patent iridectomy were present).

It is possible to conceptualize the secondary angle-closure glaucomas without pupillary block as occurring through two different mechanisms—an anterior pulling mechanism and a posterior pushing mechanism.[1] In the anterior pulling mechanism, the peripheral iris is pulled forward onto the trabecular meshwork by the contraction of a membrane, inflammatory exudate, or fibrous band (Fig. 16-1). Examples of this mechanism include neovascular glaucoma and the iridocorneal endothelial (ICE) syndrome. As the membrane, band, or inflammatory material contracts, it acts like a zipper to form permanent peripheral anterior synechiae, which can be spotty and irregular or diffuse and quite regular. Pupillary block plays little or no role in this mechanism.

In the posterior pushing mechanism, the peripheral iris is displaced forward by the lens, vitreous, or ciliary body (Fig. 16-2). An example of this mechanism occurs when gas is injected into the vitreous cavity to repair a retinal detachment, and it displaces the lens-iris diaphragm forward sufficiently to close the angle. This can happen despite the presence of a patent iridectomy. The posterior pushing mechanism is often accompanied by swelling and anterior rotation of the ciliary body, which also act to close the angle. When the anterior uvea swells from inflammation or vascular congestion, the ciliary ring is narrowed, which reduces tension on the zonules, permits the lens to come forward, and displaces the peripheral iris. When the ciliary body swells, it also rotates forward about its attachment to the scleral spur, which again loosens the zonules and displaces the root of the iris. The ciliary body is like a fan that opens about its attachment at the scleral spur as it swells.[2] Finally, ciliary body swelling is often accompanied by the accumulation of suprachoroidal and supraciliary fluid, which further rotates the ciliary body and iris root into the angle. The posterior pushing mechanism is often accompanied by varying degrees of pupillary block. In some conditions such as aqueous misdirection (ciliary-block glaucoma), pupillary block plays no role, whereas in other conditions, such as glaucoma associated with retinopathy of prematurity, pupillary block contributes to the angle closure.

When pupillary block is the major mechanism, the peripheral iris is pushed forward by aqueous humor in the posterior chamber, which is under greater pressure than the fluid in the anterior chamber (Fig. 16-3, *A*). In this situation the posterior chamber is enlarged. Pupillary block is relieved by iridectomy or pupillary dilation, which allows the pressures in the two chambers to equilibrate so that the peripheral iris is no longer bowed forward into contact with the trabecular meshwork. In the posterior pushing mechanism without pupillary block, the peripheral iris is displaced forward by direct pressure from the lens, ciliary body, vitreous, or mass lesion in the posterior segment (Fig. 16-3, *B*). This mechanism is not relieved by iridectomy or pupillary dilation because

plateau iris by Shaffer and Chandler.[5,6] Wand and co-workers[7] then divided plateau iris into two entities that they called plateau iris configuration and plateau iris syndrome.

Plateau Iris Configuration

Plateau iris configuration consists of angle-closure glaucoma in an eye with a normal central anterior chamber depth and a flat iris plane (Fig. 16-3, *C*). On gonioscopy, the iris appears flat from the pupillary margin to the midperiphery—a shape that Tornquist termed "plateau"[8]—at which point it takes a sharp turn posteriorly before inserting into the ciliary body.* This sharp turn creates a narrow angle recess and the potential for angle closure. In some cases the iris periphery has redundant folds with a prominent roll. Ultrasound biomicroscopy reveals anteriorly displaced ciliary processes that may push the peripheral iris forward or at least prevent it from falling back after iridectomy (Fig. 16-4).[9] When the pupil dilates spontaneously or in response to pharmacologic agents, the iris can bunch or crowd into the angle and cover the trabecular meshwork. This anterior segment configuration differs from the shallow central anterior chamber and iris bombé seen typically with pupillary block (see Fig. 16-3, *A*).

Plateau iris configuration is more common than recognized, although the condition is probably not common per se. In most cases the glaucoma is cured by iridectomy, which suggests that pupillary block plays a role in the development of angle closure. Iridectomy does not widen the angle substantially, even in successful cases, perhaps because there is little iris bombé preoperatively. After surgery these eyes should be examined periodically for signs of residual glaucoma. Pupillary dilation should be restricted to one eye per office visit. Mydriasis is best accomplished with either mild parasympatholytic or sympathomimetic agents, the effects of which can be readily reversed if IOP rises.

Plateau Iris Syndrome

The plateau iris syndrome resembles plateau iris configuration except that angle-closure glaucoma occurs despite the presence of a patent iridectomy. Most authorities believe that the peculiar anatomic configuration of the iris allows it to bunch in the angle and occlude the trabecular meshwork when the pupil dilates spontaneously or in response to mydriatic agents. A few early investigators postulated that angle closure occurs because the ciliary processes are rotated forward,[10,11] an

*See Figures 3-16 through 3-19 in Campbell DG, Netland PN: *Stereo atlas of glaucoma,* St Louis, 1998, Mosby.

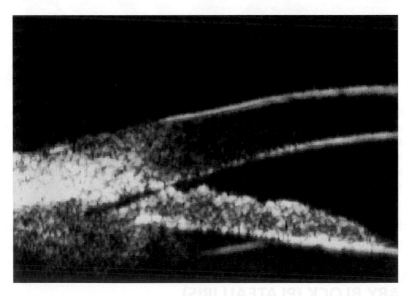

Figure 16-4   Ultrasound biomicroscopic image of plateau iris. Note anterior displacement of ciliary processes pushing iris forward and relatively straight configuration of the iris. Compare with Figure 15-2, *B* showing the forward bowing of the iris in pupillary block. (Courtesy of Robert Ritch, M.D.)

observation now confirmed by ultrasound biomicroscopy. Ultrasound biomicroscopy has also revealed several patients with multiple ciliary body cysts associated with plateau iris syndrome.[12] The plateau iris syndrome is often seen in patients aged 30 to 40 and occurs in equal numbers of men and women. This syndrome usually is seen as acute or subacute angle-closure glaucoma days to weeks after iridectomy or other intraocular surgery. This can occur spontaneously or after pharmacologic dilation of the pupil. If not diagnosed and treated properly, repeated episodes of angle closure can produce peripheral anterior synechiae and permanent elevation of IOP.[13]

Lowe and Ritch[14] proposed an "incomplete" type of plateau iris syndrome that is more common than the "complete" form of the syndrome. In the incomplete plateau iris syndrome, the iris is not as far forward as in the complete syndrome; in these patients, the IOP does not rise with dilation, but peripheral anterior synechiae may form over time. Gonioscopy and ultrasound show large and/or anteriorly positioned ciliary processes that seem to push the iris against the trabecular meshwork.[15,16]

Some investigators have stated that plateau iris syndrome is relatively common, occurring in 6% to 20% of eyes with angle closure.[17,18] However, these estimates were based on postiridectomy provocative tests that were done without gonioscopic documentation of angle closure. Plateau iris syndrome is probably much rarer than these estimates in most populations. However, in Samoans, plateau iris may be relatively common.[19]

Although it is possible to identify plateau iris before iridectomy by noting the typical iris configuration, the diagnosis is usually made by observing both elevated pressure (especially after pharmacologic dilation) and no significant opening of the chamber angle after iridotomy has been successfully performed. Obviously, if there are extensive peripheral anterior synechiae, then the diagnosis cannot be substantiated. The differential diagnosis of plateau iris syndrome includes extensive peripheral anterior synechiae due to any cause, imperforate or occluded iridectomy, multiple cysts of the iris or ciliary body (although this may be related), aqueous-misdirection (ciliary-block or malignant) glaucoma, open-angle glaucoma with anatomically narrow angles, mixed-mechanism glaucoma, and the effect of topical corticosteroids or cycloplegic agents.

The treatment for plateau iris syndrome consists of postoperative miotic agents to prevent pupillary dilation. If the response to miotics is inadequate, argon laser gonioplasty should be performed to widen the angle.[20,21] If gonioplasty plus medical therapy cannot control the IOP adequately, then trabeculectomy should be considered.

SECONDARY ANGLE-CLOSURE GLAUCOMA WITHOUT PUPILLARY BLOCK

Anterior Pulling Mechanism

Neovascular Glaucoma

Neovascular glaucoma is caused by a fibrovascular membrane that develops on the surface of the iris and the angle. At first the membrane merely covers the angle structures, but then it contracts to form peripheral anterior synechiae. Neovascular glaucoma rarely, if ever, occurs as a primary condition, but it is always associated with other abnormalities, most commonly some form of ocular ischemia. Neovascular glaucoma is an important entity because it often causes great morbidity and visual loss. A variety of other terms have been used to describe this condition, including thrombotic glaucoma, hemorrhagic glaucoma, diabetic hemorrhagic glaucoma, congestive glaucoma, and rubeotic glaucoma. The term *neovascular glaucoma* is used here because it includes all glaucoma caused by or related to a fibrovascular membrane on the iris and/or angle.[22] It is important to distinguish the terms *neovascular glaucoma* and *rubeosis iridis*. Rubeosis iridis refers to new vessels on the surface of the iris regardless of the state of the angle or the presence of glaucoma.

Neovascular glaucoma was first described in 1866 following central retinal vein occlusion.[23] Additional descriptions were provided by various observers in the latter part of the nineteenth century and early twentieth century, including Coates in 1906.[24] Nettleship[25] and Salus[26] noted the association of neovascular glaucoma and diabetes mellitus. Kurz[27] described the gonioscopic appearance of new vessels in the angle and postulated that this fibrovascular tissue contracted to form peripheral anterior synechiae. Until 1963, the condition was known mostly as "hemorrhagic glaucoma," based on the occasional association with hyphema; the term "neovascular glaucoma" was proposed by Weiss and co-workers,[28,29] and because this term better fits with the pathophysiology of the condition, it has become the accepted one.

Box 16-1
Diseases and Conditions Associated With Neovascularization of the Iris and Neovascular Glaucoma

Ocular Vascular Disease

Central retinal vein occlusion
Central retinal artery occlusion
Branch retinal vein occlusion
Branch retinal artery occlusion
Sturge-Weber syndrome with choroidal hemangioma
Leber's miliary aneurysms
Sickle cell retinopathy
Diabetes mellitus

Extraocular Disease

Carotid artery disease/ligation
Ocular ischemia
Aortic arch syndrome
Carotid-cavernous fistula
Giant cell arteritis
Pulseless disease

Assorted Ocular Diseases

Retinal detachment
Eales' disease
Coats' disease
Retinopathy of prematurity
Persistence and hyperplasia of the primary vitreous
Retinoschisis
Glaucoma
   Open-angle
   Angle-closure
   Secondary
Norrie's disease
Stickler's syndrome

Trauma

Essential iris atrophy
Neurofibromatosis
Lupus erythematosus
Marfan's syndrome
Recurrent hemorrhages
Vitreous wick syndrome

Ocular Neoplasms

Malignant melanoma
Retinoblastoma
Optic nerve glioma associated with venous stasis
Metastatic carcinoma
Reticulum cell sarcoma
Medulloepithelioma
Squamous cell carcinoma conjunctiva
Angiomatosis retinae

Ocular Inflammatory Disease

Chronic uveitis
Endophthalmitis
Sympathetic ophthalmia
Syphilitic retinitis
Vogt-Koyanagi-Harada syndrome

Ocular Therapy

Cataract excision (especially in diabetics)
Vitrectomy (especially in diabetics)
Retinal detachment surgery
Radiation
Laser coreoplasty

Modified from Gartner S, Henkind P: Neovascularization of the iris (rubeosis iridis), *Surv Ophthalmol* 22:291, 1978 and Wand M: *Neovascular glaucoma.* In: Ritch R, Shields MB, editors: *The secondary glaucomas,* St Louis, 1982, Mosby.

who suffer a central retinal vein occlusion develop neovascular glaucoma. More recent investigations have done much to clarify this association. Hayreh[87,88] deserves the credit for classifying central retinal vein occlusion into two types—ischemic and nonischemic (venous stasis retinopathy). Approximately three fourths of central retinal vein occlusions are nonischemic, and one fourth are ischemic.[89] Yet neovascular glaucoma occurs in 18% to 86% of eyes with ischemic vein occlusions, as opposed to 0% to 4% of eyes with nonischemic occlusions.[90-94] According to a large study, about 40% of patients with ischemic central retinal vein occlusion will develop neovascular glaucoma.[95] A large, multicenter study to evaluate this issue in more detail is under way. The distinction between ischemic and nonischemic vein occlusions is usually made by judging the degree of retinal capillary nonperfusion (capillary dropout) on fluorescein angiography.[96,97] Other signs of ischemia include 10 or more cotton wool spots in the retina, an absent perifoveal capillary network on fluorescein angiography, arteriovenous transit time greater than 20 seconds, leaky iris vessels on angiography, and a reduced B:A wave ratio on electroretinography. Eyes with ischemic central retinal vein occlusions should receive panretinal photocoagulation or cryoablation to reduce the incidence of neovascular glaucoma. Careful follow-up is mandated even in those with the nonischemic type because of the observation that one third of eyes with central retinal vein occlusion and good perfusion at the onset show signs of ischemia by 3 years.[98]

Neovascular glaucoma may present anywhere from 2 weeks to 2 years following a central retinal vein occlusion.[99] However, the condition often presents about 3 months after central retinal vein occlusion and thus has been called the 100-day glaucoma. Younger patients with central retinal vein occlusions often have associated vascular diseases such as hypertension or one of the collagen vascular disorders.

Older patients with central retinal vein occlusions often have associated glaucoma or elevated IOP. Elevated IOP or glaucoma has been reported in 10% to 23% of eyes that developed a central retinal vein occlusion.[100,101] In most cases the underlying glaucoma is open-angle or exfoliative in type, but there have been a few reports of central retinal vein occlusion following angle-closure glaucoma.[102] The underlying glaucoma is often masked because these eyes may have a low IOP for weeks to months following vein occlusion.[103] In addition, the low IOP may reflect transient poor perfusion of the ciliary body. A few investigators have also postulated a direct effect of an angiogenic factor on aqueous humor dynamics.[104] The presence of preexisting primary open-angle glaucoma increases the risk of neovascular glaucoma after central retinal vein occlusion despite adequate prophylactic laser treatment. Adequate treatment of the preexisting glaucoma does not prevent the onset of neovascularization. Furthermore, preexisting open-angle glaucoma may make any subsequent neovascular glaucoma more refractory to treatment.[105] It is also common for fellow eyes to have elevated IOP or to develop it at a later time. Although a true causative role for elevated IOP in central retinal vein occlusion has not been established, it is probably wise to treat fellow eyes with elevated IOP with ocular hypotensive agents. One case-control study does support elevated IOP as a risk factor in central retinal vein occlusion along with systemic hypertension and male gender.[106] Green and co-workers[107] proposed that posterior bowing of the lamina cribrosa in glaucoma creates a mechanical obstruction that impedes the venous outflow and contributes to venous stasis and/or occlusion.

Carotid Occlusive Disease. Carotid artery disease is now the third most common cause of neovascular glaucoma. Neovascular glaucoma has been reported after carotid artery ligation[108,109] and idiopathic carotid artery obstruction. The obstruction can be unilateral or bilateral and can involve the common carotid artery or the internal carotid artery.[110-113] Carotid artery obstruction does not cause neovascular glaucoma in all cases because there is usually sufficient collateral flow to prevent widespread retinal ischemia. Carotid artery palpation and auscultation should be performed in all cases of central retinal vein occlusion. Neovascular glaucoma associated with carotid artery disease often has a confusing presentation and a variable course. If anterior segment ischemia is severe, the vessels on the iris may be less visible, and the IOP may be normal or even low despite extensive neovascular closure of the angle. These eyes often suffer wide swings in IOP, depending on the perfusion to the ciliary body.[114] Patients who undergo surgery to relieve or bypass carotid artery obstruction may experience a dramatic rise in IOP when the ciliary body blood supply improves and aqueous humor formation increases. Panretinal photocoagulation may be less successful in eliminating iris neovascularization in patients with carotid artery obstruction because the anterior segment of these eyes is also ischemic and is not affected by retinal ablation techniques.

Ocular Ischemic Syndrome. Several authors have described a condition called chronic ocular ischemic syndrome that includes signs of transient ischemic attacks; ocular motor disturbances; midperipheral retinal hemorrhages; neovascularization of the iris; and late in its course, corneal striae and hypotony.[115,116] Although the term was initially used to describe obstruction of the carotid artery, extracarotid causes have also been identified, including abnormalities of carotid flow without stenosis, cranial arteritis, and coronary artery disease.[117,118] Carotid artery obstruction accounts for about 75% of these patients, with other risk factors being diabetes mellitus, systemic hypertension, and a history of cerebrovascular accident.[119] Doppler imaging of the carotids should be considered if any of the symptoms or signs associated with the ocular ischemic syndrome are manifest. Treatment proposals have included oral verapamil, panretinal photocoagulation, and carotid endarterectomy.[120,121] Sivalingam and co-workers were unable to demonstrate a significant improvement after endarterectomy.

Central Retinal Artery Occlusion. Other vascular occlusive diseases of the eye may also be associated with neovascular glaucoma. Seven percent to fifteen percent of patients with a central retinal artery occlusion will develop neovascular glaucoma.[122,125] Some, but not all, have concomitant carotid artery occlusive disease.[126] Although panretinal photocoagulation may have some effect in reducing the incidence of neovascular glaucoma, it is not as effective as in retinal vein occlusion or diabetes mellitus.[127]

Miscellaneous. Neovascular glaucoma occurs after a variety of therapeutic interventions, including radiotherapy,[128,129] microwave thermoradiotherapy,[130] and retinal detachment surgery.[131]

lation.[165-172] One can expect approximately 65% success after 1 year in controlling pressures and pain with this modality. The results seem comparable with those achieved with seton surgery. In our hands, contact cyclophotocoagulation with neodymium:yttrium-aluminum-garnet (Nd:YAG) or diode laser is a relatively safe and effective procedure for patients with poor vision or poor visual prognosis and for those for whom a seton operation may be inadvisable (e.g., previous encircling band, poor physical condition) (see Chapter 36). Retrobulbar alcohol injections and enucleation are appropriate treatments for eyes with no useful vision and pain that does not respond to medical therapy and ciliodestructive procedures.

Some have advocated direct laser treatment to new vessels in the angle, a technique referred to as goniophotocoagulation, if neovascularization of the iris is encountered before peripheral anterior synechiae have formed.[173] Low-energy argon laser treatments (0.2 seconds, 50 to 100 μm, 100 to 200 mW) are applied to the neovascular tufts as they cross the scleral spur. The laser therapy often must be repeated because these vessels may reopen minutes to days after treatment. Although goniophotocoagulation is inadequate treatment for neovascular glaucoma by itself, it may be a useful adjunct to panretinal photocoagulation in certain situations. For example, goniophotocoagulation can reduce angle neovascularization and synechia formation temporarily while panretinal photocoagulation takes effect and reduces the angiogenic stimulus. Finally, goniophotocoagulation can be applied when full panretinal photocoagulation is not totally successful in reducing the angiogenic stimulus.

In the future, therapeutic activities will be directed toward reducing or inhibiting the angiogenic stimulus. For example, inhibition of VEGF with specific antibodies will prevent the iris neovascularization produced in subhuman primates by laser occlusion of the central retinal vein.[174] Experimentally, several compounds with capabilities to inhibit VEGF have been identified. Other efforts may be directed toward finding and reversing the genetic makeup of those predisposed toward neovascular glaucoma. In another approach, experimental iris neovascularization has been treated in animal eyes using hematoporphyrin derivative and exposure to red light (630 nm).[175]

Iridocorneal Endothelial Syndrome

The iridocorneal endothelial (ICE) syndrome takes many clinical forms but usually includes some combination of iris atrophy, corneal edema, and secondary angle-closure glaucoma without pupillary block. This syndrome is caused by an abnormal corneal endothelium that forms a membrane over the anterior surface of the iris and the angle structures. When this membrane contracts, it distorts the iris and closes the angle (Fig. 16-6).[176]

Histopathology

Histopathologic examination of eyes affected by the ICE syndrome reveals a thin, abnormal corneal endothelium and Descemet's membrane separated by a thick accumulation of collagen.[177-179] These tissues form a multilayered membrane that covers the angle and extends onto the anterior surface of the iris.[180-183] The endothelial cells develop the epithelial-like characteristics of desmosomes, microvilli, tonofilaments (contractile elements), and proliferation—none of which occur in normal corneal endothelium.[184,185] Most authorities believe this to be a metaplasia of endothelium into cells with epithelial characteristics.[186] What the stimulus is for the "epithelialization" of these cells is not known. These histopathologic changes are manifest on clinical examination by a "beaten silver" appearance to the endothelium on slit-lamp examination; a loss of the normal, regular endothelial mosaic on specular reflection; and alterations in the size and shape of endothelial cells on specular microscopy.[187] The size and shape of endothelial cells show great variation—some may be necrotic, and the findings are often patchy in the early stages of the condition. Even with the variation in clinical presentation, the endothelial findings are usually there if looked for carefully enough.

Pathogenesis

The most commonly accepted theory on the pathogenesis of the ICE syndrome proposes that the fundamental defect is in the corneal endothelium. The abnormal endothelium is dysfunctional, which leads to corneal edema. Furthermore, the corneal endothelium produces a membrane that covers the angle and the anterior surface of the iris. When the membrane contracts, it causes peripheral anterior synechiae, glaucoma, corectopia, stretch holes, and iris nodules. Ischemia may be a secondary phenomenon producing melt holes. At present we do not understand what causes the corneal endothelium to behave in this unusual manner. A few investigators[188,189] postulate that there is an abnormal proliferation of neural crest cells or a fetal rest of epithelial cells.[190] Other authorities[191] suggest the endothelium proliferates because of inflammation. Electron micrographic, im-

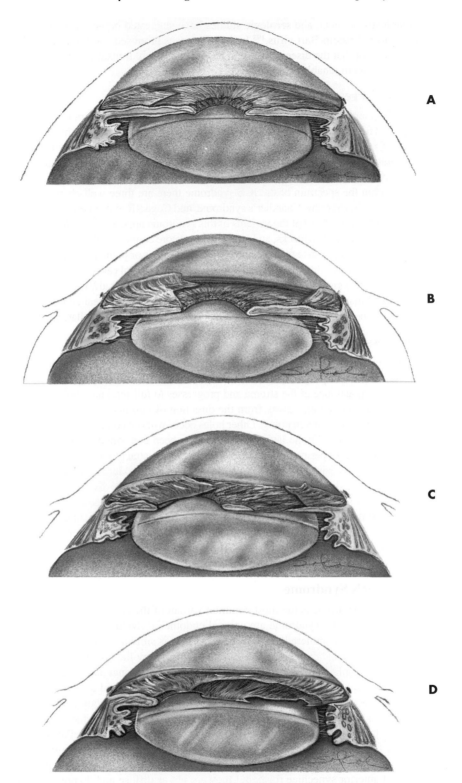

Figure 16-6 Schematic view of iridocorneal endothelial syndrome. **A,** Membrane forms in one area of angle. **B,** Additional areas of angle are involved, and contraction of membrane displaces pupil. **C,** As membrane contracts, iris thins and peripheral anterior synechiae form. **D,** Almost total closure of angle with thinning of iris, pupillary displacement, and hole formation. (Modified from Shields MB: *Surv Ophthalmol* 24:3, 1979.)

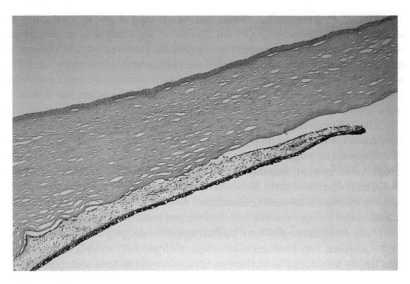

Figure 16-10   Histopathology of anterior synechia formation following postoperative flat anterior chamber. (Courtesy of William H. Spencer, M.D.)

chambers occur commonly after filtering operations, and they are often allowed to persist for a few to several days before re-formation is attempted. Flat anterior chambers also may occur in association with aqueous misdirection and penetrating keratoplasty.

Following re-formation of a flat anterior chamber, the residual secondary angle-closure glaucoma is treated with standard medical therapy. Often patients respond better to medical treatment than would have been predicted by the extent of the angle closure. This suggests that some of the trabecular meshwork is functional behind the apparent peripheral anterior synechiae; that is, the synechiae are bridging rather than closing the angle. If medical treatment is inadequate, a laser trabeculoplasty can be considered if at least one third to one half of the angle is open. However, the clinician must be aware that a sustained postlaser IOP rise may necessitate filtering surgery. Other alternatives include filtering operations, cyclodestructive procedures, and surgical lysis of the peripheral anterior synechiae.[289]

Inflammation

Inflammation can produce glaucoma through a variety of mechanisms, including increased viscosity of the aqueous humor, obstruction of the trabecular meshwork by inflammatory cells and debris, scarring of the outflow channels, elevated episcleral venous pressure, forward displacement of the lens-iris diaphragm, and pupillary block from posterior synechiae. Inflammation can also produce angle-closure glaucoma without pupillary block when the peripheral iris swells as a result of the inflammatory process, when precipitates or exudates in the angle contract to form peripheral anterior synechiae, or when there is forward rotation of the ciliary body. These can occur after surgery or trauma, in idiopathic inflammatory conditions, or with specific uveitis entities such as sarcoidosis,[290] ankylosing spondylitis,[291-292] pars planitis,[293] and juvenile rheumatoid arthritis, particularly the pauciarticular variety.[294-297] Peripheral anterior synechiae form more readily in eyes with shallow anterior chambers and in eyes afflicted with chronic granulomatous inflammatory disease.*

Secondary angle-closure glaucoma without pupillary block is usually managed with medical therapy. It is crucial that residual inflammation be suppressed with corticosteroids and cycloplegic agents. However, the ophthalmologist must keep in mind the possibility of inducing corticosteroid glaucoma. β-adrenergic antagonists, α_2-agonists, topical carbonic anhydrase inhibitors, or epinephrine derivatives are used to control IOP. Miotics may be helpful if the eye is quiet but are usually counterproductive in the presence of persistent inflammation. Similarly, prostaglandins should be used with great caution because they may precipitate an inflammatory reaction.[233] Hyperosmotic agents are administered on occasion for acute elevations of IOP.

If medical therapy fails to control IOP, filtering surgery must be considered. Because standard fil-

*See Figures 6-5 and 6-6 in Campbell DG, Netland PN: *Stereo atlas of glaucoma,* St Louis, 1998, Mosby.

tering surgery is less likely to be successful in inflamed eyes (and these patients are often young people), filtering surgery with adjunctive antimetabolite therapy or seton devices such as the Molteno, Baerveldt, or Ahmed implants should be performed. In children with inflammatory disease the prospects for successful filtering surgery are further reduced by rapid healing, low scleral rigidity, and the increased thickness of Tenon's capsule.[298] A few authorities have used a modified goniotomy procedure, trabeculodialysis, to treat children with inflammation and glaucoma. A goniotomy knife is used to depress the iris and lyse any peripheral anterior synechiae present. The trabecular meshwork is then incised below Schwalbe's line, and the trabecular tissues are retracted further.[299,300]

Penetrating Keratoplasty

Angle-closure glaucoma can develop after penetrating keratoplasty, with the mechanism being pupillary block, postoperative inflammation, or a flat anterior chamber from a wound leak. The severity of the glaucoma is generally related to the extent of the synechial closure. The incidence of postkeratoplasty angle closure is reduced by performing one or more iridectomies, closing the wound meticulously, using a graft slightly larger than the recipient bed, and administering corticosteroids postoperatively.[301-303] However, in some cases the iris becomes attached to the corneal wound, and it is pulled forward in progressive fashion. Glaucoma of one sort or another is a complication in about 20% of penetrating keratoplasties.[304]

Most cases of postkeratoplasty angle-closure glaucoma without pupillary block can be managed with standard medical treatment. Many of these eyes are aphakic and respond well to cholinesterase inhibitors, β-blockers, α-agonists, and carbonic anhydrase inhibitors. If pupillary block is contributing to the glaucoma, a laser iridotomy should be performed. Laser trabeculoplasty may be helpful provided that at least one third to one half of the angle is open.[305] When medical treatment fails to control the glaucoma, filtering surgery with mitomycin C can be successful if conjunctiva is not heavily scarred.[306] However, the surgeon must proceed with care to avoid damage to the corneal graft. Filtering surgery alone often fails.[307] Seton surgery has also been very useful in these situations.[308,309] Cyclocryotherapy and other ciliary body destructive procedures are used commonly to control IOP before or after penetrating keratoplasty.[310,311] The pressure reduction is often temporary, but the procedure can be repeated as required.

Iridoschisis

Iridoschisis is a patchy dissolution of the iris in which the anterior stroma separates from the posterior stroma and muscle layer. The anterior stroma then splits into strands that project into the anterior chamber and sometimes touch the cornea. Iridoschisis is usually bilateral and tends to involve the lower iris quadrants. This condition usually occurs in older individuals but has been reported in children.[312] Many patients have a preexisting chronic ocular disease such as uveitis. Glaucoma occurs in about 50% of the patients and is usually related to the development of peripheral anterior synechiae in the region of the iris strands.*[313,314] Pupillary block and the release of pigment and debris may also contribute to the glaucoma in some cases.[315] The cornea overlying the iris strands may develop bullous keratopathy. Angle closure may occur from forward bowing of the anterior iris stroma.[316] One report suggests that angle-closure glaucoma may actually cause iridoschisis and that any patient with the condition should have primary angle-closure glaucoma ruled out as an underlying condition.[317]

Elevated IOP and iridoschisis are usually managed by medical therapy. If pupillary block is playing a substantial role, a laser iridotomy should be performed. In some cases filtering surgery is required to control the glaucoma.

Aniridia

Aniridia produces angle-closure glaucoma without pupillary block.† This is discussed in the section devoted to glaucoma in infants and children in Chapter 21.

Posterior Pushing or Rotating Mechanism

As discussed earlier, it is possible to conceptualize secondary angle-closure glaucoma without pupillary block as occurring through two major mechanisms, the anterior pulling mechanism and the

---

*See Figure 14-5 in Campbell DG, Netland PN: *Stereo atlas of glaucoma,* St Louis, 1998, Mosby.
†See Figures 14-7 and 14-8 in Campbell DG, Netland PN: *Stereo atlas of glaucoma,* St Louis, 1998, Mosby.

If laser treatment fails to control ciliary-block glaucoma, the patient should undergo a surgical disruption of the vitreous. Traditionally this has been done by aspirating vitreous through the pars plana and then injecting fluid to re-form the anterior chamber. Use of a viscoelastic material to re-form the anterior chamber has been a useful adjunct.[355] Good results have been obtained by performing an anterior vitrectomy through the pars plana using vitreous instruments.[356-358] In aphakic eyes, ciliary-block glaucoma can be treated by an anterior vitrectomy through a limbal incision.

In the past it was common to treat ciliary-block glaucoma by lens extraction. In most cases an intracapsular cataract extraction was accompanied by vitreous loss because of back pressure. It was probably the vitreous loss rather than the lens extraction that was therapeutic in these cases.[359] If vitreous loss does not occur, the anterior vitreous face should be incised deeply. Lens extraction is now rarely required because so many other surgical approaches are available.

It should be emphasized that if one eye develops ciliary-block glaucoma after surgery, the fellow eye is likely to follow a similar course. If the fellow eye has a shallow anterior chamber, a prophylactic laser iridectomy should be performed. The fellow eye should not be treated with miotic agents, and intraocular surgery should be avoided if at all possible. If surgery must be performed, it should be done when the IOP is normal and the angle is open. Some authorities believe preoperative and prophylactic postoperative cycloplegic drugs and hyperosmotic agents are useful in this situation.

Cysts of the Iris and Ciliary Body

Primary cysts of the iris and ciliary body usually arise from the epithelial layers. The cysts can be single or multiple and involve one or both eyes. In most cases the cysts remain stationary and cause no harm.[360] In rare cases the cysts are sufficient in size and number to lift the iris forward and cause angle-closure glaucoma without pupillary block.[361,362] The syndrome of iris cysts and angle-closure glaucoma has been reported in a few families in whom it is inherited in an autosomal dominant pattern.[363]

Iris cysts are usually dark brown and may be visible through an iridectomy or at the pupillary margin, especially when the pupil is dilated. Ciliary body cysts are often less pigmented and are difficult to see unless they are quite large. The presence of the cysts gives the iris surface an undulating or irregular appearance. The anterior chamber is uneven in depth, and the angle is variable in width.

Angle-closure glaucoma associated with cysts of the iris or ciliary body may be acute, subacute, or chronic in nature. If the cysts causing angle closure are visible, they should be punctured with an argon laser. Laser settings of 50 to 100 μm, 0.1 to 0.2 seconds, and 200 to 1000 mW are used to collapse the cysts and free their fluid. It may be necessary to repeat the laser treatment if the cysts re-form.[364] If the cysts are not visible at the pupillary margin, it is possible to puncture them by first doing a laser iridotomy over the involved area. This technique is suitable when a few large cysts cause angle closure; it would not be suitable when multiple small cysts are present. Nonpigmented cysts of the ciliary body can be punctured with the Nd:YAG laser. Medical therapy may be required after cyst puncture if extensive peripheral anterior synechiae are present. In a few cases the cysts cannot be treated with a laser, and filtering surgery is necessary.

Secondary cysts of the iris and ciliary body may be caused by trauma, tumors, or congenital syphilis.[365] The cysts may cause glaucoma by the mechanism described above, or they may be associated with glaucoma on the basis of inflammation or neovascularization.

Intraocular Tumors

Ocular malignant melanoma is frequently associated with glaucoma through a variety of mechanisms, including direct extension of the tumor into the trabecular meshwork, seeding of tumor cells into the outflow channels, obstruction of the meshwork by pigment or pigment-laden macrophages,[366-369] neovascularization, peripheral anterior synechiae,[370] iridocyclitis, and hyphema.[371,372] Melanomas of the choroid and ciliary body can also displace the lens-iris diaphragm and produce angle-closure glaucoma without pupillary block.* In most cases glaucoma occurs when the melanoma is already large, and enucleation is the appropriate therapy. There have been a few reports of surgery for angle-closure glaucoma in eyes that were determined later to harbor undetected melanomas.[375-377] At times, iris melanomas invade the angle and cause secondary angle closure without pupillary block (Fig. 16-13). Generally these eyes have good vision, and the glaucoma is managed by medical treatment.

Other intraocular tumors such as adenomas and leiomyomas may push the iris forward and cause angle-closure glaucoma. One such example, a leiomyoma is shown pushing the iris forward in Figure 16-14.

---

*See Figure 10-4 in Campbell DG, Netland PN: *Stereo atlas of glaucoma,* St Louis, 1998, Mosby.

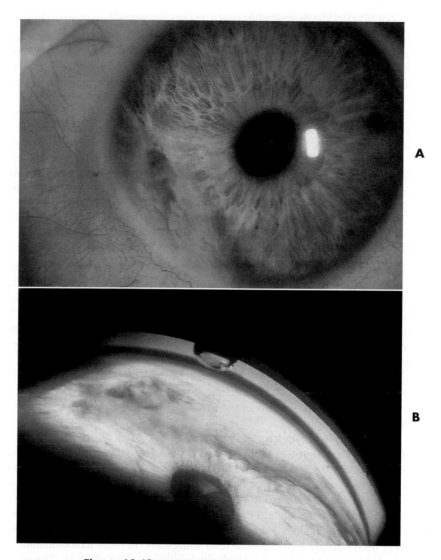

Figure 16-13 **A,** Iris melanoma. **B,** Invading angle.

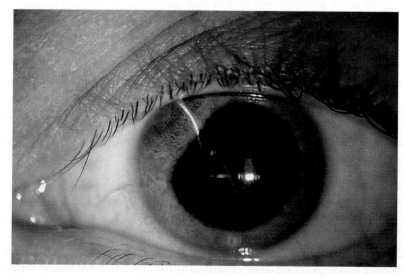

Figure 16-14 Leiomyoma pushing the peripheral iris forward and closing off the chamber angle. (Courtesy of William H. Spencer, M.D.)

80. Aiello LM, Wand M, Liang G: Neovascular glaucoma and vitreous hemorrhage following cataract surgery in patients with diabetes mellitus, *Ophthalmology* 90:814, 1983.

80a. Poliner LS, and others: Neovascular glaucoma after intracapsular and extracapular cataract extraction in diabetic patients, *Am J Ophthalmol* 100:637, 1985.

81. Francois J: La rubeose de l'iris, *Ophthalmologica* 121:313, 1951.

82. Francois J: Rubeose de l'iris et retinopathie diabetique, *Ann Ocul (Paris)* 205:1085, 1972.

83. Madsen PH: Haemorrhagic glaucoma: comparative study in diabetic and non-diabetic patients, *Br J Ophthalmol* 55:444, 1971.

84. Ohrt V: Glaucoma due to rubeosis iridis diabetica, *Ophthalmologica* 142:356, 1961.

85. Madsen PH: Ocular findings in 123 patients with proliferative diabetic retinopathy. I. Changes in the anterior segment of the eye, *Doc Ophthalmol* 29:331, 1970.

86. Madsen PH: Rubeosis of the iris and haemorrhagic glaucoma in patients with proliferative diabetic retinopathy, *Br J Ophthalmol* 55:368, 1971.

87. Hayreh SS, van Heuven WAJ, Hayreh MS: Experimental retinal vascular occlusion. I. Pathogenesis of central retinal vein occlusion, *Arch Ophthalmol* 96:311, 1978.

88. Hayreh SS: Classification of central retinal vein occlusion, *Ophthalmology* 90:458, 1983.

89. Central Retinal Vein Occlusion Study Group: Baseline and early natural history report, *Arch Ophthalmol* 111:1087, 1993.

90. Laatikainen L, Blach RK: Behavior of the iris vasculature in central retinal vein occlusion: a fluorescein angiographic study of the vascular response of the retina and the iris, *Br J Ophthalmol* 61:272, 1977.

91. Sinclair SM, Gragoudas ES: Prognosis of rubeosis iridis following central retinal vein occlusion, *Br J Ophthalmol* 63:735, 1979.

92. Zegarra H, Gutman FA, Conforto J: The natural course of central retinal vein occlusion, *Ophthalmology* 86:1931, 1979.

93. Priluck IA, Robertson DM, Hollenhorst RW: Long-term follow up of occlusion of the central retinal vein in young adults, *Am J Ophthalmol* 90:190, 1980.

94. Tasman W, Magargal LE, Augsburger JJ: Effects of argon laser photocoagulation on rubeosis iridis and angle neovascularization, *Ophthalmology* 87:400, 1980.

95. Hayreh SS, and others: Ocular neovascularization with retinal vascular occlusion. III. Incidence of ocular neovascularization with retinal vein occlusion, *Ophthalmology* 90:488, 1983.

96. Laatikainen L, Kohner EM: Fluorescein angiography and its prognostic significance in central retinal vein occlusion, *Br J Ophthalmol* 60:411, 1976.

97. Magargal LE, Donoso LA, Sanborn GE: Retinal ischemia and risk of neovascularization following central retinal vein occlusion, *Ophthalmology* 89:1241, 1982.

98. Central Vein Occlusion Study Group: Natural history and clinical management of central retinal vein occlusion, *Arch Ophthalmol* 115:486, 1997.

99. Magargal LE, Donoso LA, Sanborn GE: Retinal ischemia and risk of neovascularization following central retinal vein occlusion, *Ophthalmology* 89:1241, 1982.

100. Bertelsen TI: The relationship between thrombosis in the retinal vein and primary glaucoma, *Acta Ophthalmol Scand Suppl* 39:603, 1961.

101. Dryden RM: Central retinal vein occlusion and chronic simple glaucoma, *Arch Ophthalmol* 73:659, 1965.

102. Smith ME, Ott FT: Rubeosis iridis and primary angle closure glaucoma, *Int Ophthalmol Clin* 2:161, 1971.

103. Hayreh SS, March W, Phelps CD: Ocular hypotony following retinal vein occlusion, *Arch Ophthalmol* 96:827, 1978.

104. Cappin JM, Whitelocke R: The iris in central retinal vein thrombosis, *Proc Royal Soc Med* 67:1048, 1974.

105. Evans K, Wishart PK, McGalliard JN: Neovascular complications after central retinal vein occlusion, *Eye* 7:520, 1993.

106. Rath EZ, and others: Risk factors for retinal vein occlusions: a case-control study, *Ophthalmology* 99:509, 1992.

107. Green WR, and others: Central retinal vein occlusion: a prospective histopathologic study of 29 eyes in 28 cases, *Trans Am Ophthalmol Soc* 79:371, 1981.

108. Swan KC, Raff J: Changes in the eye and orbit following carotid ligation, *Trans Am Ophthalmol Soc* 49:435, 1951.

109. Weiss DI, Shaffer RN, Nehrenberg TR: Neovascular glaucoma complicating carotid-cavernous fistula, *Arch Ophthalmol* 69:304, 1963.

110. Smith JL: Unilateral glaucoma in carotid occlusive disease, *JAMA* 182:683, 1962.

111. Hoefnagels KLJ: Rubeosis of the iris associated with occlusion of the carotid artery, *Ophthalmologica* 148:196, 1964.

112. Hart CT, Haworth S: Bilateral common carotid occlusion with hypoxic ocular sequelae, *Br J Ophthalmol* 55:383, 1971.

113. Huckman MS, Haas J: Reversed flow through the ophthalmic artery as a cause of rubeosis iridis, *Am J Ophthalmol* 74:1094, 1972.

114. Coppeto JR, and others: Neovascular glaucoma and carotid artery obstructive disease, *Am J Ophthalmol* 99:567, 1985.

115. Sturrock GD, Mueller HR: Chronic ocular ischemia, *Br J Ophthalmol* 68:716, 1984.

116. Brown GC, Magargal LE: The ocular ischemic syndrome: clinical, fluorescein angiographic and carotid angiographic features, *Int Ophthalmol* 11:239, 1988.

117. Ward JB, Hedges TR III, Heggerick PA: Reversible abnormalities in the ophthalmic arteries detected by color Doppler imaging, *Ophthalmology* 102:1606, 1995.

118. Hamed LM, and others: Giant cell arteritis in the ocular ischemic syndrome, *Am J Ophthalmol* 113:702, 1992.

119. Mizener JB, Podhajsky P, Hayreh SS: Ocular ischemic syndrome, *Ophthalmology* 104:859, 1997.

120. Winterkorn JM, Beckman RL: Recovery from ocular ischemic syndrome after treatment with verapamil, *J Neuroophthalmol* 15:209, 1995.

121. Sivalingam A, Brown GC, Magargal LE: The ocular ischemic syndrome. III. Visual prognosis and the effect of treatment, *Int Ophthalmol* 15:15, 1991.

122. Brown GC, Magargal LE, Federman JL: Ischaemia and neovascularization, *Trans Ophthalmol Soc UK* 100:377, 1980.

123. Duker JS, Sivalingam A, Brown GC: A prospective study of acute central retinal artery obstruction: the incidence of secondary ocular neovascularization, *Arch Ophthalmol* 109:339, 1991.

124. Hayreh SS, Podhajsky P: Ocular neovascularization with retinal vascular occlusion. II. Occurrence in central and branch retinal artery occlusion, *Arch Ophthalmol* 100:1585, 1982.

125. Karjalainen K: Occlusion of the central retinal artery and retinal branch arterioles: a clinical tonographic and fluorescein angiographic study of 175 patients, *Acta Ophthalmol Scand Suppl* 109:9, 1971.

126. Jacobs NA, Trew DR: Occlusion of the central retinal artery and ocular neovascularization: an indirect association? *Eye* 6:599, 1992.

127. Duker JS, Brown GC: The efficacy of panretinal photocoagulation for neovascularization of the iris after central retinal artery obstruction, *Ophthalmology* 96:92, 1989.

128. Jones RF: Glaucoma following radiotherapy, *Br J Ophthalmol* 42:636, 1958.

129. Shields CL, and others: Reasons for enucleation after plaque radiotherapy for posterior uveal melanoma: clinical findings, *Ophthalmology* 96:919, 1989.

130. Finger PT: Microwave thermoradiotherapy for uveal melanoma: results of a 10-year study, *Ophthalmology* 104:1794, 1997.

131. Anderson DM, Morin JD, Hunter WS: Rubeosis iridis, *Can J Ophthalmol* 6:183, 1971.

132. Kim MK, and others: Neovascular glaucoma after helium ion irradiation for uveal melanoma, *Ophthalmology* 93:189, 1986.

133. Kwok SK, and others: Neovascular glaucoma developing after uncomplicated cataract surgery for heavily irradiated eyes, *Ophthalmology* 104:1112, 1997.

134. Walton DS, Grant WM: Retinoblastoma and iris neovascularization, *Am J Ophthalmol* 65:598, 1968.

135. Ehrenberg M, and others: Rubeosis iridis: preoperative iris fluorescein angiography and periocular steroids, *Ophthalmology* 91:321, 1984.

136. Verhoeff FH: Obstruction of the central retinal vein, *Arch Ophthalmol* 36:1, 1907.

137. Samuels B: Pathologic changes in the anterior half of the globe in obstruction in central vein of retina, *Arch Ophthalmol* 13:404, 1935.

138. Teich SA, Walsh JB: A grading system for iris neovascularization: prognostic implications for treatment, *Ophthalmology* 88:1102, 1981.

139. Wand M, Hutchinson BT: The surgical treatment of neovascular glaucoma, *Perspect Ophthalmol* 4:147, 1980.

140. Callahan MA, Hilton GF: Photocoagulation and rubeosis iridis *Am J Ophthalmol* 78:873, 1974.

141. Laatikainen L, and others: Panretinal photocoagulation in central retinal vein occlusion: a randomised controlled clinical study, *Br J Ophthalmol* 61:741, 1977.

142. Jacobson DR, Murphy RP, Rosenthal AR: The treatment of angle neovascularization with panretinal photocoagulation, *Ophthalmology* 86:1270, 1979.

143. May DR, and others: Xenon arc panretinal photocoagulation for central retinal vein occlusion: a randomised prospective study, *Br J Ophthalmol* 63:725, 1979.

144. Wand M, and others: Effects of panretinal photocoagulation on rubeosis iridis, angle neovascularization, and neovascular glaucoma, *Am J Ophthalmol* 86:332, 1978.

145. Allen RC, and others: Filtration surgery in the treatment of neovascular glaucoma, *Ophthalmology* 89:1181, 1982.

146. Heuer DK, and others: 5-Fluorouracil and glaucoma filtering surgery. III. Intermediate follow-up of a pilot study, *Ophthalmology* 93:1537, 1986.

147. Herschler J, Agness D: A modified filtering operation for neovascular glaucoma, *Arch Ophthalmol* 97:2339, 1979.

148. Parrish R, Herschler J: Eyes with end-stage neovascular glaucoma: natural history following successful modified filtering operation, *Arch Ophthalmol* 101: 745, 1983.

149. Molteno ACB, van Rooyen MMB, Bartholomew RS: Implants for draining neovascular glaucoma, *Br J Ophthalmol* 61:120, 1977.

150. Krupin T, and others: Filtering valve implant surgery for eyes with neovascular glaucoma, *Am J Ophthalmol* 89:338, 1980.

151. Schockett SS, Lukhanpal V, Richards R: Anterior chamber tube shunt to an encircling band in the treatment of neovascular glaucoma, *Ophthalmology* 89:1188, 1982.

152. Melamed S, Fiore PM: Molteno implant surgery in refractory glaucoma, *Surv Ophthalmol* 34:441, 1990.

153. Mills RP, and others: Long-term survival of Molteno glaucoma drainage devices, *Ophthalmology* 103:299, 1996.

154. Hodkin MJ, and others: Early clinical experience with the Baerveldt implant in complicated glaucomas, *Am J Ophthalmol* 120:32, 1995.

155. Smith MF, Doyle JW, Sherwood MB: Comparison of the Baerveldt glaucoma implant with the double-plate Molteno drainage implant, *Arch Ophthalmol* 113: 444, 1995.

156. Mermoud A, and others: Molteno tube implantation for neovascular glaucoma: long-term results and factors influencing the outcome, *Ophthalmology* 100:897, 1993.

157. Blankenship G, Cortez R, Machemer R: The lens and pars plana vitrectomy for diabetic retinopathy complications, *Arch Ophthalmol* 97:1263, 1979.

158. Drews RC: Corticosteroid management of hemorrhagic glaucoma, *Trans Am Acad Ophthalmol Otolaryngol* 78:334, 1974.

159. DeRoth A: Cryosurgery for treatment of advanced chronic simple glaucoma, *Am J Ophthalmol* 66:1034, 1968.

160. Feibel RM, Bigger JF: Rubeosis iridis and neovascular glaucoma, *Am J Ophthalmol* 74:862, 1972.

161. Bellows AR, Grant WM: Cyclocryotherapy in advanced inadequately controlled glaucoma, *Am J Ophthalmol* 75:697, 1973.

162. Krupin T, Mitchell KB, Becker B: Cyclocryotherapy in neovascular glaucoma, *Am J Ophthalmol* 86:24, 1978.

163. Ellis PP: Regression of rubeosis iridis following cyclodiathermy, *Am J Ophthalmol* 40:253, 1955.

164. DeRoth A: Cyclodiathermy in treatment of glaucoma due to rubeosis iridis diabetica, *Arch Ophthalmol* 35:20, 1946.

165. Beckman H, and others: Transscleral ruby laser irradiation of the ciliary body in the treatment of intractable glaucoma, *Trans Am Acad Ophthalmol Otolaryngol* 76: 423, 1972.

166. Schuman JS, and others: Contact transscleral Nd:YAG laser cyclophotocoagulation: midterm results, *Ophthalmology* 99:1089, 1992.

167. Shields MB, Shields SE: Noncontact transscleral Nd:YAG cyclophotocoagulation: a long-term follow-up of 500 patients, *Trans Am Ophthalmol Soc* 92:271, 1994.

168. Kivela T, and others: Clinically successful contact transscleral krypton laser cyclophotocoagulation: long-term histopathologic and immunohistochemical autopsy findings, *Arch Ophthalmol* 113:1447, 1995.

169. Kosoko O, and others: Long-term outcome of initial ciliary ablation with contact diode laser transscleral cyclophotocoagulation for severe glaucoma. The Diode Laser Ciliary Ablation Study Group, *Ophthalmology* 103:1294, 1996.

170. Dickens CJ, and others: Long-term results of noncontact transscleral neodymium:YAG cyclophotocoagulation, *Ophthalmology* 102:1777, 1995.

171. Haller JA: Transvitreal endocyclophotocoagulation, *Trans Am Ophthalmol Soc* 94:589, 1996.

172. Mora JS: Endoscopic diode laser cyclophotocoagulation with a limbal approach, *Ophthalmic Surg Lasers* 28:118, 1997.

173. Simmons RJ, Depperman SR, Dueker DK: The role of goniophotocoagulation in neovascularization of the anterior chamber angle, *Ophthalmology* 87:79, 1980.

174. Adamis AP, and others: Inhibition of vascular endothelial growth factor prevents retinal ischemia-associated iris neovascularization in a nonhuman primate, *Arch Ophthalmol* 114:66, 1996.

175. Parker AJ, and others: Hematoporphyrin photoradiation therapy for iris neovascularization: a preliminary report, *Arch Ophthalmol* 102:1193, 1984.

176. Eagle RC Jr, Shields JA: Iridocorneal endothelial syndrome with contralateral guttate endothelial dystrophy: a light and electron microscopic study, *Ophthalmology* 94:862, 1987.

177. Quigley HA, Forster RF: Histopathology of cornea and iris in Chandler's syndrome, *Arch Ophthalmol* 96:1878, 1978.

178. Rodrigues MM, and others: Glaucoma due to endothelialization of the anterior chamber angle: a comparison of posterior polymorphous dystrophy of the cornea and Chandler's syndrome, *Arch Ophthalmol* 98:688, 1980.

179. Waring GO III: Posterior collagenous layer of the cornea: ultrastructural classification of abnormal collagenous tissue posterior to Descemet's membrane in 30 cases, *Arch Ophthalmol* 100:122, 1982.

180. Campbell DG, Shields MB, Smith TR: The corneal endothelium in the spectrum of essential iris atrophy, *Am J Ophthalmol* 86:317, 1978.

181. Eagle RC Jr, and others: Proliferative endotheliopathy with iris abnormalities: the iridocorneal endothelial syndrome, *Arch Ophthalmol* 97:2104, 1979.

182. Rodrigues MM, Streeten BW, Spaeth GL: Chandler's syndrome as a variant of essential iris atrophy: a clinicopathologic study, *Arch Ophthalmol* 96:643, 1978.

183. Rodrigues MM, Stulting D, Waring GO III: Clinical, electron microscopic, and immunohistochemical study of the corneal endothelium and Descemet's membrane in the iridocorneal endothelial syndrome, *Am J Ophthalmol* 101:16, 1986.

184. Howell DN, and others: Endothelial metaplasia in the iridocorneal endothelial syndrome, *Invest Ophthalmol Vis Sci* 38:1896, 1997.

185. Levy SG, and others: The histopathology of the iridocorneal-endothelial syndrome, *Cornea* 15:46, 1996.

186. Hirst LW, and others: Immunohistochemical pathology of the corneal endothelium in iridocorneal endothelial syndrome, *Invest Ophthalmol Vis Sci* 36:820, 1995.

187. Alvarado JA, and others: Pathogenesis of Chandler's syndrome, essential iris atrophy and Cogan-Reese syndrome, *Arch Ophthalmol* 97:2104, 1979.

188. Bahn CF, and others: Classification of corneal endothelial disorders based on neural crest origin, *Ophthalmology* 91: 558, 1984.

189. Kupfer C, Kaiser-Kupfer MI: New hypothesis of developmental abnormalities of the anterior chamber associated with glaucoma, *Trans Ophthalmol Soc UK* 98:213, 1978.

190. Levy SG, and others: Pathology of the iridocorneal-endothelial syndrome: the ICE-cell, *Invest Ophthalmol Vis Sci* 36:2592, 1995.

191. Murphy C, and others: The corneal endothelium and Descemet's membrane in the ICE syndrome: a morphometric-histopathological study, *Invest Ophthalmol Vis Sci* 26(suppl):6, 1985.

192. Alvarado JA, and others: Detection of herpes simplex viral DNA in the iridocorneal endothelial syndrome, *Arch Ophthalmol* 112:1601, 1994.

193. Tsai CS, and others: Antibodies to Epstein-Barr virus in iridocorneal endothelial syndrome, *Arch Ophthalmol* 108: 1572, 1990.

194. Feingold M: Essential atrophy of the iris, *Am J Ophthalmol* 1:1, 1918.

195. Zentmayer W: Progressive atrophy of the iris, *Trans Coll Physicians Phila* 35:456, 1913.

a study has been performed in Barbados over 4 years. In this population of largely black African ancestry, the 4-year incidence of glaucoma over 40 years of age is 2.2%, with higher rates for males, those of African ancestry, those with high IOPs, and those with suspicious discs at enrollment.[6] Using data from the Framingham study, Podgor and co-workers[7] have estimated that the incidence of POAG rises from 0.2% at age 55 to 1.1% at age 70; that is, the incidence of POAG is two cases per 1000 people per year from age 55 to 60 years and 11 cases per 1000 people per year from age 70 to 75 years.

Intraocular Pressure

There is general agreement that IOP is the most important known risk factor for open-angle glaucoma development. Evidence clearly indicates that elevated IOP can cause glaucomatous optic nerve changes in experimental animals.[8,9] Even in normal-pressure glaucoma, asymmetric IOP has been noted to correlate with asymmetric cupping and field loss, with the greater damage most often occurring on the side with higher pressure.[10,11] Population surveys also support the increase in prevalence of open-angle glaucoma with increasing IOP.[12-14] Because many individuals with "elevated" IOP never develop glaucoma, and because many people with glaucoma have "normal" IOPs, IOP is obviously not the only risk factor.

Age

The prevalence of POAG increases with age (Table 17-2).[12,13,15-17] However, one should not infer from this statement that the disease is limited to middle-aged and older individuals; it occurs in children and young adults as well.[18-20] The effect of age on the prevalence of POAG holds true even after compensating for the relationship between increasing age and increasing IOP.[21]

Gender

Conflicting information exists about the effect of gender on the prevalence of POAG. In several studies males had a higher prevalence of glaucoma.[22-25] In the Barbados study, POAG was associated with older men, high IOP, positive family history, lean body mass, and low blood pressure to IOP ratio.[26]

Race

Recent studies have shown conclusively that POAG is more prevalent in blacks than in whites.[17,27] Furthermore, the disease seems to develop at an earlier age and has a more rapid progression in

Table 17-2 ————————————————————————————————————

Prevalence of Primary Open-Angle Glaucoma by Age (%)

Age (Years)	Wales (Hollows and Graham)[13]	Framingham, Mass. (Liebowitz and Co-workers)[15]	Baltimore White (Tielsch and Co-workers)*[17]	Baltimore Black (Tielsch and Co-workers)*[17]
40-49	NR	NR	0.92	1.23
50-54	0.3	NR		
55-59	0.9	0.5	0.41	4.05
60-64	0.5	0.7		
65-69	1.1	0.9	0.88	5.51
70-74	1.3	1.7		
75-79	NR	2.0	2.89	9.15
80-85	NR	4.4	2.16	11.26

Modified from Leske MC. *Am J Epidemiol* 118:166, 1983; Tielsch JM, and others: *JAMA* 266:369, 1991.
*Reported in decades (e.g., 50-59)
NR, not reported.

black patients.[7,28-30] It is estimated that the incidence and the prevalence of blindness from glaucoma are 8 to 10 times higher in black patients than in white patients in the United States.[17,31] Some have proposed that optic nerve ischemia from sickle cell anemia contributes to the high prevalence of POAG in blacks. However, this theory was not supported by one study, which found that only 2 of 40 black patients requiring filtering surgery had a positive test for sickle cell trait.[32] Black patients seem to respond to some treatment modes less favorably than do whites;[33-36] whether this explains the more virulent course has not been answered. Furthermore, some black patients may not have access to the same quality of treatment as white patients have. When compared with whites, blacks have higher levels of IOP[37-39] and larger cup:disc diameter ratios.[40]

Data on the prevalence of POAG in other ethnic and racial groups are less complete. It is stated that POAG is rare in Pacific Islanders,[41] Asians,[42-44] and certain Native American tribes. In Mongolia, the prevalence of open-angle glaucoma was found to be quite low—0.5%—with angle-closure glaucoma having a prevalence of 21.4%.[45] In Japan, the prevalence of POAG is 0.58%, with normal-pressure glaucoma having a prevalence of 2.04%.[46] In an English study, the prevalence of open-angle glaucoma was found to be similar in those of European descent and in those of Asian descent.[47] However, it is unlikely that this population living in England is representative of all Asian groups. In Tunis, the overall prevalence of open-angle glaucoma in a population over 40 years of age was 2.7%. This is similar to that found in Europeans but lower than that found in those of black African descent.[48] Further surveys using standardized techniques and definitions are needed in many population groups.

Socioeconomic Factors

Very few studies have been performed on the relationship between socioeconomic variables and the prevalence of POAG. In different reports manual laborers have an increased[49] and a decreased[50] prevalence of POAG. The Baltimore Eye Study suggested that socioeconomic factors played some role in the increased prevalence and severity of open-angle glaucoma in those of black African descent, but only a small part compared with racial factors.[17]

Little is known about the effect of life-style, vocation, geography, diet, and nutrition on glaucoma. Moderate exercise has been shown to decrease IOP in both normal volunteers and in patients with POAG.[51,52] Furthermore, moderate exercise has been shown to increase choroidal blood flow, although with some limits.[53] However, whether regular exercise results in better long-term IOP control or improved ganglion cell survival has not been demonstrated.

Refractive Error

Myopia has been associated with POAG in many studies.[54-58] It is not clear whether myopia has a direct influence on the prevalence of the disease or whether it acts through its known associations with increased IOP and larger cup:disc ratios.[59,60] It is often difficult to diagnose glaucoma in myopic individuals because they have (1) broad, shallow optic cups with less distinct margins; (2) baring of the blind spot or other refractive scotomata on visual field testing; and (3) low ocular rigidity, which makes Schiøtz readings inaccurate.

Heredity

POAG appears to have a genetic or familial component. Over the years autosomal dominant,[18,61] autosomal recessive,[62,63] and sex-linked[64] inheritance patterns have been reported. Currently most authorities believe that the genetic influence occurs through polygenic or multifactorial transmission. It is reported that 5% to 50% of cases of POAG are hereditary, with the best estimate being 20% to 25%.[65] The risk of developing POAG in first-degree relatives is 4% to 16%.[65-70] A monozygotic and dizygotic twin study estimated the inheritability to be 13%.[71] In one study, the association was higher with a sibling affected than with a parent or child.[72] Two longitudinal studies, one population-based and the other over 18 years in length, demonstrated a strong association between the development of glaucoma and positive family history.[27,73]

Recently studies have identified one gene (GLC1A) that is associated with juvenile-onset open-angle glaucoma and some (about 3% to 4%) cases of POAG in adults.[74,75] This gene is located on chromosome 1 in the q23-25 region.[76] Three different mutations of this gene have been identified in

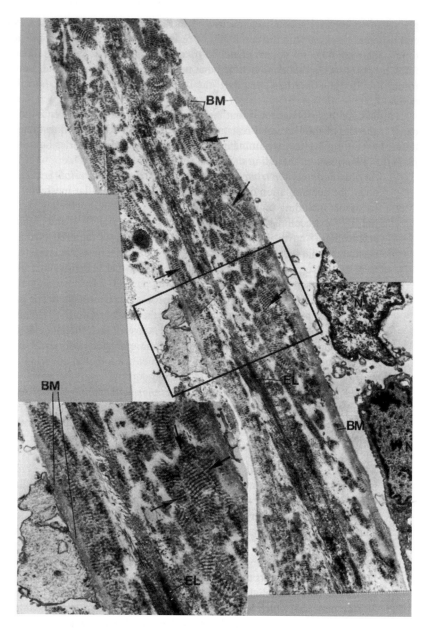

Figure 17-1   Sagittal section through trabecular meshwork in open-angle glaucoma (trabeculectomy specimen). Basement membranes are thickened, trabecular sheets are widened, and curly collagen has accumulated *(arrows). BM,* Basement membrane; *EL,* elastic fibers; *N,* nuclei. (×7500; inset ×15,000.) (From Rohen JW, Witmer R: *Graefes Arch Clin Ophthalmol* 183:251, 1972.)

10. Closure of Schlemm's canal[134,136]
11. Thickened scleral spur

However, these histopathologic changes must be interpreted with caution. Most of the glaucoma specimens are obtained at surgery; thus artifacts are common, and it is impossible to fix the tissues at their normal IOP levels. In addition, the specimens generally come from eyes with advanced damage. Furthermore, it is difficult to know whether the changes seen are primary phenomena or secondary to the effects of increased IOP or medical and surgical treatment. Finally many of the histopathologic alterations are also seen in older, normal eyes. In fact, some researchers have proposed that the outflow changes of POAG could be an acceleration of the normal aging process.[121]

Although it is impossible to be sure of the fundamental defect of aqueous humor outflow in POAG, the balance of the evidence favors the trabecular meshwork or the endothelium of Schlemm's canal as the site of the increased resistance. If we accept this hypothesis, we must still ask why outflow facility is reduced in POAG. Various investigators have linked the increased resistance to outflow with altered corticosteroid metabolism, dysfunctional adrenergic control, abnormal immunologic processes, and oxidative damage.

Altered Corticosteroid Metabolism

Soon after the early descriptions of corticosteroid-induced IOP elevations, Armaly[137] and Becker and Hahn[138] noted that patients with POAG were quite responsive to topical glucocorticoids. These researchers proposed that the IOP response to topical corticosteroids was inherited and that this inheritance was either the same as, or closely linked to, the inheritance of POAG.[137,138] The corticosteroid hypothesis was then extended to include a generalized sensitivity to the effects of glucocorticoids in patients with POAG. Various investigators noted patients with POAG had (1) increased plasma levels of cortisol,[139] (2) increased suppression of plasma cortisol with different doses of exogenous dexamethasone,[140] (3) continued suppression of plasma cortisol by dexamethasone despite concomitant administration of diphenylhydantoin (phenytoin),[141,142] (4) disturbed pituitary adrenal axis function,[143] and (5) increased inhibition of mitogen-stimulated lymphocyte transformation by glucocorticoids.[144,145] Researchers postulated that endogenous corticosteroids affected trabecular function by altering prostaglandin metabolism, glycosaminoglycan catabolism, release of lysosomal enzymes,[111] synthesis of cyclic adenosine monophosphate,[146] or inhibition of phagocytosis.[144]

The corticosteroid hypothesis came under attack as subsequent studies in glaucomatous patients failed to confirm the increased sensitivity of nonocular tissues to the effects of glucocorticoids.[147-151] In addition, the IOP response to topical corticosteroids was shown to lack reproducibility[152] and to be less controlled by inheritance than previously thought.[153-155]

Recent data have reopened the corticosteroid issue. Trabecular endothelial cells from patients with POAG have an abnormal metabolism of glucocorticoids, with increased levels of delta-4 reductase and reduced levels of 3-oxidoreductase.[156] The importance of this observation, and whether it represents a primary or a secondary change in the tissue, is unclear at present. Most recently, a gene mutation (GLC1A) has been associated with juvenile-onset glaucoma and a small fraction of adult-onset POAG.[157] Mutations of this gene (trabecular meshwork inducible glucocorticoid response [TIGR]) are associated with the production of an abnormal glucocorticoid-inducible stress-response protein (myocilin) in the trabecular meshwork that may affect glycosaminoglycan and other glycoprotein metabolism, as well as cell surface properties.[158] In addition to giving a genetic basis for some types of glaucoma, the TIGR gene could tie in a possible role for corticosteroids in the glaucomatous process. Furthermore, patients who respond to topical steroids with a very high IOP are more likely to develop visual field loss than moderate responders.[159] In this study, none of those who were low responders developed visual field loss.

Dysfunctional Adrenergic Control

In analogous fashion to the corticosteroid theory, others have proposed that the diminished outflow facility in patients with POAG could be explained by an increased sensitivity to adrenergic agonists. Various reports indicated that patients with POAG had (1) a greater IOP reduction after the administration of topical epinephrine,[160] (2) a greater response to epinephrine or theophylline in inhibiting mitogen-stimulated lymphocyte transformation,[161,162] and (3) more frequent premature ventricular contractions after topical administration of epinephrine.[160] Furthermore, ocular hypertensive subjects who demonstrated a fall in IOP greater than 5 mm Hg after topical epinephrine administration had a higher rate of developing visual field loss.[163] However, additional studies have generally failed to confirm an increased sensitivity to adrenergic agonists in patients with POAG.[164]

Abnormal Immunologic Processes

Other investigators have explained the diminished aqueous humor outflow in POAG by abnormal immune responses. Increased levels of γ-globulin and plasma cells have been detected in the trabecular meshwork of patients with POAG.[165,166] Furthermore, glaucoma patients were noted to have a high prevalence of antinuclear antibodies.[167,168] However, subsequent, more detailed studies have failed to confirm these findings.[169-171] An association between POAG and certain human lymphocyte antigens was reported[172] and then refuted by multiple studies.[173-175]

Oxidative Damage

Interest has developed in the question of whether the trabecular meshwork could be damaged by oxidative insult. The meshwork contains glutathione, which may protect the endothelial cells from the effects of hydrogen peroxide (H_2O_2) and other oxidants. This interesting hypothesis is still the subject of active research.[176,177]

In summary, the cause of the trabecular dysfunction in POAG is unclear at present. To date, no single theory explains the pathophysiology.

Optic Nerve Cupping and Atrophy

The second major issue to be addressed in the pathogenesis of POAG is the cause of the optic disc cupping and atrophy. This topic is dealt with in detail in Chapter 13. Cupping consists of backward bowing of the lamina cribrosa, elongation of the laminar beams, and loss of the ganglion cell axons in the rim of neural tissue.[178] Cupping is the hallmark of glaucomatous damage, although it is seen occasionally in ischemic states and compressive lesions in the posterior optic nerve and chiasm. Histologic studies indicate that optic nerve cupping includes the loss of all three elements of the disc—axons, blood vessels, and glial cells. Glial cells appear to atrophy as a secondary phenomenon, and some glial cells are present even in advanced stages of glaucomatous optic atrophy.[179,180] Other investigators have reported selective loss of capillaries in the disc substance[181,182] or in the peripapillary retina.[183,184] These findings have not been confirmed, however, and blood vessels actually seem to be lost in proportion to the loss of axons.[179,185]

Most authorities believe that the lamina cribrosa is the site of glaucomatous optic nerve damage.[185,186] The lamina is a relatively rigid structure that surrounds the densely packed axons. Furthermore, the lamina is the tissue that divides the higher IOP space from the lower subarachnoid pressure space. Early in glaucoma the lamina is compressed. In the later stages of the disease the laminar sheets become fused, and the entire lamina bows backward.[187]

It is commonly accepted that increased IOP either directly or indirectly causes optic nerve cupping. The evidence for this can be summarized as follows:

1. Most patients with POAG have increased IOP, which generally predates by years the development of cupping and visual field loss.
2. Elevated IOP is a major risk factor for the development of POAG in glaucoma suspects.
3. Elevated IOP is the only known common element to a wide variety of secondary glaucomas.
4. In all animal models of glaucoma, elevated IOP precedes optic nerve damage and visual loss.[178]
5. Even in normal-pressure glaucoma, in which IOPs do not exceed the statistically "normal" range, the degree of cupping is related to the level of IOP.[10,11,188]

Although IOP is certainly one risk factor, most investigators point to other factors that also affect glaucomatous cupping.[178,189,190] They point to the observations that (1) a significant percent of patients develop optic nerve cupping and visual field loss at normal levels of IOP, (2) some patients maintain normal optic nerves and visual function despite elevated IOP, and (3) the level of IOP does not correlate well with the progression of established POAG. However, these observations do not refute a linkage between IOP and optic nerve damage, rather they imply variable resistance of the optic nerve to pressure-induced damage. That is, some nerves are more sensitive to pressure than are others.

More than 130 years ago Mueller[191] proposed that elevated IOP led to direct compression and death of axons, whereas von Jaeger[192] stated that ischemia was the cause of progressive glaucomatous cupping. Although this debate continues to the present, most would agree that no one theory explains all of the observed phenomena and that each plays some role in at least some patients. The optic nerve damage from glaucoma is multifactorial and, at different times and in different eyes, may involve genetic susceptibility factors, mechanical forces, ischemia, loss of neurotrophic factors, and neurotoxicity. It also may be that actual ganglion cell death depends on the inability of astroglial cells to prevent or repair injury to the cell or its extracellular matrix regardless of the source of the initial trauma.[193]

CLINICAL FEATURES

Symptoms

POAG is usually described as an insidious, slowly progressive, bilateral condition. The adjective "insidious" is appropriate because most patients are asymptomatic until the late stages of the disease. The few exceptions to this rule include the occasional patient who notices a scotoma when performing a monocular visual task and the young patient who has sudden, severe elevations in IOP that cause corneal edema, halo vision, and discomfort. If patients are not diagnosed until they develop extensive glaucomatous damage, they become symptomatic from loss of fixation in one or both eyes or from loss of peripheral vision, which interferes with activities such as driving. The early stages of POAG usually develop slowly over months to years. As glaucoma advances, however, the pace accelerates. In a recent study from Melbourne, Australia, the prevalence of glaucoma increased from 0.1% in the 40- to 49-year-old age group to 9.7% in the 80- to 89-year-old age group; 50% of those found to have glaucoma were previously undiagnosed.[194]

Findings

POAG is generally a bilateral disease of adult onset; however, a juvenile-onset type is seen that is indistinguishable from the adult-onset variety except for a stronger genetic factor and a more aggressive course. At least one eye should have either characteristic damage to the optic nerve or retinal nerve fiber layer or characteristic visual field changes, open angles with no obvious abnormality, and absence of any other condition known to cause glaucoma. POAG often is asymmetric on presentation, however, so that one eye may have moderate or advanced damage, whereas the fellow eye may have minimal or no detectable damage. In this situation the clinician must not be fooled and mistakenly conclude that the patient has a unilateral secondary glaucoma.

Most white patients with POAG and most black patients of African ancestry with POAG have elevated IOPs in the range of 22 to 40 mm Hg. Some patients have much higher pressures, which occasionally reach levels of 60 or even 80 mm Hg. Some patients will never have IOPs over 18 mm Hg. These patients are said to have normal-tension glaucoma (low-tension glaucoma). It is important to remember that IOP fluctuates throughout the day and that patients with glaucoma undergo wider fluctuations than do normal individuals. Although most people reach their highest IOPs in the morning, others may reach their peaks in the afternoon or evening or follow no consistent pattern. Diurnal IOP measurements may be useful in some situations, including diagnosing POAG, explaining progressive damage despite apparent good pressure control, evaluating the efficacy of therapy, and distinguishing normal-tension glaucoma from POAG.

Most individuals have fairly symmetric IOP readings. When pressure is higher in one eye, that eye usually has a larger cup and a more damaged visual field than the fellow eye. Marked differences in IOPs between the two eyes should raise suspicion of exfoliative syndrome or another form of secondary glaucoma.

A reduced outflow facility is the fundamental abnormality of aqueous humor dynamics in POAG.[195] As glaucoma progresses, outflow facility declines progressively. Measurements of outflow facility by tonography are not part of the routine clinical assessment of glaucoma today. Single measurements of outflow facility do not help much in the diagnosis of POAG or in the assessment of the efficacy of treatment.

An *afferent pupillary defect* can be seen in patients with asymmetric or unilateral glaucoma. This finding, which is also referred to as *Marcus Gunn's sign,* is elicited by the swinging flashlight test. It has been noted in patients with asymmetric cupping and normal kinetic visual fields.[196]

The angles are open in patients with POAG. The angles can be narrow, but there can be no peripheral anterior synechiae (unless caused by prior laser treatment or surgery), no apposition between the iris and the trabecular meshwork, and no developmental abnormalities of the angle. Moderate pigmentation of the meshwork is often present in proportion to the patient's age and race. Heavy pigmentation is suggestive of other disorders, including pigmentary glaucoma, exfoliative syndrome, and diabetes mellitus.

The crucial clinical findings in POAG are those that occur in the optic disc and visual field. Defects in the nerve fiber layer are also seen in most patients. These matters are presented in detail in Chapters 11 and 14 and are not discussed further here. Other findings include impairment of contrast sensitivity, temporal contrast sensitivity, loss of color perception, and other psychophysical impairments as outlined in Chapter 12.

Differential Diagnosis

The differential diagnosis of POAG includes conditions that can mimic any of the cardinal features of the disease, such as elevated IOP, cupping and atrophy of the optic disc, and visual field loss. POAG must be distinguished from a variety of secondary and developmental glaucomas. These include exfoliative syndrome, pigmentary dispersion, trauma, anterior segment inflammation, sub-

eyes with normal-tension glaucoma and those with POAG are matched for the degree of visual field loss, the cupping is identical.

Patients with normal-tension glaucoma demonstrate several abnormalities on fluorescein angiography, including diffuse and focal hypofluorescence of the disc and abnormal transit time.[316-319] These abnormalities are similar to those seen in POAG. Splinter hemorrhages are noted with greater frequency in patients with normal-tension glaucoma.[279,320] Patients with normal-tension glaucoma show increased resistance of the ophthalmic artery compared with those with open-angle glaucoma as measured by a variety of indirect methods, including Doppler velocity.[321]

Some cases of normal-tension glaucoma are progressive, whereas others appear to be stable over long periods. Drance and co-workers[282,322,323] have emphasized that the stable cases are often associated with previous hemodynamic crises, such as episodes of acute blood loss, arrhythmia, and hypotension. These patients are not likely to develop further visual loss unless they experience additional hemodynamic crises. This same group has suggested that there are two groups of glaucoma patients—one associated with vasospasm (migraine or Raynaud's phenomenon) and higher IOP, and one associated with disturbed coagulation, biochemistry suggestive of vascular disease, and little association with IOP.[324] Others have identified a subgroup of normal-tension glaucoma patients (approximately one third) who have focal "ischemic" changes in the optic nerve and who are also more likely to have hypertension and other cardiovascular problems than those with "typical" high-pressure open-angle glaucoma.[325]

In most population-based studies that use perimetry and ophthalmoscopy, between one third and one half of the patients with glaucomatous visual field loss have normal IOPs on initial examination.* Some of these individuals demonstrate elevated IOP on repeat examination and are then classified as having POAG.[246,327,328] The relative prevalences of POAG and normal-tension glaucoma depend on the definition of normal IOP and the number of pressure measurements made.

As a rule, normal-tension glaucoma is seen in older individuals, especially those over age 60 although it is possible to see rare cases in those under the age of 50.[16,329-331] The disease appears to occur more often in women than in men.[279,330,332] A relatively high prevalence of normal-tension glaucoma is present in the Japanese population as compared with other racial groups.[46] The Japanese population seems to be the only ethnic/racial group with such a high prevalence of normal-tension glaucoma.[13] No clear association exists between normal-tension glaucoma and refractive error.[13] Although there have been a few descriptions of families with normal-tension glaucoma,[333] most cases appear to be sporadic. However, a family history of some form of glaucoma is reasonably common in patients with normal-tension glaucoma.[331]

Several ocular and systemic characteristics have been associated with normal-pressure glaucoma. These include abnormal immunoproteins such as anti-Ro/SS-A positivity and heat shock protein antibodies indicating a possible autoimmune mechanism.[334] Silent myocardial ischemia and ventricular extrasystoles occur more frequently in normal-tension glaucoma patients (45%), compared with 26% of patients with open-angle glaucoma and 12% of those with cataract (only slightly greater than age-adjusted normal rate).[335]

Differential Diagnosis

Many conditions can produce visual field loss and an abnormal appearance of the optic disc without an elevated IOP (Box 17-3). Some clinicians refer to these conditions as "pseudoglaucoma" or even include them under the heading of normal-tension glaucoma. This seems needlessly confusing, and as mentioned previously, the definition of normal-tension glaucoma used here excludes known ocular or systemic causes of visual loss. The term *pseudoglaucoma* should be abandoned because it adds little to our understanding of the disease process. Following are the most common entities in the differential diagnosis of normal-tension glaucoma:

1. Glaucoma. IOP readings can be misleading because of diurnal variation, low scleral rigidity, thin corneas,[336] or systemic medications that reduce pressure. Some patients demonstrate elevated IOP only in the supine position.[337,338] Elevated IOP may have caused damage in the past and now may be in remission because of hyposecretion of aqueous humor that may occur in aged and diseased eyes.[339-341] IOP may be increased at times when the patient is not evaluated.[342] The patient may be compliant with medications only on the days when he or she is seen by the ophthalmologist

*Refs: 13, 16, 46, 60, 240, 246, 326.

**Box 17-3
Differential Diagnosis of Normal-Tension Glaucoma**

I. Glaucoma
  A. Elevated intraocular pressure not detected
    1. Undetected wide diurnal variation
    2. Low scleral rigidity
    3. Systemic medication that may mask elevated intraocular pressure (IOP) (e.g., recent β-blocker treatment
    4. Past systemic medication that may have elevated IOP
    5. Elevation of IOP in supine position only
  B. Glaucoma in remission
    1. Past corticosteroid administration
    2. Pigmentary glaucoma[341]
    3. Associated with past uveitis or trauma
    4. Glaucomatocyclitic crisis
    5. Burned-out primary open-angle glaucoma
II. Optic nerve damage
  A. Congenital optic nerve conditions[9]
    1. Pits
    2. Colobomas
    3. Tilted discs
  B. Ischemic optic neuropathy
    1. Arteritic
    2. Nonarteritic
  C. Compressed lesions
    1. Tumors
    2. Aneurysms
    3. Cysts
    4. Chiasmatic arachnoiditis
  D. Optic nerve drusen
  E. Demyelinating conditions
  F. Inflammatory diseases
  G. Hereditary optic atrophy
  H. Toxic drugs or chemicals
III. Ocular disorders
  A. Myopia
  B. Retinal degeneration
  C. Myelinated nerve fibers
  D. Branch vascular occlusions
  E. Choroidal nevus or melanoma
  F. Choroidal rupture
  G. Retinoschisis
  H. Chorioretinal disease
IV. Systemic vascular conditions
  A. Anemia
  B. Carotid artery obstruction
  C. Acute blood loss
  D. Arrhythmia
  E. Hypotensive episodes
V. Miscellaneous
  A. Hysteria
  B. Artifact of visual field testing

---

2. Congenital defects of the optic disc, including pits and colobomas.
3. Ischemic optic neuropathy.
4. Compressive lesions of the optic nerve, including tumors, aneurysms, and cysts.[343]
5. Retinal diseases, including retinitis pigmentosa and branch vascular occlusion.

Work-up

A careful history is the most important part of the work-up for normal-tension glaucoma. This should include questions about previous elevations of IOP, ocular trauma or inflammation, present and past medication use, exposure to toxins, and present and past health. It is especially important to ask about corticosteroid administration systemically, to the eye, the nasal passages, or the skin. Patients must be queried about hemodynamic crises, including blood loss, anemia, arrhythmias, transfusions, and hypotensive episodes. The ocular examination should include measurements of IOP at different times of the day and evening and in the sitting and supine positions. Auscultation and palpation of the carotid arteries may reveal obstructive disease. Depending on the results of the history and physical examination, some patients should receive a general medical work-up, a neurologic examination, serologic tests for syphilis, an erythrocyte sedimentation rate, measurement of hematocrit and hemoglobin levels, antinuclear antibodies, magnetic resonance imaging, Doppler imaging of the carotid arteries, and/or carotid angiography. If the history and physical examinations are unremarkable, routine computed tomography scans or magnetic resonance imaging is rarely of benefit. Generally speaking, extensive systemic work-ups should be reserved for those patients who are under 60 years of age, whose optic discs show more pallor than cupping, whose

254. Sample PA, and others: Comparison of standard, short-wavelength, frequency doubling, and motion perimetry in eyes with glaucomatous optic neuropathy, *Invest Ophthalmol Vis Sci* 39:S656, 1998.

255. Wollstein G, and others: Identifying early glaucomatous changes: comparison between expert clinical assessment of optic disc photographs and confocal scanning ophthalmoscopy, *Invest Ophthalmol Vis Sci* 39:S1125, 1998.

256. Stromberg U: Ocular hypertension, *Acta Ophthalmol Scand Suppl* 69:7, 1962.

257. Armaly MF: *On the distribution of applanation pressure and arcuate scotoma.* In Patterson G, Miller SJH, Patterson GD, editors: *Drug mechanisms in glaucoma,* Boston, 1966, Little, Brown.

258. Hirvela H, Tuulonen A, Laatikainen L: Intraocular pressure and prevalence of glaucoma in elderly people in Finland: a population-based study, *Int Ophthalmol* 18:299, 1994-1995.

259. Sorensen PN, Nielsen NVC, Norskov K: Ocular hypertension: a 15-year follow-up, *Acta Ophthalmol* 56:363, 1978.

260. Graham PA: The definition of preglaucoma: a prospective study, *Trans Ophthalmol Soc UK* 88:153, 1968.

261. Lundberg L, Wettrell K, Linner E: Ocular hypertension: a prospective twenty-year follow-up study, *Acta Ophthalmol Scand Suppl* 65:705, 1987.

262. Armaly MF: The visual field defect and ocular pressure level in open angle glaucoma, *Invest Ophthalmol* 8:105, 1969.

263. Hart WM Jr, and others: Multivariate analysis of the risk of glaucomatous visual field loss, *Arch Ophthalmol* 97:1455, 1979.

264. Drance SM, and others: Multivariate analysis in glaucoma: use of discriminant analysis in predicting glaucomatous visual field damage, *Arch Ophthalmol* 99:1019, 1981.

265. Airaksinen PJ: Retinal nerve fiber layer and neuroretinal rim changes in ocular hypertension and early glaucoma, *Surv Ophthalmol* 33:413, 1989.

266. Quigley HA, and others: An evaluation of optic disc and nerve fiber layer examinations in monitoring progression of early glaucoma damage, *Ophthalmology* 99:19, 1992.

267. Nanba K, Schwartz B: Nerve fiber layer and optic disc fluorescein defects in glaucoma and ocular hypertension, *Ophthalmology* 95:1227, 1988.

268. Johnson CA, and others: Short-wavelength automated perimetry in low-, medium-, and high-risk ocular hypertensive eyes: initial baseline results, *Arch Ophthalmol* 113:70, 1995.

269. Silverman SE, Trick GL, Hart WM Jr: Motion perception is abnormal in primary open-angle glaucoma and ocular hypertension, *Invest Ophthalmol Vis Sci* 31:722, 1990.

270. Wall M, Jennisch CS, Munden PM: Motion perimetry identifies nerve fiber bundlelike defects in ocular hypertension, *Arch Ophthalmol* 115:26, 1997.

271. Arai M, and others: A 3-year follow-up study of ocular hypertension by pattern electroretinogram, *Ophthalmologica* 207:187, 1993.

272. Kamal DS, and others: Use of sequential Heidelberg Retina Tomograph (HRT) images to identify changes in the optic disk in ocular hypertensive (OHT) patients at risk of developing glaucoma, *Invest Ophthalmol Vis Sci* 39:S1125, 1998.

273. Anton A, and others: Nerve fiber layer measurements with scanning laser polarimetry in ocular hypertension, *Arch Ophthalmol* 115:33, 1997.

274. Tezel G, and others: Parapapillary chorioretinal atrophy in patients with ocular hypertension. I. An evaluation as a predictive factor for the development of glaucomatous damage, *Arch Ophthalmol* 115:1503, 1997.

275. Tezel G, Kolker AE, Wax MB: Parapapillary chorioretinal atrophy in patients with ocular hypertension. II. An evaluation of progressive changes, *Arch Ophthalmol* 115:1509, 1997.

276. Graham PA, Hollows FC: *A critical review of methods of detecting glaucoma.* In Hunt LB, editor: *Glaucoma: epidemiology, early diagnosis and some aspects of treatment,* Edinburgh, 1966, Churchill Livingstone.

277. Pohjanpelto PEJ, Palva J: Ocular hypertension and glaucomatous optic nerve damage, *Acta Ophthalmol* 52:194, 1974.

278. Kass MA: The ocular hypertension treatment study, *J Glaucoma* 3:97, 1994 (editorial).

279. Drance SM, and others: Studies of factors involved in the production of low tension glaucoma, *Arch Ophthalmol* 89:457, 1973.

280. Chumbley LC, Brubaker RF: Low-tension glaucoma, *Am J Ophthalmol* 81:761, 1976.

281. Caprioli J, Spaeth GL: Comparison of the optic nerve head in high-and low-tension glaucoma, *Arch Ophthalmol* 103:1145, 1985.

282. Drance SM: The visual field of low tension glaucoma and shock-induced optic neuropathy, *Arch Ophthalmol* 95:1359, 1977.

283. Hamard P, and others: Optic nerve head blood flow using a laser Doppler velocimeter and haemorheology in primary open angle glaucoma and normal pressure glaucoma, *Br J Ophthalmol* 78:449, 1994.

284. Francois J, Neetens A: The deterioration of the visual field in glaucoma and the blood pressure, *Doc Ophthalmol* 28:70, 1970.

285. Goldberg I, and others: Systemic factors in patients with low tension glaucoma, *Br J Ophthalmol* 65:56, 1981.

286. Bechetoille A, Bresson-Dumont H: Diurnal and nocturnal blood pressure drops in patients with focal ischemic glaucoma, *Graefes Arch Clin Exp Ophthalmol* 232:675, 1995.

287. Winder AF: Circulatory lipoprotein and blood glucose levels in association with low-tension and chronic simple glaucoma, *Br J Ophthalmol* 61:641, 1977.

288. Morax V: Glaucome simple au atrophie avec excavation, *Ann Ocul (Paris)* 153:25, 1916.

289. Thiel R: Glaukom ohne Hochdruck, *Ber Dtsch Ophthalmol Gessell* 48:133, 1930.

290. Gittinger JW Jr, and others: Glaucomatous cupping:sine glaucoma, *Surv Ophthalmol* 25:383, 1981.

291. Duijm HF, van den Berg TJ, Greve EL: A comparison of retinal and choroidal hemodynamics in patients with primary open-angle glaucoma and normal-pressure glaucoma. *Am J Ophthalmol* 123:644, 1997.

292. Butt Z, and others: Color Doppler imaging in untreated high- and normal-pressure open-angle glaucoma, *Invest Ophthalmol Vis Sci* 38:690, 1997.

293. Corbett JJ, and others: The neurologic evaluation of patients with low-tension glaucoma, *Invest Ophthalmol Vis Sci* 26:1101, 1985.

294. Phelps CD, Corbett JJ: Migraine and low-tension glaucoma: a case-control study, *Invest Ophthalmol Vis Sci* 26:1105, 1985.

295. Nicolela MT, Drance SM: Various glaucomatous optic nerve appearances: clinical correlations, *Ophthalmology* 103:640, 1996.

296. Leighton DA, Phillips CI: Systemic blood pressure in open-angle glaucoma, low tension glaucoma and the normal eye, *Br J Ophthalmol* 56:447, 1972.

297. Hatsuda TA: Low-tension glaucoma, *Folia Ophthalmol Jpn* 28:244, 1977.

298. Bengtsson B: Aspects of the epidemiology of chronic glaucoma, *Acta Ophthalmol Suppl Scand* 146:1, 1981.

299. Demailly P, and others: Do patients with low tension glaucoma have particular cardiovascular characteristics? *Ophthalmologica* 188:65, 1984.

300. Gramer E, Leydecker W: Glaucoma without elevated pressure: a clinical study, *Klin Mbl Augenheilk* 186:262, 1985.

301. Usui T, and others: Prevalence of migraine in low-tension glaucoma and primary open-angle glaucoma in Japanese, *Br J Ophthalmol* 75:224, 1991.

302. Klein BE, and others: Migraine headache and its association with open-angle glaucoma. The Beaver Dam Eye Study, *Invest Ophthalmol Vis Sci* 34:3024, 1993.

303. Best W: Glaucoma ohne Hohdruck, *Klin Mbl Augenheilk* 159:280, 1971.

304. Zeimer RC, and others: Association between intraocular pressure peaks and progression of visual field loss, *Ophthalmology* 98:64, 1991.

305. Ito M, Sugiura T, Mizokami K: A comparative study on visual field defect in low-tension glaucoma, *Acta Soc Ophthalmol Jpn* 95:790, 1991.

306. Shirai H, and others: Visual field change and risk factors for progression of visual field damage in low tension glaucoma, *Acta Soc Ophthalmol Jpn* 96:352, 1992.

307. Harrington DO: *Pathogenesis of the glaucomatous visual field defects: individual variations in pressure sensitivity.* In Newell FW, editor: *Conference on glaucoma. Transactions of the Fifth Josiah Macy Conference,* New York, 1960, Josiah Macy Foundation.

308. Motolko M, Drance SM, Douglas GR: Visual field defects in low-tension glaucoma: comparison of defects in low-tension glaucoma and chronic open-angle glaucoma, *Arch Ophthalmol* 100:1074, 1982.

309. Paufique L, and others: A propos du glaucôme à basse tension, *Bull Soc Oph thalmol Fr* 64:464, 1964.

310. Kriegelstein GK, Langham ME: Glaukom ohne Hochdruck ein beitrag zue Atiologie, *Klin Mbl Augenheilk* 166:18, 1975.

311. Winstanley J: Discussion on low-tension glaucoma, *Proc Royal Soc Med* 52:433, 1959.

312. Ourgard HG, Etienne R: *L'Exploration Fonctionelle de l'Oeil Glaucomateux,* Paris, 1961, Masson.

313. Tezel G, and others: Comparative optic disc analysis in normal pressure glaucoma, primary open-angle glaucoma, and ocular hypertension, *Ophthalmology* 103:2105, 1996.

314. Jonas JB, Xu L: Parapapillary chorioretinal atrophy in normal-pressure glaucoma, *Am J Ophthalmol* 115:501, 1993.

315. King D, and others: Comparison of visual field defects in normal-tension glaucoma and high-tension glaucoma, *Am J Ophthalmol* 101:204, 1986.

316. Laatikainen L: Fluorescein angiographic studies of the peripapillary and perilimbal regions in simple, capsular and low tension glaucoma, *Acta Ophthalmol Scand Suppl* 111:1, 1971.

317. Begg IS, Drance SM, Goldmann H: Fluorescein angiography in the evaluation of focal circulatory ischaemia of the optic nerve head in relation to the arcuate scotoma in glaucoma, *Can J Ophthalmol* 7:68, 1972.

318. Inoue Y, Inoue T, Shishida Y: Fluorescein angiography of the optic disc in low-tension glaucoma, *Folia Ophthalmol Jpn* 26:1400, 1975.

319. Hitchings RA, Spaeth GL: Fluorescein angiography in chronic simple glaucoma and low-tension glaucoma, *Br J Ophthalmol* 61:126, 1977.

320. Jonas JB, Xu L: Optic disk hemorrhages in glaucoma, *Am J Ophthalmol* 118:1, 1994.

321. Harris A, and others: The comprehensive ocular hemodynamic assessment in glaucoma, *Invest Ophthalmol Vis Sci* 39: S222, 1998.

322. Drance SM: Some factors in the production of low tension glaucoma, *Br J Ophthalmol* 56:229, 1972.

323. Drance SM, Morgan RW, Sweeney VP: Shock-induced optic neuropathy: a cause of nonprogressive glaucoma, *N Engl J Med* 288:392, 1973.

324. Schulzer M, and others: Biostatistical evidence for two distinct chronic open angle glaucoma populations, *Br J Ophthalmol* 74:196, 1990.

325. Geijssen HC, Greve EL: Focal ischaemic normal pressure glaucoma versus high pressure glaucoma, *Doc Ophthalmol* 75: 291, 1990.

326. Sommer A, and others: Relationship between intraocular pressure and primary open angle glaucoma among white and black Americans. The Baltimore Eye Survey, *Arch Ophthalmol* 109:1090, 1991.

327. Duke-Elder S: Fundamental concepts in glaucoma, *Arch Ophthalmol* 42:538, 1949.

328. Meyer SJ: Incomplete glaucoma, monosymptomatic glaucomatous excavation, *EENT Monthly* 29:477, 1950.

329. Sjogren H: A study of pseudoglaucoma, *Acta Ophthalmol Scand Suppl* 24:239, 1946.

330. Levene RZ: Low tension glaucoma: a critical review and new material, *Surv Ophthalmol* 24:621, 1980.

331. Geijssen HC: *Studies on normal pressure glaucoma,* Amstelveen, 1991, Kugler.

332. Nicolela MT, Drance SM: Various glaucomatous optic nerve appearances: clinical correlations, *Ophthalmology* 103: 640, 1996.

333. Sandvig K: Pseudoglaucoma of autosomal dominant inheritance: a report of 3 families. *Acta Ophthalmol* 39:33, 1961.

334. Wax MB, and others: Anti-Ro/SS-A positivity and heat shock protein antibodies in patients with normal-pressure glaucoma, *Am J Ophthalmol* 125:145, 1998.

335. Waldmann E, and others: Silent myocardial ischemia in glaucoma and cataract patients, *Graefes Arch Clin Exp Ophthalmol* 234:595, 1996.

336. Morad Y, and others: Corneal thickness and curvature in normal-tension glaucoma, *Am J Ophthalmol* 125:164, 1998.

337. Kriegelstein GK, Langham ME: Influence of body position on the intraocular pressure of normal and glaucomatous eyes, *Opthalmologica* 171:132, 1975.

338. Hyams SW, and others: Postural changes in intraocular pressure with particular reference to low tension glaucoma, *Glaucoma* 6:178, 1984.

339. Chervin M: Glaucoma por hipersecretion, glaucoma sin hipertension, seudoglaucoma, *Arch Oftalmol Buenos Aires* 42:187, 1967.

340. Sugar HS: Low tension glaucoma: a practical approach, *Ann Ophthalmol* 11: 1155, 1979.

341. Ritch R: Nonprogressive low-tension glaucoma with pigmentary dispersion, *Am J Ophthalmol* 94:190, 1982.

342. Ido T, Tomita G, Kitazawa Y: Diurnal variation of intraocular pressure of normal-tension glaucoma, *Ophthalmology* 98:296, 1991.

343. Kalenak JW, Kosmorsky GS, Hassenbusch SJ: Compression of the intracranial optic nerve mimicking unilateral normal-pressure glaucoma, *J Clin Neuroophthalmol* 12:230, 1992.

343a. Collaborative Normal-Tension Glaucoma Study Group: Comparison of glaucomatous progression between untreated patients with normal-tension glaucoma and patients with therapeutically reduced intraocular pressure, *Am J Ophthalmol* 126:487, 1998.

343b. Collaborative Normal-Tension Glaucoma Study Group: The effectiveness of intraocular pressure reduction in the treatment of normal-tension glaucoma, *Am J Ophthalmol* 126:498, 1998.

344. Rulo AH, and others: Reduction of intraocular pressure with treatment of latanoprost once daily in patients with normal-pressure glaucoma, *Ophthalmology* 103:1276, 1996.

345. Stewart WC, and others: A 90-day study of the efficacy and side effects of 0.25% and 0.5% apraclonidine vs 0.5% timolol. Apraclonidine Primary Therapy Study Group, *Arch Ophthalmol* 114:938, 1996.

346. Ito M: A study on topical treatment in low-tension glaucoma, *Jpn J Clin Ophthalmol* 45:323, 1991.

347. Kaiser HJ, and others: Longterm visual field follow-up of glaucoma patients treated with beta-blockers, *Surv Ophthalmol* 38(suppl):S156, 1994.

348. Gross RL, and others: Effects of betaxolol on glutamate- and voltage-gated currents in retinal ganglion cells, *Invest Ophthalmol Vis Sci* 39:S260, 1998.

349. Kaneko R, Ogata Y, Ueno S: Effects of 0.5% betaxolol on ocular microcirculation and whole body circulation, *Invest Ophthalmol Vis Sci* 39:S269, 1998.

350. Mitchell CK, Nguyen PT, Feldman RM: Neuroprotection of retinal ganglion cells, *Invest Ophthalmol Vis Sci* 39:S261, 1998.

351. Harris A, and others: Effects of topical dorzolamide on retinal and retrobulbar hemodynamics, *Acta Ophthalmol Scand* 74:569, 1996.

352. Schmidt KG, and others: [Ocular pulse amplitude and local carbonic anhydrase inhibition], *Ophthalmologe* 94:659, 1997.

353. Sharpe ED, Simmons RJ: Argon laser trabeculoplasty as a means of decreasing intraocular pressure from "normal" levels in glaucomatous eyes, *Am J Ophthalmol* 99:704, 1985.

354. Demailly M, Lehrer M, Kretz G: Argon laser trabeculoplasty in low-tension glaucoma: a prospective study of tonometric and perimetric results, *J Fr Ophtalmol* 3:183, 1989.

355. Schulzer M: The Normal-Tension Glaucoma Study Group: intraocular pressure reduction in normal-tension glaucoma patients, *Ophthalmology* 99:1468, 1992.

356. Chandler PA: Long-term results in glaucoma therapy, *Am J Ophthalmol* 49:221, 1960.

357. de Jong N, and others: Results of a filtering procedure in low tension glaucoma, *Int Ophthalmol* 13:131, 1989.

358. Kitazawa Y, Yamamoto T: Are POAG and NTG truly different in pathophysiology? *Invest Ophthalmol Vis Sci* 39: S222, 1998.

359. Mermoud A, Faggioni R: Treatment of normal pressure glaucoma with a serotonin S2 receptor antagonist, naftidrofuryl (Praxilen), *Klin Mbl Augenheilk* 198:332, 1991.

360. Gasser P, and others: Do vasospasms provoke ocular diseases? *Angiology* 41:213, 1990.

361. Netland PA, Chaturvedi N, Dreyer EB: Calcium channel blockers in the management of low-tension and open-angle glaucoma, *Am J Ophthalmol* 115:608, 1993.

362. Bose S, Piltz JR, Breton ME: Nimodipine, a centrally active calcium antagonist, exerts a beneficial effect on contrast sensitivity in patients with normal-tension glaucoma and in control subjects, *Ophthalmology* 102:1236, 1995.

363. Harris A, and others: Hemodynamic and visual function effects of oral nifedipine in patients with normal-tension glaucoma, *Am J Ophthalmol* 124:296, 1997.

364. Sawada A, and others: Prevention of visual field defect progression with brovincamine in eyes with normal-tension glaucoma, *Ophthalmology* 103:283, 1996.

365. Kitazawa Y, Shirai H, Go FJ: The effect of Ca2(+)-antagonist on visual field in low-tension glaucoma, *Graefes Arch Clin Exp Ophthalmol* 227:408, 1989.

366. Liu S, and others: Lack of effect of calcium channel blockers on open-angle glaucoma, *J Glaucoma* 5:187, 1996.

367. Wilson RP, and others: A color Doppler analysis of nifedipine-induced posterior ocular blood flow changes in open-angle glaucoma, *J Glaucoma* 6:231, 1997.

368. Kahn HA, and others: The Framingham Eye Study. I. Outline and major prevalence findings, *Am J Epidemiol* 106:17, 1977.

369. Bengtsson B: Findings associated with glaucomatous visual field defects, *Acta Ophthalmol Scand* 58:20, 1980.

370. Mason RP, and others: National survey of the prevalence and risk factors of glaucoma in St. Lucia, West Indies. Part I. Prevalence findings, *Ophthalmology* 96:1363, 1989.

371. Coffey M, and others: Prevalence of glaucoma in the west of Ireland, *Br J Ophthalmol* 77:17, 1993.

372. Jay JL, Allan D: The benefit of early trabeculectomy versus conventional management in primary open-angle glaucoma relative to severity of disease, *Eye* 3:528, 1989.

373. Schappert-Kimmijser J: A five-year follow-up of subjects with intraocular pressure of 22-30 mm Hg without anomalies of optic nerve and visual field typical for glaucoma at first investigation, *Ophthalmologica* 162:289, 1971.

374. Walker WM: Ocular hypertension: follow-up of 109 cases from 1963 to 1974, *Trans Ophthalmol Soc UK* 94:525, 1974.

375. Drance SM, and others: Use of discriminant analysis. II. Identification of persons with glaucomatous visual field defects, *Arch Ophthalmol* 96:57, 1978.

376. Kitazawa Y: *Clinical features of the eye in the earliest stage of primary open-angle glaucoma.* In Rehak S, Krasnov MM, Patterson GD, editors: *Recent advances in glaucoma. Proceedings of the International Glaucoma Symposium, Prague, 1976,* Prague, 1978, Avicenum Czechoslovak Medical Press.

377. Armaly MF, Krueger D, Maunder C: *Summary report of "biostatistical analysis of the Collaborative Glaucoma Study."* In Kriegelstein D, Leydhecker W, editors: *Glaucoma update. International Glaucoma Symposium, Nara, Japan, 1978,* Berlin, 1979, Springer-Verlag.

378. Trobe JD, Bergsma DR: Atypical retinitis pigmentosa masquerading as a nerve fiber bundle lesion, *Am J Ophthalmol* 79:681, 1975.

379. Trobe JD, Watson RT: Retinal degeneration without pigment alterations in progressive external ophthalmoplegia, *Am J Ophthalmol* 83:372, 1977.

380. Abedin S, Simmons RJ, Hirose T: Simulated double Bjerrum's scotomas by retinal pigment epithelium and receptor degeneration, *Ann Ophthalmol* 13:1117, 1981.

381. Krauss HR, Heckenlively JR: Visual field changes in cone-rod degenerations, *Arch Ophthalmol* 100:1784, 1982.

382. Martin WG, and others: Ocular toxoplasmosis and visual field defects, *Am J Ophthalmol* 90:25, 1980.

383. Savino PJ, Glaser JS, Rosenberg MA: A clinical analysis of pseudopapilledema. II. Visual field defects, *Arch Ophthalmol* 97:71, 1979.

384. Grehn F, Knorr-Held S, Kommerell G: Glaucomatous-like visual field defects in chronic papilledema, *Graefes Arch Clin Exp Ophthalmol* 217:99, 1981.

18

Secondary Open-Angle Glaucoma

PIGMENTARY GLAUCOMA

Pigmentary glaucoma is a secondary form of open-angle glaucoma produced by pigment dispersion in the anterior segment of the eye.[1,2] This condition constitutes 1.0% to 1.5% of the glaucomas seen in many Western countries.[3] Pigmentary glaucoma generally occurs in young adults but has been described in adolescents and older individuals as well.[1,4] The disease preferentially involves men, and the women affected usually are a decade older than the men.[4-6] Pigmentary glaucoma occurs in white individuals and is rare in blacks and Asians.[1,5,6] There is a strong association between pigmentary glaucoma and myopia; the typical pigmentary glaucoma patient is a myopic white man in his twenties or thirties. One study of black patients found that the average age of onset was 73 years, and the patients were more often hyperopic than myopic, indicating that there may be a different mechanism of disease in this subgroup.[7] Although there have been a few reports of familial pigmentary glaucoma,[1,6,8] most cases appear to be sporadic.

Pigmentary glaucoma is characterized by the release of pigment particles from the pigment epithelium of the iris. These particles are carried by the aqueous humor convection currents and then deposited on a variety of tissues in the anterior segment of the eye, including the corneal endothelium (Fig. 18-1), trabecular meshwork (Fig. 18-2), anterior iris surface, zonules (Fig. 18-3), and lens. The loss of pigment from the iris is detected as a series of radial, spoklike, midperipheral transillumination defects. These defects can range in number from 1 or 2 to 65 or 70 and can be thin slits or coalescent areas. They are best seen in a darkened room by a dark-adapted observer. The defects can be highlighted by shining a small slit beam through the pupil with the light perpendicular to the plane of the iris. On rare occasions transillumination defects are hidden by very heavy iris pigmentation. Patients with pigmentary glaucoma have very deep anterior chambers, a concave appearance of the peripheral iris, and mild iridodonesis.[9-11]

The deposition of pigment on the corneal endothelium generally takes the form of a vertically oriented spindle called *Krukenberg's spindle* (see Fig. 18-1), which can range in appearance from faint to striking. The spindle is neither pathognomonic of the disease nor invariably present, but it is a very useful sign. The spindle consists of extracellular as well as intracellular pigment granules phagocytized by the corneal endothelium.[12,13] Pigment also accumulates in the trabecular meshwork. In early cases of pigmentary glaucoma the trabecular meshwork is moderately pigmented, with pigments varying from one portion of the meshwork to another. In advanced cases the trabecular meshwork appears as a dark-brown velvet band that extends uniformly about the circumference of the angle (see Fig. 18-2). The pigment can cover the entire width of the angle from the ciliary face to the peripheral cornea; a pigment line anterior to Schwalbe's line is often referred to as *Sampaolesi's line.*

Pigment is also deposited on the zonules, posterior lens surface (Zentmayer's ring or Scheie's line), and anterior iris surface. The pigment on the anterior iris surface accumulates in the circumferential folds and can be sufficient to give a dull or even a heterochromic appearance if the pigment dispersion is asymmetric in the two eyes.[5]

The anterior chamber is very deep and the peripheral iris has a concave configuration when viewed at the slit lamp or with gonioscopy (Fig.18-4). With the exception of pigmentary dispersion, pigmentary glaucoma resembles primary open-angle glaucoma (POAG) in most aspects, includ-

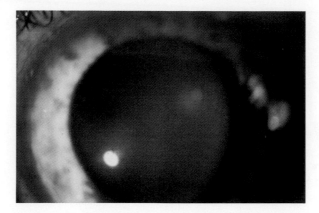

Figure 18-1 Deposition of pigment on the corneal endothelium, referred to as *Krukenberg's spindle.* (From Alward WLM: *Color atlas of gonioscopy,* St Louis, 1994, Mosby.)

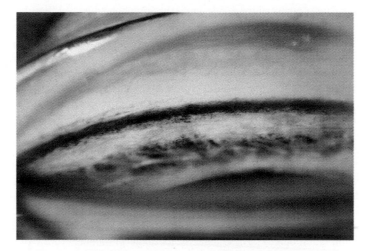

Figure 18-2 Goniophotograph of dense pigment in the anterior chamber angle.

Figure 18-3 Pigment deposit on the zonules. (From Campbell DG, Netland PN: *Stereo atlas of glaucoma,* St Louis, 1998, Mosby.)

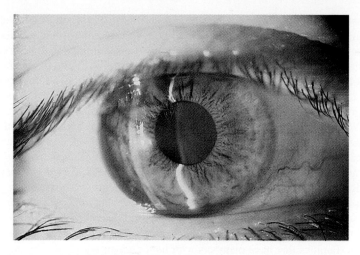

Figure 18-4   Concave peripheral iris illustrated by an inferior slit beam in a patient with pigmentary glaucoma.

ing elevated intraocular pressure (IOP), decreased outflow facility, optic nerve cupping, and visual field loss. Large diurnal IOP fluctuations are thought to occur more often in pigmentary glaucoma and can be sufficient to cause corneal edema, blurring, and halo vision. Patients with pigmentary glaucoma can have a sudden release of pigment with severe IOP elevations after pupillary dilation or exercise.[14-18] At times this release of pigment can be confused with active anterior segment inflammation. Pigment release and marked IOP elevation after exercise can be blocked by topical pilocarpine therapy.[19]

Several reports have indicated that pigment dispersion lessens with time so that Krukenberg's spindles and trabecular pigmentation become less prominent.[4,5] In some cases this is accompanied by an improvement in aqueous humor dynamics. Ritch[20] has proposed that this disappearance of pigment may explain some nonprogressive cases of normal-tension glaucoma. That is, a patient who has optic nerve cupping, visual field loss, and normal IOP may have had pigmentary glaucoma and elevated IOP in the past. Remission of pigmentary dispersion also has been reported after glaucoma surgery[6] and lens subluxation.[21]

The differential diagnosis of pigmentary glaucoma includes any condition that produces pigmentation of the trabecular meshwork. These include normal eyes with aging, POAG, uveitis, cysts of the iris and ciliary body, pigmented intraocular tumors, previous surgery (including laser surgery), trauma, angle-closure glaucoma, amyloidosis, diabetes mellitus, herpes zoster, megalocornea, radiation, siderosis, and hemosiderosis. These conditions should be readily distinguished from pigmentary glaucoma by the history and physical examination. The condition most likely to be confused with pigmentary glaucoma is exfoliation syndrome. However, the pattern of iris atrophy in exfoliation syndrome is usually central and geographic, and the pigment accumulation in the trabecular meshwork consists of larger particles that are unevenly distributed about the angle.

It is important to emphasize that many individuals have pigment dispersion without glaucoma or abnormal aqueous humor dynamics.[22] The true prevalence of the pigmentary dispersion syndrome in the population is not known; most cases of mild pigment dispersion are probably never detected. Pigment dispersion appears to be at least as common as pigmentary glaucoma and occurs with equal frequency in both sexes. In some cases pigment dispersion progresses to pigmentary glaucoma over time, which can be as long as 12 to 20 years.[1] However, most individuals with pigmentary dispersion syndrome maintain normal visual fields and aqueous humor dynamics, even on long-term follow-up. This good prognosis is especially likely if the patient has a normal tonographic outflow facility when first seen.[14] Generally the degree of pigment dispersion does not correlate well with the presence or future development of glaucoma.[6] Patients with pigment dispersion syndrome and normal IOPs should receive a careful initial examination, including visual field examinations and optic nerve photographs. These individuals should then be followed up periodically without treatment.

Any theory about the pathogenesis of pigmentary glaucoma must explain two phenomena: pigment release and diminished outflow facility. Campbell[9] has proposed a mechanical theory to explain pigment dispersion. He postulated that the concave shape of the peripheral iris allows it to rub against the zonules, causing pigment release and dispersion. Campbell noted that the pattern of iris transillumination defects corresponds with the arrangement of the anterior zonular packets.[9] He also noted that the number and extent of the iris transillumination defects correlates with the progression of pigmentary glaucoma.[9] When patients receive miotic treatment, the ensuing pupillary block lifts the peripheral iris off the zonules and allows the transillumination defects to fill in and even disappear. Although this theory explains pigment dispersion, it does not explain why some individuals with pigment dispersion develop pigmentary glaucoma while others do not.

When iris pigment is infused into animal or enucleated human eyes, outflow facility decreases and IOP increases.[16,23] Repeated infusions of pigment, however, do not produce chronic glaucoma in animal eyes.[24] Some authorities believe that patients with pigmentary glaucoma must have an underlying developmental abnormality of the outflow channels. As evidence for this theory, they cite (1) the high prevalence of prominent iris processes in patients with pigmentary glaucoma,[5] (2) patients with pigmentary glaucoma who have angles that resemble infantile glaucoma, and (3) families who have some members with pigmentary glaucoma and other members with congenital glaucoma.

Other authorities propose that pigmentary glaucoma is a variant of POAG. These investigators point to families that have members with both pigmentary glaucoma and POAG.[5] However, patients with pigmentary glaucoma do not resemble those with POAG when corticosteroid testing is considered.[25]

Histopathologic examination of specimens from eyes with pigmentary glaucoma demonstrates pigment and debris in the trabecular meshwork cells.[26-28] With advanced disease the trabecular cells degenerate and wander from their beams, allowing sclerosis and eventual fusion of the trabecular meshwork.[26,28] Some propose that excessive phagocytosis of foreign material damages the trabecular endothelial cells and causes them to migrate.[29]

The treatment of pigmentary glaucoma resembles that of POAG in that the usual progression is from medical therapy to argon laser trabeculoplasty (ALT) to filtering surgery. β-Adrenergic antagonists, epinephrine, dipivefrin, and carbonic anhydrase inhibitors (CAIs) are useful in the management of pigmentary glaucoma. Miotic agents reduce IOP in pigmentary glaucoma and are theoretically appealing because they increase pupillary block and lift the peripheral iris from the zonules. However, cholinergic drugs are generally poorly tolerated by these young patients. Some reports also indicate that patients with pigmentary glaucoma have a high incidence of retinal detachment[6]; thus a careful peripheral retinal examination is mandatory before cholinergic agents can be prescribed. Thymoxamine, an α-adrenergic antagonist, might be useful in this situation because it constricts the pupil without inducing a myopic shift in refraction.[30]

The most intriguing therapy for pigmentary glaucoma is peripheral iridectomy to cure the "reverse" pupillary block that is responsible for the characteristic peripheral iris concavity.[31] Ultrasonic biomicroscopy is helpful in indicating those eyes that are most likely to benefit from iridectomy.[11] In eyes with deep peripheral concavity the effects of peripheral iridectomy are almost immediate. Within seconds of completing the iridectomy the peripheral iris moves forward and assumes a more normal configuration (Fig. 18-5). The long-term effects of peripheral iridectomy are

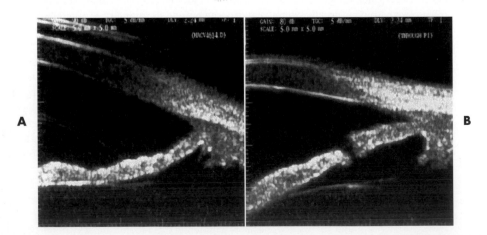

Figure 18-5 Ultrasonic biomicroscopy of the anterior segment showing the iris before (**A**) and after (**B**) peripheral iridectomy in the same patient as in Figure 18-1. The iris configuration changes from concave to slightly convex.

unclear. Ideally peripheral iridectomy would provide effective prophylaxis for patients with pigment dispersion syndrome before they develop glaucomatous visual field loss. Although it is impossible to determine exactly which patients with pigmentary dispersion syndrome will develop glaucoma,[22] it may be most appropriate to treat patients at the first sign of significant IOP elevation. Patients who show elevation following exercise may also be good candidates for peripheral iridectomy.[18] Pilocarpine and other miotics can reduce exercise-induced pressure rises, but parasympathetics routinely cause significant ocular side effects in the young adults most likely to have pigmentary glaucoma. Peripheral iridectomy has the same beneficial effects and is well tolerated by patients of all ages.

If medical management does not control IOP, ALT should be performed.[33] Because of the heavy pigmentation of the angle, ALT is done with relatively low-energy settings in the range of 200 to 600 mW.

Many individuals with pigmentary glaucoma eventually require filtering surgery. Despite the young age of these patients, the results of surgery are generally successful.

As mentioned previously, pigment dispersion may diminish with age. Some patients require less medical therapy and eventually discontinue therapy as they reach 60 or 70 years of age. This does not occur invariably, however, and some individuals with pigmentary glaucoma require lifelong treatment.

There have been several reports of pigment dispersion and secondary glaucoma from posterior chamber intraocular lenses (IOLs). This subject is discussed in the section on glaucoma after cataract surgery.

EXFOLIATION SYNDROME

Exfoliation syndrome occurs when several ocular tissues synthesize an abnormal protein. This protein may obstruct the trabecular meshwork and cause glaucoma. At one time most cases of exfoliation syndrome were diagnosed in Scandinavia. Although it is now clear that this condition occurs throughout the world, some areas seem to have a higher prevalence of the disease than do others.[34,35] It is difficult to compare the published prevalences of exfoliation syndrome because various studies used different techniques and definitions and did not match the patients for age. The prevalence of exfoliation syndrome is closely linked to age, reaching a maximum in the seventh to ninth decades of life.[36-38] The prevalence of exfoliation syndrome in the Framingham study was 0.6% in patients younger than 65 years of age, 2.6% in patients 65 to 74 years of age and 5.0% in patients 75 to 85 years of age.[39] Others have reported that exfoliation syndrome occurs in 3% to 28% of patients with open-angle glaucoma in the United States, with the best estimates in the range of 3% to 10%.[36-38,40] In contrast, in some areas of Scandinavia more than 50% of patients with open-angle glaucoma have evidence of exfoliation.

Exfoliation syndrome is more common in women than in men, but the combination of exfoliation syndrome and glaucoma occurs equally in both sexes.[41] Most cases appear to be sporadic rather than familial.[34] One third to one half of the cases of exfoliation syndrome are unilateral at detection, but 14% to 43% of these cases become bilateral over 5 to 10 years.[41,42] The prevalence of glaucoma in exfoliation syndrome is reportedly 0% to 93%.[41] However, many of these studies diagnosed glaucoma on the basis of elevated IOP or even abnormal provocative tests. Using strict definitions, recent studies detected glaucoma in 6% to 7% of patients with exfoliation syndrome and detected elevated IOP in an additional 15%.[41,43,44] In patients who had exfoliation syndrome and normal IOPs at diagnosis, glaucoma developed in 3% to 15% over 3 to 15 years.[35,41,42]

Exfoliation syndrome is not associated with any known systemic disorder. Exfoliation syndrome and its associated glaucoma are known by a variety of other names, including pseudoexfoliation, senile exfoliation, senile uveal exfoliation, glaucoma capsulare, and iridociliary exfoliation.[45]

The clinical presentation of exfoliation syndrome includes a classic pattern on the anterior lens surface consisting of a central translucent disc surrounded by a clear zone, which in turn is surrounded by a granular grey-white ring with scalloped edges (Fig. 18-6). This is best appreciated when the lens is examined with the slit lamp after pupillary dilation; if the pupil is not dilated, many cases can be missed because the characteristic ring may not be visible within a small pupil. The central and peripheral zones can be entirely separate or can be joined by bridges of material. It has been postulated that the movement of the central iris polishes the lens and produces the clear zone. In some cases the central disc is not present. The peripheral zone may have radial striations and

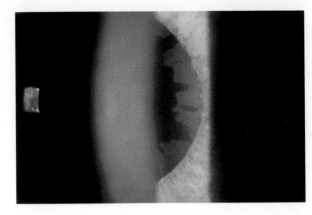

Figure 18-6   Exfoliation material on the lens. (From Alward WLM: *Color atlas of gonioscopy,* St Louis, 1994, Mosby.)

raised edges. Dandrufflike flakes of exfoliation material are deposited on the corneal endothelium, trabecular meshwork, anterior and posterior iris, pupillary margin, zonules, and ciliary processes as well as the anterior hyaloid face in aphakic eyes. The peripupillary iris has an irregular, moth-eaten pattern of transillumination. This is often the finding that alerts the examiner to the possibility of exfoliation syndrome. The pigment released from the iris is deposited in the trabecular meshwork, in the anterior iris, and to a lesser extent on the corneal endothelium. The angle pigmentation is moderate to heavy in amount and somewhat patchy in distribution. A wavy pigmented line (Sampaolesi's line) may be seen anterior to Schwalbe's line. When the pupil is dilated, a shower of pigment may be released. Fluorescein angiography of the iris reveals a decreased number of vessels, neovascularization, and leakage from the vessels.[46,47]

The treatment of glaucoma associated with exfoliation syndrome is similar to that of POAG. IOP is usually higher in exfoliation syndrome, however, and the response to medical treatment is less favorable.[48] ALT has its greatest pressure-lowering effect in exfoliation syndrome.[49,50] Somewhat paradoxically, however, the ultimate success rate of ALT in patients with exfoliation syndrome may be lower than that in other conditions because the initial pressures are higher and because adjunctive medical therapy is less effective. Further, in many successfully treated eyes the IOP rises again in 12 to 36 months. Filtering surgery has a high rate of success in this condition.[44] It has been reported that eyes with exfoliation syndrome have fragile zonules and a greater incidence of vitreous loss during cataract surgery.[51-53]

On microscopy the exfoliation material appears as a fibrillar protein arranged in an irregular meshwork.[54,55] Evidence of exfoliation syndrome is widely distributed in the ocular tissues and may affect the rigidity of the lamina cribrosa.[56] This material has been compared to zonules, basement membrane,[57-59] microtubular constituents,[60,61] and amyloid.[54,62] At one time many thought that all of the exfoliation material came from the lens capsule and epithelium. However, the material has a multifocal origin and has been found in the iris, ciliary epithelium, and conjunctiva as well as in ocular and orbital blood vessels.[58,62-66]

Exfoliation syndrome with glaucoma appears to be a secondary glaucoma in which exfoliation material and pigment obstruct the trabecular meshwork.[27,67-69] A few authorities have postulated an underlying defect of the outflow channels and supported this theory by finding a few patients with unilateral exfoliation and bilateral glaucoma.[36-38, 68] However, many patients with apparent unilateral disease have bilateral exfoliation that can be demonstrated by conjunctival biopsy.[70] In addition, most patients with unilateral exfoliation syndrome have more abnormal aqueous humor dynamics in the affected eye.[71] Finally, patients with exfoliation syndrome and glaucoma resemble the normal population rather than patients with POAG in their corticosteroid responsiveness. One investigator has postulated a developmental defect in eyes with exfoliation syndrome and glaucoma,[72] but this has not been confirmed.

CORTICOSTEROID GLAUCOMA

Corticosteroid administration can produce a clinical picture that closely resembles that of POAG, with elevated IOP, decreased outflow facility, open angles, and eventually optic nerve cupping and visual field loss. Classic studies by Armaly[73,74] and Becker[75] indicate that 5% to 6% of normal people develop marked IOP rises after 4 to 6 weeks of topical dexamethasone or betamethasone administration. However, an even higher percentage of normal individuals develop substantially increased IOPs if the glucocorticoid is administered in greater frequency or for a longer period. Certain groups in the population are particularly susceptible to the pressure-raising effects of glucocorticoids. These groups include patients with POAG,[73,76] their first-degree relatives,[75,77,78] diabetic patients,[79] and highly myopic individuals.

Most cases of corticosteroid glaucoma are caused by drops or ointments instilled in the eye for therapeutic purposes. However, glucocorticoid creams, lotions, and ointments applied to the face or eyelids may reach the eye in sufficient quantity to raise IOP,[80,81] as may systemically administered corticosteroids.[82-84] This latter category includes glucocorticoids used topically on the skin that may be absorbed and produce systemic and ocular effects. In addition, periocular corticosteroid injections, especially those involving repository or "depot" preparations, are capable of raising IOP.[85-87] There have been several case reports of increased IOP following use of a corticosteroid inhaler for asthma,[88,89] and we have seen at least two cases in which intractable IOP elevation followed the use of a corticosteroid nasal spray for allergic rhinitis. In rare cases glaucoma is produced by endogenous glucocorticoids associated with adrenal hyperplasia or adenoma.[90,91]

The rise in IOP from corticosteroids may occur within a week of initiating treatment or may be delayed for years. Patients undergoing long-term glucocorticoid treatment must be examined periodically because no time limit exists for this problem. Tragically, many cases of corticosteroid glaucoma are produced by treatment for trivial conditions such as contact lens discomfort or red eyes. In part because of their widespread availability and general effectiveness, combination steroid–antibiotic eyedrops are prescribed routinely by the general medical community for red eyes. In many such cases the IOP is neither measured nor followed. The overwhelming majority of patients tolerate a short course of these medications quite well, but a small percentage are unusually susceptible to steroid-induced pressure elevation or are allowed to refill the drops for an extended period of time. These patients are at significant risk of developing a dangerous elevation of IOP.

As stated, corticosteroid glaucoma usually resembles POAG. However, the clinical picture may be altered by the age of the patient. Infants treated with corticosteroids may develop a condition that resembles congenital glaucoma.[92-94] In contrast, elderly patients who received corticosteroid treatment in the past may have normal-tension glaucoma. The clinical picture of corticosteroid glaucoma may also be confounded by the presence of other ocular diseases. For example, a patient with shallow anterior chambers and corticosteroid glaucoma may appear to have chronic angle-closure glaucoma.

Glucocorticoids raise IOP by lowering outflow facility through an unknown mechanism.[73] The most common explanation for this phenomenon has been that glucocorticoids cause an accumulation of glycosaminoglycans in the trabecular meshwork,[95] perhaps by stabilizing lysosomal membranes and inhibiting the release of catabolic enzymes. Cultured human trabecular cells secrete a wide variety of substances that contribute to the extracellular matrix. Treating cultured trabecular cells with steroid induces the secretion of elastin, which may have a role in trabecular obstruction *in vivo*.[96] Other explanations for corticosteroid glaucoma include an inhibition of the phagocytosis of foreign matter by trabecular endothelial cells[97] and decreased synthesis of prostaglandins that regulate aqueous humor outflow.[98] Southren and co-workers[99,100] and Weinstein and co-workers[101] found abnormal glucocorticoid metabolism in trabecular tissue from patients with POAG. This finding may explain the increased susceptibility of patients with POAG to the ocular hypertensive effects of glucocorticoids. Alternatively, if steroids cause changes that would tend to result in a reduced outflow facility in most or all human eyes, those individuals with marginal or compromised outflow facility to begin with would be expected to show the greatest rise in IOP.

The first step in managing corticosteroid glaucoma is to discontinue the drug. In most cases IOP returns to normal over a few days to several weeks. During this period, antiglaucoma medications may be used to control IOP. If medication is unsuccessful in controlling IOP and the optic nerve is threatened, filtering surgery should be considered. Caution should be exercised, however, before performing an irreversible procedure in what is usually a time-limited condition. It may be most appropriate to confirm progression in glaucomatous damage before operating.

If glucocorticoid treatment is necessary for the patient's life or well-being, therapy should be altered to the weakest possible drug at the lowest possible dose. The residual glaucoma is then treated in the same fashion as is POAG. In the cases that require topical ocular corticosteroid therapy, the patient should be treated if possible with drugs such as medrysone or fluorometholone because these drugs have less of a tendency to raise IOP.

In rare cases IOP remains elevated months to years after the corticosteroid has been discontinued.[102] In these situations it may be impossible to determine whether this is a residual effect of glucocorticoid treatment or whether the patient has had underlying open-angle glaucoma unmasked by the treatment. In either case the patient is treated in similar fashion. If IOP is elevated because of a periocular glucocorticoid injection and medical therapy is unsuccessful in controlling the pressure and protecting the optic nerve, the repository material should be excised.[85]

LENS-INDUCED GLAUCOMA

There are a variety of lens-induced glaucomas. In the past great controversy surrounded the pathogenesis and nomenclature of these disorders. This chapter uses the following classification system:[103]

1. *Phacomorphic glaucoma:* A swollen lens causes increased pupillary block and secondary angle closure.
2. *Dislocated lens:* A dislocated lens causes increased pupillary block and secondary angle closure.
3. *Phacolytic glaucoma:* Lens protein leaks from an intact cataract and obstructs the trabecular meshwork.
4. *Lens-particle glaucoma:* Lens material liberated by trauma or surgery obstructs the outflow channels.
5. *Phacoanaphylaxis:* Sensitization to lens protein produces granulomatous inflammation and occasionally secondary glaucoma.

Phacomorphic glaucoma and dislocated lens are discussed in Chapter 15. The remainder of this section is devoted to the other three conditions.

Phacolytic Glaucoma

Lens protein is normally sequestered within the lens capsule. With age and the development of cataract, the protein composition of the lens is altered to components with heavier molecular weight.[104] If these soluble molecules leak through what grossly appears to be an intact capsule, they can obstruct the trabecular meshwork.[105,106] The lens protein also stimulates inflammation and a macrophage response. The macrophages engulf the lens protein and may further obstruct the outflow channels[107] (Fig. 18-7). Protein of heavy molecular weight is not seen in infants and children, possibly explaining the absence of phacolytic glaucoma in young patients with cataract.

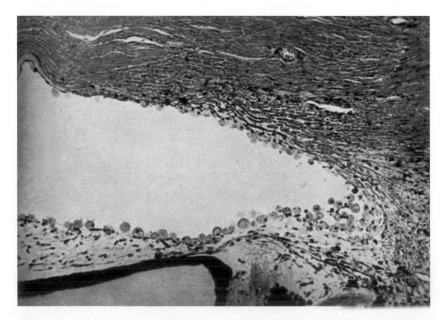

Figure 18-7   Phacolytic glaucoma with bloated macrophages and lens material obstructing the trabecular meshwork.

Phacolytic glaucoma is usually seen in older patients, who usually have a history of poor vision in the eye for months or years. The patients we have seen with this condition have often been from areas with little access to health care such as inner cities or developing nations. The disease typically appears with an acute onset of monocular pain, redness, and perhaps a further decrease in vision. Examination reveals a severe IOP elevation, corneal edema, ciliary injection, open angles, and heavy cell and flare. The cells appear larger than white blood cells and somewhat iridescent. The cells may precipitate on the corneal endothelium, but no true keratic precipitates or hypopyon is seen. Ultrastructural analysis of aqueous humor and trabeculectomy specimens in phacolytic glaucoma have revealed melanin-laden macrophages, red blood cells (RBCs), ghost RBCs, macrophages showing erythrophagocytosis, and free cell debris in addition to the lens material–laden macrophages that are traditionally associated with this condition.[108] The flare may be so heavy that the aqueous humor appears yellow. An important physical finding is the appearance of white particles on the anterior lens surface and in the aqueous; these particles are thought to be cellular aggregates or clumps of insoluble lens protein. Visual acuity is reduced in this condition, sometimes to the level of inaccurate light perception. The lens has a mature, hypermature, or even morgagnian cataract[109] (Fig. 18-8). Rarely this disease is produced by an immature cataract with a zone of liquefied cortex.

On rare occasions phacolytic glaucoma has a subacute course, with intermittent leakage of protein producing recurrent episodes of glaucoma, hyperemia, and inflammation. This appearance is more likely if the cataract has been dislocated into the vitreous. The diagnosis of phacolytic glaucoma is usually made on clinical grounds. If the diagnosis is in doubt, an anterior chamber paracentesis should be performed to detect macrophages engorged with lens material. Aqueous humor is examined by phase-contrast microscopy or Millipore filtration and staining.

Cataract extraction is the definitive treatment for phacolytic glaucoma.[110] Before surgery IOP and inflammation should be reduced by medical treatment, including hyperosmotic agents, topical adrenergic agents, CAIs, cycloplegic drugs, and topical corticosteroids. Traditionally most surgeons have removed these cataracts by an intracapsular technique. Microscopic examination of the lens reveals characteristic calcium oxalate crystals (Figs. 18-9 and 18-10). Because the lens capsule is quite fragile, a sector iridectomy and α-chymotrypsin are employed. If the capsule ruptures during delivery, the anterior chamber should be irrigated copiously to remove any residual protein. Other surgeons have used extracapsular cataract extraction in patients with this condition with good results.[111-113] Because of the friability of the zonules and the brittleness of the capsule, the anterior capsulorrhexis may be performed by Vannas scissors or some other means that minimizes zonular and capsular stress. Lens delivery and residual cortical aspiration are also performed in an unusually delicate manner. In successful cases posterior chamber IOL placement is possible and yields excellent results. As the last generation of surgeons trained in intracapsular surgery ages, the extracapsular technique will most likely replace the intracapsular approach. Regardless of approach, most patients have good visual acuity postoperatively and total remission of the glaucoma.

If phacolytic glaucoma is caused by a dislocated lens, the lens should be removed by vitrec-

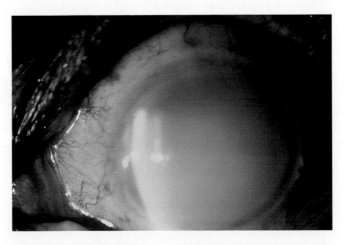

Figure 18-8 Hypermature cataract.

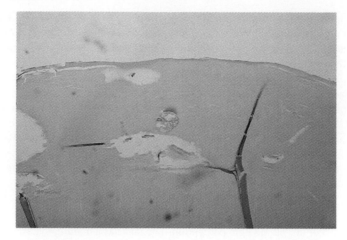

Figure 18-9 Calcium oxalate crystal in the lens of a patient with glaucoma associated with hypermature cataract. (Hematoxylin and eosin stain)

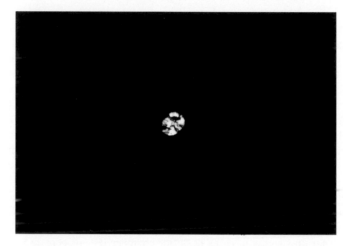

Figure 18-10 In the same lens as Figure 18-9, the calcium oxalate crystal is birefringent when viewed through polarized light.

tomy instruments. Occasionally a dislocated lens can be floated into the anterior chamber with a stream of irrigation fluid and then removed through a limbal incision.

In the rare situation when phacolytic glaucoma is caused by an immature cataract and the eye has good vision, attempts should be made to control IOP and inflammation by medical means. If this fails, the lens should be removed.

Lens-Particle Glaucoma

Disruption of the lens capsule by penetrating trauma or surgery liberates lens material, which can obstruct the trabecular meshwork. The resulting glaucoma depends on the amount of lens material liberated, the inflammatory response of the eye, and the ability of the trabecular meshwork to clear the foreign matter.[105,106] Generally the glaucoma has its onset a few days after the precipitating event. In rare cases the lens material can be released long after surgery or trauma.

Patients with lens-particle glaucoma usually have significant pain, redness, and decreased vision. Examination reveals corneal edema, elevated IOP, open angles, heavy cell and flare, and chunky white particles in the aqueous humor. An hypopyon may be present, as may fluffy cortical material. If the condition has existed for some time, peripheral anterior synechiae and posterior synechiae may be present.

Generally the diagnosis of lens-particle glaucoma is suggested by the sequence of events. It is more difficult to diagnose delayed cases or cases with spontaneous rupture of the lens capsule, which may be confused with phacolytic glaucoma, phacoanaphylactic glaucoma, or other conditions. Anterior chamber paracentesis in this condition reveals macrophages and free lens material.[103]

The elevated IOP and inflammation associated with lens-particle glaucoma are treated medically in the same fashion as phacolytic glaucoma. If this is not adequate, the residual lens material should be removed. Although fluffy cortical material can be aspirated easily, it is more difficult to remove solid lens material trapped in membranes behind the iris. Sometimes the entire lens mass can be teased from the eye after intracameral infusion of α-chymotrypsin. Lens particles in the vitreous can be removed with vitrectomy instruments. Surgery should not be delayed unduly in this disease or complications may occur, including posterior synechiae, peripheral anterior synechiae, cystoid macular edema, retinal detachment, and corneal decompensation.

Phacoanaphylaxis

Phacoanaphylaxis is an uncommon condition that is thought to occur when patients become sensitized to their own lens protein. Phacoanaphylaxis typically develops after penetrating trauma or extracapsular cataract extraction.[114,115] Histopathologically these eyes have a granulomatous inflammation of the lens with polymorphonuclear leukocytes, lymphocytes, epithelioid cells, and giant cells. Occasionally the inflammation involves the trabecular meshwork and leads to a rise in IOP.

Phacoanaphylaxis is treated with medication to reduce inflammation and control IOP. If this is unsuccessful, residual lens material should be removed.

GLAUCOMA AFTER CATARACT SURGERY

Elevated IOP often occurs after cataract surgery through a variety of mechanisms (Box 18-1). Many of these clinical problems are presented elsewhere, so the discussion here is restricted to the entities that are peculiar to cataract surgery.

A transient rise in IOP has been reported in 33% to almost 100% of eyes after cataract extraction, depending on the method of extraction and the surgeon involved.[115a] This pressure rise may be undetected because it occurs several hours after surgery, and the pressure may return to near-normal levels by the next morning or whenever the patient is seen for the first postoperative visit. The ocular hypertension may be sufficient to cause pain, nausea and vomiting, corneal edema, and optic nerve damage, especially in patients with preexisting glaucoma. The elevated IOP usually abates spontaneously over 2 to 4 days. During this period the patients are treated with topical and systemic antiglaucoma medications, including hyperosmotic agents as needed to control IOP. The mechanism of the IOP rise appears to be complex and includes the following:

1. Inflammation with the release of active substances, including prostaglandins and the formation of secondary aqueous humor
2. A watertight wound closure with multiple fine sutures limiting the "safety valve" leak of aqueous humor
3. Deformation of the limbal area, reducing trabecular outflow. On gonioscopy, Kirsch and co-workers[116] noted a white ridge internal to limbal cataract wounds. This ridge, attributed to tight sutures[117] and to operative edema and swelling, is associated with reduced trabecular function.
4. Obstruction of the trabecular meshwork by pigment, blood, lens particles, inflammatory cells, and viscoelastic substances

α-Chymotrypsin Glaucoma

α-Chymotrypsin fragments zonules and has been used widely to facilitate intracapsular cataract extraction. However, elevated IOP often occurs within 1 to 5 days after using this drug.[118-120] When examined, these eyes have open angles, decreased outflow facility,[118] and increased IOP, which can be sufficient to cause corneal edema, wound disruption, and optic nerve damage. This entity is self-limited, lasting for 2 to 4 days and leaving no permanent abnormalities of aqueous humor dynamics.[121]

The generally accepted mechanism for α-chymotrypsin glaucoma is that zonular fragments obstruct the outflow channels. This theory is supported by scanning electron microscopy, which shows

---

Box 18-1
Glaucoma in Aphakic and Pseudophakic Eyes

I. Open-angle glaucoma
  A. Early onset (within first postoperative week)
    1. Preexisting chronic open-angle glaucoma
    2. α-Chymotrypsin-induced glaucoma
    3. Hyphema/debris
    4. Viscoelastic material
    5. Idiopathic pressure elevation
  B. Intermediate onset (after first postoperative week)
    1. Preexisting chronic open-angle glaucoma
    2. Vitreous in the anterior chamber
    3. Hyphema
    4. Inflammation
    5. Lens particle glaucoma
    6. Corticosteroid-induced glaucoma
    7. Ghost cell glaucoma
  C. Late onset (more than 2 months postoperatively)
    1. Preexisting chronic open-angle glaucoma
    2. Ghost cell glaucoma
    3. Neodymium:yttrium-aluminum-garnet (Nd:YAG) laser capsulotomy
    4. Vitreous in the anterior chamber
    5. Late-occurring hemorrhage
    6. Chronic inflammation
II. Angle-closure glaucoma
  A. With pupillary block
    1. Anterior hyaloid face
    2. Posterior lens capsule
    3. Intraocular lens
    4. Posterior synechiae
    5. Silicone oil
  B. Aqueous misdirection (malignant glaucoma)
  C. Without pupillary block
    1. Preexisting angle-closure glaucoma
    2. Inflammation/hyphema
    3. Prolonged anterior chamber shallowing
    4. Iris incarceration in cataract incision
    5. Intraocular lens haptics
    6. Neovascular glaucoma
    7. Epithelial ingrowth
    8. Fibrous ingrowth
    9. Endothelial proliferation
    10. Proliferation of iris melanocytes across the trabecular meshwork

Modified from Tomey KF, Traverso CE: *Glaucoma associated with aphakia and pseudophakia.* In Ritch R, Shields MB, Krupin T: *The glaucomas,* ed 2, St Louis, 1996, Mosby.

---

zonular fragments in the trabecular meshwork, and by experimental studies in monkeys[122-124] (Fig. 18-11). A few investigators have proposed alternative mechanisms for the glaucoma, including inflammation or a direct toxic effect on the meshwork, but direct infusion of α-chymotrypsin into the anterior chamber of monkeys actually produced an increase in outflow facility.[125] During the period of elevated IOP, patients are treated with topical and systemic glaucoma medications as needed. Patients with preexisting optic nerve damage must be watched very closely because the pressure may rise to extremely high levels. The incidence and severity of the pressure rise can be reduced by using a lesser concentration of the drug (1:10,000 instead of 1:5000) in a lower volume (0.25 to 0.5 ml instead of 2 ml).[119,126] The anterior chamber should be irrigated before lens extraction to remove

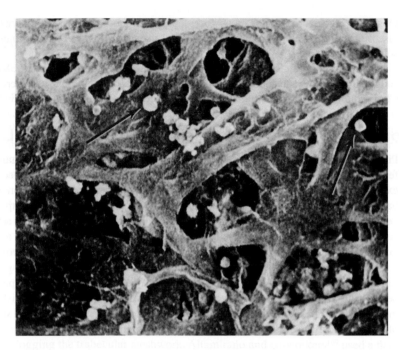

Figure 18-11 Scanning electron micrograph of the zonular fragments obstructing the trabecular meshwork after α-chymotrypsin administration. (Courtesy of Douglas Anderson, Miami.)

zonular fragments. Prophylactic treatment with a variety of agents has generally failed to block this IOP rise,[118] although one group found prophylactic timolol and acetazolamide useful in this situation. α-Chymotrypsin–associated IOP elevation is seen rarely today because intracapsular cataract extraction is performed infrequently.

Glaucoma From Viscoelastic Substances

Viscoelastic substances often are employed in cataract surgery to protect the corneal endothelium and to facilitate IOL insertion. Sodium hyaluronate, the agent with the widest clinical use, frequently causes marked postoperative IOP elevations.[127-131] When examined, these eyes demonstrate elevated IOP, deep anterior chambers, and corneal edema. Cellular and particulate matter in the aqueous humor may appear suspended and almost immobile if large amounts of viscoelastic remain in the anterior chamber, but IOP elevations may occur even in the absence of clinically detectable viscoelastic. It is sometimes possible to see tiny rubylike globs of hemorrhage on the iris surface or suspended in the anterior chamber. These isolated blood droplets indicate the presence of retained viscoelastic. The IOP reaches a maximum in 12 to 16 hours and then abates spontaneously over the next 72 hours. During this period patients are treated with topical and systemic glaucoma medications and hyperosmotic agents as needed to control IOP. The postoperative IOP rise can apparently be limited by removing as much of the sodium hyaluronate as possible at the end of the surgery,[129] although some studies have failed to show a significant difference in IOP between eyes that have had the viscoelastic removed and those in which it was left in place at the end of surgery.[132,133] Because it is difficult to standardize all of the variables that can affect the pressure rise in a given patient, it has been difficult to determine the effectiveness of various prophylactic treatment regimens on preventing the postoperative IOP rise seen after viscoelastic use. Some of these variables include the viscoelastic agent used, the surgeon, the surgical technique, the completeness of viscoelastic removal at the end of the procedure, and the rate at which the patient's eye clears itself of retained viscoelastic.

It is postulated that viscoelastic substances obstruct the trabecular meshwork. This theory is supported by experiments showing that sodium hyaluronate causes elevated IOP in animal eyes[134] and reduces outflow facility in enucleated human eyes.[135] The latter is reversed by intracameral infusion of hyaluronidase. Hyaluronidase is normally present in the anterior segment of the eye but not in sufficient quantity to metabolize the large volume of sodium hyaluronate infused at surgery.

GLAUCOMA AFTER TRAUMA

Chemical Burns

Chemical burns are often associated with a complex pattern of IOP alterations that include an immediate IOP rise followed by a period of hypotony, which in turn is followed by an elevation in the intermediate or late phases of the disease process. Glaucoma is more common after alkali burns but can also be seen after severe acid burns.[175] The diagnosis of glaucoma is often difficult in patients with chemical injuries because opacities of the media may interfere with optic nerve and visual field assessment. Also, external swelling, scarring, and corneal irregularity may interfere with standard methods of tonometry. IOP measurements may be more accurate with the pneumatic or MacKay-Marg tonometers than with the Goldmann applanation tonometer.[176]

IOP elevations in the early phase of disease are caused by scleral shrinkage and release of active substances, including prostaglandins.[177,178] This situation is managed by topical and systemic medications, including β-adrenergic antagonists, α-adrenergic agonists, CAIs, and hyperosmotic agents as needed.

Elevated IOP in the intermediate phase is usually caused by inflammation.[179] These eyes are treated with aqueous suppressants, hyperosmotic agents, and cycloplegic drugs. Topical and systemic corticosteroids are also used, but the patients must be monitored closely to avoid corneal melting. At times sufficient posterior synechiae form to produce pupillary block, which requires vigorous pupillary dilation and/or iridectomy. Acute lens swelling can also produce pupillary block.[179]

Late elevations of IOP are usually caused by trabecular damage and formation of peripheral anterior synechiae or other intraocular scarring.[180] This situation is usually managed by standard medical therapy. Filtering surgery may be required but can be technically difficult if there is extensive scarring of the conjunctiva and episcleral tissues. If extensive scarring is present, a cyclodestructive procedure or a seton procedure such as an Ahmed or Molteno valve should be considered.[181-185]

Electric Shock

Transient IOP elevations have been reported after electric injury, cardioversion, and electroshock therapy. Various investigators have attributed the pressure rise to venous dilation, contraction of the extraocular muscles, and pigment dispersion.[186-188] Because the IOP elevation is usually transient, no therapy is administered.

Radiation

Radiation can cause elevated IOP through a variety of mechanisms, including neovascularization, open-angle glaucoma associated with diffuse conjunctival telangiectasia, and ghost-cell glaucoma associated with radiation retinopathy and vitreous hemorrhage.[189] In many cases the widespread ocular disease and radiation damage indicate a poor prognosis.

Penetrating Injuries

Penetrating injuries can produce elevated IOP through various mechanisms, including flat anterior chamber with formation of peripheral anterior synechiae; inflammation, including sympathetic ophthalmia; intraocular hemorrhage, including hyphema and ghost-cell glaucoma; lens swelling with pupillary block; lens subluxation with pupillary block; lens-particle glaucoma; phacoanaphylaxis; posterior synechiae with pupillary block; epithelial downgrowth; and fibrous ingrowth. When penetrating trauma includes retained organic material, severe inflammation and secondary glaucoma often follow. When blunt and penetrating trauma are combined, angle recession or other forms of direct trabecular damage may produce elevated IOP.

Retained metallic foreign bodies can produce open-angle glaucoma months to years after the injury. It is postulated that iron released from the foreign body is toxic to several ocular tissues, including the retina and the trabecular meshwork. This condition, known as *siderosis,* is similar to hemosiderosis, which results from the release of iron from blood. When examined, eyes with siderosis demonstrate heterochromia, mydriasis, elevated IOP, decreased outflow facility, and a diminished electroretinogram.[190] The deep cornea, trabecular meshwork, and anterior subcapsular region of the lens all have a rust-brown color. In some eyes a previous corneal scar and an iris transillumination defect indicate the path of injury.

Prevention is the key to treating ocular siderosis. Traumatized eyes must be examined carefully with indirect ophthalmoscopy, gonioscopy, ultrasound, radiography, and computed tomography (CT) studies to detect metallic foreign bodies. Whenever possible, the foreign bodies should be removed to prevent this occurrence. Once glaucoma is present, the foreign body may be so encapsulated that standard extraction techniques may not be possible.[191] Furthermore, at this stage the prognosis may be limited by extensive retinal damage. Standard medical and surgical means are used to treat the glaucoma. Glaucoma and retinal changes are also seen in chalcosis, which is caused by copper-containing foreign bodies.

Contusion Injuries

Contusion injuries occur most frequently in young men[192,193] and can cause hyphema, iridocyclitis, iris sphincter tears, iridodialysis, cyclodialysis, lens subluxation, retinal tear or dialysis, retinal detachment, vitreous hemorrhage, choroidal rupture, and glaucoma. Postcontusion glaucoma can occur immediately after the injury or be delayed for months to years.[194] Uveal effusion and angle closure can occur rarely after blunt trauma.[195]

The pressure rise that occurs immediately after nonpenetrating trauma can be severe but is usually limited in duration to days or weeks. During this period patients are treated with topical β-adrenergic antagonists, CAIs, and hyperosmotic agents as needed to control IOP. The cause of the early pressure elevation is often complex and includes trauma to the trabecular meshwork as well as obstruction of the outflow channels by RBCs, leukocytes, pigment, and inflammatory debris. Tears in the trabecular meshwork typically occur after contusions but often are not recognized because gonioscopy is not performed routinely (Fig. 18-13). The tears have the appearance of a hinged flap, with the cut edge posterior to Schwalbe's line. The tear in the meshwork heals within several weeks to months, leaving an area of scarring that is sometimes combined with peripheral anterior synechiae.

In some cases IOP is low after trauma and then becomes elevated weeks to months later. The likely explanation for this phenomenon is that both outflow facility and aqueous production are reduced immediately after trauma, and then aqueous production recovers first. An alternative explanation is the closing of a tear in the trabecular meshwork or a traumatic cyclodialysis cleft. The

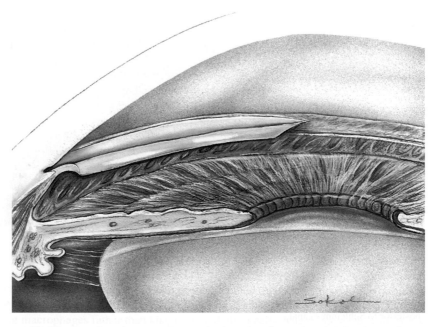

Figure 18-13 Drawing of an acute flap tear in the trabecular meshwork following ocular trauma.

molytic glaucoma shows the trabecular meshwork to be occluded by RBCs, debris, and macrophages laden with pigment.[218] Hemolytic glaucoma is usually a self-limited condition that responds to management with topical and systemic pressure-lowering medications. If IOP is not controlled, an anterior chamber washout should be performed. If this is not successful a filtration or cyclodestructive procedure may be indicated.

Hemosiderosis

Hemosiderotic glaucoma is a rare entity associated with intraocular hemorrhage. Hemosiderosis is similar to siderosis, except that the source of iron in hemosiderosis is degenerating RBCs rather than a retained foreign body. Hemoglobin released by degenerated RBCs is phagocytized by trabecular endothelial cells. The iron liberated from the hemoglobin causes siderosis and discoloration of the meshwork.[174,219]

Hyphema

Blunt trauma to the globe can produce a tear in the ciliary face and bleeding into the anterior chamber. Traumatic hyphemas can occur in patients of any age or either gender but are typically seen in young men.[220,221] Patients with hyphemas complain of redness and blurred vision, if IOP is elevated, patients may also complain of pain, nausea, and vomiting. The history of the injury reveals trauma that seems severe in some cases and trivial in others. In all cases, however, the object causing the trauma must have been small enough or sufficiently deferrable to fit inside the rim of the orbit in order to strike the globe.

When examined, patients with hyphemas demonstrate diminished vision, conjunctival injection, RBCs floating in the aqueous humor, a variable amount of blood settled to the bottom of the anterior chamber, and normal or low IOPs. Children with traumatic hyphemas often appear somnolent. In most patients the blood clears spontaneously in a few days with no immediate complications. A few weeks after the injury these patients should have a careful dilated examination to search for retinal tears, retinal dialyses, and choroidal ruptures. They should also undergo gonioscopy to determine whether angle recession is present.

Unfortunately some patients with traumatic hyphemas have recurrent episodes of hemorrhage into the anterior chamber, or rebleeds. Most episodes of rebleeding occur within a few days of the trauma. It is postulated that additional bleeding occurs when the blood clot closing the vessel torn in the original injury undergoes lysis and retraction.[222] Reports indicate that rebleeding after traumatic hyphema occurs in 4% to 35% of patients.[222-232] There is reasonable evidence linking aspirin use to rebleeding.[224,233,234] Some authorities also believe that rebleeding is more common in blacks and in individuals with larger hyphemas and hypotony.[227,230]

Rebleeding is important because it is often associated with complications, including corneal blood staining (Fig. 18-16), optic atrophy, and elevated IOP. In most cases elevated IOP is caused by RBCs obstructing the trabecular meshwork.[235] Less often the blood clot may produce pupillary block. Glaucoma is more frequent when the hyphema is total. A total hyphema changing color from red to black (*black-ball* or *eightball hyphema*) is an ominous sign of impending complications. The exact reason for this is obscure, but it is assumed that the underlying injury is more severe in many eyes with eightball hyphema compared with eyes with subtotal hyphema.

The management of traumatic hyphema has been controversial.[236] Typical practice in the past was to hospitalize all patients for bedrest, sedation, and bilateral patching. However, there is evidence that bedrest and patching are not necessary and that equally good results can be obtained by limiting activity.[225,229,237] If there is a stable family situation, some patients can be managed at home and checked daily in the physician's office. Despite widespread use, no evidence suggests that either cycloplegics or miotics facilitate the clearing of blood.[238,239] The antifibrinolytic agents epsilon–aminocaproic acid (Amicar) and tranexamic acid have been found to decrease the incidence of rebleeding.[222,223,228,240-244] The reported track record of tranexamic acid remains fairly good, although its use is not entirely without risk. The effectiveness of aminocaproic acid has been questioned by some investigators, who found no significant difference in rebleed rates between patients treated with aminocaproic acid and those treated with either corticosteroids or placebo.[245-248]

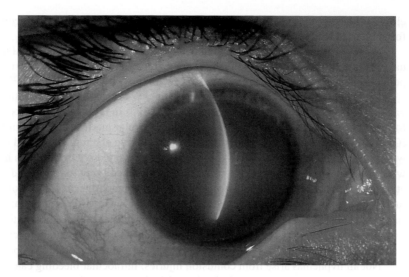

Figure 18-16   Blood staining of a cornea that is beginning to clear in the periphery.

This has been a difficult issue to study. The rebleed rate of the control groups in these studies ranges from less than 5% to over 25%. In several cases the patients in the study group were collected over periods of 10 years or more, and it is difficult to be certain that identical diagnostic criteria and treatment regimens were employed. For the most part the studies with high rates of rebleeding in the control group found the medications helpful.[249-251] Other studies with seemingly similar entry criteria and treatment plans had low rebleed rates in the control group and showed no benefit from aminocaproic acid.[247] Some authorities recommend that all patients with traumatic hyphemas be treated with an antifibrinolytic agent, assuming no contraindication.[224,229,244] Other authorities use these agents only after severe trauma or in patients with large initial hyphemas. The best available data support using these agents in circumstances in which the rebleed rate is likely to exceed about 10%. If this is the case in the experience of a particular hospital or practice it would also seem prudent to carefully review the entire treatment regimen as well as the circumstances and extent of the injury causing the hyphema and the support services available to the patient during convalescence.[252] A few reports indicate that systemic corticosteroids reduce the rate of rebleeding,[253] although this was not confirmed in other studies.[230,254] Again, patient demographics, the circumstances of injury, and other critical factors are difficult to compare. Elevated IOP associated with a traumatic hyphema is managed by topical and systemic glaucoma medications as needed. Topical corticosteroids are administered if the eye is significantly inflamed, independent of any potential positive effect on rebleeding rates.

Nonclearing total or subtotal hyphema is a serious condition. In addition to other damage to the eye caused by the event that produced the hyphema, the hyphema itself can cause corneal blood staining, persistent inflammation, and dramatically elevated IOP. Tissue plasminogen activator (t-PA) is a fibrin-specific fibrinolytic agent that has shown promise in experimental[255] and limited clinical use.[256,257] Current experience remains limited, at least partially because appropriate cases are rare. Early case reports have been favorable, however.

Surgical removal of blood from the anterior chamber is indicated for persistent pain, corneal blood staining, or IOP elevations threatening the optic nerve. It is difficult to know what IOP level will be tolerated by young healthy patients who have no preexisting optic nerve disease. One proposed guideline is that an IOP of 60 mm Hg for 2 days, 50 mm Hg for 5 days, or 35 mm Hg for 7 days requires intervention.[229] If possible, evacuation of blood should be delayed until the fourth day because at this time the clot is somewhat retracted and less adherent to the surrounding tissues. Removal of blood can be done as a washout through a peripheral corneal puncture using saline or a fibrinolytic agent such as urokinase,[192,258,259] fibrinolysin, or, when available, t-PA. Liquid blood is irrigated from the eye during this maneuver; it is neither necessary nor wise to remove the entire

GLAUCOMA WITH UVEITIS

Inflammation can produce glaucoma through a variety of mechanisms, including (1) increased viscosity of aqueous humor, (2) obstruction of the trabecular meshwork by inflammatory cells and debris, (3) swelling and dysfunction of the trabecular meshwork, (4) liberation of active substances such as prostaglandins, (5) scarring of the outflow channels, (6) development of a cuticular endothelial membrane over the angle, (7) neovascularization, (8) elevation of episcleral venous pressure, (9) forward displacement of the lens–iris diaphragm (uveal effusion), (10) pupillary block, and (11) formation of peripheral anterior synechiae. Elevated IOP can occur with any type of ocular inflammatory disease but is more common in the chronic forms than in the acute forms. In most ocular inflammatory diseases, aqueous humor formation is reduced and IOP is low.[293] If outflow facility is reduced as well, however, IOP can be elevated. Because of this dual involvement of aqueous humor inflow and outflow, eyes with active inflammatory disease often suffer wide swings of IOP, and glaucoma may be missed if only occasional pressure measurements are made. Additionally, these patients can be extremely sensitive to medications (e.g., acetazolamide) that decrease aqueous production. In sensitive patients the pressure can drop from over 50 mm Hg to under 5 mm Hg with a single dose. Careful individual titration is needed to arrive at the proper medication regimen.

The treatment of glaucoma associated with ocular inflammatory disease depends on the underlying condition, but in most situations inflammation is suppressed by some combination of topical, systemic, and periocular corticosteroids. During this treatment the ophthalmologist must be aware of the possibility of corticosteroid-induced IOP elevations. Steroid glaucoma is a particular problem in patients on long-term corticosteroid therapy for chronic or recurrent uveitis. A variety of other medications may be employed to reduce inflammation, including cycloplegic agents, nonsteroidal antiinflammatory drugs, and immunomodulators such as methotrexate, azathioprine, and chlorambucil. Elevated IOP is generally managed by topical and systemic glaucoma medications as needed. Miotics are usually avoided because they increase pain and congestion and may promote the development of posterior synechiae. Prostaglandins such as latanoprost are used with caution in uveitic patients because they could theoretically exacerbate signs and symptoms that might be confused with the underlying inflammatory condition.

ALT is not very helpful in eyes with active inflammation. ALT may cause a mild acute anterior uveitis in some patients and may also lead to peripheral anterior synechiae. For this and other reasons most surgeons avoid ALT in patients with uveitis. Surgery should be avoided in eyes with active inflammation, but if a filtering procedure is required inflammation should be suppressed as much as possible by topical and systemic corticosteroid treatment. Inhibitors of scarring such as mitomycin-C[294] or 5-fluorouracil (5-FU)[295] are often useful in this situation, as are seton devices such as the Ahmed[183] or Molteno valve.[294] Eyes with active inflammation sometimes require cyclodestructive procedures, although the risk of exacerbating inflammation makes this option worrisome.[296]

A wide variety of inflammatory diseases are associated with secondary open-angle glaucoma. This section discusses a few of the more common entities

Fuchs' Heterochromic Iridocyclitis

Fuchs' heterochromic iridocyclitis is a chronic but relatively mild form of anterior uveitis associated with cataract and glaucoma.[297-300] Approximately 90% of the cases are unilateral, and the disease has its onset in the third and fourth decades of life.[301] Men and women are affected in equal numbers. Patients are generally asymptomatic until they develop cataract or vitreous opacities. The physical findings in this syndrome include minimal cell and flare, fine round or stellate keratic precipitates, fine filaments on the endothelium between the keratic precipitates, a patchy loss of the iris pigment epithelium, hypochromia, grey-white nodules on the anterior iris, a few opacities in the anterior vitreous, and chorioretinal scars that resemble toxoplasmosis.[301-304] Gonioscopy reveals fine vessels that bridge the angle and can bleed with minimal trauma, such as paracentesis.[305] Fluorescein angiography of the iris demonstrates ischemia, leakage, neovascularization, and delayed filling of the vessels.[306,307]

Increased IOP has been reported in 13% to 59% of patients with Fuchs' heterochromic iridocyclitis.[304,308] One study, albeit with fairly small numbers, reported an increased glaucoma prevalence among black patients, with 38% (5 of 13) of blacks having glaucoma compared with only 11% (6 of 54) of whites.[309] The cause of the glaucoma is not clear, but the angle is open and no peripheral anterior synechiae are seen. It is postulated that the inflammation eventually produces scarring and dysfunction of the outflow channels. Histologic examination of a few surgical specimens has confirmed the inflammation and scarring of the trabecular meshwork and revealed an inflammatory membrane over the angle.[310,311]

Glaucoma may also be seen following cataract surgery, neovascularization, or overzealous treatment with corticosteroids. The inflammatory component of Fuchs' heterochromic iridocyclitis is generally unresponsive to corticosteroid treatment. Elevated IOP is treated with medical therapy, but the results are often disappointing, with only about a quarter of patients achieving satisfactory control.[312] In the past, the results of conventional filtration surgery were also poor, with less than half of patients achieving control.[304,313] Use of wound-healing retardants such as 5-FU and mitomycin-C has improved surgical outcomes considerably, with success rates as high as 72%.[312]

Glaucomatocyclitic Crisis

Glaucomatocyclitic crisis, also called the *Posner-Schlossman syndrome,* is usually seen in young to middle-aged adults and consists of recurrent episodes of mild anterior uveitis and marked elevations of IOP.[314-319] Generally this condition is unilateral, but both eyes can be affected at different times.[317] Patients have relatively few symptoms considering the height of their IOPs, but they may complain of slight discomfort, slight blurring of vision, or halo vision.

The physical findings during an episode of glaucomatocyclitic crisis include mild ciliary flush, a dilated or sluggishly reactive pupil, corneal epithelial edema, IOP in the range of 40 to 60 mm Hg, decreased outflow facility, open angles, faint flare, and 1 to 20 fine keratic precipitates. The keratic precipitates may not appear for 2 or 3 days after the IOP has risen, which may obscure the diagnosis. It is postulated that the elevated IOP is caused by inflammation of the trabecular meshwork, perhaps mediated by prostaglandins.[320] There is also evidence of an association between herpes simplex virus and glaucomatocyclitic crisis, but the significance of this association is unknown.[321] The crises last several hours to a few weeks. Some patients experience one or two episodes in their lives, whereas other patients experience recurrent crises for many years. As a rule, the frequency of recurrences diminishes with age.

For many years it was accepted that glaucomatocyclitic crisis never caused optic nerve cupping or visual field loss and that aqueous humor dynamics were normal between episodes. It is now clear, however, that some patients with glaucomatocyclitic crisis have abnormal aqueous humor dynamics between episodes and that some have underlying POAG.[317,319] Furthermore, some patients develop optic nerve cupping and visual field loss because of repeated crises or underlying POAG.[316,317,319]

Glaucomatocyclitic crisis is usually treated with topical corticosteroids and topical and systemic glaucoma medications. As with all types of uveitis, miotics are avoided. Apraclonidine 1% has been found to be particularly effective.[322] Some authorities recommend the administration of systemic or topical nonsteroidal antiinflammatory agents because of increased aqueous humor prostaglandin levels. Because the episodes are self-limited, moderate elevations of IOP should be well tolerated. An occasional patient requires filtering surgery because of progressive cupping and visual field loss. Successful filtering surgery prevents IOP elevations but does not prevent recurrent episodes of inflammation.

Precipitates on the Trabecular Meshwork

Inflammatory precipitates on the trabecular meshwork can cause a clinical picture that is easily mistaken for POAG. In this condition the eyes are white and quiet, and the only signs of inflammation are a few grey or slightly yellow precipitates on the trabecular meshwork associated with irregular peripheral anterior synechiae. Most of these patients have idiopathic disorders, although some later develop a recognizable inflammatory condition such as sarcoidosis, rheumatoid arthritis, or ankylosing spondylitis.[323] The precipitates and the elevated IOP are responsive to topical corticosteroid treatment. While waiting for this effect, aqueous humor suppressants may be useful to control IOP. This uncommon condition may be recurrent and asymptomatic, and these patients should be examined periodically to monitor IOP. Inflammatory precipitates have been reported as a cause of increased IOP following ALT.[324] As with idiopathic cases this condition responded to treatment with topical corticosteroids.

Herpes Simplex

Elevated IOP is common when herpes simplex causes iridocyclitis, disciform keratitis, or stromal ulcer.[325] The increased IOP is caused by inflammation, swelling, and obstruction of the trabecular meshwork. Herpetic keratouveitis is usually treated with antiviral agents, cycloplegics, and topical corticosteroids. The IOP is controlled with aqueous humor suppressants. Glaucoma may be quite severe in these cases and filtration surgery with wound-healing retardants such as 5-FU or mitomycin-C may be necessary to control pressure.[326] ALT has been implicated as a trigger for recurrent herpes simplex keratitis in at least one case and thus is not an attractive treatment option.[327] Cyclodestructive procedures have been attempted in many cases, but serious complications have occurred in several eyes and these procedures are best considered as a last resort.[328]

Herpes Zoster

When herpes zoster involves the ophthalmic division of the trigeminal nerve, especially the nasociliary branch, there is often associated keratitis, iridocyclitis, and secondary glaucoma. The anterior uveitis can be severe, and secondary open-angle glaucoma occurs in 11% to 25% of patients.[329] The inflammation is treated with acyclovir and cycloplegic agents; the IOP is controlled by aqueous humor suppressants.[330] Topical steroids are used routinely, although there are differences of opinion regarding the optimum timing and intensity of steroid treatment.[331,332] Surgery in actively inflamed eyes is challenging, although some authors have reported excellent results.[333] Mitomycin-C– and/or 5-FU–enhanced filtering operations are the procedures of choice.[334]

Sarcoidosis

Approximately 10% of patients with sarcoidosis develop elevated IOP.[335] This occurs through a variety of mechanisms, including swelling and dysfunction of the trabecular meshwork, obstruction of the trabecular meshwork by inflammatory cells and debris, peripheral anterior synechiae, posterior synechiae with pupillary block, and neovascular glaucoma.[323,336,337] These cases can be extremely difficult to manage because of the continual battle between therapy aimed at controlling the underlying pathology and that used to control the glaucoma.[338] Patients with ocular sarcoidosis frequently develop thick broad-based peripheral anterior synechiae that can lead to a scarred and dysfunctional anterior segment well after the inflammatory episode is over. Valve (e.g., Molteno, Ahmed) implantation with adjunctive 5-FU or mitomycin-C may be necessary to control severe cases. HLA typing suggests a molecular basis for some of the clinical heterogeneity seen in sarcoid patients.[339]

Juvenile Rheumatoid Arthritis

Severe acute and chronic eye disease is an unfortunate but common component of juvenile rheumatoid arthritis.[340-342] Elevated IOP can occur in any of the forms of juvenile rheumatoid arthritis but is most common in young girls with iridocyclitis and monoarticular or pauciarticular involvement.[343,344] Glaucoma can result from posterior synechiae and pupillary block or inflammation of the trabecular meshwork.[345-348] The response to medical treatment and filtering surgery is often disappointing in this condition. A few physicians have reported long-term IOP reductions in these children with a modified goniotomy procedure called *trabeculodialysis*[345,346,349] (see Chapter 39). Treating these patients is often complicated further by concomitant visually significant pathology as well as a host of psychosocial issues related to treating children with a painful chronic systemic disease.[350,351] Close ophthalmic follow-up and prompt treatment of ocular pathology are important in maintaining vision. Genetic typing may allow more precise and earlier diagnosis, which should facilitate early intervention in select cases.[352]

Syphilis

Glaucoma often occurs in individuals with congenital or acquired syphilis. Secondary open-angle glaucoma can occur in any of the active inflammatory phases of the disease, including acute interstitial keratitis. Iridoschisis occurs rarely but may be associated with glaucoma in 50% of cases.[353-355]

A late form of secondary open-angle glaucoma occurs in 15% to 20% of patients.[356] In these cases gonioscopy reveals occasional peripheral anterior synechiae and irregular pigmentation of the trabecular meshwork.[357,358] These patients respond poorly to medical treatment, and it is postulated that there may be an endothelial membrane covering the angle.[359,360] Filtering surgery with wound-healing retardants or drainage valve implantation is often required for this condition.

Syphilis is also associated with angle-closure glaucoma. Some patients with congenital syphilis have small anterior segments and develop acute or chronic angle closure in later years. Elevated IOP has also been reported in association with other inflammatory conditions, including ankylosing spondylitis, pars planitis,[289] Behçet's syndrome, sympathetic ophthalmia,[361] onchocerciasis,[362,363] leprosy,[364] and mumps.[365]

INTRAOCULAR TUMORS AND GLAUCOMA

A variety of ocular tumors can produce glaucoma through various mechanisms. Because the tumors producing glaucoma in children are presented in Chapter 20, the discussion here is limited to tumors in adults.

Malignant melanoma can be associated with normal, elevated, or depressed IOP. Elevated IOP is reported more frequently with melanomas of the anterior uveal tract than with choroidal melanomas.[366] Glaucoma can occur through several mechanisms, including the following: (1) Direct extension of the tumor into the trabecular meshwork (Fig. 18-17); (2) seeding of tumor cells into the outflow channels; (3) pigment dispersion; (4) inflammation; (5) hemorrhage, inducing hemolytic glaucoma, and suprachoroidal hemorrhage, leading to angle closure; (6) neovascularization of the angle; (7) angle closure from anterior displacement of the lens–iris diaphragm, peripheral anterior synechiae, or posterior synechiae; and (8) obstruction of the trabecular meshwork by macrophages containing melanin released by a necrotic tumor (melanomalytic glaucoma).

Most eyes with advanced melanomas are treated with enucleation or radiation.[367-373] In some cases local excisional surgery may be a viable option.[374,375] If the eye is retained, medical therapy is used to attempt to control IOP. Unfortunately many irradiated eyes develop neovascular glaucoma. In a 5-year study of helium ion irradiation, for example, Decker and co-workers[369] found that 43% of patients developed neovascularization. Neovascular glaucoma was often not responsive to treatment and was a prominent contributing factor in the subsequent decision to perform enucleation. Metastatic tumors to the eye may cause glaucoma, especially if the metastasis involves the anterior segment.[376-378] The mechanisms producing glaucoma are similar to those described for malignant melanoma. There is one report of a metastatic tumor invading Schlemm's canal and the collector channels.[379] Many metastatic tumors are treated with radiation and/or chemotherapy. Medical treatment for glaucoma is indicated to retain vision and reduce discomfort.

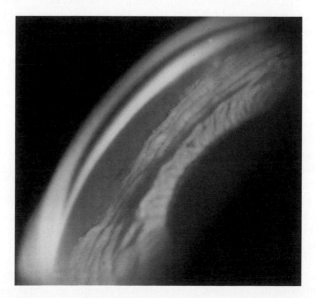

Figure 18-17 Choroidal melanoma invading the ciliary body and angle.

Intraocular lymphoma and leukemia can produce glaucoma by seeding the outflow channels or by producing angle closure.[378] Several benign ocular tumors can also produce glaucoma. Melanocytomas of the iris can invade the angle[380] or cause sufficient pigment dispersion to obstruct the trabecular meshwork.[378] Pigment dispersion and glaucoma are also reported with adenomas of the pigment epithelium,[284,381] melanosis oculi,[382] and nevus of Ota.[383-385] These conditions generally respond well to medical therapy or to ALT. Medulloepithelioma can displace the lens–iris diaphragm or produce neovascularization of the angle.[366]

AMYLOIDOSIS

The hereditary systemic amyloidoses are a group of diseases in which amyloid is deposited in tissues throughout the body, leading to cardiovascular, renal, endocrine, muscular, gastrointestinal, and neurologic deficits. The ocular findings include vitreous opacification, proptosis, lid abnormalities, extraocular muscle weakness, anisocoria, internal ophthalmoplegia, and retinal vasculitis.[386,387]

Secondary open-angle glaucoma develops in approximately 25% of the patients with the hereditary systemic amyloidoses. The glaucoma somewhat resembles pigmentary glaucoma because modest pigment exists in the trabecular meshwork and on the corneal endothelium. There is also a resemblance to the exfoliation syndrome because white flecks are seen on the iris near the pupil and on the anterior lens capsule.[388] Histologic examination of these eyes reveals heavy accumulation of amyloid in the trabecular meshwork.[387] Anatomic changes and amyloid deposition involve the ciliary body as well.[389] This accumulation most likely causes glaucoma by obstructing aqueous humor outflow.[390]

Another form of familial systemic amyloidosis and secondary open-angle glaucoma has been reported that includes lattice dystrophy of the cornea, cranial neuropathy, and no vitreous opacities.[391] These patients may require multiple penetrating keratoplasties over the years, and unresponsive glaucoma is a frequent sequela.[392] There is also a report of nonfamilial systemic amyloidosis associated with secondary open-angle glaucoma.[393]

The treatment of glaucoma in amyloidosis is similar to the treatment of POAG. It has been reported that filtering surgery is successful initially but that the blebs fail over several months to a few years because of the accumulation of amyloid material.[394]

ELEVATED EPISCLERAL VENOUS PRESSURE

Any condition that raises episcleral venous pressure also raises IOP by obstructing the posttrabecular flow of aqueous humor. In acute experiments, when a pressure cuff is placed around a patient's neck and episcleral venous pressure is raised 1 mm Hg, IOP increases approximately 0.8 mm Hg.[395,396] In a study of IOP and episcleral venous pressure in patients who were placed in a vertically inverted posture (i.e., upside down), Friberg and co-workers[397] found that when the episcleral venous pressure increased 0.83 ± 0.21 mm Hg the IOP rose 1 mm Hg. The difference between these pressure increases has been attributed to fluid being forced from the eye[398] or to *pseudofacility* (i.e., a pressure-related reduction in aqueous humor formation).[396] Recently, however, the concept of pseudofacility has been questioned. It is difficult to interpret acute experiments such as the one just described because IOP, outflow facility, and episcleral venous pressure never reach steady state. Furthermore, acute experimental increases of episcleral venous pressure do not mimic the clinical situation of chronically elevated episcleral venous pressure. For example, acute elevations of episcleral venous pressure increase the total outflow facility,[398] whereas chronic elevations often decrease outflow facility.[399] Thus no reliable method exists for predicting the change in IOP that will accompany a specific rise in episcleral venous pressure. The two pressure changes are often of similar magnitude, but the IOP may be less than or even greater than the rise in episcleral venous pressure.[400]

The physical signs of elevated episcleral venous pressure depend on the underlying disease or condition and include chemosis, proptosis, orbital bruit, and pulsating exophthalmos. Generally the episcleral veins are dilated, tortuous, and have a corkscrew appearance, although this can vary from mild to severe.[401] The retinal veins are usually not dilated because the rise in venous pressure is counterbalanced by a rise in IOP. The angles are open, and blood is often present in Schlemm's canal. The elevated IOP may produce typical glaucomatous optic nerve cupping and visual field loss. Outflow facility is normal in most cases of elevated episcleral venous pressure. In longstanding cases, however, secondary changes in the trabecular meshwork may reduce outflow facility.[399]

Elevated episcleral venous pressure can be confused with any condition that produces dilated extraocular vessels, including conjunctivitis, episcleritis, scleritis, and general orbital inflammation. Usually the venous pressure is normal in these inflammatory conditions. Furthermore, the most common of these entities, conjunctivitis, affects the superficial vessels and spares the deeper episcleral vessels. This distinction can be made by observing the vessels during slit-lamp examination while moving the conjunctiva with a moist swab. In addition, dilated superficial vessels constrict in response to topical agents such as phenylephrine 2.5%, whereas deeper vessels do not.

Many conditions can produce elevated episcleral venous pressure. These conditions are usually divided into three major categories: obstruction of venous drainage, arteriovenous fistulas, and idiopathic elevations (Box 18-3). The discussion here is restricted to the more common entities.

Superior Vena Cava Obstructions

Various conditions can obstruct the superior vena cava, including tumors, aortic aneurysms, mediastinal masses, hilar adenopathy, and intrathoracic goiter.[402-404] This obstruction produces edema and cyanosis of the face and neck (pumpkinhead appearance) as well as dilated vessels in the head, neck, chest, and upper extremities.[405] Obstruction of the superior vena cava increases intracranial pressure, which leads to headache, stupor, vertigo, seizures, and mental changes. The associated ocular findings include exophthalmos, papilledema, and prominent blood vessels in the conjunctiva, episclera, and retina. IOP is elevated, and the IOP increase is greater when the patient is in the supine position.[406] There is a clinical impression that glaucomatous cupping occurs infrequently with superior vena cava obstruction despite the elevated IOP. Some researchers propose that cupping does not occur because the IOP is counterbalanced by elevated intracranial pressure.[407] Therapy in this situation is directed toward relieving the obstruction.[408] During this period the IOP elevation is treated primarily with medications that decrease aqueous production, such as β-blockers and topical or systemic CAIs.

Thyroid Eye Disease

Thyroid eye disease is known by a variety of names, including endocrine exophthalmos, thyrotropic exophthalmos, and Graves' disease. The hormonal defect of this condition is unclear, and patients can be hypothyroid, euthyroid, or hyperthyroid when their eye problems begin.[409,410] The physical findings are variable and include exophthalmos, chemosis, lid retraction, lid lag, a staring or startled appearance, dilated conjunctival and episcleral vessels, corneal exposure, restriction of ocular motility, optic atrophy, and diminished retropulsion of the globe. IOP can be increased for several reasons, including elevated episcleral venous pressure. Ocular rigidity is reduced in thyroid eye disease, and thus IOP measurements should be taken with applanation rather than Schiøtz tonometry. In addition, because of restricted ocular motility, pressure measurements should be taken with

---

Box 18-3
Etiology of Elevated Episcleral Venous Pressure

I. Obstruction of venous drainage
  A. Episcleral
    1. Chemical burns
    2. Radiation
  B. Orbital
    1. Retrobulbar tumors
    2. Thyroid eye disease
    3. Pseudotumor
    4. Phlebitis
  C. Cavernous sinus thrombosis
  D. Jugular vein obstruction
  E. Superior vena cava obstruction
  F. Pulmonary venous obstruction
II. Arteriovenous fistulas
  A. Orbital
  B. Intracranial
    1. Carotid-cavernous fistula
    2. Dural fistula
    3. Venous varix
    4. Sturge-Weber syndrome
III. Idiopathic

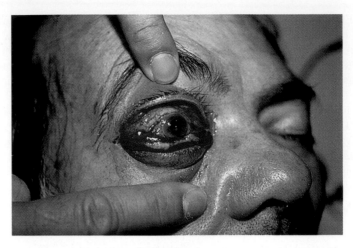

Figure 18-18 Carotid-cavernous fistula. (Courtesy of Randall T. Higashida, M.D., UCSF Medical Center, San Francisco.)

the patient gazing down slightly to minimize a potential transient IOP rise.[411] In this situation elevated IOP is treated with aqueous humor suppressants. Corticosteroids, radiation, and surgical decompression have been employed to protect the optic nerve, limit corneal exposure, and improve cosmetic appearance.[412-418]

Arteriovenous Fistulas

Carotid-cavernous fistulas provide a free communication between the internal carotid artery and the surrounding cavernous sinus, resulting in high blood flow and high mean pressure in the shunt. The reversal of blood flow in the vessels leads to congestion of the orbital veins and soft tissues. The shunting of the blood may produce ocular ischemia[419] and may transmit arterial pulsations to the globe. Patients with carotid-cavernous fistulas often give a history of previous trauma.[420-421] Many of these patients have a dramatic appearance, with pulsating exophthalmos, chemosis, lid edema, vascular engorgement, and restriction of ocular motility[422,423] (Fig. 18-18). The conjunctival and episcleral veins have a tortuous, corkscrew appearance.[401] The physical findings usually occur on the same side as the fistula. Because of the connections between the cavernous sinuses, however, the findings may be bilateral or even alternating.[424,425] Patients with carotid-cavernous fistula often complain of a noise in their head or ears; a bruit is often present over the frontal or temporal regions or over the globe. IOP is usually elevated because of increased episcleral venous pressure, although angle closure and neovascular glaucoma have also been reported.[426,427] Skull and orbital radiography, ultrasonography, and CT or MRI confirm the diagnosis, but arteriography provides the most detailed information about the fistula.[424] Treatment of these fistulas can be difficult and is usually reserved for individuals who have severe pain, incapacitating bruit, progressive glaucomatous visual loss, or other serious complications. A variety of embolization and balloon catheter techniques have been employed with increasing success.[428-431]

Dural fistulas are communications between the cavernous sinus and an extradural branch of the external or internal carotid artery. These fistulas generally have lower blood flow and lower mean pressure.[432-435] The clinical appearance of these patients is far less dramatic than that of patients with carotid-cavernous fistulas (Fig. 18-19). Patients with dural fistulas lack bruits and have variable exophthalmos and variable limitation of ocular motility. The conjunctival and episcleral vessels have the same corkscrew, arterialized appearance, and IOP is elevated. This condition is often seen in elderly women who have no history of trauma.[436] At times the findings are so subtle that only the dilated vessels distinguish this entity from POAG. This condition has been referred to as the "red-eyed shunt syndrome" by Phelps and co-workers.[435] Low-flow or dural fistulas can close spontaneously and may not require treatment. High-flow shunts re-

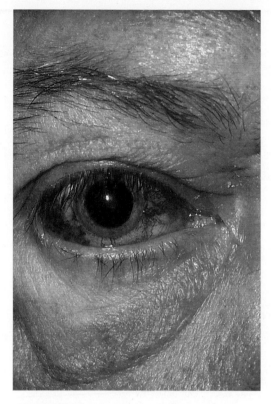

Figure 18-19   Dural shunt with engorged vessels.

spond well to interventional approaches in experienced hands.[431] Elevated IOP generally responds to topical β-adrenergic antagonists and CAIs. Glaucoma associated with neovasculariation may respond to local laser treatment.[436]

Sturge-Weber Syndrome

Sturge-Weber syndrome is a rare oculocutaneous disorder that produces increased IOP through a variety of mechanisms, including elevated episcleral venous pressure.[437-441] This condition is discussed in Chapter 20.

Idiopathic Elevations

Several cases of unexplained or idiopathic elevations of episcleral venous pressure and IOP have been described.[339,442-445] This condition can be unilateral or bilateral and sporadic or familial. The IOP elevations can lead to glaucomatous cupping and visual field loss. The treatment of elevated episcleral venous pressure depends greatly on the underlying condition. Elevated IOP is treated with topical and systemic medications to reduce aqueous production.

Cholinergic agents may be useful, especially in patients with reduced outflow facility. ALT may also be helpful in these patients. One study reports lowering IOP with the topical administration of vasodilators.[446]

Many of these patients eventually require filtering surgery, but ophthalmologists must be aware of the increased possibility of complications. The high venous pressure favors the development of intraoperative choroidal effusion, expulsive hemorrhage, and flat anterior chamber.[444,447,448] It is recommended that prophylactic sclerotomies be made in one or two inferior quadrants at the beginning of filtering surgery. The sclerotomies are then left open at the end of surgery and covered only by conjunctiva to allow continued drainage of suprachoroidal fluid.[447]

REFERENCES

1. Sugar HS: Pigmentary glaucoma: a 25 year review, *Am J Ophthalmol* 62:499, 1966.
2. Sugar HS, Barbour FA: Pigmentary glaucoma: rare clinical entity, *Am J Ophthalmol* 32:90, 1949.
3. Mapstone R: Pigment release, *Br J Ophthalmol* 65:258, 1981.
4. Speakman JS: Pigmentary dispersion, *Br J Ophthalmol* 65:249, 1981.
5. Lichter PR, Shaffer RN: Diagnosis and prognostic signs in pigmentary glaucoma, *Trans Am Acad Ophthalmol Otolaryngol* 74:984, 1970.
6. Scheie HG, Cameron JD: Pigment dispersion syndrome: a clinical study, *Br J Ophthalmol* 65:264, 1981.
7. Semple HC, Ball SF: Pigmentary glaucoma in the black population, *Am J Ophthalmol* 109:518, 1990.
8. Paglinauan C, and others: Exclusion of chromosome 1q21-q31 from linkage to three pedigrees affected by the pigment-dispersion syndrome, *Am J Hum Genet* 56:1240, 1995.
9. Campbell DG: Pigmentary dispersion and glaucoma, *Arch Ophthalmol* 97:1667, 1979.
10. Davidson JA, Brubaker RF, Ilstrup DM: Dimensions of the anterior chamber in pigment dispersion syndrome, *Arch Ophthalmol* 10:81, 1983.
11. Pavlin CJ, and others: Ultrasound biomicroscopic features of pigmentary glaucoma, *Can J Ophthalmol* 29:187, 1994.
12. Iwamoto T, Witmer R, Landolt E: Light and electron microscopy in absolute glaucoma with pigment dispersion phenomena and contusion angle deformity, *Am J Ophthalmol* 72:420, 1971.
13. Korobova V: On the etiology of Krukenberg's spindle, *Russkii Ophthalmol J* 12:476, 1929.
14. Epstein DL, Boger WP III, Grant WM: Phenylephrine provocative testing in the pigmentary dispersion syndrome, *Am J Ophthalmol* 85:43, 1978.
15. Kristensen P: Mydriasis-induced pigment liberation in the anterior chamber associated with acute rise in intraocular pressure in open-angle glaucoma, *Acta Ophthalmol Scand* 43:714,1965.
16. Peterson HP: Can pigmentary deposits on the trabecular meshwork increase the resistance of the aqueous outflow? *Acta Ophthalmol (Copenh)* 47:743, 1969.
17. Haynes WL, and others: Effects of jogging exercise on patients with the pigmentary dispersion syndrome and pigmentary glaucoma, *Ophthalmology* 99:1096, 1992.
18. Jensen PK, and others: Exercise and reversed pupillary block in pigmentary glaucoma, *Am J Ophthalmol* 120:110, 1995.
19. Shenker HI, and others: Exercise-induced increase of intraocular pressure in the pigmentary dispersion syndrome, *Am J Ophthalmol* 89:598, 1980.
20. Ritch R: Nonprogressive low-tension glaucoma with pigmentary dispersion, *Am J Ophthalmol* 94:190, 1982.

21. Ritch R, Manusow D, Podos SM: Remission of pigmentary glaucoma in a patient with subluxated lenses, *Am J Ophthalmol* 94:812, 1982.
22. Herpel JK: Prevalence of pigment dispersion syndrome in a population undergoing glaucoma screening, *Am J Ophthalmol* 117:123, 1994 (letter; comment).
23. Grant WM: Experimental aqueous perfusion in enucleated human eyes, *Arch Ophthalmol* 69:783, 1963.
24. Epstein DL: *Chandler and Grant's glaucoma,* Philadelphia, 1986, Lea & Febiger.
25. Zink HA, and others: Comparison of in vitro corticosteroid response in pigmentary glaucoma and primary open-angle glaucoma, *Am J Ophthalmol* 80:478, 1975.
26. Richardson TM, Hutchinson BT, Grant WM: The outflow tract in pigmentary glaucoma: a light and electron microscopic study, *Arch Ophthalmol* 95:1015, 1977.
27. Rodrigues MM, and others: Value of trabeculectomy specimens in glaucoma, *Ophthalmic Surg* 9:29, 1978.
28. Shimuza T, Hara K, Futa R: Fine structure of trabecular meshwork and iris in pigmentary glaucoma, *Graefes Arch Clin Exp Ophthalmol* 215:171, 1981.
29. Rohen JW, van der Zypen EP: The phagocytic activity of the trabecular meshwork endothelium: an electron microscopic study of the vervet *(Ceropithecus aethiops), Graefes Arch Clin Exp Ophthalmol* 175:143, 1968.
30. Wand M, Grant WM: Thymoxamine hydrochloride: an alpha-adrenergic blocker, *Surv Ophthalmol* 25:75, 1980.
31. Lagreze WD, Funk J: Iridotomy in the treatment of pigmentary glaucoma: documentation with high resolution ultrasound, *Ger J Ophthalmol* 4:162, 1995.
32. Farrar SM, and others: Risk factors for the development and severity of glaucoma in the pigment dispersion syndrome, *Am J Ophthalmol* 108:223, 1989.
33. Ritch R, and others: Argon laser trabeculoplasty in pigmentary glaucoma, *Ophthalmology* 100:909, 1993.
34. Luntz HM: Prevalence of pseudo-exfoliation syndrome in urban South African clinic population, *Am J Ophthalmol* 74:581, 1972.
35. Meyer E, Haim T, Zonis S: Pseudoexfoliation: epidemiology, clinical and scanning electron microscopic study, *Ophthalmologica* 188:141, 1984.
36. Layden WE, Shaffer RN: Exfoliation syndrome, *Am J Ophthalmol* 78:835, 1974.
37. Layden WE, Shaffer RN: The exfoliation syndrome, *Trans Am Acad Ophthalmol Otolaryngol* 78:326, 1974.
38. Roth M, Epstein DL: Exfoliation syndrome, *Am J Ophthalmol* 89:477, 1980.
39. Hiller R, Sperduto RO, Krueger DE: Pseudoexfoliation, intraocular pressure, and senile lens changes in a population-based survey, *Arch Ophthalmol* 100:1080, 1982.
40. Horven I: Exfoliation syndrome, *Arch Ophthalmol* 76:505, 1966.

41. Henry JC, and others: Long-term follow-up of pseudoexfoliation and the development of elevated intraocular pressure, *Ophthalmology* 94:545, 1987.
42. Aasved H: The frequency of fibrillopathia epitheliocapsularis (so-called senile exfoliation or pseudoexfoliation) in patients with open-angle glaucoma, *Acta Ophthalmol Scand* 49:194, 1971.
43. Kozart DM, Yanoff M: Intraocular pressure status in 100 consecutive patients with exfoliation syndrome, *Ophthalmology* 89:214, 1982.
44. Konstas AG, and others: Prevalence, diagnostic features, and response to trabeculectomy in exfoliation glaucoma, *Ophthalmology* 100:619, 1993.
45. Layden WE: *Exfoliation syndrome.* In Ritch R, Shields MB, editors: *The secondary glaucomas,* St Louis, 1982, Mosby.
46. Brooks AMV, Gillies WE: Fluorescein angiography and fluorophotometry of the iris in pseudoexfoliation of the lens capsule, *Br J Ophthalmol* 67:429, 1983.
47. Friedburg D, Bischof G: Fluorescein angiographic features of the pseudoexfoliation syndrome, *Glaucoma* 4:13, 1982.
48. Olivius E, Thornburn W: Prognosis of glaucoma simplex and glaucoma capsulare: a comparative study, *Acta Ophthalmol Scand* 56:291, 1978.
49. Psilas K, and others: Comparative study of argon laser trabeculoplasty in primary open-angle and pseudoexfoliation glaucoma, *Ophthalmologica* 198:57, 1989.
50. Rouhianen H, and others: The effect of some treatment variables on long-term results of argon laser trabeculoplasty, *Ophthalmologica* 209:21, 1995.
51. Lumme P, Laatikainen L: Exfoliation syndrome and cataract extraction, *Am J Ophthalmol* 116:51, 1993.
52. Schlotzer-Schrehardt U, Naumann GO: A histopathologic study of zonular instability in pseudoexfoliation syndrome, *Am J Ophthalmol* 118:730, 1994.
53. Skuta G, Parrish RK, Hodapp E: Zonular dialysis during extracapsular cataract extraction in pseudoexfoliation syndrome, *Arch Ophthalmol* 105:632, 1987.
54. Dark AJ, Streeten BW, Cornwall CC: Pseudoexfoliative disease of the lens: a study in electron microscopy and histochemistry, *Br J Ophthalmol* 61:462, 1977.
55. Davanger M: The pseudo-exfoliation syndrome: a scanning electron microscopic study: I. The anterior lens surface, *Acta Ophthalmol Scand* 53:809, 1975.
56. Netland PA, and others: Elastosis of the lamina cribrosa in pseudoexfoliation syndrome with glaucoma, *Ophthalmology* 102:878, 1995.
57. Bertelsen TI, Drablos PA, Flood PR: The so-called senile exfoliation (pseudoexfoliation) of the anterior lens capsule, a product of the lens epithelium, fibrillopathia epitheliocapsularis: a microscopic, histochemical and electron microscopic investigation, *Acta Ophthalmol Scand* 2:1096, 1964.

58. Eagle RC Jr, Font RL, Fine BS: The basement membrane exfoliation syndrome, *Arch Ophthalmol* 97:510, 1979.

59. Harnisch JP, and others: Identification of a basement membrane proteoglycan in exfoliation material, *Graefes Arch Clin Exp Ophthalmol* 214:273, 1981.

60. Garner A, Alexander RA: Pseudoexfoliative disease: histochemical evidence of an affinity with zonular fibres, *Br J Ophthalmol* 68:574, 1984.

61. Streeten BW, Dark AJ, Barnes CW: Pseudoexfoliative material and oxytalan fibers, *Exp Eye Res* 38:523, 1984.

62. Ringvold A, Davanger M: Notes on the distribution of pseudo-exfoliation material with particular reference to the uveoscleral route of aqueous humor, *Acta Ophthalmol Scand* 55:807, 1977.

63. Bergmanson JPG, Jones WL, Chu LW-F: Ultrastructural observations on (pseudo-) exfoliation of the lens capsule: a re-examination of the involvement of the lens epithelium, *Br J Ophthalmol* 68:118, 1984.

64. Ghosh M, Speakman JS: The iris in senile exfoliation of the lens, *Can J Ophthalmol* 9:289, 1974.

65. Speakman JS, Ghosh M: The conjunctiva in senile lens exfoliation, *Arch Ophthalmol* 94:1757, 1976.

66. Karjalainen K, and others: Exfoliation syndrome in enucleated haemorrhagic and absolute glaucoma, *Acta Ophthalmol (Copenh)* 65:320, 1987.

67. Benedikt O, Roll P: The trabecular meshwork of a non-glaucomatous eye with the exfoliation syndrome: electron-microscopic study, *Virchows Arch A* 384:347, 1979.

68. Sampaolesi R, Argento C: Scanning electron microscopy of the trabecular meshwork in normal and glaucomatous eyes, *Invest Ophthalmol Vis Sci* 16:302, 1977.

69. Sampaolesi R, and others: The chamber angle in exfoliation syndrome: clinical and pathological findings, *Acta Ophthalmol Scand Suppl* 184:48, 1988.

70. Prince A, Streeten BW, Ritch R: Preclinical diagnosis of pseudoexfoliation syndrome, *Arch Ophthalmol* 105:1076, 1987.

71. Johnson DH, Brubaker RF: Dynamics of aqueous humor in the syndrome of exfoliation with glaucoma, *Am J Ophthalmol* 93:629, 1982.

72. Jerndal T, Svedbergh B: Goniodysgenesis in exfoliation glaucoma, *Adv Ophthalmol* 35:45, 1978.

73. Armaly MF: Effects of corticosteroids on intraocular pressure and fluid dynamics. I. The effect of dexamethasone in the normal eye, *Arch Ophthalmol* 70:482, 1963.

74. Armaly MF: Effect of corticosteroids on intraocular pressure and fluid dynamics. II. The effect of dexamethasone in the glaucomatous eye, *Arch Ophthalmol* 70:492, 1963.

75. Becker B: Intraocular pressure response to topical corticosteroids, *Invest Ophthalmol Vis Sci* 4:198, 1965.

76. Becker B, Mills DW: Corticosteroids and intraocular pressure, *Arch Ophthalmol* 70:500,1963.

77. Becker B, Hahn KA: Topical corticosteroids and heredity in primary open-angle glaucoma, *Am J Ophthalmol* 57:543, 1964.

78. Davies TG: Tonographic survey of the close relatives of patients with simple glaucoma, *Br J Ophthalmol* 52:32, 1968.

79. Becker B: Diabetes mellitus and primary open-angle glaucoma: the XXVII Edward Jackson Memorial lecture, *Am J Ophthalmol* 77:1, 1971.

80. Tukey RB: Glaucoma following the application of corticosteroid to the skin of the eyelid, *Br J Dermatol* 95:207, 1976.

81. Zugerman C, Saunders D, Levit F: Glaucoma from topically applied steroids, *Arch Dermatol* 112:1326, 1976.

82. Alfano JE: Changes in the intraocular pressure associated with systemic steroid therapy, *Am J Ophthalmol* 56:346, 1963.

83. Bernstein NH, Schwartz B: Effects of long-term systemic steroids on intraocular pressure, *Arch Ophthalmol* 69:742, 1962.

84. Kitazawa Y: Acute glaucoma due to systemic corticosteroid administration, *Acta Soc Ophthalmol Jpn* 70:2197, 1966.

85. Herschler J: Intractable intraocular hypertension induced by repository triamcinolone acetonide, *Am J Ophthalmol* 74:501, 1972.

86. Nozik RA: Periocular injection of steroids, *Trans Am Acad Ophthalmol Otolaryngol* 76:695,1972.

87. Perkins ES: Steroid-induced glaucoma, *Proc R Soc Med* 58:531, 1965.

88. Dreyer EB: Inhaled steroid use and glaucoma, *N Engl J Med* 329:1822, 1993 (letter).

89. Opatowsky I, and others: Intraocular pressure elevation associated with inhalation and nasal corticosteroids, *Ophthalmology* 102:177, 1995.

90. Bayer JM: Ergebnisse und Beurteilund der subtotalen Adrenalektomie beim hyperfunctions-Cushing, *Langenbecks Arch Chir* 291:531, 1959.

91. Haas JS, Nootens RH: Glaucoma secondary to benign adrenal adenoma, *Am J Ophthalmol* 78:497, 1974.

92. Kass MA, Kolker AE, Becker B: Chronic topical corticosteroid use simulating congenital glaucoma, *J Pediatr* 81:1175, 1972.

93. Scheie HG, Rubinstein RA, Albert DM: Congenital glaucoma and other ocular abnormalities with idiopathic infantile hypoglycemia, *J Pediatr Ophthalmol* 1:45, 1964.

94. Turner JB: A clinical review of congenital glaucoma, *South Med J* 64:1362, 1971.

95. Francois J: The importance of the mucopolysaccharides in intraocular pressure regulation, *Invest Ophthalmol Vis Sci* 14:173, 1975.

96. Yun AJ, and others: Proteins secreted by human trabecular cells: glucocorticoid and other effects, *Invest Ophthalmol Vis Sci* 30:2012, 1989.

97. Bill A: The drainage of aqueous humor, *Invest Ophthalmol Vis Sci* 14:1, 1975.

98. Weinreb RN, Mitchell ME, Polansky JR: Prostaglandin production by human trabecular cells: in vitro inhibition by dexamethasone, *Invest Ophthalmol Vis Sci* 24:1541, 1983.

99. Southren AL, and others: 5-Beta-dihydrocortisol: possible mediator of the ocular hypertension in glaucoma, *Invest Ophthalmol Vis Sci* 26:393, 1985.

100. Southren AL, and others: Altered cortisol metabolism in cells cultured from trabecular meshwork specimens obtained from patients with primary open-angle glaucoma, *Invest Ophthalmol Vis Sci* 24:1413, 1983.

101. Weinstein BI, and others: Defects in cortisol-metabolizing enzymes in primary open-angle glaucoma, *Invest Ophthalmol Vis Sci* 26:890, 1985.

102. Spaeth GL, Rodrigues MM, Weinreb S: Steroid-induced glaucoma. A. Persistent elevation of intraocular pressure. B. Histopathologic aspects, *Trans Am Ophthalmol Soc* 75:535, 1977.

103. Epstein DL: Diagnosis and management of lens-induced glaucoma, *Ophthalmology* 89:227, 1982.

104. Jedziniak JA, and others: The concentration and localization of heavy molecular weight aggregates in aging, normal, and cataractous human lenses, *Exp Eye Res* 20:367, 1975.

105. Epstein DL, Jedziniak JA, Grant WM: Identification of heavy-molecular-weight soluble protein in aqueous humor in human phacolytic glaucoma, *Invest Ophthalmol Vis Sci* 17:398, 1978.

106. Epstein DL, Jedziniak JA, Grant WM: Obstruction of aqueous outflow by lens particles and by heavy-molecular-weight soluble lens proteins, *Invest Ophthalmol Vis Sci* 17:272,1978.

107. Flocks M, Lettwin CS, Zimmerman LE: Phacolytic glaucoma: a clinicopathologic study of one hundred thirty-eight cases of glaucoma associated with hypermature cataract, *Arch Ophthalmol* 54:37, 1955.

108. Ueno H, and others: Electron microscopic observation of the cells floating in the anterior chamber in a case of phacolytic glaucoma, *Jpn J Ophthalmol* 33:103, 1989.

109. Irvine SR, Irvine AR Jr: Lens-induced uveitis and glaucoma. Part III. "Phacolytic-glaucoma": lens-induced glaucoma; mature or hypermature cataract; open iridocorneal angle, *Am J Ophthalmol* 35:489, 1952.

110. Chandler PA: Problems in the diagnosis and treatment of lens-induced uveitis and glaucoma, *Arch Ophthalmol* 60:828, 1958.

111. Lane SS, and others: Treatment of phacolytic glaucoma with extracapsular cataract extraction, *Ophthalmology* 95:749, 1988.

112. Mandal AK: Endocapsular surgery and capsular bag fixation of intraocular lenses in phacolytic glaucoma, *J Cataract Refract Surg* 22:288, 1996.

113. Singh G, and others: Phacolytic glaucoma: its treatment by planned extracapsular cataract extraction with posterior chamber intraocular lens implantation, *Indian J Ophthalmol* 42:145, 1994.

114. Perlman EM, Albert DM: Clinically unsuspected phacoanaphylaxis after ocular trauma, *Arch Ophthalmol* 95:244, 1977.

115. Ellant JP, Obstbaum SA: Lens-induced glaucoma, *Doc Ophthalmol* 81:317, 1992.

115a. Tuberville A, and others: Post surgical intraocular pressure elevation, *Am Intra Ocular Implant Soc J* 9:309, 1983.

116. Kirsch RE, Levine O, Singer JA: Ridge at internal edge of cataract incision, *Arch Ophthalmol* 94:2098, 1976.

117. Campbell DG, Grant WM: Trabecular deformation and reduction of outflow facility due to cataract and penetrating keratoplasty sutures, *Invest Ophthalmol Vis Sci* 16:126,1977.

118. Galin MA, Barasch KR, Harris LS: Enzymatic zonulolysis and intraocular pressure, *Am J Ophthalmol* 61:690, 1966.

119. Kirsch RE: Dose relationship of alpha-chymotrypsin in production of glaucoma after cataract extraction, *Arch Ophthalmol* 75:774, 1966.

120. Lantz JM, Quigley JH: Intraocular pressure after cataract extraction: effects of alpha-chymotrypsin, *Can J Ophthalmol* 8:339, 1973.

121. Jocsin VL: Tonography and gonioscopy: before and after cataract extraction with alpha chymotrpysin, *Am J Ophthalmol* 60:318, 1965.

122. Anderson DR: Experimental alpha chymotrypsin glaucoma studied by scanning electron microscopy, *Am J Ophthalmol* 71:470, 1971.

123. Anderson DR: Scanning electron microscopy of zonulolysis by alpha chymotrypsin, *Am J Ophthalmol* 71:619, 1971.

124. Kalvin NH, Hamasaki DI, Gass JDM: Experimental glaucoma in monkeys. I. Relationship between intraocular pressure and cupping of the optic disc and cavernous atrophy of the optic nerve, *Arch Ophthalmol* 76:82, 1968.

125. Hamanaka T, Bill A: Effects of alpha-chymotrypsin on the outflow routes for aqueous humor, *Exp Eye Res* 46:323, 1988.

126. Barraquer J, Rutlan J: Enzymatic zonulolysis and postoperative ocular hypertension, *Am J Ophthalmol* 63:159, 1967.

127. Barron BA, and others: Comparison of the effects of Viscoat and Healon on postoperative intraocular pressure, *Am J Ophthalmol* 100:377, 1985.

128. Binkhorst CD: Inflammation and intraocular pressure after the use of Healon in intraocular lens surgery, *Am Intraocular Implant Soc J* 6:340, 1980.

129. Cherfan GM, Ritch WJ, Wright G: Raised intraocular pressure and other problems with sodium hyaluronate and cataract surgery, *Trans Ophthalmol Soc UK* 103:277,1983.

130. Lazenby GW, Brocker G: The use of sodium hyaluronate (Healon) in intracapsular cataract extraction with insertion of anterior chamber intraocular lenses, *Ophthalmic Surg* 12:646, 1981.

131. Passo MS, Earnest JT, Goldstick TK: Hyaluronate increases intraocular pressure when used on cataract extraction, *Br J Ophthalmol* 69:572, 1985.

132. Stamper RL, and others: Effect of intraocular aspiration of sodium hyaluronate on postoperative intraocular pressure, *Ophthalmic Surg* 21:486, 1990.

133. Probst LE, and others: Phacoemulsification with aspirated or retained Viscoat, *J Cataract Refract Surg* 20:145, 1994.

134. MacRae SM, and others: The effects of sodium hyaluronate, chondroitin sulfate, and methylcellulose on the corneal endothelium and intraocular pressure, *Am J Ophthalmol* 95:332, 1983.

135. Berson FG, Patterson MM, Epstein DL: Obstruction of aqueous outflow by sodium hyaluronate in enucleated human eyes, *Am J Ophthalmol* 95:668, 1983.

136. Schubert H, Denlinger JL, Balazs EA: Na-hyaluronate injected into the anterior chamber of the owl monkey: effect on intraocular pressure and rate of disappearance, *Invest Ophthalmol Vis Sci* 21:1181, 1981.

137. Aron-Rosa P, and others: Methylcellulose instead of Healon in extracapsular surgery with intraocular lens implantation, *Ophthalmology* 90:1235,1983.

138. Carty JB: Chondroitin sulfate in anterior segment surgery, *Trans Ophthalmol Soc UK* 103:263, 1983.

139. Soll DB, Harrison SE: The use of chondroitin sulfate in protection of the corneal endothelium, *Ophthalmology* 88:51, 1981.

140. Ballin N, Weiss DM: Pigment dispersion and intraocular pressure elevation in pseudophakia, *Ann Ophthalmol* 14:627, 1982.

141. Huber C: The gray iris syndrome: an iatrogenic form of pigmentary glaucoma, *Arch Ophthalmol* 102:397, 1984.

142. Samples JR, Van Buskirk EM: Pigmentary glaucoma associated with posterior chamber intraocular lenses, *Am Ophthalmol* 100:385, 1985.

143. Smith JP: Pigmentary open-angle glaucoma secondary to posterior chamber intraocular lens implantation and erosion of the iris pigment epithelium, *Am Intraocular Implant Soc J* 11:174, 1985.

144. Woodhams JT, Lester JC: Pigmentary dispersion glaucoma secondary to posterior chamber intra-ocular lens, *Ann Ophthalmol* 16:852, 1984.

145. Percival SBP, Das K: UGH syndrome after posterior chamber lens implantation, *Am Intraocular Implant Soc J* 9:200, 1983.

146. Van Liefferinge T, and others: Uveitis-glaucoma-hyphema syndrome: a late complication of posterior chamber lenses, *Bull Soc Belge Ophthalmol* 252:61, 1994.

147. Ellingson FT: The uveitis-glaucoma-hyphema syndrome associated with the Mark-VII Choyce anterior chamber lens implant, *Am Intraocular Implant Soc J* 4:50, 1978.

148. Hagan JC: A comparative study of the 91Z and other anterior chamber intraocular lenses, *Am Intraocular Implant Soc J* 10:324, 1984.

149. Johnson SH, Kratz RP, Olson PF: Iris transillumination defect and microhyphema syndrome, *Am Intraocular Implant Soc J* 10:425, 1984.

156. Miller D, Doone MG: High-speed photographic evaluation of intraocular lens movements, *Am J Ophthalmol* 97:752, 1984.

157. Doren GS, and others: Indications for and results of intraocular lens explanation, *J Cataract Refract Surg* 18:79, 1993.

158. Channell MM, Beckman H: Intraocular pressure changes after Nd:YAG laser posterior capsulotomy, *Arch Ophthalmol* 102:1024, 1984.

159. Keates RH, and others: Long-term follow-up of Nd:YAG laser posterior capsulotomy, *Am Intraocular Implant Soc J* 10: 164, 1984.

160. Kurata F, and others: Progressive glaucomatous visual field loss after neodymium-YAG laser capsulotomy, *Am J Ophthalmol* 98:632, 1984.

161. Richter CV, and others: Intraocular pressure elevation following Nd:YAG laser posterior capsulotomy, *Ophthalmology* 92:636, 1985.

162. Shrader CE: Acute glaucoma following Nd:YAG laser membranectomy, *Ophthalmic Surg* 14:1015, 1983.

163. Stark WJ, and others: Neodymium:YAG lasers an FDA report, *Ophthalmology* 92:209, 1985.

164. Terry AC, and others: Neodymium:YAG for posterior capsulotomies, *Am J Ophthalmol* 96:716, 1983.

165. Slomovic AR, Parrish RK: Acute elevations of intraocular pressure following Nd:YAG laser posterior capsulotomy, *Ophthalmology* 92:973, 1985.

166. Pollack IP, and others: Prevention of the rise in intraocular pressure following neodymium-YAG posterior capsulotomy using topical 1% apraclonidine, *Arch Ophthalmol* 106:754, 1988.

167. Cullom RD Jr, Schwartz LW: The effect of apraclonidine on the intraocular pressure of glaucoma patients following Nd:YAG laser posterior capsulotomy, *Ophthalmic Surg* 24:623, 1993.

168. Nesher R, Kolker AE: Failure of apraclonidine to prevent delayed IOP elevation after Nd:YAG laser posterior capsulotomy, *Trans Am Ophthalmol Soc* 88:229, 1990.

169. Altamirano D, and others: Aqueous humor analysis after Nd:YAG laser capsulotomy with the laser flare-cell meter, *J Cataract Refract Surg* 18:554, 1992.

170. Lynch MG, and others: The effect of neodymium:YAG laser capsulotomy on aqueous humor dynamics in the monkey eye, *Ophthalmology* 93:1270, 1986.

171. Schubert HD, and others: The role of the vitreous in the intraocular pressure rise after neodymium-YAG laser capsulotomy, *Arch Ophthalmol* 103:1538, 1985.

172. Grant WM: Open-angle glaucoma associated with vitreous filling the anterior chamber, *Trans Am Ophthalmol Soc* 61:196, 1963.

173. Iuglio N, Tieri O: Glaucoma ad angolo aperto da vitreo in camera anteriore, *Arch Ophthalmol* 68:481, 1964.

174. Simmons RJ: The vitreous in glaucoma, *Trans Ophthalmol Soc UK* 95:422, 1975.

175. Nelson JD, Kopietz LA: Chemical injuries to the eyes: emergency, intermediate, and long-term care, *Postgrad Med* 81:62, 1987.

176. Richter RC, and others: Tonometry on eyes with abnormal corneas, *Glaucoma* 2:508, 1980.

177. Green K, Paterson CA, Siddiqui A: Ocular blood flow after experimental alkali burns and prostaglandin administration, *Arch Ophthalmol* 103:569, 1985.

178. Paterson CA, Pfister RR: Intraocular pressure changes after alkali burns, *Arch Ophthalmol* 91:211, 1974.

179. Brown SI, Tragakis MP, Pearce DB: Treatment of the alkali burned cornea, *Am J Ophthalmol* 74:316, 1972.

180. Girard LJ, and others: Severe alkali burns, *Trans Am Acad Ophthalmol Otolaryngol* 74:788, 1970.

181. Zaidman GW, Wandel T: Transscleral YAG laser photocoagulation for uncontrollable glaucoma in corneal patients, *Cornea* 7:112, 1988.

182. Melamed S, Fiore PM: Molteno implant surgery in refractory glaucoma, *Surv Ophthalmol* 34:441, 1990.

183. Coleman AL, and others: Initial clinical experience with the Ahmed Glaucoma Valve implant [published erratum appears in *Am J Ophthalmol* 120:684, 1995], *Am J Ophthalmol* 120:23, 1995.

184. Leen MM, and others: Anatomic considerations in the implantation of the Ahmed glaucoma valve, *Arch Ophthalmol* 114:223, 1996 (letter).

185. White TC: Aqueous shunt implant surgery for refractory glaucoma, *J Ophthalmic Nurs Technol* 15:7, 1996.

186. Berger RO: Ocular complications of cardioversion, *Ann Ophthalmol* 10:161, 1978.

187. Berger RO: Ocular complications of electroconvulsive therapy, *Ann Ophthalmol* 10:737, 1978.

188. McClellen JW, Mills M, Markson J: Measurement of intraocular tension in insulin and electroconvulsive therapy, *Bull Menniger Clin* 14:220, 1950.

189. Barron A, McDonald JE, Hughes WF: Long-term complications of beta radiation therapy in ophthalmology, *Trans Am Ophthalmol Soc* 68:112, 1970.

190. Hope-Ross MJ, and others: Ocular siderosis, *Eye* 7:419, 1993.

191. Sneed SR, Weingeist TA: Management of siderosis bulbi due to a retained iron-containing intraocular foreign body, *Ophthalmology* 97:375, 1990.

192. Canavan YM, Archer DB: Anterior segment consequences of blunt ocular injury, *Br J Ophthalmol* 66:549, 1982.

193. Salmon JF, and others: The detection of post-traumatic angle recession by gonioscopy in a population-based glaucoma survey, *Ophthalmology* 101:1844, 1994.

194. Chi TS, Netland PA: Angle-recession glaucoma, *Int Ophthalmol Clin* 35:117, 1995.

195. Dotan S, Oliver M: Shallow anterior chamber and uveal effusion after nonperforating trauma to the eye, *Am J Ophthalmol* 94:782, 1982.

196. Collins ET: On the pathological examination of three eyes lost from concussion, *Trans Ophthalmol Soc UK* 12:180, 1892.

197. Blanton FM: Anterior chamber angle recession and secondary glaucoma: a study of the after effects of traumatic hyphema, *Arch Ophthalmol* 72:39, 1964.

198. Kaufman JH, Tolpin DW: Glaucoma after traumatic angle recession, *Am J Ophthalmol* 78:648, 1974.

199. Thiel H-J, Aden G, Pulhorn G: Changes in the chamber angle following ocular contusions, *Klin Monatsbl Augenheilkd* 177:165, 1980.

200. Armaly MF: *Steroids and glaucoma.* In *Transactions of the New Orleans Academy of Ophthalmology Symposium on Glaucoma,* St Louis, 1967, Mosby.

201. Melamed S, and others: Nd:YAG laser trabeculopuncture in angle-recession glaucoma, *Ophthalmic Surg* 23:31, 1992.

202. Fukuchi T, and others: Nd:YAG laser trabeculopuncture (YLT) for glaucoma with traumatic angle recession, *Graefes Arch Clin Exp Ophthalmol* 231:571, 1993.

203. Mermoud A, and others: Surgical management of post-traumatic angle recession glaucoma, *Ophthalmology* 100:634, 1993.

204. Mermoud A, and others: Post-traumatic angle recession glaucoma: a risk factor for bleb failure after trabeculectomy, *Br J Ophthalmol* 77:631, 1993.

205. Campbell DG, Simmons RJ, Grant WM: Ghost cells as a cause of glaucoma, *Am J Ophthalmol* 81:441, 1976.

206. Montenegro MH, Simmons RJ: Ghost cell glaucoma, *Int Ophthalmol Clin* 35: 111, 1995.

207. Campbell DG, and others: Glaucoma occurring after closed vitrectomy, *Am J Ophthalmol* 83:63, 1977.

208. Summers CG, Lindstrom RL: Ghost cell glaucoma following lens implantation, *Am Intraocular Implant Soc J* 9:429, 1983.

209. Frazer DG, and others: Ghost cell glaucoma in phakic eyes, *Int Ophthalmol* 11: 51, 1987.

210. Quigley HA, Addicks EM: Chronic experimental glaucoma in primates, *Invest Ophthalmol Vis Sci* 19:126, 1980.

211. Campbell DG, Essigman EM: Hemolytic ghost cell glaucoma: further studies, *Arch Ophthalmol* 97:2141, 1979.

212. Cameron JD, Havener VR: Histologic confirmation of ghost cell glaucoma by routine light microscopy, *Am J Ophthalmol* 96:251, 1983.

213. Summers CG, Lindstrom RL, Cameron JD: Phase contrast microscopy: diagnosis of ghost cell glaucoma following cataract extraction, *Surv Ophthalmol* 28:342, 1984.

214. Singh H, Grand MG: Treatment of blood-induced glaucoma by trans pars plana vitrectomy, *Retina* 1:255, 1981.

215. Abu el-Asrar AM, al-Obeidan SA: Pars plana vitrectomy in the management of ghost cell glaucoma, *Int Ophthalmol Vis Sci* 19:121, 1995.

216. Fenton RH, Zimmerman LE: Hemolytic glaucoma, *Arch Ophthalmol* 70:236, 1963.

217. Phelps CD, Watzke RC: Hemolytic glaucoma, *Am J Ophthalmol* 80:690, 1975.

218. Grierson I, Lee WR: Further observations on the process of haemophagocytosis in the human outflow system, *Graefes Arch Clin Exp Ophthalmol* 208:49, 1978.

219. Benson WE, Spalter HF: Vitreous hemorrhage, *Surv Ophthalmol* 15:297, 2971.

220. Schein OD, and others: The spectrum and burden of ocular injury, *Ophthalmology* 95:300, 1988.

221. Berrios, RR, Dreyer EB: Traumatic hyphema, *Int Ophthalmol Clin* 35:93, 1995.

222. Crouch ER Jr, Frankel M: Aminocaproic acid in the treatment of traumatic hyphema, *Am J Ophthalmol* 81:255, 1976.

223. Bramsen T: Traumatic hyphaema treated with the antifibrinolytic drug tranexamic acid, *Acta Ophthalmol Scand* 54:250, 1976.

224. Crawford JS, Lewandowski RL, Chan W: The effect of aspirin on rebleeding in traumatic hyphema, *Am J Ophthalmol* 80:543, 1975.

225. Edwards WC, Layden WE: Traumatic hyphema: a report of 184 consecutive cases, *Am J Ophthalmol* 76:110, 1973.

226. Fritch CD: Traumatic hyphema, *Ann Ophthalmol* 8:1223, 1976.

227. Giles CL, Bromley WG: Traumatic hyphema: a retrospective analysis from the University of Michigan Teaching Hospitals, *J Pediatr Ophthalmol* 9:90, 1972.

228. Mortensen KK, Sjolie AK: Secondary haemorrhage following traumatic hyphaema: a comparative study of conservative and tranexamic acid treatment, *Acta Ophthalmol (Copenh)* 56:763, 1978.

229. Read J, Goldberg MF: Comparison of medical treatment for traumatic hyphema, *Trans Am Acad Ophthalmol Otolaryngol* 78:799, 1974.

230. Spoor TC, Hammer M, Belloso H: Traumatic hyphema failure rate of steroids to alter its course: a double-blind prospective study, *Arch Ophthalmol* 98:116, 1980.

231. Thomas MA, Parrish RK II, Feuer WJ: Rebleeding after traumatic hyphema, *Arch Ophthalmol* 104:206, 1986.

232. Thygeson P, Beard C: Observations of traumatic hyphema, *Am J Ophthalmol* 35:977, 1952.

233. Ganley JP, and others: Aspirin and recurrent hyphema after blunt ocular trauma, *Am J Ophthalmol* 96:797, 1983.

234. Gorn RA: The detrimental effect of aspirin on hyphema rebleed, *Ann Ophthalmol* 11:351, 1979.

235. Sternberg P Jr, and others: Changes in outflow facility in experimental hyphema, *Invest Ophthalmol Vis Sci* 19: l388, 1980.

236. Little BC, Aylward GW: The medical management of traumatic hyphaema: a survey of opinion among ophthalmologists in the UK, *J R Soc Med* 86:458, 1993.

237. Edwards WC, Layden WE: Monocular versus binocular patching in traumatic hyphema, *Am J Ophthalmol* 76:359, 1973.

238. Masket S, and others: Therapy in experimental hyphema, *Arch Ophthalmol* 85: 329, 1971.

239. Rose SW, and others: Experimental hyphema clearance in rabbits: drug trials with 1% atropine and 2% and 4% pilocarpine, *Arch Ophthalmol* 95:1442, 1977.

240. Sukumaran K: The role of tranexamic acid (Cyklokapron) in the treatment of traumatic hyphaema, *Med J Malaysia* 43:155, 1988.

241. Deans R, and others: Oral administration of tranexamic acid in the management of traumatic hyphema in children, *Can J Ophthalmol* 27:181, 1992.

242. Clarke WN, Noel LP: Outpatient treatment of microscopic and rim hyphemas in children with tranexamic acid, *Can J Ophthalmol* 28:325, 1993.

367. Fries PD, and others: Sympathetic ophthalmia complicating helium ion irradiation of a choroidal melanoma, *Arch Ophthalmol* 105:1561, 1987.

368. Char DH, and others: Five-year follow-up of helium ion therapy for uveal melanoma, *Arch Ophthalmol* 108:209, 1990.

369. Decker M, and others: Ciliary body melanoma treated with helium particle irradiation, *Int J Radiat Oncol Biol Phys* 19:243, 1990.

370. Shields JA, Shields CL: Current management of posterior uveal melanoma, *Mayo Clin Proc* 68:1196, 1993.

371. Meecham WJ, and others: Anterior segment complications after helium ion radiation therapy for uveal melanoma: radiation cataract, *Arch Ophthalmol* 112:197, 1994.

372. Schachat AP: Management of uveal melanoma: a continuing dilemma: Collaborative Ocular Melanoma Study Group, *Cancer* 74:3073, 1994 (letter; comment).

373. Char DH, and others: Long term visual outcome of radiated uveal melanomas in eyes eligible for randomisation to enucleation versus brachytherapy, *Br J Ophthalmol* 80:117, 1996.

374. Waterhouse WJ, and others: Bilateral ciliary body melanomas, *Can J Ophthalmol* 24:125, 1989.

375. Memmen JE, McLean IW: The long-term outcome of patients undergoing iridocyclectomy, *Ophthalmology* 97:429, 1990.

376. Ferry AP, Font RL: Carcinoma metastatic to the eye and orbit. I. A clinicopathologic study of 227 cases, *Arch Ophthalmol* 92:276, 1974.

377. Ferry AP, Font RL: Carcinoma metastatic to the eye and orbit. II. A clinicopathological study of 26 patients with carcinoma metastatic to the anterior segment of the eye, *Arch Ophthalmol* 93:472, 1975.

378. Shields CL, and others: Prevalence and mechanisms of secondary intraocular pressure elevations in eyes with intraocular tumors, *Ophthalmology* 94:839, 1987.

379. Johnson BL: Bilateral glaucoma caused by nasal carcinoma obstructing Schlemm's canal, *Am J Ophthalmol* 96:550, 1983.

380. Nakazawa M, Tamai M: Iris melanocytoma with secondary glaucoma, *Am J Ophthalmol* 97:797, 1984.

381. Shields JA, and others: Adenoma of the iris-pigment epithelium, *Ophthalmology* 90:735, 1983.

382. Goncalves V, Sandler T, O'Donnell FE Jr: Open angle glaucoma in melanosis oculi: response to laser trabeculoplasty, *Ann Ophthalmol* 17:33, 1985.

383. Fishman GRA, Anderson R: Nevus of Ota: report of two cases, one with open angle glaucoma, *Am J Ophthalmol* 54:453, 1962.

384. Foulks GN, Shields MB: Glaucoma in oculodermal melanocytosis, *Ann Ophthalmol* 9:1299, 1977.

385. Futa R, Shimizu T, Okura F, Yasutake T: A case of open-angle glaucoma associated with nevus of Ota: electron microscopic study of the anterior chamber angle and iris, *Folia Ophthalmol Jpn* 35:501, 1984.

386. Kaufman HE: Primary familial amyloidosis, *Arch Ophthalmol* 60:1036, 1958.

387. Paton D, Duke JR: Primary familial amyloidosis (ocular manifestations with histopathologic observations), *Am J Ophthalmol* 61:736, 1966.

388. Plane C, and others: Manifestations oculaires de l'amylose Portugaise de Corino de Andrade, *Bull Soc Ophtalmol Fr* 77:123, 1977.

389. Kivela T, and others: Ocular amyloid deposition in familial amyloidosis, Finnish: an analysis of native and variant gelsolin in Meretoja's syndrome, *Invest Ophthalmol Vis Sci* 35:3759, 1994.

390. Silva-Araujo AC, and others: Aqueous outflow system in familial amyloidotic polyneuropathy, Portuguese type, *Graefes Arch Clin Exp Ophthalmol* 231:131, 1993.

391. Meretoja J: Comparative histological and clinical findings in eyes with lattice corneal dystrophy of two different types, *Ophthalmologica* 165:15, 1972.

392. Shimazaki J, and others: Long-term follow-up of patients with familial subepithelial amyloidosis of the cornea, *Ophthalmology* 102:139, 1995.

393. Schwartz MF, and others: An unusual case of ocular involvement in primary systemic nonfamilial amyloidosis, *Ophthalmology* 98:394, 1982.

394. Epstein DL: *Chandler and Grant's glaucoma,* Philadelphia, 1986, Lea & Febiger.

395. Kupfer C: Pseudofacility in the human eye, *Trans Am Ophthalmol Soc* 69:383, 1971.

396. Kupfer C, Ross K: Studies of aqueous humor dynamics in man: I. Measurements in young normal subjects, *Invest Ophthalmol Vis Sci* 10:518, 1971.

397. Friberg TR, and others: Intraocular and episcleral venous pressure increase during inverted posture, *Am J Ophthalmol* 103:523, 1987.

398. Barany EH: The influence of extraocular venous pressure on outflow facility in *Cercopithecus ethiops* and *Macaca fascicularis, Invest Ophthalmol Vis Sci* 17:711, 1978.

399. Minas TF, Podos SM: Familial glaucoma associated with elevated episcleral venous pressure, *Arch Ophthalmol* 80:201, 1968.

400. Kollarits CR, and others: Management of a patient with orbital varices, visual loss and ipsilateral glaucoma, *Ophthalmic Surg* 8:54,1977.

401. DeKeiyer RJW: Spontaneous carticocavernous fistulas: the importance of the typical limbal vascular loops for the diagnosis, the recognition of glaucoma and the use of conservative therapy in this condition, *Doc Ophthalmol* 46:403, 1979.

402. Lockich JJ, Goodman R: Superior vena cava syndrome, *JAMA* 231:58, 1975.

403. Meister FL, and others: Urokinase: a cost-effective alternative treatment of superior vena cava thrombosis and obstruction, *Arch Intern Med* 149:1209, 1989.

404. Downes AJ, and others: Intimal sarcoma of the superior vena cava, *Postgrad Med J* 69:155, 1993.

405. Alfano JE, Alfano PA: Glaucoma and the superior vena cava obstruction syndrome, *Am J Ophthalmol* 42:685, 1956.

406. Brolin ES: Ocular tension changes imposed by rapid intentionally varied venous pressure in a case of pulmonary tumor, *Acta Ophthalmol Scand* 27:394, 1949.

407. Yablonski ME, Podos SM: *Glaucoma secondary to elevated episcleral venous pressure.* In Ritch R, Shields MB, editors: *The secondary glaucomas,* St Louis, 1982, Mosby.

408. Robinson I, Jackson J: New approach to superior vena caval obstruction [clinical conference], *BMJ* 308:1697, 1994.

409. Wiersinga WM, and others: Temporal relationship between onset of Graves' ophthalmopathy and onset of thyroidal Graves' disease, *J Endocrinol Invest* 11:615, 1988.

410. Wall JR, and others: Pathogenesis of thyroid-associated ophthalmopathy: an autoimmune disorder of the eye muscle associated with Graves' hyperthyroidism and Hashimoto's thyroiditis, *Clin Immunol Immunopathol* 68:1, 1993.

411. Currie ZI, and others: Dysthyroid eye disease masquerading as glaucoma, *Ophthalmic Physiol Opt* 11:176, 1991.

412. Kendall-Taylor P, and others: Intravenous methylprednisolone in the treatment of Graves' ophthalmopathy *BMJ* 297: 1574, 1988.

413. Leone CR Jr, and others: Medial and lateral wall decompression for thyroid ophthalmopathy, *Am J Ophthalmol* 108:160, 1989.

414. Sandler HM, and others: Results of radiotherapy for thyroid ophthalmopathy, *Int J Radiat Oncol Biol Phys* 17:823, 1989.

415. Burch HB, Wartofsky L: Graves' ophthalmopathy: current concepts regarding pathogenesis and management, *Endocr Rev* 14:747, 1993.

416. Girod DA, and others: Orbital decompression for preservation of vision in Graves' ophthalmopathy, *Arch Otolaryngol Head Neck Surg* 119:229, 1993.

417. Trokel S, and others: Orbital fat removal: decompression for Graves orbitopathy, *Ophthalmology* 100:674, 1993.

418. Lyons CJ, Rootman J: Orbital decompression for disfiguring exophthalmos in thyroid orbitopathy, *Ophthalmology* 101:223, 1994.

419. Spencer WH, Thompson HS, Hoyt W: Ischaemic ocular necrosis from carotid-cavernous fistula, *Br J Ophthalmol* 57:145, 1973.

420. Keiser GJ, and others: Carotid cavernous fistula after minimal facial trauma: report of a case, *Oral Surg Oral Med Oral Pathol Oral Radiol Endod* 71:549, 1991.

421. Kim JK, and others: Traumatic bilateral carotid-cavernous fistulas treated with detachable balloon: a case report, *Acta Radiol* 37:46, 1996.

422. Brosnahan D, and others: Neuro-ophthalmic features of carotid cavernous fistulas and their treatment by endoarterial balloon embolisation, *J Neurol Neurosurg Psychiatry* 55:553, 1992.

423. Acierno MD, and others: Painful oculomotor palsy caused by posterior-draining dural carotid cavernous fistulas, *Arch Ophthalmol* 113:1045, 1995.

424. Martin TJ, and others: Left dural to right cavernous sinus fistula: a case report, *J Neuroophthalmol* 15:31, 1995.

425. Sugar HS, Meyer SJ: Pulsating exophthalmos, *Arch Ophthalmol* 23:1288, 1939.

426. Harris GT, Rice PR: Angle closure in carotid-cavernous fistula, *Ophthalmology* 86:1512, 1979.

427. Sanders M, Hoyt W: Hypoxic ocular sequelae of carotid-cavernous fistulae: study of the causes of visual failure before and after neurosurgical treatment in a series of 25 cases, *Br J Ophthalmol* 53:82, 1969.

428. Barker FGN, and others: Transethmoidal transsphenoidal approach for embolization of a carotid-cavernous fistula: case report, *J Neurosurg* 81:921, 1994.

429. Lewis AI, and others: Management of 100 consecutive direct carotid-cavernous fistulas: results of treatment with detachable balloons: *Neurosurgery* 36:239, 1995.

430. Teng MM, and others: Embolization of carotid cavernous fistula by means of direct puncture through the superior orbital fissure, *Radiology* 194:705, 1995.

431. Goldberg RA, and others: Management of cavernous sinus-dural fistula: indications and techniques for primary embolization via the superior ophthalmic vein, *Arch Ophthalmol* 114:707, 1996.

432. Keltner JL, and others: Dural and carotid cavernous sinus fistulas: diagnosis, management, and complications, *Ophthalmology* 94:1585, 1987.

433. Grove AS Jr: The dural shunt syndrome: pathophysiology and clinical course, *Ophthalmology* 90:31, 1983.

434. Harbison JW, Guerry D, Wiesenger H: Dural arteriovenous fistula and spontaneous choroidal detachment: new cause of an old disease, *Br J Ophthalmol* 62:483,1978.

435. Phelps CD, Thompson HS, Ossoinig KC: The diagnosis and prognosis of atypical carotid-cavernous fistula (red-eyed shunt syndrome), *Am J Ophthalmol* 93:423, 1982.

436. Fiore PM, and others: The dural shunt syndrome. I. Management of glaucoma *Ophthalmology* 97:56, 1990.

437. Wagner RS, and others: Trabeculectomy with cyclocryotherapy for infantile glaucoma in the Sturge-Weber syndrome, *Ann Ophthalmol* 20:289, 1988.

438. Iwach AG, and others: Analysis of surgical and medical management of glaucoma in Sturge-Weber syndrome, *Ophthalmology* 97:904, 1990.

439. Sullivan TJ, and others: The ocular manifestations of the Sturge-Weber syndrome, *J Pediatr Ophthalmol Strabismus* 29:349, 1992.

440. Sujansky E, Conradi S: Outcome of Sturge-Weber syndrome in 52 adults, *Am J Med Genet* 57:35, 1995.

441. Phelps CD: The pathogenesis of glaucoma in Sturge-Weber syndrome, *Ophthalmology* 85:276, 1978.

442. Lanzl IM, and others: Unilateral open-angle glaucoma secondary to idiopathic dilated episcleral vein, *Am J Ophthalmol* 121:587, 1996.

443. Benedikt O, Roll P: Dilation and tortuosity of episcleral vessels in open-angle glaucoma. I. Clinical picture, *Klin Monatsbl Augenheilkd* 176:292, 1980.

444. Bigger JF: Glaucoma with elevated episcleral venous pressure, *South Med J* 68:1444, 1975.

445. Radius RL, Maumenee AE: Dilated episcleral vessels and open-angle glaucoma, *Am J Ophthalmol* 86:31, 1978.

446. Kandarakis A, and others: The effect of nitrates on intraocular pressure in Sturge Weber syndrome, *Glaucoma* 7:120, 1985.

446. Talusan ED, Fishbein SL, Schwartz B: Increased pressure of dilated episcleral veins with open-angle glaucoma without exophthalmos, *Ophthalmology* 90:257, 1983.

447. Bellows RA, and others: Choroidal effusion during glaucoma surgery in patients with prominent episcleral vessels, *Arch Ophthalmol* 97:493,1979.

448. Christensen GR, Records RE: Glaucoma and expulsive hemorrhage mechanisms in the Sturge-Weber syndrome, *Ophthalmology* 86:1360, 1979.

or a pseudophakos. When this occurs it is important to suppress inflammation with topical, periocular, and systemic corticosteroid therapy. If pupillary block is contributing to the glaucoma, a laser iridectomy or surgical iridectomy should be performed. These eyes are among the few in which a YAG laser iridectomy may close. Residual glaucoma is then treated with medical therapy and filtering surgery as required. Argon laser trabeculoplasty may be attempted, but results have been mixed.[21,22]

Neovascular Glaucoma After Central Retinal Vein Occlusion

It is possible to find underlying open-angle glaucoma in eyes that develop neovascular glaucoma after ischemic central retinal vein occlusions.[23,24] Chronic elevations of IOP may impede vascular flow to the eye and cause secondary degeneration in the blood vessels of the optic nerve. When faced with this situation, the physician should rapidly perform panretinal photocoagulation or cryoablation to cause regression of the new vessels and save open portions of the angle from being obliterated by the fibrovascular membrane.[25] Residual glaucoma is treated with medical therapy, goniophotocoagulation, and filtering surgery as needed.[26] Fellow eyes should also be checked carefully for signs of open-angle glaucoma.

PRIMARY ANGLE-CLOSURE GLAUCOMA WITH TRABECULAR DAMAGE

Following acute, subacute, or chronic angle-closure glaucoma, tonographic facility of outflow may be much poorer than would be expected from the appearance of the angle; that is, outflow facility may be very low despite an open angle with minimal or no peripheral anterior synechiae. In the absence of tonographic data this is seen as an elevated IOP even after the angle-closure component of the glaucoma has been eliminated. It is postulated that apposition between the iris and the trabecular meshwork damages the outflow channels even in the absence of permanent adhesions. A patient in this situation should have a laser iridectomy if one is not already present. The IOP usually falls somewhat after iridectomy but may remain elevated above the acceptable range. Residual glaucoma is then treated with medical therapy, argon laser trabeculoplasty, and filtering surgery as required.

SECONDARY OPEN-ANGLE GLAUCOMA WITH SUPERIMPOSED SECONDARY ANGLE-CLOSURE GLAUCOMA

Idiopathic, uveitic, or posttraumatic inflammation can damage the trabecular meshwork, leading to secondary open-angle glaucoma. If intraocular inflammation recurs, peripheral anterior synechiae and secondary angle-closure glaucoma can develop with or without pupillary block. In these situations it is important to suppress active inflammation with topical, periocular, and systemic corticosteroid therapy. In chronic uveitis the steroid therapy itself can be the cause of secondary open-angle glaucoma. Uncontrolled inflammation can lead to secondary angle-closure glaucoma as well. The physician is faced with the dilemma of increasing the steroid dosage to try to control the inflammation—which may worsen the secondary open-angle glaucoma—or decreasing the steroid dose only to have inflammation close the angle further.

Cytotoxic agents may be a reasonable alternative for controlling uveitis in some steroid-responsive patients.[32] If posterior synechiae are forming, they should be broken by vigorous pupillary dilation. In some cases a laser or surgical iridectomy is required to eliminate any element of pupillary block. When the inflammatory process subsides, residual glaucoma is treated with medical therapy, argon laser trabeculoplasty, and filtering surgery as required.

PRIMARY OPEN-ANGLE GLAUCOMA WITH SUPERIMPOSED SECONDARY OPEN-ANGLE GLAUCOMA

An individual with POAG may develop any form of secondary open-angle glaucoma as well, such as secondary glaucoma from trauma or inflammation. One interesting variant of this situation is the patient who has apparent unilateral secondary open-angle glaucoma but also has a borderline IOP and outflow facility in the fellow eye. The fellow eye may eventually develop POAG without any contribution from the factor that precipitated glaucoma in the first eye. This suggests that the patient had an underlying tendency to develop POAG in both eyes and that the trauma or inflammation superimposed a secondary form of glaucoma in the initially affected eye. This concept is supported by studies that demonstrate increased corticosteroid responsiveness in the fellow eyes of patients with apparent unilateral, posttraumatic, angle-recession glaucoma[33] and the high incidence of abnormal outflow facility (56%) in the fellow eyes of patients with unilateral acute uveitis and ocular hypertension.[34] In this situation glaucoma is managed as in any other form of open-angle glaucoma, using medical therapy, argon laser trabeculoplasty, and filtering surgery as needed. Physicians should watch carefully the fellow eyes of patients who have what appears to be unilateral secondary open-angle glaucoma.

ELEVATED EPISCLERAL VENOUS PRESSURE CAUSING SECONDARY IMPAIRMENT OF OUTFLOW FACILITY

A variety of conditions, including thyroid ophthalmopathy, carotid–cavernous fistula, and Sturge-Weber syndrome, are associated with increased episcleral venous pressure and secondary glaucoma (see Chapter 18). Typically the tonographic facility of outflow in an affected eye is normal because the obstruction to aqueous humor flow lies beyond the trabecular meshwork. In a few eyes, however, the facility of outflow diminishes over time despite open angles and the absence of neovascular glaucoma. Investigators postulate that the decline in outflow facility represents secondary trabecular damage from chronically elevated episcleral venous pressure.[27,28] It may be difficult to determine whether the decreased outflow facility in a given patient is caused by the effects of increased episcleral venous pressure rather than by the effects of age or by the coincident development of POAG. Nevertheless the progressive decline in outflow facility in eyes with increased episcleral venous pressure seems to occur more often than would be predicted by chance. In many cases the impaired outflow facility persists after treatment has reduced episcleral venous pressure to normal levels.

Some patients with secondary glaucoma and elevated episcleral venous pressure have underlying diseases that are amenable to treatment. Following such treatment the residual glaucoma can be managed with medical therapy, argon laser trabeculoplasty, and filtering surgery as needed. In other cases treatment of the underlying disease is difficult or dangerous. IOP is best reduced by drugs that act on aqueous humor production, such as topical β-adrenergic antagonists and systemic carbonic anhydrase inhibitors. Miotic agents and argon laser trabeculoplasty are less effective in reducing IOP in this situation, although they are somewhat helpful if there is a reduction in outflow facility.

Some patients with increased episcleral venous pressure and glaucoma eventually require filtering surgery. The physician must be wary, however, because intraocular surgery in these eyes is associated with a high rate of complications, including bleeding, uveal effusion, and a flat anterior chamber.[28-31] Some of these complications can be prevented by performing posterior sclerotomies in one or two quadrants before opening the eye.[29]

REFERENCES

1. Firoiu I: [Mixed glaucoma: a separate entity?], *Oftalmologia* 34:27, 1990.
2. Teikari J, O'Donnell J: Epidemiologic data on adult glaucomas, *Acta Opthalmologica* 67:184, 1989.
3. Wilson MR: Epidemiologic features of glaucoma, *Int Opthalmol Clin* 30:153, 1990.
4. Congdon N, Wang F, Trelsh J: Issues in the epidemology and population-based screening of primary angle-closure glaucoma, *Surv Ophthalmol* 36:411, 1992.
5. Shiose Y, and others: Epidemiology of glaucoma in Japan–a nationwide glaucoma survey, *Jpn J Ophthalmol* 35:133, 1991.
6. Abrams JD: Mixed glaucoma, *Br J Ophthalmol* 45:503, 1961.
7. Hyams WE, Keroub C, Pokotilo E: Mixed glaucoma, *Br J Ophthalmol* 61:105, 1977.
8. Lowe R: Acute angle-closure glaucoma precipitated by miotics plus adrenaline eyedrops, *Med J Aust* 2:1037, 1966.
9. Langerhorst CT, and others: Effect of peripheral iridectomy on intraocular pressure in chronic primary angle closure glaucoma, *Doc Ophthalmol* 85:51, 1993.
10. Wang N, and others: Mechanism and etiology of primary chronic angle closure glaucoma, *Yen Ko Hsueh Pao* 10:186, 1994.
11. Wand M, Grant WM: Thymoxamine test: differentiating, angle-closure glaucoma from open-angle glaucoma with narrow angles, *Arch Ophthalmol* 96:1009, 1978.
12. McGalliard JN, Wishart PK: The effect of Nd: YAG iridotomy on intraocular pressure in hypertensive eyes with shallow anterior chambers, *Eye* 4(Pt6):823, 1990.
13. Abramson DH, and others: Pilocarpine-induced lens changes: an ultrasonic biometric evaluation of dose responses, *Arch Ophthalmol* 92:464, 1974.
14. Abramson DH, and others: Pilocarpine: effect on the anterior chamber and lens thickness, *Arch Ophthalmol* 87:615, 1972.
15. Lowe RF: Persistent symptoms after peripheral iridectomy for angle-closure glaucoma, *Aust N Z J Ophthalmol* 15:83, 1987.
16. Ritch R: *Glaucoma secondary to lens intumescence and dislocation.* In Ritch R, Shields MB, editors: *The secondary glaucomas,* St Louis, 1982, Mosby.

17. Richardson LE: Argon laser trabeculoplasty: a review, *J Am Optom Assoc* 63: 252, 1992.
18. Rouhiainen HJ, and others: Peripheral anterior synechiae formation after trabeculoplasty, *Arch Ophthalmol* 106:189, 1988.
19. Wilensky JT, Weinreb RN: Early and later failure of argon laser trabeculoplasty, *Arch Ophthalmol* 101:895, 1983.
20. West RH: The effect of topical corticosteroids on laser-induced peripheral anterior synechiae, *Aust N Z J Ophthalmol* 20:305, 1992.
21. Shirakashi M, and others: Argon laser trabeculoplasty for chronic angle-closure glaucoma uncontrolled by iridotomy, *Acta Ophthalmol Scand* 67:265, 1989.
22. Wishart PK: Argon laser trabeculoplasty in narrow angle glaucoma, *Eye* 1(Pt 5):567, 1987.

23. Bertelson TI: The relationship between thrombosis in the retinal vein and primary glaucoma, *Acta Ophthalmol* 39:603, 1961.
24. Dryden RM: Central retinal vein occlusion and chronic simple glaucoma, *Arch Ophthalmol* 73:659, 1965.
25. Duker JS, Brown GC: The efficacy of panretinal photocoagulation for neovascularization of the iris after central retinal artery obstruction, *Ophthalmology* 96:92, 1989.
26. Katz LJ, Spaeth GL: Surgical management of the secondary glaucomas: part I, *Ophthalmic Surg* 18:826, 1987.
27. Minas TF, Podos SM: Familial glaucoma associated with elevated episcleral venous pressure, *Arch Ophthalmol* 80:201, 1968.
28. Yablonski ME, Podos SM: *Glaucoma secondary to elevated episcleral venous pressure.* In Ritch R, Shields MB, editors: *The secondary glaucomas,* St Louis, 1982, Mosby.

29. Bellows RA, and others: Choroidal effusion during glaucoma surgery in patients with prominent episcleral vessels, *Arch Ophthalmol* 97:493, 1979.
30. Bigger JF: Glaucoma with elevated episcleral venous pressure, *South Med J* 68: 1444, 1975.
31. Christensen GR, Records RE: Glaucoma and expulsive hemorrhage mechanism in the Sturge-Weber syndrome, *Ophthalmology* 86:1360, 1979.
32. Shah SS, and others: Low-dose methotrexate therapy for ocular inflammatory disease, *Ophthalmology* 99:1419, 1992.
33. Spaeth GL: Traumatic hyphema, angle recession, dexamethasone hypertension, and glaucoma, *Arch Ophthalmol* 78:714, 1967.
34. Calugaru M: [Factors determining the occurrence of intraocular hypertension in uveitis], *J Fr Ophthalmol* 10:233, 1987.

20

Developmental and Childhood Glaucoma

The developmental glaucomas are a group of disorders characterized by improper development of the eye's aqueous outflow system. Although the glaucoma may not manifest itself until adulthood, most developmental glaucomas are seen in infancy and childhood. Glaucoma in the infant is an uncommon disease, but the impact on visual development can be significant. Early recognition of and appropriate therapy for the glaucoma can significantly improve a child's visual future. Preservation of any vision during a child's formative years is important, even if, in severe cases, the vision is ultimately lost.

The childhood glaucomas are divided into three major categories: (1) primary congenital glaucoma, in which the developmental anomaly is restricted to a maldevelopment of the trabecular meshwork; (2) glaucoma associated with other ocular or systemic congenital anomalies; and (3) glaucoma secondary to other ocular diseases, such as inflammation, trauma, or tumors.

TERMINOLOGY

Previously, the terminology of the glaucomas affecting infants was inconsistent and, at times, confusing. More precise terminology has arisen with developments in the field and should be used whenever possible.

The term *developmental glaucoma* refers to those glaucomas associated with developmental anomalies that are present at birth, including primary congenital glaucoma and glaucoma associated with other developmental anomalies, either ocular or systemic.

- *Congenital glaucoma* is a term synonymous with developmental glaucoma. Secondary glaucoma in infants refers to glaucoma resulting from acquired ocular diseases.
- *Primary congenital glaucoma* is a specific term referring to eyes that have an isolated maldevelopment of the trabecular meshwork without other developmental ocular anomalies or diseases that can raise intraocular pressure (IOP).
- *Infantile glaucoma* is a term that has been used in a variety of contexts. Some use this term as a synonym for primary congenital glaucoma, whereas others apply it to any glaucoma occurring during the first several years of life. Its meaning, therefore, should be specified or its use avoided. Primary infantile glaucoma is synonymous with primary congenital glaucoma.
- *Juvenile glaucoma* is a nonspecific term referring to any type of glaucoma occurring later in childhood (after 5 years of age) and through the third to fourth decades. Sometimes a syndrome is implied and is associated with myopia, autosomal dominant family history, and characteristic clinical course; this condition has been linked to the short arm of the first (1q) human chromosome.[1-3]
- *Buphthalmos* and *hydrophthalmia* are archaic descriptive terms. Buphthalmos literally means "ox eye" and refers to the marked enlargement that can result from any type of glaucoma present in infancy. Hydrophthalmia refers to the high fluid content of buphthalmic eyes (Fig. 20-1).

Box 20-1
Syndrome Classification of Congenital Glaucoma

I. Primary glaucoma
  A. Congenital open-angle glaucoma
    1. Presenting age: 0 to 5 years
    2. Later recognized
  B. Autosomal dominant juvenile glaucoma
  C. Glaucoma associated with systemic abnormalities
    1. Axenfeld-Rieger syndrome
    2. Chromosomal disorders
    3. Congenital rubella
    4. Fetal alcohol syndrome
    5. Mucopolysaccharidosis
    6. Neurofibromatosis
    7. Oculocerebrorenal (Lowe) syndrome
    8. Hepatocerebrorenal (Zellweger) syndrome
    9. Oculodermal vascular malformations
      a. Sturge-Weber syndrome
      b. Klippel-Trenaunay-Weber syndrome
      c. Oculodermal melanocytosis
      d. Phakomatosis pigmentovascularis
      e. Cutis marmorata telangiectasia congenita
    10. Prader-Willi syndrome
    11. Rubenstein-Taybi (broad-thumb) syndrome
    12. Pierre Robin and Stickler syndromes
    13. Skeletal dysplastic syndromes
      a. Kniest syndrome
      b. Michel syndrome
      c. Oculodentodigital syndrome
  D. Glaucoma associated with ocular abnormalities
    1. Aniridia
    2. Axenfeld-Rieger syndrome
    3. Congenital ectropion uveae
    4. Congenital hereditary endothelial dystrophy
    5. Microcornea syndromes
    6. Familial iris hypoplasia
    7. Peters syndrome
    8. Posterior polymorphous dystrophy
    9. Sclerocornea
II. Secondary glaucoma
  A. Traumatic glaucoma
    1. Acute-onset
      a. Hyphema and angle recession
      b. Lens debris or vitreal blockade of trabeculum

Data from Shaffer RN, Weiss DI: *Congenital and pediatric glaucomas,* St Louis, 1970, Mosby and Walton DS: *Childhood glaucoma.* In Roy FH, editor: *Master techniques in ophthalmic surgery,* Baltimore, 1995, Williams and Wilkins.

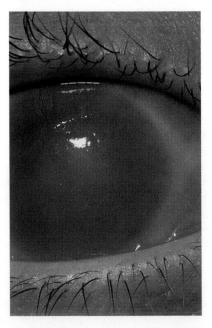

Figure 20-1   Advanced developmental glaucoma with extensive enlargement and scarring of the cornea. The anterior segment structures are not visible. This is classic buphthalmos.

Box 20-1
Syndrome Classification of Congenital Glaucoma—cont'd

II. Secondary glaucoma—cont'd
  B. Glaucoma secondary to intraocular
    neoplasm
    1. Retinoblastoma
    2. Juvenile xanthogranuloma
    3. Leukemia
    4. Iris rhabdomyosarcoma
  C. Uveitic glaucoma
    1. Open-angle
    2. Angle-closure
      a. Synechial closure
      b. Iris bombé with pupillary block
  D. Lens-induced glaucoma
    1. Subluxation–dislocation with pupillary
      block
      a. Marfan syndrome
      b. Homocystinuria
    2. Spherophakia with pupillary block
      a. Weill-Marchesani syndrome
        (autosomal recessive)
      b. GEMSS syndrome (autosomal
        dominant)
  E. Glaucoma after congenital cataract surgery
    1. Chronic open-angle (aphakic or
      pseudophakic)
    2. Lens debris or uveitic blockade of
      trabeculum
    3. Pupillary blockade
  F. Steroid-induced glaucoma

  G. Neovascular glaucoma
    1. Retinoblastoma
    2. Coats' disease
    3. Medulloepithelioma
    4. Familial exudative vitreoretinopathy
  H. Secondary angle-closure glaucoma
    1. Retinopathy of prematurity
    2. Microphthalmos
    3. Nanophthalmos
    4. Retinoblastoma
    5. Persistent hyperplastic primary vitreous
    6. Congenital pupillary–iris lens
      membrane
    7. Aniridia
    8. Iridoschisis
    9. Cornea plana
  I. Glaucoma with increased episcleral venous
    pressure
    1. Sturge-Weber syndrome
    2. Idiopathic or familial elevated epi-
      scleral venous pressure
    3. Orbital vascular malformations
  J. Glaucoma secondary to intraocular
    infections
    1. Acute recurrent toxoplasmosis
    2. Acute herpetic iritis
    3. Opportunistic infections seen with
      AIDS
    4. Congenital rubella

CLASSIFICATION

Syndrome Classification

The developmental glaucomas have been classified in various ways (Box 20-1).[4-11] The Shaffer-Weiss classification is based on syndromes that divide patients into those with primary congenital glaucoma, glaucoma associated with other congenital ocular or systemic anomalies, and secondary glaucomas in infants.[8]

PRIMARY GLAUCOMA

Because not all cases fit precisely into a specific syndrome, an anatomic classification of these glaucomas has been developed.[5,6] These findings have been grouped according to their clinical manifestations rather than to categories based on pathogenetic mechanisms or genetic linkage.[12]

Clinical Anatomic Classification

Maldevelopment of the anterior segment is present in all forms of congenital glaucoma. Clinically, gonioscopy and biomicroscopy of the anterior segment provide the crucial information to determine the therapy and prognosis for the infant.[13,14] Maldevelopment of the anterior segment may involve the trabecular meshwork alone or the trabecular meshwork in combination with the iris,

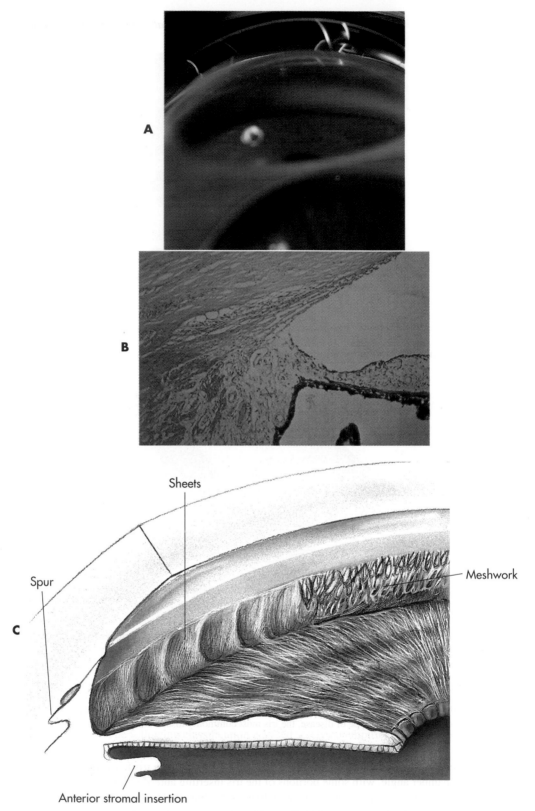

A

B

C

Sheets

Spur

Meshwork

Anterior stromal insertion

Figure 20-5   **A,** Goniophotograph of a young patient with primary congenital glaucoma revealing a flat iris with peripheral thinning and peripheral radial vessels. A high insertion to the level of the scleral spur is not visible above but is visible below. The trabecular meshwork is slightly greyish, and there is no definition to Schwalbe's line. There is no pigmentation within the trabecular meshwork, which is normal for young people. **B,** Histopathology of primary infantile glaucoma. The iris and anterior ciliary body cover the scleral spur and posterior trabecular meshwork. The intratrabecular spaces are compacted. **C,** Concave iris insertion in isolated trabeculodysgenesis. Iris may sweep up over trabecular meshwork as dense sheet or loose syncytium. Glaucoma associated with this type of iris insertion will respond to goniotomy in infants. (**A** from Campbell DG, Netland PN: *Stereo atlas of glaucoma,* St Louis, 1998, Mosby. **B** from Armed Forces Institute of Pathology. In Alward WLM: *Color atlas of gonioscopy,* St Louis, 1994, Mosby.)

anterior flat iris insertion and the "wrap-around" configuration may appear in later "juvenile" forms of open-angle glaucoma through the third or fourth decade of life.[2]

Isolated trabeculodysgenesis must be differentiated from the gonioscopic appearance of the anterior chamber angle in a normal newborn eye. In a normal newborn, a flat insertion of the iris into the angle wall just posterior to the scleral spur is present. The normal angle recess forms during the first 6 to 12 months of life. The ciliary body is seen as a distinct band anterior to this iris insertion. The more narrow the ciliary body band, the more developmentally immature is the angle.[16]

Isolated trabeculodysgenesis usually presents with symptoms of elevated IOP after the first month of life. A key point in the surgical management of glaucoma infants: if examination reveals isolated trabeculodysgenesis, a prompt goniotomy is highly successful.[17]

Iridodysgenesis

Congenital anomalies of the iris are associated with maldevelopment of the trabecular meshwork, the anterior stroma, the full thickness of the iris, the iris vessels, or any combination of these structures. In these disorders the appearance of the trabecular meshwork may be similar to that found in isolated trabeculodysgenesis. In some cases, additional changes may be seen in the angle, such as irregular clumping of tissue, abnormal vessels, or iridocorneal adhesions.

Anterior Stromal Defects

Hypoplasia of the anterior iris stroma is the most common iris defect associated with developmental glaucoma. True hypoplasia of the anterior stroma, as opposed to atrophy or thinning, is diagnosed only when there is clear malformation of the collarette with absence or marked reduction of the crypts. This condition is to be distinguished from the stretching of the iris from elevated IOP, which can thin the anterior stroma. The pupillary sphincter may be quite prominent and can have a distinct ring appearance or a "feathered" outer border (Fig. 20-6; see Fig. 20-32).

Iris hyperplasia causes a thickened, velvety, pebbled appearance of the anterior iris stroma. Hyperplasia is uncommon and is sometimes seen in association with Sturge-Weber syndrome.

Developmental anomalies of the iris vasculature can occur as a persistent tunica vasculosa lentis or as irregularly wandering superficial iris vessels. In persistence of the tunica vasculosa lentis (Fig. 20-7), a regular arrangement of vessels is seen looping into the pupillary axis either in front of or behind the lens. Over time attenuation and involution of the vascular veil occur, and continued clinical surveillance is usually sufficient.

Superficial anomalous iris vessels wander irregularly over the iris surface (Fig. 20-8) and do not conform to the normal radial configuration of the iris vasculature. The pupil is usually distorted, and the iris surface has a whorled appearance, often with areas of hypoplastic anterior iris stroma. Present at birth, it is unclear whether these vessels represent an earlier onset of primary congenital

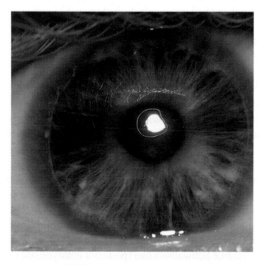

Figure 20-6   Anterior segment photograph of a patient with Axenfeld's anomaly showing a prominent, centrally displaced Schwalbe's ring with peripheral iris attachments. There is iris hypoplasia with loss of iris stroma. (From Campbell DG, Netland PN: *Stereo atlas of glaucoma,* St Louis, 1998, Mosby.)

tinct ring around the pupil. Glaucoma may occur at any time from birth until late adulthood; the striking iris appearance correlates with eventual glaucoma in 100% of cases. Childhood cases respond well to goniotomy or trabeculotomy. Cases with later onset have been managed successfully with medical therapy, argon laser trabeculoplasty, trabeculotomy, or trabeculectomy.

Its hereditary pattern is autosomal dominant.[138] Recent studies have found genetic linkage of iris hypoplasia to the Rieger's syndrome locus at 4q25,[139] but this association is not consistent.[140] Moreover, there is little overlap of anterior segment findings between classic Rieger's syndrome and iris hypoplasia. This is of interest because it illustrates that there may be a significant difference in the *clinical* classification of the developmental glaucomas (i.e., autosomal dominant iris hypoplasia and autosomal dominant juvenile glaucoma share a common clinical presentation but different chromosomal defects) and the *genetic* associations discovered by molecular biology (i.e., iris hypoplasia and Rieger's syndrome are linked on chromosome 4 but appear very different from one another).[12]

Developmental Glaucoma With Anomalous Superficial Iris Vessels

Irregularly wandering superficial iris vessels with distortion or absence of the superficial iris stroma and distortion of the pupil are commonly seen in newborn children with glaucoma (see Fig. 20-8). The cornea usually is hazy, and the vessels may be difficult to see. These vessels can be differentiated easily from the normal radial iris vessels, which are straight and have no associated distortion of the iris tissue. The normal radial iris vessels frequently are visible at birth, before the anterior stroma and its pigmentation have developed completely.

Superficial anomalous iris vessels in children are usually bilateral and resistant to therapy. Early trabeculotomy offers the most hope. Goniotomy can be performed in the least cloudy eye during the same surgery. If the cornea has not cleared dramatically, trabeculotomy or goniotomy should be repeated after 3 or 4 weeks.

Most of these eyes require multiple surgeries and long-term medical therapy. With aggressive management, many can be saved, although vision is rarely normal.

Aniridia

Aniridia (Fig. 20-24) is a bilateral congenital anomaly in which there is profound hypoplasia of the iris in frequent association with multiple ocular anomalies, such as peripheral corneal pannus and keratopathy, foveal hypoplasia, diffuse retinal dysfunction as seen on electroretinography, impaired acuity with nystagmus, cataract and ectopia lentis, and optic nerve hypoplasia.[141] The combination of these defects usually causes a formidable barrier to normal visual function. In addition, 50% to 75% of aniridics develop glaucoma.[142]

Two thirds of patients with aniridia have an affected parent (autosomal dominant form) and one

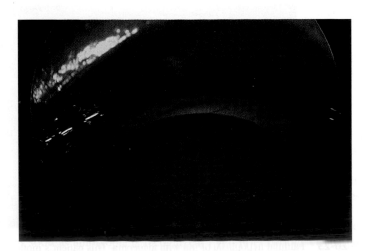

Figure 20-24   Edge of lens seen in aniridia shows absence of iris. Epithelial keratopathy is clearly visible in lower nasal portion, and a dense cataract is dislocated superiorly.

third represent isolated new mutations.[12] In these sporadic cases, approximately 20% of patients have been found to have Wilms tumor as part of the multisystem WAGR syndrome (Wilms' tumor + aniridia + genitourinary anomalies + retardation).[139] Thus aniridic children without a family history require comanagement with a pediatrician for surveillance of neoplasm and other complications.

The genetic locus of this syndrome for both the sporadic and familial forms is a mutation of the PAX6 gene on the 11p13 chromosome.[143,144] Curiously this is the same defective gene seen in one case of Peter's anomaly, although the two clinical syndromes are usually distinct and show little overlap.[12,145]

Although the defective iris is readily apparent at birth, in most cases glaucoma does not develop until later childhood or early adulthood and sometimes does not develop at all.[146] In the less frequent infantile onset cases, the glaucoma is thought to be due to a trabeculodysgenic anomaly of the anterior chamber angle. Because large corneas are rarely seen in aniridic glaucoma, the IOP elevation is presumed to occur at a later developmental stage, usually after age 5 and often into adolescence. Walton[142] directly correlates the severity of the glaucoma with the extent of progressive synechial angle closure by the pulled-up residual iris stump.[146a]

The iris is never completely absent; it may vary from being fairly well developed in some areas to being only a rudimentary stump in others. Most commonly, the anterior stroma sweeps up and over the meshwork like concave trabeculodysgenesis.

Corneal dystrophy initially presents as a circumferential and peripheral opacification of the epithelial and subepithelial layers, with vessels advancing into these areas from the limbus. Over many years, this pannus can extend centrally and eventually completely opacify the cornea.

Cataracts develop in most aniridic patients, and the lens may be displaced, with a segmental absence of zonules. Foveal hypoplasia is present in most cases and is clinically appreciated by the appearance of meandering small retinal vessels in what should be the normal avascular zone of the macular region. Vision is usually limited to no better than 20/200, with an accompanying pendular nystagmus. Cases of families with aniridia but normal macular development, no nystagmus, and good vision do occur, which implies that the foveal hypoplasia is genetically determined rather than acquired as a result of light damage from lack of iris tissue.[147]

If the glaucoma occurs in infancy, a trabeculotomy is the procedure of choice because goniotomies are usually unsuccessful.[142] In older children, medical therapy is indicated as the initial treatment. Surgical complications include direct lens injury and lens or vitreous incarceration in filtration sites; these problems are considerably reduced with the use of intracameral viscoelastic at the time of surgery.

Preventive goniotomy to prevent progressive adherence of the peripheral iris to the trabecular meshwork has been proposed by Walton,[148] with 32 of 34 treated eyes retaining normal IOPs over a long-term follow-up. However, such a prophylactic maneuver is still investigational. Many such patients with mild IOP elevations may be well managed by medicines alone. In cases of failed trabecular surgery, glaucoma implants (e.g., Molteno) or ciliodestructive procedures have been used, often with more than two procedures per eye required.[149]

The cornea may become sufficiently opaque so that penetrating keratoplasty is needed, although the visual results are marginal (one to two lines improvement in Snellen acuity).[150] Lens opacification may require cataract extraction. Before operating, however, the ophthalmologist should attempt refraction through the aphakic portion of the pupil if the lens is subluxated. Either extracapsular or phacoemulsification surgery may be used, depending on the stability of the zonules. Cataract extraction can be difficult and often is accompanied by vitreous loss or further deterioration of the cornea. The use of intraocular lens implants in children is an evolving field,[151] and their utility in aniridic eyes is unknown.

Sturge-Weber Syndrome (Encephalofacial Angiomatosis, Encephalotrigeminal Angiomatosis)

Sturge-Weber syndrome[152,153] is seen with a flat facial hemangioma that follows the distribution of the fifth cranial nerve (Fig. 20-25). A meningeal hemangioma, which can produce a seizure disorder in the child, may be present. The meningeal hemangioma may be associated with calcification, which can be revealed by radiographic examination after the child is 1 year of age. The facial hemangioma is usually unilateral but occasionally may be bilateral. Choroidal hemangiomas and episcleral hemangiomas are commonly seen, and leakage from the choroidal hemangioma may cause retinal edema (Fig. 20-26). The genetic transmission of this disease is unclear.

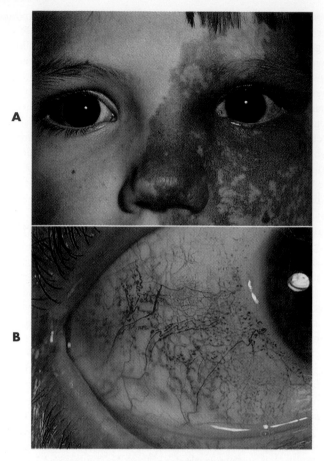

Figure 20-25 Sturge-Weber manifestion on face (**A**) and as a vascular congestion of the episclera (**B**).

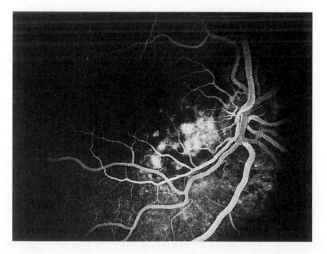

Figure 20-26 Hemangioma of the choroid is almost always present in eyes with Sturge-Weber syndrome. In this case, leakage reduced macular acuity.

Whereas pediatric glaucoma in aniridia can occur as an infantile trabeculodysgenesis but is more likely to occur later as a secondary glaucoma (progressive angle closure), the glaucoma associated with Sturge-Weber syndrome is more likely to appear in infancy and less often manifests in late childhood or adolescence from secondary causes. Sturge-Weber glaucoma is present when the facial hemangioma involves the lids or conjunctiva. Two different mechanisms are thought to be involved. If the glaucoma occurs in infancy, an isolated trabeculodysgenesis type of angle anomaly

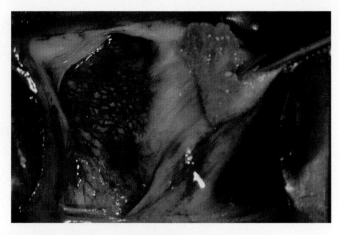

Figure 20-27 Note the dense episcleral anastomosis found in surgery. These were not visible until Tenon's capsule was elevated. Anastomoses can be cauterized easily and usually do not represent a significant bleeding problem at surgery.

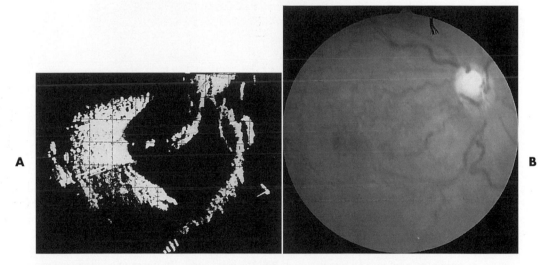

A

B

Figure 20-28 **A,** On opening this eye for trabeculectomy, the anterior chamber collapsed and could not be reformed by injection of balanced salt solution. The flap was closed. Postoperative ultrasonography revealed this large choroidal elevation extending almost to the optic nerve posteriorly. **B,** Serous retinal detachment overlying choroidal expansion in a Sturge-Weber patient following postsurgical choroidal expansion. There was no retinal hole in this patient and the detachment resolved spontaneously.

usually is present. Some claim that this is responsive to goniotomy,[154] whereas others disagree.[142,155] As the child ages, the elevated IOP is due to an elevation of episcleral venous pressure that occurs as a result of arteriovenous shunts through the episcleral hemangiomas (Fig. 20-27).[156-157] In older children, medical therapy is the initial treatment. If medical therapy is unsuccessful, trabeculectomy alone or trabeculectomy combined with trabeculotomy is more likely to succeed than trabeculotomy alone.[154]

In approximately 25% of trabeculectomies, intraoperative or early postoperative choroidal detachment results from a rapid expansion of the choroidal hemangioma with effusion of fluid into the suprachoroidal and subretinal spaces (Fig. 20-28). Careful attention to maintaining a normal-to-high IOP, through the use of an anterior chamber infusion or generous amounts of viscoelastic, may forestall intraoperative complications. The anterior chamber can precipitously flatten and may be impossible to re-form through the surgical site or paracentesis site. Posterior sclerotomy followed by anterior chamber reformation should be performed in an attempt to drain fluid from the suprachoroidal space. Extreme caution is advised: the choroid must not be penetrated because a disastrous hemorrhage could occur.

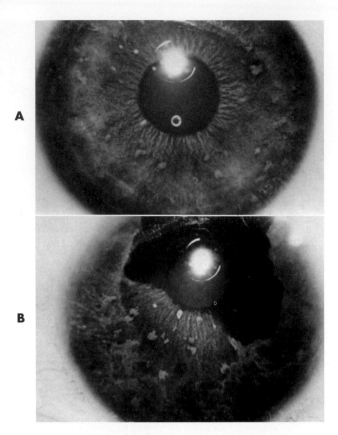

Figure 20-29   A 22-year-old patient with neurofibromatosis. **A,** External appearance of iris nodules. **B,** External view of abnormally pigmented iris.   *Continued*

If these efforts are not fully successful, usually in a few days the expansion subsides as the IOP increases. Repeat filtering surgery can be reconsidered at a later time because the choroidal hemangioma may scar, sometimes enabling the surgeon to successfully perform the procedure without recurrence of the expansion. Some surgeons recommend preplacement of two or three posterior sclerotomies to prevent this anticipated expansion. Similarly the use of a glaucoma valve or shunt, inserting the tube into an eye in which IOP has been carefully maintained by an anterior chamber full of viscoelastic, may be considered as an alternative to a failed filtering surgery.

A recent classification of neural crest disorders that involve episceral vascular malformations plus ocular hyperpigmentation groups together the Sturge-Weber syndrome, Klippel-Trénaunay-Weber syndrome, oculodermal melanocytosis (nevus of Ota), and phakomatosis pigmentovascularis (a combination of oculodermal melanocytosis and nevus flammeus that is found almost exclusively in Asians).[158] When oculodermal melanocytosis and nevus flammeus (phakomatosis pigmentovascularis) occur together, with each extensively involving the globe, there is a strong predisposition for congenital glaucoma. When one or both are present with only partial globe involvement, elevated IOP could develop later in life, and long-term glaucoma surveillance is advised. The vascular malformations appear to play a more important role in the predisposition to glaucoma than the oculodermal melanocytosis.

A related syndrome called cutis marmorata telangiectatica congenita involves periocular vascular anomalies associated either with regional or generalized cutaneous marbling.[159] It has also been associated with infantile trabeculodysgenic glaucoma[160-163] and in one report, with intraoperative suprachoroidal hemorrhage.[150]

Neurofibromatosis (von Recklinghausen's Disease)

Neurofibromatosis (Fig. 20-29) is an autosomal dominant disorder with variable expressivity, manifesting as anomalies of the neuroectoderm and the development of active hamartomas throughout the

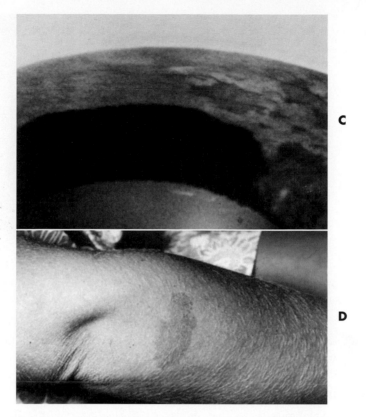

Figure 20-29, cont'd   C, Goniophotograph. Note the round pupil, absence of angle recess, and high iris insertion. **D,** Café au lait spot.

body.[164] The most common form, neurofibromatosis type 1 (NF-1) (von Recklinghausen's disease), has seven possible manifestations, requiring two for diagnosis: six or more large café-au-lait macules; plexiform neurofibromata; inguinal or axillary freckling; optic glioma; Lisch nodules (melanocytic hamartomas of the iris); distinctive osseous lesions of the sphenoid or long bones; and a first-degree relative with NF-1. Neurofibromatosis type 2 is a rarer disorder associated with bilateral acoustic neuromas or other neural proliferative lesions, such as meningioma, schwannoma, and glioma.

Ocular involvement of NF-1 includes neurofibromatous nodules on the iris and eyelids, with ectropion uvea;[165] optic nerve gliomas in as many as 15% of asymptomatic children under age 6;[166] and a variety of complications resulting from mass-occupying lesions in the orbit, such as pulsating exophthalmos to sphenoid bone maldevelopment, herniation of brain tissue into the orbit, or proptosis resulting from optic nerve gliomas. Multiple retinal tumors can be seen, including large retinal astrocytic hamartomas, multiple retinal capillary hemangiomas, and combined hamartomas of the retina and retinal pigment epithelium, resulting in rubeotic glaucoma, vitreous hemorrhage, and retinal detachment.[167]

Glaucoma may appear up to 50% of the time when neurofibromas involve the upper eyelid or the eye itself (Fig. 20-30). The anterior chamber angle may take on several appearances.[168] Isolated trabeculodysgenesis may be evident. Synechial closure caused by neurofibromatous tissue posterior to the iris or neurofibromatous infiltration of the angle itself, which may be accompanied by synechial closure, may be present. A sheet of avascular, opaque, dense tissue may arise from the periphery of the iris and extend anteriorly into the angle. Later onset glaucoma in neurofibromatosis can be associated with unilateral ectropion uvea at the pupillary margin.[142,169,170] Usually there is accompanying unilateral ptosis without a palpable neurofibroma; the pupil appears larger due to the static iris hyperplasia of the central iris pigment epithelium. This form of iris ectropion glaucoma may also appear as a distinct form, independent of NF-1 or other anterior segment anomalies.[171]

The preferred treatment in infants is usually goniotomy, with trabeculotomy recommended if iris adhesions are prominent. In older children, medical therapy should be tried first, followed by the

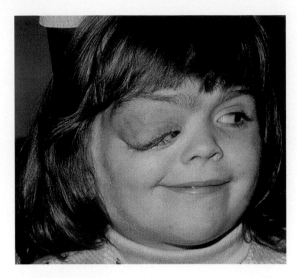

Figure 20-30   Plexiform neuroma of the upper lid in this patient with neurofibromatosis. Eye beneath plexiform neuroma had severe glaucoma that had not been diagnosed.

usual escalation of surgical interventions of trabeculotomy, trabeculectomy with antimetabolites, and glaucoma shunt.

Pierre Robin and Stickler Syndromes

Pierre Robin syndrome was originally characterized by micrognathia, glossoptosis, cleft palate, and cardiac and ocular anomalies.[172] Recent studies emphasize the triad of retrognathia, cleft palate, and respiratory distress both from airway and brainstem abnormalities.[173] Ocular disorders manifest as developmental glaucoma, cataracts, high myopia, retinal detachments, and occasional microphthalmos. There is some overlap of symptoms with Stickler syndrome.[174,175] The glaucoma in both Stickler and Pierre Robin syndromes is due to isolated trabeculodysgenesis, and goniotomy is the preferred initial procedure.

Skeletal Dysplastic Syndromes

This category embraces an enormous variety of systemic abnormalities with variable ocular manifestations that can include trabeculodysgenic infantile glaucoma. Such disorders include Kniest syndrome,[176,177] Michel syndrome,[178] and the oculodentaldigital syndrome.[179]

Corneodysgenesis

Axenfeld's anomaly and Rieger's anomaly and syndrome involve corneodysgenesis of the peripheral (Axenfeld's) and midperipheral (Rieger's) cornea and iris. These disorders appear to represent a spectrum of developmental variations rather than distinctive diseases.[19,180]

Axenfeld's Anomaly

Axenfeld's anomaly (Figs. 20-31 and 20-32) is characterized by a prominent anteriorly displaced Schwalbe's line termed *posterior embryotoxon*. This finding differs from isolated posterior embryotoxon occurring in normal eyes in that in this condition, bands of iris tissue extend across the anterior chamber angle and attach to Schwalbe's line. Some patients have mild hypoplasia of the anterior iris stroma, but more severe defects of the iris are not present. The disease usually is bilateral, and the inheritance pattern is autosomal dominant.

Approximately 50% of patients with Axenfeld's anomaly develop glaucoma. The glaucoma may occur in infancy and responds to goniotomy or trabeculotomy. If it occurs in later childhood, medical therapy should be tried initially, with trabeculotomy or trabeculectomy considered as surgical procedures.

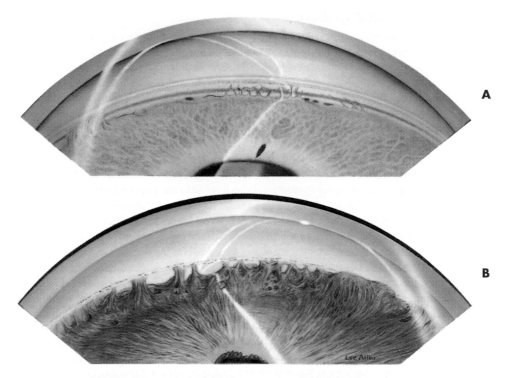

Figure 20-31   **A,** Axenfeld's anomaly. Multiple iris processes have formed between the iris and a prominent Schwalbe's line. There is a broad area of iris adhesion to Schwalbe's line *(left).* **B,** Axenfeld's anomaly with dense iris adhesions that almost completely cover the trabecular meshwork. Particles of pigment are deposited along a very prominent Schwalbe's ring. (From Hermann M, and others: Published courtesy of *Arch Ophthalmol* 53:767, 1955. Copyright the American Medical Association, 1955.)

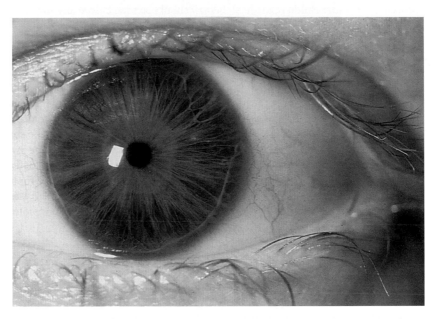

Figure 20-32   Axenfeld's syndrome with peripheral posterior embryotoxon and hypoplasia of anterior stroma. Note the prominent sphincter present with hypoplasia.

180. Shields M, and others: Axenfeld-Rieger syndrome, *Surv Ophthalmol* 29:387, 1985.

181. Weiss JS, and others: Specular microscopy in aniridia, *Cornea* 6:27, 1987.

182. Fitch N, Kaback M: The Axenfeld syndrome and the Rieger syndrome, *J Med Genet* 15:30, 1978.

183. Alward W: *Axenfeld-Rieger syndrome.* In Wiggs JL, editor: *Molecular genetics of ocular disease,* New York, 1995, Wiley-Liss.

184. Legius E, and others: Genetic heterogeneity in Rieger eye malformations, *J Med Genet* 31:340, 1994.

185. Pollack IM, Graue EL: Scanning electron microscopy of congenital corneal leukomas (Peter's anomaly), *Am J Ophthalmol* 88:169, 1979.

186. Heon E, and others: Peters' anomaly: the spectrum of associated ocular and systemic malformations, *Ophthalmic Paediatr Genet* 13:137, 1992.

187. Mayer UM: Peters' anomaly and combination with other malformations (series of 16 patients), *Ophthalmic Paediatr Genet* 13:131, 1992.

188. Traboulsi EI, Maumenee IH: Peters' anomaly and associated congenital malformations, *Arch Ophthalmol* 110:1739, 1992.

189. Thompson EM, and others: Kivlin syndrome and Peters'-plus syndrome: are they the same disorder? *Clin Dysmorphol* 2:301, 1993.

190. Gollamudi SR, and others: Visual outcome after surgery for Peters' anomaly, *Ophthalmic Genet* 15:31, 1994.

191. Cameron JA: Good visual result following early penetrating keratoplasty for Peters' anomaly, *J Pediatr Ophthalmol Strabismus* 30:109, 1993.

191a. Curtin VT, Joyce EE, Ballin N: Ocular pathology in oculo-cerebro-renal syndrome of Lowe, *Am J Ophthalmol* 64:533, 1967.

192. Charnas LR, and others: Clinical and laboratory findings in the oculocerebrorenal syndrome of Lowe, with special reference to growth and renal function, *N Engl J Med* 324:1318, 1991.

193. Charnas LR, Gahl WA: The oculocerebrorenal syndrome of Lowe, *Adv Pediatr* 38:75, 1991.

194. Wadelius C, and others: Lowe oculocerebrorenal syndrome: DNA-based linkage of the gene to Xq24-q26, using tightly linked flanking markers and the correlation to lens examination in carrier diagnosis, *Am J Hum Genet* 44:241, 1989.

195. Nussbaum RL, and others: Physical mapping and genomic structure of the Lowe syndrome gene *OCRL1, Hum Genet* 99:145, 1997.

196. Folz SJ, Trobe JD: The peroxisome and the eye, *Surv Ophthalmol* 35:353, 1991.

197. Weiss AH, and others: Simple microphthalmos, *Arch Ophthalmol* 107:1625, 1989.

198. Chattopadhyay A, and others: Microcornea, glaucoma, and absent frontal sinus, *J Pediatr* 127:333, 1995 (letter).

199. Mills MD, Robb RM: Glaucoma following childhood cataract surgery, *J Pediatr Ophthalmol Strabismus* 31:355, 1994.

200. Wallace DK, Plager DA: Corneal diameter in childhood aphakic glaucoma, *J Pediatr Ophthalmol Strabismus* 33:230, 1996.

201. Givens KT, and others: Congenital rubella syndrome: ophthalmic manifestations and associated systemic disorders, *Br J Ophthalmol* 77:358, 1993.

202. Wolff SM: The ocular manifestations of congenital rubella: a prospective study of 328 cases of congenital rubella, *J Pediatr Ophthalmol* 10:101, 1973.

203. Traboulsi EI, and others: Infantile glaucoma in Down's syndrome (trisomy 21), *Am J Ophthalmol* 105:389, 1988.

204. Izquierdo NJ, and others: Anterior segment malformations in 18q- (de Grouchy) syndrome, *Ophthalmic Paediatr Genet* 14:91, 1993.

205. Johnson BL, Cheng KP: Congenital aphakia: a clinicopathologic report of three cases, *J Pediatr Ophthalmol Strabismus* 34:35, 1997.

206. Mears AJ, and others: Autosomal dominant iridogoniodysgenesis anomaly maps to 6p25, *Am J Hum Genet* 59:1321, 1996.

207. Mirzayans F, and others: Identification of the human chromosomal region containing the iridogoniodysgenesis anomaly locus by genomic-mismatch scanning, *Am J Hum Genet* 61:111, 1997.

208. Chrousos GA, and others: Ocular findings in partial trisomy 3q: a case report and review of the literature, *Ophthalmic Paediatr Genet* 9:127, 1988.

209. Roy FH, and others: Ocular manifestations of the Rubenstein-Taybi syndrome, *Arch Ophthalmol* 79:272, 1968.

210. Brei TJ, and others: Glaucoma and findings simulating glaucoma in the Rubinstein-Taybi syndrome, *J Pediatr Ophthalmol Strabismus* 32:248, 1995.

211. Goldberg M: Persistent fetal vasculature (PVF): an integrated interpretation of signs and symptoms associated with persistent hyperplastic primary vitreous (PHPV), *Am J Ophthalmol* 124:587, 1997.

212. Mafee MF, and others: Magnetic resonance imaging versus computed tomography of leukocoric eyes and use of in vitro proton magnetic resonance spectroscopy of retinoblastoma, *Ophthalmology* 96:965, 1989.

213. Scott WE, and others: Management and visual acuity results of monocular congenital cataracts and persistent hyperplastic primary vitreous, *Aust N Z J Ophthalmol* 17:143, 1989.

214. Pollard ZF: Results of treatment of persistent hyperplastic primary vitreous, *Ophthalmic Surg* 22:48, 1991.

214a. Smith J, Shivitz I: Angle-closure glaucoma in adults with cicatricial retinopathy of prematurity, *Arch Ophthalmol* 102:371, 1984.

215. Pollard ZF: Secondary angle-closure glaucoma in cicatricial retrolental fibroplasia, *Am J Ophthalmol* 89:651, 1980.

216. Hartnett ME, and others: Glaucoma as a cause of poor vision in severe retinopathy of prematurity, *Graefes Arch Clin Exp Ophthalmol* 231:433, 1993.

217. Michael AJ, and others: Management of late-onset angle-closure glaucoma associated with retinopathy of prematurity, *Ophthalmology* 98:1093, 1991.

218. Tsipouras P, and others: Genetic linkage of the Marfan syndrome, ectopia lentis, and congenital contractural arachnodactyly to the fibrillin genes on chromosomes 15 and 5, *New Engl J Med* 326:905, 1992.

219. Kainulainen K, and others: Mutations in the fibrillin gene responsible for dominant ectopia lentis and neonatal Marfan syndrome, *Nat Genet* 6:64, 1994.

220. Maumenee I: The eye in Marfan's syndrome, *Trans Am Ophthalmol Soc* 79:696, 1981.

221. Allen RA, and others: Ocular manifestations of Marfan's syndrome, *Trans Am Acad Ophthalmol Otolaryngol* 71:1, 1967.

222. Cross HE, Jensen AD: Ocular manifestations in Marfan's syndrome and homocystinuria, *Am J Ophthalmol* 75:405, 1973.

223. Izquierdo NJ, and others: Glaucoma in the Marfan syndrome, *Trans Am Ophthalmol Soc* 90:111, 1992.

224. Burian HM, Allen L: Histologic study of the chamber angle of patients with Marfan's syndrome, *Arch Ophthalmol* 65:323, 1961.

225. Tsai MY, and others: Molecular and biochemical approaches in the identification of heterozygotes for homocystinuria, *Atherosclerosis* 122:69, 1996.

226. Borota J, and others: Homocystinuria: biochemical, clinical and genetic aspects, *Med Pregl* 50:187, 1997.

227. Kaur M, and others: Clinical and biochemical studies in homocystinuria, *Indian Pediatr* 32:1067, 1995.

228. Wilcken DE, Wilcken B: The natural history of vascular disease in homocystinuria and the effects of treatment, *J Inherit Metab Dis* 20:295, 1997.

229. Lieberman TW, Podos SM, Hartstein J: Acute glaucoma, ectopia lentis and homocystinuria, *Am J Ophthalmol* 61:252, 1966.

230. Traboulsi E: *Ectopia lentis and associated systemic disease.* In Wiggs JL, editor: *Molecular genetics of ocular disease,* New York, 1995, Wiley-Liss.

231. Ramsey M, Dickson D: Lens fringe in homocystinuria, *Br J Ophthalmol* 59:338, 1975.

232. Burke JP, and others: Ocular complications in homocystinuria: early and late treated, *Br J Ophthalmol* 73:427, 1989.

233. Wirtz MK, and others: Weill-Marchesani syndrome: possible linkage of the autosomal dominant form to 15q21.1, *Am J Med Genet* 65:68, 1996.

234. Jensen AD, Cross HE, Paton D: Ocular complications in the Weill-Marchesani syndrome, *Am J Ophthalmol* 77:261, 1974.

235. Wright K, Chrousos G: Weill-Marchesani syndrome with bilateral angle-closure glaucoma, *J Pediatr Ophthalmol Strabismus* 22:129, 1985.

236. Ritch R, Solomon L: Argon laser peripheral iridoplasty for angle-closure glaucoma in siblings with Weill-Marchesani syndrome, *J Glaucoma* 1:243, 1992.

237. Verloes A, and others: Glaucoma-lens ectopia microspherophakia-stiffness shortness (GEMSS) syndrome: a dominant disease with manifestations of Weill-Marchesani syndromes, *Am J Med Genet* 44:48, 1992.

238. Pe'er J, and others: Panuveal malignant mesenchymoma, *Arch Pathol Lab Med* 119:844, 1995.

239. Katsushima H, and others: Non-rubeotic angle-closure glaucoma associated with ciliary medulloepithelioma, *Jpn J Oph-thalmol* 40:244, 1996.

240. Shields CL, and others: Prevalence and mechanisms of secondary intraocular pressure elevation in eyes with intraocular tumors, *Ophthalmology* 94:839, 1987.

241. Hernandez-Martin A, and others: Juvenile xanthogranuloma, *J Am Acad Dermatol* 36:355-367; quiz 368, 1997.

242. Chang MW, and others: The risk of intraocular juvenile xanthogranuloma: survey of current practices and assessment of risk, *J Am Acad Dermatol* 34:445, 1996.

243. Borne MJ, and others: Juvenile xanthogranuloma of the iris with bilateral spontaneous hyphema, *J Pediatr Ophthalmol Strabismus* 33:196, 1996.

244. Casteels I, and others: Early treatment of juvenile xanthogranuloma of the iris with subconjunctival steroids, *Br J Ophthalmol* 77:57, 1993.

245. Andersson Gare B, and others: Incidence and prevalence of juvenile chronic arthritis: a population survey, *Ann Rheum Dis* 46:277, 1987.

246. Kanski JJ: Juvenile arthritis and uveitis, *Surv Ophthalmol* 34:253, 1990.

247. Cabral DA, and others: Visual prognosis in children with chronic anterior uveitis and arthritis, *J Rheumatol* 21:2370, 1994.

248. Yaldo M, Lieberman M: *Management of secondary glaucoma in the uveitis patient.* In Nozick R, Michelson J, editors: *Ophthalmology clinicis of North America: uveitis,* Philadelphia, 1993, WB Saunders.

249. Canski JJ, McAllister JA: Trabeculodialysis for inflammatory glaucoma in children and young adults, *Ophthalmology* 92:927, 1985.

250. Williams RD, and others: Trabeculodialysis for inflammatory glaucoma: a review of 25 cases, *Ophthalmic Surg* 23:36, 1992.

251. Wand M: *Neovascular glaucoma.* In Ritch R, Shields M, Krupin T, editors: *The glaucomas,* ed 2, St Louis, 1996, Mosby.

252. Wand M: *Neovascular glaucoma: you've come a long way, baby.* In van Buskirk E, Shields M, editors: *100 years of progress in glaucoma,* Philadelphia, 1997, Lippincott-Raven.

253. Silodor SW, and others: Natural history and management of advanced Coats' disease, *Ophthalmic Surg* 19:89, 1988.

254. Plager DA, and others: X-linked recessive familial exudative vitreoretinopathy, *Am J Ophthalmol* 114:145, 1992.

255. Fullwood P, and others: X-linked exudative vitreoretinopathy: clinical features and genetic linkage analysis, *Br J Ophthalmol* 77:168, 1993.

256. Mintz-Hittner HA, and others: Peripheral retinopathy in offspring of carriers of Norrie disease gene mutations: possible transplacental effect of abnormal Norrin, *Ophthalmology* 103:2128, 1996.

257. Sihota R, and others: Traumatic glaucoma, *Acta Ophthalmol Scand* 73:252, 1995.

258. Jaafar MS, Kazi GA: Normal intraocular pressure in children: a comparative study of the Perkins applanation tonometer and the pneumatonometer, *J Pediatr Ophthalmol Strabismus* 30:284, 1993.

259. Spierer A, and others: Normal intraocular pressure in premature infants, *Am J Ophthalmol* 117:801, 1994 (letter).

260. Murphy D: Anesthesia and intraocular pressure, *Anesth Analg* 71:181, 1985.

261. Watcha MF, and others: Effects of halothane on intraocular pressure in anesthetized children, *Anesth Analg* 71:181, 1990.

262. Fledelius HC, Christensen AC: Reappraisal of the human ocular growth curve in fetal life, infancy, and early childhood, *Br J Ophthalmol* 80:918, 1996.

263. Hoskins HD, and others: *Developmental glaucomas: diagnosis and classification.* In *The New Orleans Academy of Ophthalmology-Symposium on glaucoma,* St Louis, 1981, Mosby.

PART V

Medical Treatment

21

Medical Treatment of Glaucoma: General Principles

The ultimate goal of glaucoma treatment is to delay, stop,[1] and sometimes reverse[2] the damage to the optic nerve and ganglion cell layer caused by the glaucomatous process. The only way to accomplish this at present is by reducing intraocular pressure (IOP) below the level that will cause continued damage to the optic nerve. Although a medication that would directly protect the optic nerve or reverse the damage from glaucoma would be most welcome, no such medication has yet been proven to be effective. Medications that have some promise in this regard are discussed in a later chapter.

One recent study has called into question whether lowering IOP truly helps prevent or reduce glaucomatous damage.[3] However, the vast majority of studies produce evidence that lowering IOP is indeed beneficial.[4,5] As has been noted in chapters 2 and 17, animal studies and secondary glaucomas clearly point to IOP as an important risk factor, if not a causal factor. Other studies strongly suggest that the lower the IOP, the less likely optic nerve damage is to develop or progress.[6-8] Some of these same data indicate that past efforts to lower IOP into the "normal" range of 21 mm Hg or lower may have been inadequate and that "control" really means an IOP of less than 15 or 16 mm Hg, especially in advanced glaucoma. One recent long-term study showed that lowering IOP in normal-pressure glaucoma by at least 30% protects at least some patients from progression.[8a] Most physicians today try to tailor therapy to the individual patient and his or her situation (i.e., to estimate and then aim for a "target pressure").

TARGET PRESSURE

The concept of target pressure arose from the observation that progression in advanced glaucoma and occasionally even in early glaucoma, often occurs at what are thought to be "physiologic" pressures. An IOP of 21 mm Hg or lower—the previously sought goal—may not be low enough for many glaucomatous eyes. The goal should be to lower the IOP to a level that is "safe" for that particular eye. Because our current knowledge does not indicate with any certainty what a safe IOP level may be for any given patient, the target pressure is estimated for each patient based on initial IOP and degree of existing damage. It is then continually reassessed and reset based on the clinical course.

The less the initial pretreatment of IOP, the more advanced the optic nerve damage, and the older the patient, the lower the target pressure should be set. The presence of a vasculopathy such as diabetes or arteriosclerotic cardiovascular disease should also lower the target pressure. A young person with glaucoma secondary to trauma with a pretreatment IOP of 32 mm Hg and a 0.5 cup:disc ratio with early visual field loss may do quite well with an initial target IOP of 25 mm Hg. An elderly patient with a pretreatment IOP of 22 mm Hg, a cup:disc ratio of 0.9, and advanced visual field loss may require a target pressure of 15 mm Hg or lower.

The currently available approaches to lower IOP include medical therapy, laser trabeculoplasty, filtering surgery, and cyclodestructive procedures—each of these has its own risk:benefit ratios. Whichever method is chosen, it should ideally be predictable, safe, and easy for the patient to use. Unfortunately, there is no ideal treatment for glaucoma. Because the risk:benefit ratio for medical therapy seems to be lowest, both historical and current practice has been to attempt medical treatment before resorting to other alternatives. However, this approach has been called into question in recent years.[9]

MEDICAL THERAPY
Advantages

Medical therapy has been the mainstay of initial glaucoma treatment for over a century. The vast majority of patients respond to a simple regimen with a desirable reduction in IOP. Side effects are usually few and tolerable. When they do occur, side effects are often easily reversible by stopping the medication. Only rarely are vision- or life-threatening side effects seen. Medical therapy is less costly over the short-term, and because many glaucoma patients are elderly, the cost of medical treatment may never exceed that of surgery. Finally, most patients expect a trial of medical therapy first and are likely to be somewhat suspicious of a too rapid suggestion for surgery.

Disadvantages

Over the last decade, the disadvantages of medical therapy have been increasingly highlighted. Several prospective studies have pointed to medical therapy as less effective in lowering IOP and perhaps in preventing further visual field loss than either laser trabeculoplasty or filtering surgery.[10-12] However, some of the differences between the medically and surgically treated groups in these studies may be the result of not setting the target IOP low enough in the medically treated group (the surgically treated groups had pressures "automatically" set at low levels). The Glaucoma Laser Trial showed that after 2 years only 30% of patients initially treated with medications were still being controlled with a single topical β-blocker.[13]

Medically treated eyes may not have as good a success rate from subsequent filtering surgery compared with eyes treated with surgery from the outset.[14] This may be due to an increased number of inflammatory cells and a decreased number of goblet cells in the conjunctiva of medically treated eyes compared with eyes treated initially with surgery.[15,16] Medical treatment has the potential for significant and serious side effects, not all of which may be obvious to the patient or physician. During an 8-year period (1978 to 1985) in the United States, 32 deaths (of about 2 million glaucoma patients) were attributed to complications arising from the use of topical timolol maleate.[17] Carbonic anhydrase inhibitors also can produce rare fatal reactions.[18]

Less dramatic side effects of topical medications include allergic reactions, toxic corneal changes, induced refractive errors, cataract formation, asthma, tachycardia, bradycardia, orthostatic hypotension, gastrointestinal symptoms, decreased libido, impotence, mood changes, possible memory loss, and alopecia. Systemic carbonic anhydrase inhibitors are notorious for significant side effects such as lethargy, depression, diarrhea, and loss of appetite. All of these may have subtle or profound effects on the patient's quality of life.

In addition, many older patients are also taking a number of other medications, which may add to the potential for cross-reaction and confusing side effects. Patients and their primary care physicians often do not associate systemic side effects with topical eye medications, and the ophthalmologist may fail to ask about systemic symptoms; in these cases the cause of a systemic problem induced by antiglaucoma medications may go undetected.

A further complication of antiglaucoma medications is their high cost. Retail prices for any one type of topical eyedrop may run as high as $80 for a month's supply. If the patient is using multiple glaucoma medications, the cost of antiglaucoma therapy could well be over $120 per month.[19] For someone whose only source of income is a modest pension or social security, this may mean choosing between eating and taking needed medication. Because glaucoma is a chronic, lifetime condition, the cost of medications over the long term may be astronomic both personally and from a public health–medical economics point of view. This is a major factor in nations with limited resources and can be a significant factor even in the most wealthy countries.

Finally, the issue of compliance must be addressed. It is probably unrealistic to think that a typical elderly patient who is taking medications for hypertension, diabetes, arthritis, and hiatal hernia is going to be able to accurately stick to a regimen that includes two or three topical medications and a carbonic anhydrase inhibitor. Kass and co-workers[20] have shown that compliance is surprisingly poor, even with just one medication used four times a day.

124. Alfredsson LS, Norell SE: Spacing between doses on a thrice-daily regimen, *BMJ* 282:1036, 1981.
125. Kass MA, Gordon M: The effect of a generic drug law on the retail cost of antiglaucoma medication, *Am J Ophthalmol* 92:273, 1981.
126. Steinert RF, Thomas JV, Boger WP III: Long-term drift and continued efficacy after multiyear timolol therapy, *Arch Ophthalmol* 99:100, 1981.
127. Hong YJ, and others: Intraocular pressure after a two-week washout following long-term timolol or levobunolol, *J Ocul Pharmacol Ther* 11:107, 1995.
128. Kass MA, and others: *The retail cost of antiglaucoma medication.* In Leopold IH, Burns RP, editors: *Symposium on Ocular Therapy, Vol. 10,* New York, 1977, John Wiley & Sons.
129. Ritch R, and others: Retail cost of antiglaucoma drugs in two cities, *Am J Ophthalmol* 86:1, 1978.

22

Cholinergic Drugs

The cholinergic drugs are the oldest effective medical treatment for glaucoma. More than 100 years ago, Laqueur[1] used physostigmine (eserine), an extract from the Calabar or ordeal bean, for the treatment of glaucoma, and Weber[2] described the effects of pilocarpine, an extract from the leaf of a South American plant, on the pupil. The cholinergic drugs mimic the effects of acetylcholine, which is a transmitter at postganglionic parasympathetic junctions, some postganglionic sympathetic endings (e.g., sweat glands), autonomic ganglia, somatic motor nerve endings (i.e., skeletal muscle), and some central nervous system synapses. Acetylcholine is synthesized by the enzyme choline acetyltransferase and produces its effects by binding to cholinergic receptors in various tissues. Cholinergic drugs are applied topically for the treatment of glaucoma because of their effect on parasympathetic receptors in the iris and ciliary body. However, topical miotics absorbed systemically can produce side effects by stimulating cholinergic receptors in other sites.

Drugs that mimic the effects of acetylcholine act at muscarinic and/or nicotinic receptors, the latter being subdivided into N_1 and N_2 types. This classification system is based on the relative potency of various agonists and antagonists at the different receptor sites. As a rule, muscarinic receptors are found in smooth muscle and glands, stimulated by muscarine and inhibited by atropine. N_1 nicotinic receptors are found in autonomic ganglia, stimulated by dimethylphenylpiperazine and inhibited by hexamethonium and d-tubocurarine. N_2 receptors are found in striated muscle, stimulated by paratrimethylammonium and inhibited by decamethonium or d-tubocurarine. Nicotine stimulates N_1 and N_2 receptors at low doses and inhibits them at high doses.

Acetylcholine is released from vesicles in nerve terminals and then hydrolyzed within a few milliseconds by acetylcholinesterase. The rapid destruction of acetylcholine permits the cholinergic receptors to repolarize and prepare for the next stimulation. Cholinergic drugs act either directly by stimulating cholinergic receptors or indirectly by inhibiting the enzyme cholinesterase, thereby potentiating and prolonging the effects of endogenous acetylcholine.

Strictly speaking, the words *cholinergic, parasympathomimetic,* and *miotic* are not synonymous; cholinergic refers to acetylcholine, parasympathomimetic refers to the parasympathetic nervous system, and miotic refers to a constricted pupil. However, we will follow common ophthalmic usage in this text and use the three words interchangeably to refer to this entire class of drugs.

MECHANISMS OF ACTION

Angle-Closure Glaucoma

Cholinergic drugs are useful for the short-term management of angle-closure glaucoma associated with pupillary block. Miotic agents help prepare an eye for iridotomy and are not a substitute for it in angle-closure glaucoma. Cholinergic drugs constrict the pupillary sphincter, tighten the iris, decrease the volume of iris tissue in the angle, and pull the peripheral iris away from the trabecular meshwork. These changes reduce intraocular pressure (IOP) by allowing aqueous humor to reach the outflow channels. If the IOP is quite elevated (i.e., above 45 or 50 mm Hg), the pupillary sphincter may be ischemic and may not respond to cholinergic stimulation.[3] In this situation other drugs (i.e., a topical α-adrenergic antagonist, topical apraclonidine or brimonidine, possibly a topical or systemic carbonic anhydrase inhibitor, and, if necessary, a systemic hyperosmotic agent) are used to reduce IOP sufficiently so that a parasympathomimetic agent can produce miosis.

It is important to emphasize that miotic agents are capable of narrowing the angle in some

The gel prolongs contact time between the drug and the tear film, enhances drug penetration, and reduces the frequency of drug administration. A single dose of 4% pilocarpine gel applied at bedtime is approximately equal in effect to 4% pilocarpine eyedrops applied 4 tin. , daily.[61] Some patients prefer the gel because it is more convenient, whereas others prefer it because of lessened side effects. However, it is not clear whether the gel applied once daily can control IOP for 24 hours in all patients. Some studies suggest a diminishing effect of the gel after 18 hours.[60] In addition, in one study 20% of the patients treated with pilocarpine gel for several months developed reversible anterior stromal haze of the cornea.[62]

Pilocarpine Polymer (Piloplex). Piloplex represents another attempt to obtain a prolonged drug effect from a single administration of pilocarpine. Piloplex is an aqueous emulsion consisting of a polymeric material to which pilocarpine base is chemically bound. The drug is released over a period of hours as the polymer is hydrolyzed. Piloplex appears to be effective in preliminary trials and may provide better control of IOP when administered twice daily than pilocarpine eyedrops do when administered 4 times daily.[63-65] Despite the positive reports, Piloplex has failed to make any inroads in the United States.

Methacholine (Mecholyl)

Methacholine chloride is a synthetic derivative of acetylcholine. In the past, 10% to 20% methacholine was administered every 5 to 10 minutes to treat angle-closure glaucoma, and 2% to 10% methacholine was given alone or combined with neostigmine to treat open-angle glaucoma. The drug is rarely used anymore because it is unstable in solution and is short acting, and it penetrates the cornea poorly. Its major use today is in the diagnosis of Adie's pupil.

Carbachol

Carbachol, a synthetic derivative of choline, acts primarily by stimulating muscarinic receptors. It also releases acetylcholine at certain neuroeffector junctions and ganglia.[66] Carbachol is manufactured in aqueous solutions of 0.75% to 3% and is administered 3 to 4 times daily (i.e., every 6 to 8 hours). It is more powerful than pilocarpine on a concentration basis (e.g., 1.5% carbachol has the same ocular effect as 2% pilocarpine) and has a more prolonged effect.[67] However, carbachol penetrates the cornea poorly and must be combined with a wetting agent or a preservative such as benzalkonium chloride to reach an effective intraocular concentration.[68] Like pilocarpine, carbachol is not destroyed by cholinesterase.

Carbachol is an excellent miotic agent that could be used more frequently for the treatment of glaucoma. It can be used to initiate cholinergic treatment or to substitute for pilocarpine and other miotics when the patient develops resistance or intolerance.[69] Carbachol has a greater tendency than pilocarpine to produce headache and accommodative spasm, especially during the first few days of treatment. It is also a more potent miotic that can cause more interference with vision than pilocarpine for those patients with lens opacities.

The use of carbachol has declined with the general decline in the use of miotics. Today, it finds its widest use intracamerally to reduce the postoperative IOP and especially to prevent a significant pressure spike in glaucoma patients whose optic nerves might be further damaged.

Aceclidine (Glaucostat)

Aceclidine, a synthetic cholinergic drug, is used extensively in Europe for the treatment of glaucoma.[70,71] Aceclidine stimulates muscarinic receptors directly and inhibits cholinesterase weakly. It is less effective than pilocarpine on a concentration basis (e.g., 4% aceclidine has the same ocular hypotensive effect as 2% pilocarpine). Aceclidine is thought to induce less ciliary muscle spasm and accommodation than pilocarpine.[72]

Indirect (Anticholinesterase) Agents

Anticholinesterase drugs inhibit the enzyme acetylcholinesterase, thereby potentiating the effects of endogenous acetylcholine. In general, these agents produce more side effects than the direct-acting cholinergic drugs, including hyperemia, irritation, vascular congestion, and spasm of the orbicularis, ciliary, and iris sphincter muscles.[73] Cholinesterase inhibitors are rarely administered to eyes with narrow angles before iridectomy; the drug-induced miosis, forward movement of the lens, and vascular congestion can precipitate or aggravate angle closure. In the past, anticholinesterase drugs were classified as reversible (e.g., physostigmine, neostigmine) or irreversible (e.g., isoflurophate, echothiophate) enzyme inhibitors. It is probably more accurate to classify these drugs as weak/short-acting or strong/long-acting inhibitors of cholinesterase.

Echothiophate Iodide (Phospholine Iodide)

Echothiophate, a potent inhibitor of both true cholinesterase and pseudocholinesterase, is manufactured as a white crystalline solid that is mixed with a diluent at the time of dispensing. Because of limited stability, solutions of the drug should be refrigerated. Echothiophate is administered as an aqueous solution in concentrations of 0.03% to 0.25% every 12 to 48 hours (Fig. 22-3). The 0.06% concentration produces the maximum IOP reduction in most patients and is roughly equivalent in peak effect to 4% pilocarpine.[74,75] Echothiophate, however, has a much longer duration of action than pilocarpine[76] and controls IOP in some eyes that have not responded adequately to direct-acting cholinergic agents.[77] However, the benefits of echothiophate are offset by the systemic and ocular

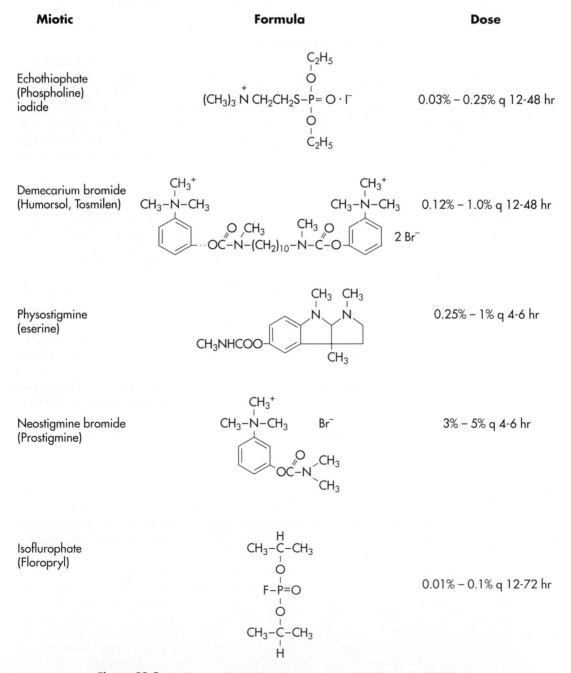

Miotic	Formula	Dose
Echothiophate (Phospholine) iodide		0.03% – 0.25% q 12-48 hr
Demecarium bromide (Humorsol, Tosmilen)		0.12% – 1.0% q 12-48 hr
Physostigmine (eserine)		0.25% – 1% q 4-6 hr
Neostigmine bromide (Prostigmine)		3% – 5% q 4-6 hr
Isoflurophate (Floropryl)		0.01% – 0.1% q 12-72 hr

Figure 22-3   Indirect-acting cholinergic agents (acetylcholinesterase inhibitors).

side effects, particularly cataract formation. Because of these side effects, echothiophate and the other strong inhibitors of cholinesterase are used mostly in aphakic and pseudophakic eyes and in eyes that have not responded adequately to standard medical and surgical treatment for glaucoma.

Demecarium Bromide (Humorsol, Tosmilen)

Demecarium is a potent, stable, long-acting cholinesterase inhibitor with considerable specificity for acetylcholinesterase. It is usually administered in aqueous solutions of 0.12% to 0.25% every 12 to 48 hours. The resulting IOP reduction occurs 30 minutes after administration, reaches a maximum at 24 hours, and lasts for 1 to several days.[78] Demecarium is less effective than echothiophate on a concentration basis (e.g., 0.12% demecarium is equal in effect to 0.06% echothiophate). However, demecarium is effective in some patients who have not responded adequately to echothiophate. Demecarium is said to produce tolerance more quickly than the other potent cholinesterase inhibitors. Demecarium is available in a stable solution that does not need refrigeration and therefore may be used as a short-term substitute for echothiophate when a patient is travelling or otherwise does not have convenient access to refrigeration.

Isoflurophate (Floropryl, Diisopropyl Fluorophosphate, Dyflos)

Isoflurophate, an extremely potent cholinesterase inhibitor, is more active against nonspecific or pseudocholinesterase than against acetylcholinesterase. Isoflurophate is usually administered as an ointment (0.025%) every 12 to 72 hours.[79] The drug is also available as a 0.01% to 0.1% solution in anhydrous peanut oil. The oil frequently causes allergic reactions and must be refrigerated. Isoflurophate produces intense miosis, ciliary spasm, and headache and is hydrolyzed so rapidly that touching the lids with the eyedropper during application may inactivate the drug. Isoflurophate has largely been replaced by the more stable anticholinesterase agents echothiophate and demecarium and is not used in the United States.

Physostigmine (Eserine)

Physostigmine is a short-acting inhibitor of cholinesterase. It is administered in aqueous solution as a salicylate (0.25% to 1%) every 4 to 6 hours, or as an alkaloid in an oily vehicle (0.25% to 0.5%) once or twice daily. Topical administration of physostigmine produces an IOP reduction that begins in 10 to 30 minutes, reaches a maximum in 1 to 2 hours, and lasts for 4 to 6 hours. Physostigmine solutions are unstable and decompose with pH changes or on exposure to light. Patients should be cautioned that discolored solutions are irritating and less effective. Physostigmine can rarely be used for long periods of time because it produces irritation and follicular hypertrophy of the conjunctiva. It also can cause depigmentation of the eyelids in black patients.[80] This agent is rarely used for chronic glaucoma therapy.

Neostigmine (Prostigmine)

Neostigmine is a short-acting anticholinesterase agent similar in effect to physostigmine. It is administered in 3% to 5% aqueous solutions every 4 to 6 hours. Neostigmine is more stable and more potent than physostigmine and causes less vascular congestion and conjunctival follicular hypertrophy. However, neostigmine is ultimately less effective because of poor corneal penetration.

SIDE EFFECTS

Ocular

Miotic drugs commonly produce ocular side effects, including conjunctival injection, ocular and periocular pain (headache), twitching of the eyelids, fluctuating myopic shift in refraction, and decreased vision in dim illumination. Almost all of the ocular side effects are more common and more severe with the anticholinesterase agents (Box 22-1). Patients are more likely to accept the side effects if the physician provides encouragement, explains that the symptoms improve spontaneously over the first several days, and initiates treatment with a low concentration of the cholinergic drug. Pain and headache can be relieved by salicylates. Older patients, particularly those with lens opacities, often complain of decreased vision in dim illumination. They should be warned about the dangers of driving at night. Some of these patients may be helped by concomitant treatment with phenylephrine. Other alternatives include β-adrenergic antagonists, an α-adrenergic agonist, a topical carbonic anhydrase inhibitor, the Ocusert delivery system, and pilocarpine gel.

Box 22-1
Ocular Side Effects of Topical Cholinergic Drugs*

Miosis, decreased vision in dim illumination
Ciliary muscle spasm, fluctuating vision, headache
Orbicularis muscle spasm, lid twitching, periocular pain
Vascular dilation, conjunctival and iris hyperemia
Increased vascular permeability, formation of posterior synechiae, postoperative inflammation
Production or enhancement of angle-closure glaucoma
Temporary increase in intraocular pressure
Cataract formation
Stinging, irritation
Tearing
Allergic blepharoconjunctivitis[112]†
Cyst of the iris pigment epithelium
Retinal hole, retinal detachment, vitreous hemorrhage
Lacrimal obstruction, ocular pseudopemphigoid[113]
Corneal epithelial staining, vascularization†
Atypical band keratopathy caused by phenylmercuric nitrate preservative[114]

*Almost all ocular side effects are more common and more severe with the anticholinesterase drugs.
†These side effects are an exception.

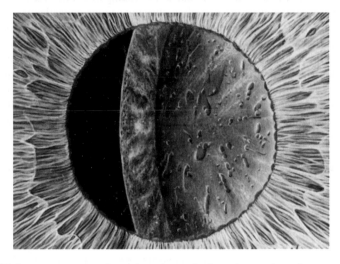

Figure 22-4   Slit-lamp appearance of anterior subcapsular lens changes in patient treated with echothiophate. (From Shaffer RN, Hetherington J Jr: *Am J Ophthalmol* 62:613, 1966. Published with permission from the American Journal of Ophthalmology. Copyright by the Ophthalmic Publishing Company.)

Younger patients often complain of a fluctuating myopic shift in refraction that may be 12 to 15 D in magnitude. Younger patients often prefer pilocarpine gel or the Ocusert system to standard miotic eyedrops 4 times daily. Other alternatives include β-adrenergic antagonists, α-agonists, and topical carbonic anhydrase inhibitors.

Anticholinesterase drugs initiate and speed the development of cataracts, especially in patients over age 50.[81-84] The initial lens changes consist of small anterior subcapsular vacuoles arranged in a cluster, giving a characteristic mossy appearance (Fig. 22-4).[81,85] Such changes are noted in approximately 10% of nonglaucomatous eyes and 30% to 50% of eyes treated with echothiophate or demecarium for 6 months.[86,87] Visual acuity is not affected at this stage, and most cases do not progress if treatment is stopped. If anticholinesterase treatment is continued for 3 years, approximately 50% of patients over age 50 have a decrease in visual acuity of two lines or more because of cataract.[88] Progressive drug-related cataract involves all layers and zones of the lens. If cataract (or any other kind of intraocular) surgery becomes necessary, anticholinesterase drugs should be dis-

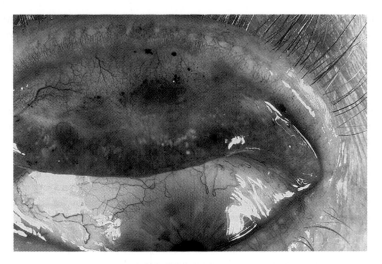

Figure 23-2 Adrenochrome deposits in conjunctiva from epinephrine.

Adrenochrome material is frequently deposited in the lacrimal sac[136] and nasolacrimal ducts[137]; this can be responsible for nasolacrimal system obstruction and epiphora, especially after long-term use. Actual adrenochrome calculi may be found or felt in the lacrimal drainage system. Stopping the epinephrine product may help, but resolution may take years or may require removal or dacryocystorhinostomy. Adrenochrome deposits occur more commonly when patients use old, discolored epinephrine solutions and when they have been applying the medication for prolonged periods of time.

Epinephrine drugs can produce a hypersensitivity blepharoconjunctivitis, including lid erythema, lichenification, and conjunctival chemosis; vascular engorgement; and follicular hypertrophy[138,139] (Fig. 23-3). Occasionally this is accompanied by mild iridocyclitis and subepithelial infiltration of the cornea.[140] Some patients who develop hypersensitivity blepharoconjunctivitis with epinephrine treatment can tolerate dipivefrin indefinitely.[141] Some have cross-reactivity.[142] Other patients can continue epinephrine treatment if a weak topical corticosteroid such as 1% medrysone is administered concurrently. Medrysone is unlikely to elevate IOP, even with long-term administration.[143]

Epinephrine solutions stain soft contact lenses.[144] The stain can be removed by soaking the lenses for 5 hours in 3% hydrogen peroxide.[145] Dipivefrin is much less likely than epinephrine to produce a stain in soft contact lenses,[146] but patients should still be cautioned to remove the lenses before instilling the drops.

Topical epinephrine treatment produces macular edema in 10% to 20% of aphakic eyes.[147,148] Dipivefrin can also cause cystoid macular edema, but perhaps less commonly.[149] The mechanism for this condition is unknown; speculation has centered around ultraviolet radiation and, more recently, the possible release into the eye of prostaglandin analogs by the epinephrine and their interaction on the retinal vasculature.[150] The combination of an adrenergic agonist and prostaglandin has been shown to disrupt the blood-retinal barrier in experimental animals.[151]

The macular edema occurs after months to years of treatment. It is manifested by a gradual decline in visual acuity that may reach the level of 20/200. The condition appears to be reversible if the drug is discontinued, although resolution may require several months. If epinephrine treatment is not stopped, structural damage of the retina can produce permanent loss of central vision. The retinal findings and the appearance on fluorescein angiography resemble the petaloid pattern of aphakic cystoid macular edema.

Occasionally the area of edema is surrounded by fine retinal hemorrhages. The relatively high incidence of epinephrine-induced macular edema suggests that epinephrine drugs are not the first choice for aphakic eyes. However, epinephrine can be used if needed in aphakic eyes provided that the patients test their vision weekly at home and the clinician is particularly careful to note any loss of vision. Even a small decrease in vision in an aphakic eye receiving epinephrine or dipivefrin treatment requires a careful examination to determine if cystoid macular edema is present; if so, epinephrine treatment should be discontinued. Unfortunately, this condition is often not recognized

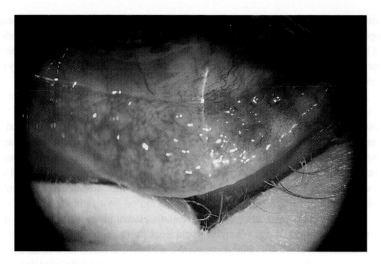

Figure 23-3   Follicular conjunctival reaction typical of adrenergic agonists.

because of the gradual nature of its clinical onset; the reduction in vision may be ascribed to other causes. It is unclear whether epinephrine-induced macular edema occurs as commonly after extracapsular cataract extraction as after intracapsular cataract extraction because the decline in the use of intracapsular surgery has paralleled a decline in the use of epinephrine. An intact posterior capsule may be a mechanical barrier to posterior movement of small molecules such as epinephrine.[152]

A few patients receiving epinephrine may develop corneal haze or even frank edema despite good IOP control, causing complaints of halos and blurred vision. The symptoms and corneal findings abate after discontinuing the drug. In rabbits, epinephrine administered intramuscularly or by iontophoresis activates latent herpes simplex virus.[153,154] There is no evidence that topical epinephrine treatment influences herpetic disease in humans.

There is some concern that epinephrine-induced vasoconstriction may compromise optic nerve perfusion. Some postulate that this effect is worse with unilateral treatment because the fellow untreated eye does not have a lowered IOP to offset any decrease in perfusion. Further studies of the effects of topical and systemic medication on optic-nerve blood flow are required to resolve this issue.

There are a number of approaches to reduce or control the side effects related to epinephrine treatment. Systemic side effects can be reduced by using low concentrations of the drug, instilling only one drop in each eye, using punctal occlusion, and having the patient sit quietly with the eyelids closed for 2 minutes. Using a different salt or using a concomitant weak topical corticosteroid that does not cross the cornea such as medrysone can reduce a number of local side effects. Another approach to reducing side effects is to prescribe dipivefrin. Dipivefrin is stable in solution and produces a lower incidence of external irritation than standard epinephrine preparations. As noted previously, administering concomitant topical medrysone twice daily can allow continued use of epinephrine products in the face of mild to moderate blepharoconjunctivitis.

Because dipivefrin produces a similar intraocular concentration of epinephrine, it is just as likely to produce macular edema in aphakic eyes or angle closure in eyes with narrow angles. However, because of the lower concentration of drug administered and the localized ability to convert it to epinephrine, dipivefrin produces fewer systemic side effects than epinephrine. Therefore dipivefrin is the drug of choice in this group of agents for any patient with substantial cardiovascular disease, poorly controlled hypertension, or any other condition in which systemic administration of adrenaline might be inadvisable.

α_2-Agonists

The α_2-agonists are relatively new antiglaucoma agents. Their mechanism(s) of action include decreasing aqueous formation, increasing trabecular outflow (apraclonidine), and increasing uveoscleral outflow (brimonidine). Apraclonidine is the agent that has been in clinical use in the United

---

Box 23-2
Side Effects of α_2-Agonists

Systemic	Ocular
Dry mouth	Allergy
Fatigue	Blurred vision
Drowsiness	Burning/stinging
Headache	Follicular conjunctival response
Hypotension	Hyperemia
Bradycardia in neonates	Itching
Hypothermia in neonates	Photophobia

---

ously, clonidine reduces blood pressure by as much as 30 mm Hg in up to 48% of subjects.[58] Some of this may be centrally mediated; however, the newer agents, apraclonidine and brimonidine, do not cross the blood-brain barrier and would be expected to have less cardiovascular effects.[188] In fact, apraclonidine and brimonidine have much less of an effect on blood pressure; although a statistically significant effect can be measured, it is rarely of clinical significance.[189] Unlike timolol and the other nonselective β-blocking agents, brimonidine and apraclonidine have little effect on heart rate either while resting or during exercise. The α_2-agonists have no effect on pulmonary function. No teratogenic, reproductive, fertility, or other organ effects were noted in rats.[188] Another systemic side effect noted with these agents is dry mouth, which may be experienced by up to 30% of patients (compared with 17% of those on timolol therapy) but is rarely serious enough to require discontinuing the drug. Fatigue and drowsiness are seen with brimonidine and are dose dependent and occasionally severe enough to require cessation of therapy.[190] The use of brimonidine has been associated with bradycardia, hypotension, and apnea in two neonates; therefore it should be used with great caution or not at all in infants under 1 year of age.[191]

Ocular allergy is relatively common with these agents, as it is with all adrenergic agonists. Because conjunctival follicular response may be correlated with the oxidative potential of the agent and the reactivity of oxidative metabolites, the more stable agents like dipivefrin and brimonidine have a lower rate of local reaction. Stinging and burning on application are also seen, but to a lesser degree than with betaxolol and timolol.[178] Foreign body sensation occurred in about 3%. Blurred vision with brimonidine is less than with timolol. Rebound hyperemia is common with clonidine and apraclonidine and may be a cosmetic problem. Patients using brimonidine may display hyperemia, but it is less common than with the other agents and is rarely cause for discontinuing the medication. Overall, brimonidine seems to have the least propensity for ocular side effects in this group of drugs.[192]

Suggestions for Use

At the present time, it appears that 0.5% apraclonidine given within 30 minutes before, and/or immediately after, anterior segment laser treatment has the most published support as the prophylactic drug of choice because 0.5% brimonidine is not commercially available. Because 0.5% apraclonidine is effective in preventing the IOP spikes after anterior segment laser, there is little reason to use the 1% solution. However, as noted previously, one study and the authors' experience support the efficacy of 0.2% brimonidine for this application. The α_1 effects of apraclonidine may be beneficial to prevent or reduce bleeding in the particular instance of Nd:YAG laser iridotomy. Side effects from this regimen with either agent are rare.

Apraclonidine 0.5% is also useful to help reduce IOP in acute glaucomas such as angle-closure, inflammatory, postsurgical, and traumatic. The drug is administered every 8 hours when used alone or may be used every 12 hours when used in combination with other antiglaucoma medications.

For chronic glaucoma, brimonidine is the α_2-agent of first choice. It is effective as monotherapy in those patients in whom use of a β-blocker is contraindicated or inadvisable; it is also useful in those intolerant of, or unresponsive to, β-blockers or other antiglaucoma medications. As monotherapy or adjunctive therapy, brimonidine 0.2% is effective in a twice daily dosage. When used as monotherapy, dosage 3 times daily may be slightly more effective than twice daily. Brimonidine has been a very important addition to the glaucoma armamentarium.

SUMMARY

Topical adrenergic agonist agents have a long history of effectiveness in the treatment of glaucoma. The nonselective α-/β-agonists epinephrine and dipivefrin have a relatively high rate of local side effects, with epinephrine causing significant systemic effects in some patients. In the recent past, the more selective α_2-agonist agents apraclonidine and brimonidine have had increasing use for prophylaxis against pressure spikes in laser surgery. Most recently, the highly selective α_2-agonist brimonidine has found an important place in the management of chronic glaucoma because of its lower rate of local side effects, sustained IOP lowering, and better additivity to other antiglaucoma medications.

REFERENCES

1. Darier A: De l'extrait de capsule surrenales en therapeutique oculaire, *Lab Clin Ophthalmol* 6:141, 1900.
2. Hamburger K: Experimentelle glaucomtherapie, *Klin Mbl Augenheilk* 7:810, 1923.
3. Ahlquist RP: A study of the adrenotropic receptors, *Am J Physiol* 153:586, 1948.
4. Lands AM, and others: Differentiation of receptor systems activated by sympathomimetic amines, *Nature* 214:597, 1967.
5. Gluchowski C, and others: Use of recombinant human alpha adrenergic receptors for the pharmacological evaluation of alpha adrenergic ocular hypotensive agents, *Invest Ophthalmol Vis Sci* 35(suppl): 1399, 1994.
6. Huang Y, and others: Localization of alpha$_2$-adrenergic receptor subtypes in the anterior segment of the human eye with selective antibodies, *Invest Ophthalmol Vis Sci* 36:2729, 1995.
7. Kobilka BK, and others: Cloning, sequencing, and expression of the gene coding for the human platelet alpha$_2$-adrenergic receptor, *Science* 238:650, 1987.
8. Minneman KP, Puttman RN, Molinoff PB: Beta-adrenergic receptor subtypes: properties, distribution and regulation, *Annu Rev Neurosci* 4:419, 1981.
9. Jakobs FH, and others: *Inhibition of adenylate cyclase*. In Cooper DMF, Seamon R, editors: *Advances in cyclic nucleotide and protein phosphorylation research, vol 19*, New York, 1985, Raven Press.
10. Fain JN, Garcia-Sainz JS: Role of phosphatidylinositol turnover in alpha$_1$ and adenylate cyclase inhibition in alpha$_2$ effects of catecholamines, *Life Sci* 26: 1183, 1980.
11. Hokin LE: Receptors and phosphoinositide-generated second messengers, *Annu Rev Biochem* 54:205, 1985.
12. Neufeld AH, and others: Influences on the density of beta-adrenergic receptors in the cornea and iris ciliary body of the rabbit, *Invest Ophthalmol Vis Sci* 17: 1069, 1980.
13. Becker B, Ley AP: Epinephrine and acetazolamide in the therapy of the glaucomas, *Am J Ophthalmol* 45:639, 1958.

14. Weekers R, Delmarcelle Y, Gustin J: Treatment of ocular hypertension by adrenaline, and diverse sympathomimetic amines, *Am J Ophthalmol* 40:666, 1955.
15. Ballintine EJ, Garner LL: Improvement of the coefficient of outflow in glaucomatous eyes: prolonged local treatment with epinephrine, *Arch Ophthalmol* 66:314, 1961.
16. Becker B, Pettit TH, Gay AJ: Topical epinephrine therapy of glaucoma, *Arch Ophthalmol* 66:219, 1961.
17. Shenker HE, and others: Fluorophotometric study of epinephrine and timolol in human subjects, *Arch Ophthalmol* 99:1212, 1981.
18. Townsend DJ, Brubaker RF: Immediate effect of epinephrine on aqueous formation in the normal human eye as measured by fluorophotometry, *Invest Ophthalmol Vis Sci* 19:256, 1980.
19. Thomas JV, Epstein DL: Transient additive effect of timolol and epinephrine in primary open angle glaucoma, *Arch Ophthalmol* 99:91, 1981.
20. Erickson K, and others: Adrenergic regulation of aqueous outflow, *J Ocul Pharmacol* 10:241, 1994.
21. Neufeld AH, Sears ML: Adenosine 3,5-monophosphate analogue increases the outflow facility of the primate eye, *Invest Ophthalmol* 14:688, 1975.
22. Robinson JC, Kaufman PL: Effects and interactions of epinephrine, norepinephrine, timolol, and betaxolol on outflow facility in the cynomolgus monkey, *Am J Ophthalmol* 109:189, 1990.
23. Crawford KS, and others: Indomethacin and epinephrine effects on outflow facility and cyclic adenosine monophosphate formation in monkeys, *Invest Ophthalmol Vis Sci* 37:1348, 1996.
24. Kaufman PL, Barany EN: Adrenergic drug effects on aqueous outflow following ciliary muscle displacement in the cynomolgus monkey, *Invest Ophthalmol Vis Sci* 20:644, 1981.
25. Bill A: Early effects of epinephrine on aqueous humor dynamics in vervet monkeys (Cercopithecus ethiops), *Exp Eye Res* 8:35, 1969.
26. Araie M, Takase M: Effects of various drugs on aqueous humor dynamics in man, *Jpn J Ophthalmol* 25:91, 1981.

27. Higgins RG, Brubaker RF: Acute effect of epinephrine on aqueous humor formation in the timolol-treated normal eye as measured by fluorophotometry, *Invest Ophthalmol Vis Sci* 19:420, 1980.
28. Lee DA, Brubaker RF, Nagataki S: Acute effects of thymoxamine on aqueous humor formation in the epinephrine treated normal eye as measured by fluorophotometry, *Invest Ophthalmol Vis Sci* 24:165, 1983.
29. Schneider TL, Brubaker RF: Effect of chronic epinephrine on aqueous humor flow during the day and during sleep in normal healthy subjects, *Invest Ophthalmol Vis Sci* 32:2507, 1991.
30. Kupfer C, Gaasterland D, Ross K: Studies of aqueous humor dynamics in man. II. Measurements in young normal subjects using acetazolamide and l-epinephrine, *Invest Ophthalmol* 10:523, 1971.
31. Langham ME, Krieglstein GK: Biphasic intraocular response of conscious rabbits to epinephrine, *Invest Ophthalmol* 15: 119, 1976.
32. Mittag TW, Tormay A: Desensitization of the beta-adrenergic receptor adenylate cyclase complex in rabbit iris-ciliary body induced by topical epinephrine, *Exp Eye Res* 33:497, 1981.
33. Flach AJ, Donahue ME, Wood IS: Nerve terminal degeneration in the rat iris observed following chronic topical 2% epinephrine and 0.1% dipivalyl epinephrine: a quantitative comparison of electron microscopic observations and tissue norepinephrine levels, *Graefes Arch Clin Exp Ophthalmol* 230:575, 1992.
34. Neufeld AH, Page ED: In vitro determination of the ability of drugs to bind to adrenergic receptors, *Invest Ophthalmol Vis Sci* 16:1118, 1979.
35. Flach AJ, Kramer SG: Supersensitivity to topical epinephrine after long-term epinephrine therapy, *Arch Ophthalmol* 98: 482, 1980.
36. Camras C, and others: Inhibition of the epinephrine-induced reduction of intraocular pressure by systemic indomethacin in humans, *Am J Ophthalmol* 100:169, 1985.

cape" by Boger and co-workers[49] and may relate to an increase in the number of β-adrenergic receptors in the ciliary processes under the condition of prolonged β-adrenergic blockade.[50] Unfortunately, the response to timolol at 1 month is not predicted by the response to a single administration given in the office.[51] After this initial adjustment process, most patients maintain a reduction in IOP for months to years. However, 10% to 20% of patients demonstrate some loss of drug effect over subsequent months.[52,53] Fluorophotometric studies indicate that aqueous humor production is reduced 47% after 1 week of timolol treatment but only 25% after 1 year of treatment.[54] This process has been termed the "long-term drift" by Steinert and co-workers[53] and may be explained by a time-dependent decrease in cellular sensitivity to adrenergic antagonists.

Over the short-term, timolol is more effective in reducing IOP than is pilocarpine[55-57] or epinephrine.[58] The ocular hypotensive effect of timolol is additive to that of the miotics[49-60] and the carbonic anhydrase inhibitors (CAIs).[49,61-63] It should be emphasized that timolol and the CAIs are only somewhat additive in their effects on IOP.[62,63] In one study, timolol alone reduced aqueous humor formation by 33%, acetazolamide alone reduced aqueous formation by 27%, and the combination reduced aqueous humor formation by 44%[64] (i.e., the combination was more effective than either agent alone but less effective than the sum of the two drugs).

The effectiveness of combining timolol and epinephrine (or dipivefrin) is controversial. Some studies suggest that the drugs are additive in their ocular hypotensive effects,[49,60,65,66] but others deny this effect.[26,67] When epinephrine or dipivefrin is added to timolol treatment, there is little additional reduction of IOP.[26,59] When timolol is added to epinephrine treatment there is an initial decrease in IOP,[26,65,67] but this reduction declines rapidly over a few weeks.[26,68] It appears that only a minority of patients experience a substantial long-term reduction in IOP when timolol is added to epinephrine treatment or vice versa.[68] The best way to determine the efficacy of combined therapy in a specific patient is to use a therapeutic trial in one eye for several weeks. Some investigators believe that the order of administration or the interval between the drugs affects the additivity of timolol and epinephrine.[69] However, most physicians believe that these factors make little difference.[68] The poor additivity of the two drugs may reflect the fact that timolol blocks the effect of epinephrine on outflow facility.[26] Timolol reduces IOP in patients who are receiving otherwise maximum tolerated medical therapy.[70,71] This additional IOP reduction may persist for months to years and may prevent or delay the necessity for surgery.

The question arises as to whether topical timolol reduces IOP in patients treated with systemically administered β-adrenergic antagonists. The IOP response depends on the dose of the systemic agent. Topical timolol reduces IOP in patients treated with lower doses of the oral β-adrenergic antagonists (e.g., propranolol, 10 to 80 mg/day).[72] However, there is little additional reduction in IOP when topical timolol is administered to patients treated with larger doses of the systemic drugs (e.g., propranolol, 160 mg/day, or oral timolol, 20 mg/day).[73] The value of prescribing topical timolol in this situation is best determined in a therapeutic trial in one eye.

Timolol Hemihydrate

Timolol hemihydrate (Betimol, Ciba Vision, Duluth, Ga) is a recently introduced new salt of timolol. Its clinical effectiveness and side effects are similar to those of timolol maleate.[74] The major advantage of this formulation seems to lie in its cost, which may be less than Timoptic but usually more than generic timolol maleate. Timolol hemihydrate is available in 0.25% and 0.5% solutions for use once or twice daily.[48]

Betaxolol

Betaxolol (Betoptic, Alcon Laboratories, Fort Worth, Texas) is a relatively selective β$_1$-adrenergic antagonist that lacks intrinsic sympathomimetic activity and membrane-stabilizing properties (see Table 24-1). It is puzzling why a β$_1$-adrenergic antagonist should lower IOP because the β-receptors in the ciliary epithelium are thought to be β$_2$ in type.[28,30] The most likely explanation is that betaxolol reaches the ciliary epithelium in sufficient concentration to inhibit β$_2$-receptors. Other possible explanations include the presence of β$_1$ receptors in the ciliary body or a nonadrenergic effect of betaxolol on IOP.[75] Betaxolol is supplied either in a 0.5% solution or a 0.25% microsuspension for administration every 12 hours. The drug reduces IOP[75-77] by decreasing aqueous humor formation.[15] Although a few studies indicate that betaxolol and timolol are equipotent,[78,79] most physicians believe timolol is more effective at lowering IOP.[80] The latter impression is supported by experiments indicating that selective β-adrenergic antagonists are less effective than are nonselective antagonists in reducing IOP in animal models of ocular hypertension.[81] Some clinical and animal studies further suggest that tachyphylaxis is common with selective β-adrenergic antagonists;[7] this has not been a major problem with long-term betaxolol treatment, although it does occur to some extent. Betaxolol appears to be additive in its ocular hypotensive effect with the miotics and the CAIs.[82] Because of its relative β_1-specificity, betaxolol may not block the effect of epinephrine on aqueous outflow. A few studies suggest that betaxolol and epinephrine are more additive in their ocular hypotensive effects than are timolol or levobunolol and epinephrine.[83,84]

Evidence is beginning to accumulate that betaxolol may be more "neuroprotective" than its more nonselective cousins despite a weaker effect on IOP lowering. Betaxolol seems to reduce the progression of visual field defects compared with timolol[85] and may even increase retinal sensitivity.[86] Betaxolol relaxes the smooth muscle in the walls of retinal microarterioles.[87] Using Doppler color imaging of retinal vessels, which is an indirect measure of blood flow, topical betaxolol seems to increase retinal blood flow.[88] This appears to be particularly true in patients with normal-pressure glaucoma.[89] The clinical significance of these observations remains unknown, but the implication is that some property of betaxolol other than its pressure-lowering effect may improve blood flow and/or nerve function.

Betaxolol is less likely than is timolol to induce β_2-adrenergic–mediated bronchial constriction and therefore is a better choice for patients with reactive airway disease.[90] It must be emphasized that the β-adrenergic specificity of betaxolol is relative, and the drug can induce or exacerbate pulmonary problems in susceptible patients. Some investigators postulate that betaxolol is less likely than is timolol to produce cardiovascular and central nervous system side effects, perhaps because of decreased systemic effectiveness or more rapid metabolism.[91] This impression requires further study. Betaxolol is less likely than is timolol to interfere with exercise tolerance.[92] Betaxolol in solution form produces more burning and stinging on instillation than does timolol,[93] whereas the microsuspension form has an ocular discomfort profile more like timolol.[94]

Levobunolol

Levobunolol (Betagan, Allergan, Irvine, Calif) is a nonselective β_1- and β_2-adrenergic antagonist that lacks intrinsic sympathomimetic activity and local anesthetic properties.[95,96] The drug is used systemically to treat hypertension, ventricular arrhythmias, and angina. Levobunolol is supplied as either a 0.25% or a 0.5% solution, which is administered every 12 to 24 hours. The drug appears to be similar to timolol with regard to both efficacy and safety.[97-100] It has been suggested that levobunolol is more likely than is timolol to control IOP with once-daily administration.[101] However, the two drugs seem to have similar durations of action.[102] Levobunolol produces blepharoconjunctivitis more frequently than does timolol.[103,104] The metabolites of levobunolol also appear to have ocular hypotensive effects.

Carteolol

Carteolol (Ocupress, Otsuka America Pharmaceutical, Inc, Seattle) is a nonselective, β-adrenergic antagonist. It is chemically related to timolol, metipranolol, levobunolol, and betaxolol with a potency 10 times that of propranolol; it has partial intrinsic agonist properties toward both β_1- and β_2-adrenoreceptors but no local anesthetic activity.[105] Carteolol is available as a 1% or 2% solution for use every 12 hours; the drug has a significant effect on IOP by 1 hour after administration and reaches its peak effect at about 4 hours after administration.[106] Carteolol 1% appears to produce a pressure-lowering effect similar to that of timolol 0.5% when administered every 12 hours.[107,108] Carteolol seemed to produce fewer local side effects than does timolol.[102]

Because of its intrinsic sympathomimetic activity, carteolol might be expected to produce fewer cardiovascular side effects such as bradycardia and systemic hypotension and perhaps fewer pulmonary effects. Carteolol produced less bradycardia, lowering of blood pressure, dizziness, and headache and had less of an effect on pulmonary function studies than did topical timolol.[102,109] However, the differences are small and may be of only modest clinical significance. All of these side effects tend to occur more frequently with any of the nonselective β-blocking agents in a general population and with longer-term use compared to the carefully selected patients in formal studies.

Long-term use of topical timolol maleate has been shown to increase plasma triglycerides by an average of 12% and decrease high-density lipoprotein (good) cholesterol levels by 9%.[110] The authors[110] estimated that over a period of years this could result in an increase of coronary heart dis-

and found to have satisfactory but not impressive effectiveness.[56,61,62] Finally, dorzolamide (formerly known as L-671, 152, then MK-507) was found to have the right balance of effectiveness and minimal local side effects.[63-65]

Dorzolamide

Dorzolamide (Trusopt, Merck, West Point, Penn) differs from the oral agents in that it has both a free sulfonamide group and a second amine group, which adds the right amount of lipid and aqueous solubility for good corneal penetration.[66] Dorzolamide is effective in inhibiting isoenzymes II and IV, with a somewhat weaker effect on isoenzyme I.[66] There is little crossover effect on the other eye, confirming its local rather than systemic action. The drug is excreted by the kidneys largely unmetabolized, but a small amount is metabolized by the liver to the *des*-ethyl form.[68]

The *des*-ethyl form has a significant inhibitory effect on isoenzyme I.[67] Both dorzolamide and its metabolite are largely bound to RBC cholinesterase and are not present to any extent as free molecules in plasma. Systemic effects are minimal, but RBC CA is depressed to 21% of normal levels.[65] After 8 days of topical therapy, virtually all of the RBC CA is inhibited.[67] After 18 months of use, only about 1/200th of the concentration needed to induce significant systemic side effects is found in plasma.[67] The depression of CA in the RBCs may be seen for months after the drug has been discontinued.

Dose–response studies of 0.7%, 1.4%, and 2.0% have shown that the 2% solution is the most effective, producing peak and trough IOP reductions of 21% and 13%, respectively, with twice-daily usage and slightly better trough reduction with dosing three times daily.[64] Topical dorzolamide reaches a peak effect on IOP at about 3 hours after dosing compared with 2 hours with oral acetazolamide.[68] At its peak, dorzolamide lowers IOP as well as does timolol maleate, but the effect does not last as long.[69] In monkeys, dorzolamide 2.0% will produce a 38% reduction in aqueous inflow.[57] In a 1-year study, topical dorzolamide 2.0% appeared to be as effective and as well tolerated as topical betaxolol 0.5%.[70] Long-term studies have shown tolerability similar to or better than other topical agents such as timolol and pilocarpine.[71] Dorzolamide is available commercially as a 2% solution to be used every 8 hours as monotherapy and every 12 hours as adjunctive therapy.

Dorzolamide is additive to other aqueous suppressants such as timolol[72] and to drugs acting on the outflow system such as pilocarpine.[71] Dorzolamide has been used successfully in a fixed combination with timolol (Cosopt, Merck, West Point, Penn).[73]

The corneal endothelium is rich in CA; this fact caused concern that CA inhibition by topical agents might interfere with endothelial function. Using ultrasonic pachymetry, Wilkerson and co-workers[65] showed that topical dorzolamide administered over 4 weeks increases the corneal thickness very slightly compared with placebo; however, it is unlikely that this small change is clinically significant. Furthermore, Serle and co-workers[74] failed to show any change in corneal thickness after 6 weeks of application.

Brinzolamide

Another promising topical agent, brinzolamide (Azopt, Alcon Laboratories, Fort Worth, Texas), is currently available.[66] Brinzolamide was a known CAI that was irritating when used topically in solution because of its low pH and had a disappointing effect due to poor corneal penetration. Placing the compound in a suspension rather than in the traditional solution was found to improve its ability to get across the cornea, reduce the surface irritation, increase its pressure-reducing activity, and prolong the duration of action.[75] In fact, topical brinzolamide 1% given three times daily to patients with glaucoma or ocular hypertension was shown in two masked studies to be at least as effective as dorzolamide 2% administered three times daily, with less discomfort on administration.[76,77] In addition, twice-daily dosing with brinzolamide was equal in pressure-lowering efficacy to thrice-daily dorzolamide and twice-daily timolol maleate.[71] Finally, brinzolamide three times daily lowered IOP an additional 13% to 16% when added to twice-daily timolol maleate therapy.[78] Long-term studies are under way and will determine the usefulness of this agent in the management of glaucoma.

Systemic Carbonic Anhydrase Inhibitors

All of the commonly used oral CAIs produce similar IOP reductions and similar types of side effects when administered in equipotent doses. The various oral agents differ in potency and to some extent in efficacy; that is, they all produce a similar IOP reduction but at different doses. All of the compounds have a similar range of activity *in vitro* except for ethoxzolamide, which is 5 to 10 times more active. The difference in potency of the various drugs *in vivo* reflects differences in lipid solubility and protein binding that affect body distribution (Table 25-1).

Acetazolamide

Acetazolamide (Diamox, Storz Ophthalmics, St. Louis; Ak-Zol, Akorn, Inc., Abita Springs, La) was the first CAI to receive widespread use in ophthalmology, and it remains the agent with which we have the greatest experience. It is supplied in 125- and 250-mg tablets and as a 500-mg sustained-release (SR) preparation. The 250-mg tablet administered four times daily produces an IOP reduction similar to that seen with the 500-mg SR preparation administered twice daily. The SR preparation is more convenient, not significantly more expensive per day, and better tolerated than are the tablets.[79,80] In fact, the SR capsules are the fastest-acting, most effective, and best tolerated at full dosage of the oral CAIs.[81] It is rarely useful to prescribe acetazolamide in doses greater than 1000 mg/day.

After oral tablet administration, IOP begins to drop in 1 to 2 hours, reaches a minimum in 2 to 4 hours, and returns to baseline in 4 to 12 hours. After oral administration of a 500-mg SR preparation, IOP begins to drop in 2 to 4 hours, reaches a minimum in 8 hours, and returns to baseline in 12 to 24 hours. However, one study suggested that the SR preparation may be faster acting than previously thought.[81]

Oral acetazolamide can be administered to infants in a dose of 5 to 10 mg/kg every 6 hours. To prepare the medication the pharmacist must crush the tablets and suspend the powder in flavored syrup.

Acetazolamide is also available in 500-mg emergency ampules. The drug is dissolved in 5 to 10 ml of distilled water and then intravenously or intramuscularly administered in a dose of 250 to 500 mg. After intravenous injection, IOP begins to fall within minutes, reaches a minimum in 15 to 30 minutes, and returns to baseline in 4 to 6 hours. Parenteral injection is indicated in conditions associated with nausea and vomiting (e.g., acute angle-closure glaucoma) or when maximum IOP lowering is immediately imperative.

Acetazolamide penetrates the eye poorly because of high plasma binding and ready ionization. The serum half-life of the drug is approximately 4 hours. Acetazolamide is not metabolized and is actively secreted by the renal tubules and then passively resorbed by nonionic diffusion.[24,82] Older patients have a lower clearance of unbound acetazolamide, but this is mostly offset by a lower percentage of binding.[83]

The IOP reduction produced by acetazolamide generally parallels the plasma level of the drug. The maximum IOP reduction is generally obtained with plasma acetazolamide concentrations of 4 to 20 μg/ml.[18,84,85] Initially, acetazolamide causes a loss of sodium, potassium, and bicarbonate in the urine. The mild metabolic acidosis that develops with acetazolamide therapy is a consequence of the initial bicarbonate loss. However, the electrolyte balance soon reaches a new steady state de-

Table 25-1

The Chemical and Pharmacologic Properties of the Systemic Carbonic Anhydrase Inhibitors in Clinical Use

Name	$K_1 \times 10^{-9}$	pK$_a$	Unionized in Plasma pH 7.4 (%)	Unbound in Plasma (%)	Half-life in Humans (hours)
Acetazolamide	6	7.4	50	5	4
Methazolamide	8	7.2	39	45	15
Ethoxzolamide	1	8.1	83	4	6
Dichlorphenamide	18	8.3	89	—	2

Modified from Friedland BR, Maren TH: *Carbonic anhydrase: pharmacology of inhibitors and treatment of glaucoma.* In Sears ML, editor: *Pharmacology of the eye: handbook of experimental ophthalmology,* vol 69, Berlin, 1984, Springer-Verlag.

spite continued treatment. Bicarbonate resorption independent of carbonic anhydrase prevents further loss of this ion and progressive acidosis.[84]

Methazolamide

Methazolamide (Neptazane, Storz Ophthalmics, St. Louis; Glauctabs, Akorn, Inc., Abita Springs, La; MZM, Ciba Vision Ophthalmics, Duluth, Ga) is supplied in 25- and 50-mg tablets. It is best to initiate methazolamide therapy with a low dose of the drug (e.g., 25 mg twice daily) and to increase this dose as required to control IOP. Low doses of methazolamide often reduce IOP while producing minimal acidosis and electrolyte disturbance as well as a low incidence of side effects.[18,21] Higher doses of the drug produce greater IOP reductions but also greater acidosis and a higher incidence of side effects.[21,85] The most common treatment regimen for methazolamide is 50 to 100 mg twice daily. Methazolamide, 50 mg twice daily, is slightly less effective than is acetazolamide, 250 mg four times daily or 500-mg SR preparations twice daily.[21,85] After administration of a 50-mg tablet, IOP begins to drop in 1 to 2 hours, reaches a minimum in 4 to 6 hours, and returns to baseline in 12 to 24 hours. Because methazolamide has a serum half-life of 14 hours, it is unnecessary to administer the drug more frequently than twice daily.[18]

Methazolamide is not actively secreted by the kidneys. Approximately 25% of the drug appears unchanged in the urine. The metabolic fate of the remainder is unknown, although some appears to be converted by glutathione.[86] The metabolism of methazolamide makes it a safer choice than acetazolamide for patients with advanced renal disease (e.g., a diabetic patient with neovascular glaucoma). Methazolamide has some advantages over acetazolamide. First, methazolamide diffuses into the eye more easily than does acetazolamide. This probably reflects in part the fact that methazolamide is less bound to plasma protein. Second, methazolamide is not actively taken up by the renal tubules as is the case with acetazolamide. Third, its duration of action makes it more convenient to use (twice daily) than acetazolamide tablets (four times daily). Some authorities postulate that methazolamide is less likely than is acetazolamide to produce urolithiasis because it produces less suppression of urinary citrate and less urine alkalinization.[85] However, methazolamide therapy has been reported to cause urinary tract stones.[87,88] Whether methazolamide actually has a lower incidence of urinary calculi than does acetazolamide has not been established, but most authorities prefer methazolamide to acetazolamide in patients with a history of renal lithiasis. Methazolamide diffuses more easily into the eye and CNS.[82,89] Thus it is more likely than acetazolamide to produce such CNS-related symptoms as fatigue, depression, and drowsiness.

Ethoxzolamide

Ethoxzolamide is the most potent of the clinically used CAIs *in vitro*. However, its *in vivo* activity is reduced by high plasma protein binding. Ethoxzolamide is supplied in a 125-mg tablet and prescribed in doses of 62.5 to 250 mg every 4 to 8 hours. The most commonly prescribed dose is 125 mg every 6 hours. After administration of a 125-mg tablet, IOP begins to fall in 2 hours, reaches a minimum in 5 hours, and returns to baseline in 12 hours.

Ethoxzolamide is a weak organic acid that is secreted slightly by the renal tubules. Forty percent of the drug appears unchanged in the urine. The metabolic fate of the remainder is not entirely known, but some is converted by glutathione. Ethoxzolamide was the first CAI to be successfully used topically. This agent has essentially disappeared from current use in the United States.

Dichlorphenamide

Dichlorphenamide (Daranide, Merck, West Point, Penn) is supplied in a 50-mg tablet and prescribed in doses of 25 to 200 mg every 6 to 8 hours. After oral administration of a 50-mg tablet, IOP begins to fall in 30 minutes, reaches a minimum in 2 to 4 hours, and returns to baseline in 6 to 12 hours.

Despite the fact that the dichlorphenamide molecule contains two sulfonamide groups, it is no more effective than the other CAIs. Dichlorphenamide produces less metabolic acidosis because it has inherent chloruretic activity.[90] However, the continued loss of chloride sometimes produces sustained diuresis and potassium depletion. Dichlorphenamide produced more symptoms and side effects than did the other CAIs in one trial.[91] It is little used at this time.

SIDE EFFECTS

Topical Carbonic Anhydrase Inhibitors

The side effects of the topical CAIs are largely ocular in nature (Box 25-1). Stinging on administration is the most common. Presumably because of their sulfonamide derivation, the topical agents are associated with a relatively high rate of allergic reactions (about 10%), as are the oral agents. Superficial punctate keratopathy is seen in about 10% of cases. Transient myopia has been reported. Although systemic side effects are not common, some do occur. A metallic taste in the mouth, especially associated with carbonated beverages, is relatively common (25%). Gastrointestinal distress may occur particularly in the first few days of use. Urticaria and dizziness have also been reported in rare instances. Although RBC CA is depressed with topical dorzolamide, no symptoms appear to be associated with this finding.

Obviously, systemic side effects can be reduced by having the patient use simple eyelid closure and punctal occlusion immediately after administering the drops. Some of the more serious side effects associated with the oral agents (e.g., aplastic anemia and Stevens-Johnson syndrome) have not been reported with topical agents; however, anecdotal reports of neutropenia suggest that it may only be a matter of time before the rare case is actually seen.[91a] Other side effects, especially those associated with systemic agents, may be seen as the topical agents are used in more patients for longer periods.

Oral Carbonic Anhydrase Inhibitors

It is estimated that 50% of glaucoma patients cannot tolerate long-term treatment with oral CAIs because of the associated side effects (Box 25-2). The etiology of many of the side effects is unclear but may be related to acidosis or carbon dioxide retention. It is important to emphasize that the incidence and severity of side effects can be reduced greatly by using the medication in the lowest dose and frequency necessary for IOP control. Patients should be warned of potential side effects and told that many side effects will diminish in severity after a few days to a few weeks of treatment. Patients prepared in this manner are more trusting of the physician and are more ready to accept problems when they occur. Older patients are generally less tolerant of oral CAIs.[92]

One important study found that patient tolerance to the various CAIs in fixed doses is as follows (in order of decreasing tolerance): acetazolamide, 500 mg SR preparation twice daily; methazolamide, 50 mg every 6 hours; ethoxzolamide, 125 mg every 6 hours; acetazolamide, 250 mg every 6 hours; and dichlorphenamide, 50 mg every 6 hours.[91] Although no study has placed methazolamide, 25 mg every 12 hours, in this tolerance ranking, in the authors' experience it is often effective and the best tolerated of the oral CAIs. A patient who is intolerant of one CAI may be more tolerant of another. Generally, however, the side effects are more closely linked to the dose than to the specific drug.

Box 25-1
Side Effects of Topical Carbonic Anhydrase Inhibitors

Ocular	Systemic
Stinging	Metallic taste
Allergy	Urticaria
Dryness	Neutropenia
Superficial punctate keratopathy	Headache
Induced myopia	Gastrointestinal distress
	Dizziness
	Paresthesias
	?Aplastic anemia
	?Stevens-Johnson syndrome

may be helpful to detect early changes. Patients with gray-brown, blue-brown, hazel, or green-brown irides should be warned about iris color change and its permanence. If cosmesis is a concern to the patient, consideration should be given to alternative medications if possible. Similarly, patients should be warned that their eyelashes may grow longer and darker and may proliferate. Most patients will not mind this at all, but, again, if it may be a problem, consideration should be given to an alternative. Because an increase of eyelid hair is also a potential side effect, this should be included in the warnings.

Because systemic side effects may be subtle and not usually associated with topical eyedrop medications, the patient should be asked specifically about myalgia, joint pain, headache, and bitter taste. Rarely are the systemic symptoms enough to warrant discontinuation. If systemic side effects become significant, eyelid closure and punctal occlusion should be tried before discontinuing.

Latanoprost has not been tested in children or infants, although there is little reason to withhold its use if vision is threatened. Data regarding its use in pregnancy are absent. Given the fact that prostaglandins are used to initiate labor, latanoprost should probably be avoided during the last phases of pregnancy.[75]

REFERENCES

1. Ambache N: Irin, a smooth-muscle contracting substance present in rabbit iris, *J Physiol (Lond)* 129:65P, 1955.
2. Amache N: Properties of irin, a physiological constituent of the rabbit iris, *J Physiol (Lond)* 135:114, 1957.
3. Toris CB, Camras CB: Prostaglandins: a new class of aqueous outflow agents, *Ophthalmol Clin North Am* 10:335, 1997.
4. Eakins KE: Prostaglandin and non-prostaglandin mediated breakdown of the blood-aqueous barrier, *Exp Eye Res* 25:483, 1977.
5. Weinreb RN, and others: *Glucocorticoid regulation of eicosanoid biosynthesis in cultured human trabecular cells.* In Ticho U, editor: *Recent advances in glaucoma,* New York, 1984, Elsevier Science.
6. Matsumoto S, and others: Endothelin-induced changes of second messengers in cultured human ciliary muscle cells, *Invest Ophthalmol Vis Sci* 37:1058, 1996.
7. Bazan NG, Allan G: Signal transduction and gene expression in the eye: a contemporary view of the pro-inflammatory, anti-inflammatory and modulatory roles of prostaglandins and other bioactive lipids, *Surv Ophthalmol* 41(supp 2):S23, 1997.
8. Gabelt BT, Kaufman PL: *Pharmacologic enhancement of aqueous humor outflow.* In Van Buskirk EM, Shields MB, editors: *100 years of progress in glaucoma,* Philadelphia, 1997, Lippincott-Raven.
9. Starr MS: Further studies on the effect of prostaglandin on intraocular pressure in the rabbit, *Exp Eye Res* 11:170, 1971.
10. Camras CB, Bito LZ, Eakins KE: Reduction of intraocular pressure by prostaglandins applied topically to the eyes of conscious rabbits, *Invest Ophthalmol Vis Sci* 16:1125, 1977.
11. Camras CB, Bito LZ: Reduction of intraocular pressure in normal and glaucomatous primate *(Aotus trivirgatus)* eyes by topically applied prostaglandin F_2, *Curr Eye Res* 1:205, 1981.
12. Crawford KS, Kaufman PL, Gabelt BT: Effects of topical PGF_2 on aqueous humor dynamics in cynomolgus monkeys, *Curr Eye Res* 6:1035, 1987.
13. Gabelt BT, Kaufman PL: The effect of prostaglandin F_2 on trabecular outflow facility in cynomolgus monkeys, *Exp Eye Res* 51:87, 1990.
14. Hayashi M, Yablonski ME, Bito LZ: Eicosanoids as a new class of ocular hypotensive agents. 2. Comparison of the apparent mechanism of the ocular hypotensive effects of A and F type prostaglandins, *Invest Ophthalmol Vis Sci* 28:1639, 1987.
15. Crawford KS, Kaufman PL: Dose-related effects of prostaglandin F_2 isopropylester on intraocular pressure, refraction and pupil diameter in monkeys, *Invest Ophthalmol Vis Sci* 32:510, 1991.
16. Woodward DF, and others: The molecular biology and ocular distribution of prostanoid receptors, *Surv Ophthalmol* (suppl 2):S15, 1997.
17. Woodward DF, and others: Marked species differences in the pharmacology of prostanoid induced ocular hypotension, *Invest Ophthalmol Vis Sci* 32:1257, 1994.
18. Bito LZ: Species differences in the responses of the eye to irritation and trauma: a hypothesis of divergence in ocular defense mechanisms, and the choice of experimental animals for eye research, *Exp Eye Res* 38:131, 1984.
19. Nilsson SFE, and others: Increased uveoscleral outflow as a possible mechanism of ocular hypotension caused by prostaglandin F_2-1-isopropylester in the cynomolgus monkey, *Exp Eye Res* 48:707, 1989.
20. Gabelt BT, Kaufman PL: Prostaglandin F_2 increases uveoscleral outflow in the cynomolgus monkey, *Exp Eye Res* 49:389, 1989.
21. Selen G, and others: Effects of PHXA34 and PhDH100A, two phenyl substituted prostaglandin esters, on aqueous humor dynamics and microcirculation in the monkey eye, *Invest Ophthalmol Vis Sci* 32:869, 1991.
22. Ziai N, and others: The effects on aqueous dynamics of PHXA41, a new prostaglandin F_2 alpha analogue, after topical application in normal and ocular hypertensive human eyes, *Arch Ophthalmol* 111:1351, 1993.
23. Lutjen-Drecoll E, Tamm E: Morphological study of the anterior segments of cynomolgus monkey eyes following treatment with prostaglandin F_2, *Exp Eye Res* 47:761, 1988.
24. Tamm E, Rittig M, Lutjen-Drecoll E: Elektronenmikroskopische and immuno-histochemische Untersuchungen zur augendruckensenkenden Wirkung von Prostaglandin F_2, *Fortschr Ophthalmol* 87:623, 1990.
25. Lindsey JD, and others: Prostaglandin action on ciliary smooth muscle extracellular matrix metabolism: implications for uveoscleral outflow, *Surv Ophthalmol* 41(suppl 2):S53, 1997.
26. Giuffre G: The effects of prostaglandin F_2, in the human eye, *Graefes Arch Clin Exp Ophthalmol* 222:139, 1985.
27. Lee P, and others: The effect of prostaglandin F_2 on intraocular pressure in normotensive human subjects, *Invest Ophthalmol Vis Sci* 29:1474, 1988.
28. Nakjima M, and others: Effects of prostaglandin D_2 and its analog, BW245C, on intraocular pressure in humans, *Graefes Arch Clin Exp Ophthalmol* 229:411, 1991.
29. Flach AJ, Eliason JA: Topical prostaglandin E_2 effects on normal human intraocular pressure, *J Ocul Pharmacol* 4:13, 1988.
30. Vilumseb J, Alm A: Prostaglandin F_2-1-isopropylester eye drops: effects in normal human eyes, *Br J Ophthalmol* 73:419, 1989.
31. Takase M, and others: Ocular effects of topical instillation of UF-021 ophthalmic solution in healthy volunteers, *Nippon Ganka Gakkai Zasshi* 96:1261, 1992.
32. Takase M, and others: Ocular effects of continuous topical instillations of UF-021 ophthalmic solution in healthy volunteers, *Atarashii Ganka J Eye* 9:1055, 1992.

33. Stjernschantz J, and others: Phenyl substituted prostaglandin esters: effects in the eye, *Invest Ophthalmol Vis Sci* 32:1257, 1991.

34. Justin N, and others: Effect of PHXA34, a new prostaglandin (PG) derivative, on intaocular pressure (IOP) after topical application to glaucomatous monkey eyes, *Invest Ophthalmol Vis Sci* 32:947, 1991.

35. Alm A, and others: PHXA34, a new potent ocular hypotensive drug: a study on dose-response relationship and on aqueous humor dynamics in healthy volunteers, *Arch Ophthalmol* 109:1564, 1991.

36. Camras CB, and others: Intraocular pressure reduction with PHXA34, a new prostaglandin analogue, in patients with ocular hypertension, *Arch Ophthalmol* 110:1733, 1992.

37. Camras CB, Podos SM: *Reduction of intraocular pressure by exogenous and endogenous prostaglandins.* In Drance SM, Van Buskirk EM, Neufeld AH, editors: *Pharmacology of glaucoma,* Baltimore, 1992, Williams & Wilkins.

38. Alm A, and others: Intraocular pressure-reducing effect of PHXA41 in patients with increased eye pressure: a one month study, *Ophthalmology* 100:1312, 1993.

39. Hotehana Y, and others: Ocular hypotensive effect of PHXA41 in patients with ocular hypertension or primary open-angle glaucoma, *Jpn J Ophthalmol* 37: 270, 1993.

40. Nagasubramanian S, and others: Intraocular pressure-reducing effect of PHXA41 in ocular hypertension: comparison of dose regimens, *Ophthalmology* 100:1305, 1993.

41. Racz P, and others: Maintained intraocular pressure reduction with once-a-day application of a new prostaglandin F_2 analogue (PHXA41): an in-hospital placebo-controlled study, *Arch Ophthalmol* 111: 657, 1993.

42. Alm A, Stjernschantz J, Scandinavian Latanoprost Study Group: Effects of intraocular pressure and side-effects of 0.005% latanoprost applied once daily, evening or morning: a comparison with timolol, *Ophthalmology* 102:1743, 1995.

43. Camras CB, US Latanoprost Study Group: Comparison of latanoprost and timolol in patients with ocular hypertension and glaucoma: a six-month, masked, multicenter trial in the United States, *Ophthalmology* 103:138, 1996.

44. Watson PG, Stjernschantz J, Latanoprost Study Group: A six-month, randomized, double-masked study comparing latanoprost with timolol in open angle glaucoma and ocular hypertension, *Ophthalmology* 103:126, 1996.

45. Mishima HK, and others: A comparison of latanoprost and timolol in primary open angle glaucoma and ocular hypertension: a 12-week study, *Arch Ophthalmol* 114: 929, 1996.

46. Hedner J, and others: The lack of respiratory effects of the ocular hypotensive drug latanoprost in patients with moderate-steroid treated asthma, *Surv Ophthalmol* 41(suppl 2):S111, 1997.

47. Racz P, and others: Around-the-clock intraocular pressure reduction with once-daily application of latanoprost by itself or in combination with timolol, *Ophthalmology* 114:268, 1996.

48. Mishima HK, and others: The effects of latanoprost on diurnal and nocturnal IOP and aqueous humor dynamics, *Surv Ophthalmol* 41(suppl 2):S139, 1997.

49. Camras CB, and others: Latanoprost, a prostaglandin analog, for glaucoma therapy: efficacy and safety after 1 year of treatment in 198 patients. Latanoprost Study Groups, *Ophthalmology* 103:1916, 1996.

50. Linden C, Nuija E, Alm A: Effects on IOP restoration and blood-aqueous barrier after long-term treatment with latanoprost in open angle glaucoma and ocular hypertension, *Br J Ophthalmol* 81:370, 1997.

51. Diestelhorst M, Roters S, Kriegelstein GK: The effect of latanoprost (PHXA41) on the intraocular pressure and aqueous humor protein concentration: a randomized, double-masked comparison of 50 g/ml vs 15 g/ml with timolol 0.5% as control, *Invest Ophthalmol Vis Sci* 36(suppl): S823, 1995.

52. Diestelhorst M, and others: Clinical dose-regimen studies with latanoprost, a new ocular hypotensive PGF analogue, *Surv Ophthalmol* 41(suppl 2):S77, 1977.

53. Nicolela MT, and others: A comparative study of the effects of timolol and latanoprost on blood flow velocity of the retrobulbar vessels, *Am J Ophthalmol* 122:784, 1996.

54. Greve EI., and others: Reduced intraocular pressure and increased ocular perfusion pressure in normal tension glaucoma: a review of short-term studies with three dose regimens of latanoprost treatment, *Surv Ophthalmol* 41(suppl 2):S89, 1997.

55. Villumsen J, Alm A: The effect of adding prostaglandin F_2 alpha-isopropylester to timolol in patients with open angle glaucoma, *Arch Ophthalmol* 108:1102, 1990.

56. Lee PY, and others: Additivity of prostaglandin F_2 alpha-1-isopropyl ester to timolol in glaucoma patients, *Ophthalmology* 98:1079, 1991.

57. Rulo AH, Greve EL, Hoyng PF: Additive effect of latanoprost, a prostaglandin F_2 alpha analogue, and timolol in patients with elevated intraocular pressure, *Br J Ophthalmol* 78:899, 1994.

58. Alm A, and others: Latanoprost administered once daily caused a maintained reduction of intraocular pressure in glaucoma patients treated concomitantly with timolol, *Br J Ophthalmol* 79:12, 1955.

59. Hoyng PF, and others: The additive intraocular pressure-lowering effect of latanoprost in combined therapy with other ocular hypotensive agents, *Surv Ophthalmol* 41(suppl 2):S93, 1997.

60. Bill A: *Uveoscleral drainage of aqueous humor: physiology and pharmacology.* In Bito LZ, Stjernschantz J, editors: *The ocular effects of prostaglandins and other eicosanoids,* New York, 1989, Alan R Liss.

61. Villumsen J, Alm A: Effect of prostaglandin$_2$ analogue PHXA41 in eyes treated with pilocarpine and timolol, *Invest Ophthalmol Vis Sci* 33:1248, 1992.

62. Fristrom B, Nilsson SE: Interaction of PhXA41, a new prostaglandin analogue, with pilocarpine: a study on patients with elevated intraocular pressure, *Arch Ophthalmol* 111:662, 1993.

63. Linden C, Alm A; Latanoprost and physostigmine have mostly additive ocular hypotensive effects in human eyes, *Arch Ophthalmol* 115:857, 1997.

64. Sakurai M, and others: Effects of topical application of UF-021, a novel prostaglandin-related compound, on aqueous humor dynamics in rabbit, *Jpn J Ophthalmol* 37:252, 1993.

65. Azuma I, and others: Double-masked comparative study of UF-021 and timolol opthalmic solutions in patients with primary open angle glaucoma or ocular hypertension, *Jpn J Ophthalmol* 37:514, 1993.

66. Yamamoto T, and others: Clinical evaluation of UF-021 (Rescula; isopropyl unoprostone), *Surv Ophthalmol* 41(suppl 2):S99, 1997.

67. Kitaya N, and others: Effect of timolol and UF-021 (a prostaglandin-related compound) on pulsatile ocular blood flow in normal volunteers, *Ophthalmic Res* 29: 139, 1997.

68. Alm A, Camras CB, Watson PG: Phase III latanoprost studies in Scandinavia, the United Kingdom and the United States, *Surv Ophthalmol* 41(suppl 2):S105, 1997.

69. Selen G, Stjernschantz J, Resul B: Prostaglandin-induced iridial pigmentation in primates, *Surv Ophthalmol* 41(suppl 2):S125, 1997.

70. Wistrand PJ, Stjernschantz J, Olsson K; The incidence and time-course of latanoprost-induced iridial pigmentation as a function of eye color, *Surv Ophthalmol* 00:(suppl 2):S129, 1997.

71. Yamamoto T, Kitazawa Y: Iris-color change developed after topical isopropyl unoprostone treatment, *J Glaucoma* 6: 430, 1997.

72. Imesch PD, Wallow IH, Albert DM: The color of the human eye: a review of morphologic correlates and of some conditions that affect iridial pigmentation, *Surv Ophthalmol* 41(suppl 2):S117, 1997.

73. Warwar RE, Bullock JD, Ballal D: Cystoid macular edema and anterior uveitis associated with latanoprost use: experience and incidence in a retrospective review of 94 patients, *Ophthalmology* 105: 263, 1998.

74. Johnstone MA: Hypertrichosis and increased pigmentation of eyelashes and adjacent hair in the region of the ipsilateral eyelids of patients treated with unilateral topical latanoprost, *Am J Ophthalmol* 124: 544, 1997.

75. Hannah ME, and others: Induction of labor compared with expectant management for prelabor rupture of the membranes at term. TERMPROM Study Group, *N Engl J Med* 334:1005, 1996.

27

Hyperosmotic Agents

Although the effect of hyperosmotic agents on intraocular pressure (IOP) has been known for almost a century,[1-3] these agents have been widely used in ophthalmology only for the past 35 years. Hyperosmotic agents are useful for the short-term management of acute glaucoma. These drugs can prevent the need for surgery in transient glaucoma conditions, such as occurs with traumatic hyphema. They are also used for lowering IOP preoperatively. Hyperosmotic agents have greatly reduced the necessity for surgically decompressing eyes with markedly elevated IOPs. In addition, they are used in cases of acute cerebral edema and (topically) for corneal edema.

MECHANISMS OF ACTION

Hyperosmotic agents reduce IOP by increasing the osmolality of the plasma and drawing water from the eye into the circulation via the blood vessels of the retina and uveal tract.[4] This transient effect lasts until osmotic equilibrium is reestablished. Within a few hours, the hyperosmotic agent may penetrate the eye. If the agent has already cleared the plasma,[5] reversal of the osmotic gradient occurs (i.e., plasma osmolality decreases to a level below that of the dehydrated tissues), with a rebound increase in IOP. For most agents in clinical use, effective IOP lowering is achieved when plasma osmolality is increased by 20 to 30 mOsm/l. Most of the fluid drawn from the eye comes from the vitreous; vitreous weight is reduced by 2.7% to 3.9% in experimental animals after administration of hyperosmotic agents in doses equivalent to those used clinically.[6] Glaucomatous eyes appear to get a proportionately greater IOP-lowering effect from an osmotic challenge than do normal eyes.[7]

Hyperosmotic agents also appear to lower IOP by a second mechanism; they decrease aqueous humor production via a central nervous system (CNS) pathway involving osmoreceptors in the hypothalamus. The evidence for this second mechanism is summarized as follows: (1) After the administration of hyperosmotic agents, the decrease in IOP and the increase in plasma osmolality are not correlated closely in terms of magnitude of effect or time course.[8] (2) Small doses of hyperosmotic agents administered intravenously can reduce IOP without changing plasma osmolality.[9] (3) Intracarotid injections of hyperosmotic and hypoosmotic solutions alter electric activity in regions of the hypothalamus that are known to affect fluid balance in the body.[10,11] (4) Destruction of the supraoptic nuclei abolishes the IOP response to hypoosmotic solutions.[12] (5) Injections of hyperosmotic and hypoosmotic agents into the third ventricle alter IOP without affecting plasma osmolality.[13]

It has been postulated that the osmoreceptors in the hypothalamus alter aqueous humor production via efferent fibers in the optic nerve. This theory was stimulated by the observation that human eyes with optic nerve lesions develop less elevation of IOP after water loading.[8] Furthermore, some investigators have noted that unilateral optic nerve transection in experimental animals diminishes the IOP response to hyperosmotic and hypoosmotic agents administered intravenously or into the third ventricle.[8,14,15] However, other researchers have failed to confirm the effect of optic nerve transection and have questioned the existence of osmoregulatory efferent fibers in the optic nerve.[16,17]

Intraarterial injections of hyperosmotic agents lead to breakdown of the blood-aqueous barrier and destruction of the nonpigmented ciliary epithelium.[18,19] However, intravenous injections do not have the same effect.[19] Thus it is unlikely that this mechanism plays a role in the clinical response to hyperosmotic agents.

Hyperosmotic agents pull water from the eye along an osmotic gradient and reduce aqueous humor formation via osmoreceptors in the hypothalamus. The specifics of this latter mechanism remain unknown.

DRUGS IN CLINICAL USE

A number of factors are important in determining the osmotic gradient induced between plasma and the ocular fluids. Because the change in plasma osmolality depends on the number of milliosmols of substance administered, agents of low molecular weight (e.g., urea) have a greater effect per gram administered than do compounds of high molecular weight (e.g., mannitol) at the same dose.[20,21] Agents confined to the extracellular fluid space (e.g., mannitol) produce a greater effect on plasma osmolality than do agents distributed in total body water (e.g., urea). This latter factor has a larger effect than that associated with molecular weight. Some drugs rapidly enter the eye (e.g., alcohol), thereby producing less of an osmotic gradient than do those that penetrate slowly (e.g., glycerol). Agents administered intravenously bypass gastrointestinal absorption and produce a more rapid and a slightly greater rise in plasma osmolality.[22]

Other factors that affect the osmotic gradient include the rate of elimination of the agent from the circulation, the production of hypoosmotic diuresis (e.g., alcohol), the condition of the ocular vessels, and the state of the blood-aqueous and blood retinal barriers (e.g., inflammation).[23,24] It is peculiar that these many factors tend to balance each other sufficiently so that most hyperosmotic drugs in clinical use are effective in doses of 1 to 2 g/kg. Patients should be cautioned not to drink water or other fluids after administration of the agent because doing so may reduce the osmotic gradient.[24]

Oral Agents

Orally administered hyperosmotic agents are slightly less effective and have a slower onset of action than do the intravenous agents.[24] Variable absorption from the gastrointestinal tract makes their effect less predictable. These differences are not great, however, and the oral agents are safer and less likely to produce volumetric overload in patients with borderline cardiac status. Oral agents are not well tolerated by patients with nausea and vomiting.

Glycerol

Glycerol (Glyrol, Osmoglyn), the most commonly prescribed hyperosmotic agent, is usually administered as a 50% solution in a dose of 1.5 to 3 ml/kg[7,25] (Table 27-1). (Glycerol is also available as a 75% solution.) It begins to lower IOP in 10 to 30 minutes, reaches a maximum effect in 45 to 120 minutes, and has a duration of effect of 4 to 5 hours.[7,25,26] Glycerol has an intense, sweet taste and is more palatable when given in an iced unsweetened fruit juice or cola base. If necessary, glycerol can be administered repeatedly because it penetrates the eye and other tissues poorly and is confined to the extracellular water.

The major disadvantage of glycerol is the relatively high frequency of associated nausea and vomiting. Glycerol is metabolized in the liver and produces 4.32 kcal/g of energy. The caloric value of glycerol and its metabolites as well as the osmotic dehydration it produces can lead to ketoacidosis and other problems in diabetic patients.[27,28]

Isosorbide

Isosorbide (Ismotic, Hydronol) is a dihydric alcohol formed by the removal of two molecules of water from sorbitol. It is an effective oral hyperosmotic agent, administered as a 45% solution in doses of 1.5 to 4 ml/kg[29-31] (see Table 27-1). Its time of onset and duration of action are similar to those of glycerol.[32] Isosorbide is absorbed rapidly from the gastrointestinal tract and is excreted unchanged in the urine. It must be given in somewhat larger doses than glycerol to produce a comparable effect on IOP. Isosorbide is more expensive than glycerol.

Isosorbide is less likely to produce nausea and vomiting but more likely to produce diarrhea than is glycerol.[33,34] Because isosorbide is not metabolized and is excreted unchanged in the urine, it does not produce any calories and is thus a better choice for diabetic patients.[34] It is possible to confuse isosorbide with isosorbide dinitrate (Isordil), which is used to treat angina.[35]

Ethyl Alcohol

Ethyl alcohol may be an effective oral hyperosmotic agent when administered as straight spirits or diluted with appropriate mixers to a final dose of about 1.0 to 1.8 ml/kg of absolute alcohol (about 1 to 2 ml/kg of a 40% to 50% solution [80 to 100 proof]). Alcohol also induces hypotonic diuresis by inhibiting production of antidiuretic hormone. This prolongs and increases the osmotic gradient. Alcohol enters the eye rapidly, but vitreous penetration is sufficiently delayed to create an osmotic

Table 27-1

Hyperosmotic Agents

Agents	Molecular Weight	Distribution	Ocular Penetration	Usual Dose (gm/kg)	Excreted	Other
Oral						
Glycerol	92	Extracellular	Poor	1-1.5 (1.5-3 ml/kg 50% solution)	Urine and metabolized	May cause nausea and vomiting; source of calories
Isosorbide	146	Total body water	Good	1-2 (1.5-4 ml/kg 45% solution)	Urine	May cause diarrhea
Ethanol	46	Total body water	Good	0.8-1.5 (2-3 ml/kg 40-50% solution)	Metabolized	Hypotonic diuresis, source of calories, may cause nausea, vomiting, central nervous system and gastrointestinal effects
Intravenous						
Urea	60	Total body water	Good	1-2 (2-7 ml/kg 30% solution, 60 drops/min)	Urine	Unstable solution Skin slough Increases BUN Not very soluble
Mannitol	182	Extracellular	Poor	1-2 (2.5-7 ml/kg, 20% solution, 60 drops/min)	Urine	Large volume of solution Dehydration

gradient. The effects of alcohol on the CNS as well as on the gastric mucosa limit its chronic use. It is important to know about alcohol's effect on IOP because a low IOP after a three martini lunch may not be representative of other afternoon pressures. Like glycerol, ethyl alcohol is metabolized, producing calories that may be a problem for diabetic patients. Its use in this context is limited to emergency situations in which other, more appropriate agents are not available.

Intravenous Agents

Intravenously administered hyperosmotic agents produce a more rapid onset of action and a slightly greater effect than do agents administered orally.[24] The intravenous drugs are usually administered over a period of 45 to 60 minutes.

Mannitol

Mannitol (Osmitrol) is an effective hyperosmotic drug that is currently the agent of choice for intravenous administration. The usual dose is 2.5 to 7.0 ml/kg of the 20% solution (see Table 27-1). The drug begins to lower IOP in 15 to 30 minutes, reaches a maximum effect in 30 to 60 minutes, and has a duration of action of approximately 6 hours.[30,36-38] It is not necessary to administer the full dose of the drug; when IOP falls to the desired level, the infusion can be terminated. Mannitol is excreted unchanged in the urine (i.e., it is not metabolized). Because it penetrates the eye poorly, mannitol is especially useful as a hypotensive agent in the presence of ocular inflammation.[24] The 20% solution is stable and less irritating to blood vessels and subcutaneous tissue than is urea.[36]

The major disadvantages of mannitol are the greater likelihood of cellular dehydration because of its confinement to extracellular water and the larger volume of fluid required because of its limited solubility.[39] Cellular dehydration in the CNS may produce symptoms of dementia and disorientation, especially in the elderly. Great caution should be observed in patients with renal failure because they may be unable to excrete the large quantity of fluid extracted from the cells. Similarly, the increased blood volume may place an intolerable load on patients with congestive heart failure. The 20% solution should be warmed to dissolve crystals, and a blood administration filter should be used in the intravenous line. An anaphylactic reaction to mannitol has been reported.[40]

Urea

Urea (Urevert, Ureaphil) was the first intravenous agent used for the treatment of glaucoma. Administered intravenously as a 30% solution in a dose of 2.0 to 7.0 ml/kg (see Table 27-1), urea begins to lower IOP in 15 to 30 minutes, reaches a maximum effect in 60 minutes, and has a duration of action of 4 to 6 hours.[41-44] Urea is slightly less effective than is mannitol because urea diffuses more freely through body water and penetrates the eye more readily. The latter is especially true in inflamed eyes.[23] The drug is prepared in a 10% invert sugar solution to prevent hemolysis. Urea is not metabolized and is excreted rapidly in urine.

As urea is cleared from the circulation, the plasma osmolality may fall below that of the vitreous, resulting in a rebound increase in IOP. Only fresh urea solutions should be administered because old solutions decompose to ammonia. However, fresh solutions must be warmed to compensate for the endothermic reaction of dissolving the drug. The physician should be aware that warming the solution to 50° C or higher produces ammonia. Extravasation of urea results in thrombophlebitis and skin necrosis.[43] Because of these side effects, urea is rarely used.

SIDE EFFECTS

Side effects from hyperosmotic agents are relatively common (Box 27-1). Although most of the associated side effects are relatively mild, some are serious and even potentially fatal. These drugs should be administered with caution in patients with cardiac, renal, and hepatic disease. Headache, nausea, vomiting, and diuresis are the most frequent side effects and are seen with all of the agents in clinical use.[29,43] Intense diuresis after hyperosmotic therapy may lead to urinary retention and a need for catheterization, especially in older men with prostatic enlargement. Nausea, vomiting, and a desire to void may interfere with the calm conditions desired for surgery. For this reason, patients should void before coming to the operating room.

Hyperosmotic agents, especially those restricted to extracellular water, may precipitate pulmonary edema and congestive heart failure in elderly patients with borderline cardiac and renal

75. Carter CJ, and others: Investigations into a vascular etiology for low-tension glaucoma, *Ophthalmology* 97:49, 1990.

76. Kitazawa Y, Shirai H, Go FJ: The effect of Ca-antagonist on visual field in low-tension glaucoma, *Graefes Arch Clin Exp Ophthalmol* 227:408, 1989.

77. Sawada A, and others: Prevention of visual field defect progression with brovincamine in eyes with normal-tension glaucoma, *Ophthalmology* 103:283, 1996.

78. Gasser P, Flammer J: Short- and long-term effect of nifedipine on the visual field in patients with presumed vasospasm, *J Int Med Res* 18:334, 1990.

79. Netland PA, Chaturvedi N, Dreyer EB: Calcium channel blockers in the management of low-tension and open-angle glaucoma, *Am J Ophthalmol* 115:608, 1993.

80. Harino S, Riva CE, Petrig BL: Intravenous nicardipine in cats increases optic nerve head but not retinal blood flow, *Invest Ophthalmol Vis Sci* 33:2885, 1992.

81. Schmidt KG, and others: Influence of physical exercise and nifedipine on ocular pulse amplitude, *Graefes Arch Clin Exp Ophthalmol* 234:527, 1996.

82. Schmidt KG, and others: Effect of nifedipine on ocular pulse amplitude in normal pressure glaucoma, *Klin Monatsbl Augenheilkd* 210:355, 1997.

83. Geyer O, and others: Effect of oral nifedipine on ocular blood flow in patients with low-tension glaucoma, *Br J Ophthalmol* 80:1060, 1996.

84. Wilson RP, and others: A color Doppler analysis of nifedipine-induced posterior ocular blood flow changes in open-angle glaucoma, *J Glaucoma* 6:231, 1997.

85. Harris A, and others: Hemodynamic and visual function effects of oral nifedipine in patients with normal-tension glaucoma, *Am J Ophthalmol* 124:296, 1997.

86. Liu S, and others: Lack of effect of calcium channel blockers on open-angle glaucoma, *J Glaucoma* 5:187, 1996.

PART VI

Laser Therapy

Light Brown Iris

The surgeon can usually recognize a thin area in the anterior stroma, often in the base of a crypt, and can actually see into the depths of the iris. The laser beam should be aimed away from the posterior pole, especially while enlarging the perforation. When the laser energy strikes the iris, a deep pit is produced. These signs indicate that the iris is relatively soft and absorbs the laser energy well so that iridotomy will be easily accomplished.

Initial power settings should be 600 to 1000 mW with a spot size of 50 μm and a shutter speed of 0.05 second. Repeated applications of the laser in the center of the pit produced by the first shot will result in a 200- to 300-μm crater in the iris stroma. When the pigment epithelium is penetrated, a cloud of pigment will come out of the pit. Shutter speed can then be reduced to 0.02 second to remove the pigment epithelium from the depths of the pit and create an opening that is at least 0.2 mm in diameter. This is best done by chipping away at the edges of the small initial opening in the pigment epithelium by aiming the laser beam so that two thirds of the beam is on the pigment epithelium and one third is in the opening. The surgeon should avoid aiming the laser toward the posterior pole by asking the patient to look up.

This technique usually produces a complete iridotomy with 30 to 50 shots in a light brown iris.

Dark Brown Iris

The densely pigmented dark brown iris has a uniform surface with no apparent thin areas. Charring of the surface occurs frequently with exposure times of longer than 0.05 second. This char appears as black shiny material (possibly carbon) at the laser application site. Additional laser applications do not penetrate the char, and instead of forming a coherent single bubble, multiple tiny bubbles spray off the surface after each application. After such charring occurs, it is very difficult, if not impossible, to penetrate that area, and a new location must be chosen.

To avoid charring, short exposure times of 0.02 to 0.05 second should be used with initial power settings of 400 to 1000 mW and a spot size of 50 μm. If a reasonable pit develops in the iris, these settings can be continued, striking the same spot until perforation of the pigment epithelium is recognized by formation of the typical pigment cloud. The hole is then enlarged in the same manner as with light brown irides.

If a pit does not develop or is very small, power can be increased in 200-mW increments until an effective power is obtained. It is rarely necessary to go above 1000 mW. Exposure times should not be increased above 0.10 second because charring is very likely with longer exposures. Completion of iridotomy can usually be accomplished with 60 to 100 applications.

Light Blue Iris

The chromophore for laser iridotomy is in the iris pigment epithelium posterior to the stroma. Blue or pale grey irides have insufficient stromal pigment to absorb laser energy. The energy can pass directly through the stroma, leaving it intact, and separate the pigment epithelium from the back of the iris. This can be recognized as a transillumination defect in the iris with intact overlying stroma. Subsequent shots simply pass through the iris stroma without creating a hole (Fig. 30-6).

Occasionally a small pigmented area, which will respond much like a light brown iris, may be found in an appropriate site for iridotomy. If there is no pigmented area, longer exposures will generate heat in the pigment epithelium; the heat is then transmitted into the stroma and destroys it. The surgeon's goal is to create a bubble at the laser site before the pigment epithelium is destroyed. Then, by firing additional shots through the apex of the bubble, the stroma is destroyed, exposing the underlying pigment epithelium.[37]

The initial setting should be a 200-μm spot, 200 to 400 mW, 0.1 second duration to anneal the pigment epithelium to the stroma. Then the spot size is reduced to 50-μm and the power increased to 600 to 1000 mW at 0.02 to 0.1 second to perforate. If the stroma is clearly being treated, as evidenced by its clumping and opacification, then these settings can be continued. If penetration has not occurred in 20 to 40 shots, then a new spot should be treated with an alternative technique.

One alternative technique requires higher energy (1200 to 1500 mW), with exposure times of 0.3 to 0.4 second and a 50-μm spot size. The shutter speed is set at 0.5 second. As the firing pedal is depressed a bubble will form. When the bubble is about 0.5 mm in diameter the pedal is released. Before the bubble can float away, a second laser application is fired directly through the apex of the bubble (Fig. 30-7). Occasionally a third such application is required. These initial high-energy shots will create a crater whose base is the pigment epithelium. It is then a simple matter to remove the

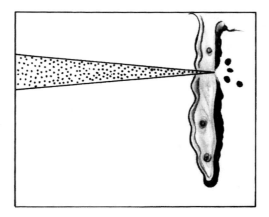

Figure 30-6 Argon laser peripheral iridotomy in a light blue iris. The argon beam may pass directly through the light blue stroma and blast the pigment off the back of the iris. Subsequent laser applications will pass through the stroma without destroying it because there is no pigmented material left to absorb the energy.

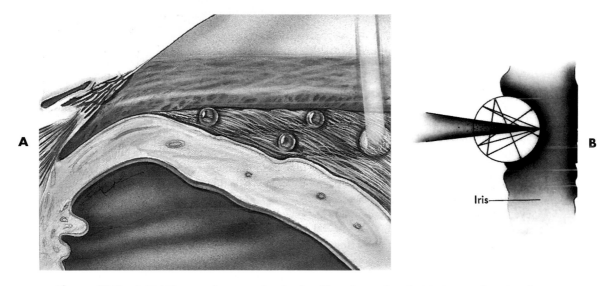

Figure 30-7 **A,** Bubbles are often created at the site of laser impact into the iris tissue and can be advantageous, transferring greater energy from each application into the iridotomy site. **B,** A bubble captured in the iris stroma acts much like a concave mirror redirecting reflected energy back into the iris stroma. Where the iris is in contact with the stroma, the laser energy escapes from the bubble and is absorbed by the tissue. The bubble enhances the effect of the laser energy, allowing development of a crater in the iris surface with fewer applications. If the bubble is in contact with the corneal endothelium, the laser energy will be absorbed by the endothelium and cause an endothelial burn.

pigment epithelium by using shorter exposures (0.05 to 0.1 second) at lower energies (400 to 600 mW), as described for brown irides.

Another alternative uses low-energy "stretch" burns of 200 mW and a 200-μm spot size for 0.1 to 0.2 second on either side of (or surrounding) the site to be perforated. The concept behind this technique is to tighten the iris between the stretch burns, making iris perforation easier. Most iridectomies can be performed without this additional trauma.

Complications of Laser Iridotomy

Iritis

Some degree of iritis always follows laser iridotomy. Iritis can be minimized by topical corticosteroid eyedrops (e.g., prednisolone acetate 1% hourly until bedtime on the day of laser treatment and four times daily for the following day or two), but most patients do quite well without treatment.

500 mW for 0.1 to 0.2 second. It is important to begin with very low energy levels and increase power until the desired effect is seen. Dark brown irides absorb much more energy than do light blue irides, so the treatment level must be titrated to the individual patient. The applications should be placed in a row close to the pupillary border and peripheral to the sphincter. Another laser series at a 500-μm spot size should then be placed just peripheral to the first row. Their effect, however, may not be permanent if miotics are resumed. Care must be taken to avoid burning or vaporizing tissue and to avoid retinal injury.

REFERENCES

1. Suzuki Y, and others: Transscleral Nd:YAG laser cyclophotocoagulation versus cyclocryotherapy, *Graefes Arch Clin Exp Ophthalmol* 229:33, 1991.

2. Simmons RB, and others: Transscleral Nd:YAG laser cyclophotocoagulation with a contact lens, *Am J Ophthalmol* 112:671, 1991.

3. Beckman H, Sugar HS: Neodymium laser cyclocoagulation, *Arch Ophthalmol* 90:27, 1973.

4. Beckman H, and others: Transscleral ruby laser irradiation of the ciliary body in the treatment of intractable glaucoma, *Trans Am Acad Ophthalmol Otolaryngol* 76:423, 1972.

5. Cohn HC, Aron-Rosa D: Reopening blocked trabeculectomy sites with the YAG laser, *Am J Ophthalmol* 95:293, 1983.

6. Shields S, and others: Transpupillary argon laser cyclophotocoagulation in the treatment of glaucoma, *Ophthalmic Surg* 19:171, 1988.

7. Kim JY, Fanous MM: Comparison of treatment results of noncontact transscleral Nd:YAG and diode laser cyclophotocoagulation in patients with refractory glaucoma, *Invest Ophthal Vis Sci* 38:846, 1997.

8. Ulbig MW, and others: Clinical comparison of semiconductor diode versus neodymium:YAG non-contact cyclophotocoagulation, *Br J Ophthalmol* 79:569, 1995.

9. Schuman JS, and others: Experimetal use of semiconductor diode laser in contact transscleral cyclophotocoagulation in rabbits, *Arch Ophthalmol* 108:1152, 1990.

10. Assia EI, and others: A comparison of neodymium:yttrium aluminum garnet and diode laser transscleral cyclophotocoagulation and cyclocryotherapy, *Invest Ophthalmol Vis Sci* 32:2774, 1991.

11. Brancato R, and others: Histopathology of continuous wave neodymium:yttrium aluminum garnet and diode laser contact transscleral lesions in rabbit ciliary body: a comparative study, *Invest Ophthalmol Vis Sci* 32:1586, 1991.

12. Brancato R, and others: Diode and Nd:YAG laser contact transscleral cyclophotocoagulation in a human eye: a comparative histopathologic study of the lesions produced using a new fiber optic probe, *Ophthalmic Surg* 25:607, 1994.

13. Fankhauser F, and others: Transscleral cyclophotocoagulation using a neodymium YAG laser, *Ophthalmic Surg* 17:94, 1986.

14. Schwartz LW, Moster MR: Neodymium: YAG laser transscleral cyclodiathermy, *Ophthalmic Laser Ther* 1:135, 1986.

15. Wilensky JT, Welch D, Mirolovich M: Transscleral cyclocoagulation using a neodymium: YAG laser, *Ophthalmic Surg* 16:95, 1985.

16. Shields MB, and others: A contact lens for transscleral Nd:YAG cyclophotocoagulation, *Am J Ophthalmol* 108:457, 1989 (letter).

17. Simmons RB, and others: Comparison of transscleral neodymium:YAG cyclophotocoagulation with and without a contact lens in human autopsy eyes, *Am J Ophthalmol* 109:174, 1990.

18. Crymes BM, Gross RL: Laser placement in noncontact Nd:YAG cyclophotocoagulation, *Am J Ophthalmol* 110:670, 1990.

19. Hardten DR, Brown JD: Transscleral neodymium:YAG cyclophotocoagulation: comparison of 180-degree and 360-degree intial treatments [published erratum appears in *Ophthalmic Surg* 24:417, 1993], *Ophthalmic Surg* 24:181, 1993.

20. Schuman JS, and others: Contact transscleral continuous wave neodymium:YAG laser cyclophotocoagulation, *Ophthalmology* 97:571, 1990.

21. Gaasterland DE, and others: A multicenter study of contact diode laser transscleral cyclophotocoagulation in glaucoma patients, *Invest Ophthalmol Vis Sci* 33(suppl):1019. 1992.

22. Stewart WC, Brindley GO, Shields MB: *Cyclodestructive procedures.* In Ritch R, Shields MB, Krupin T, editors: *The glaucomas: glaucoma therapy,* St Louis, 1996, Mosby.

23. Hennis HL, Stewart WC: Semiconductor diode laser transscleral cyclophotocoagulation in patients with glaucoma, *Am J Ophthalmol* 113:81, 1992.

24. Moriarty AP: Diode lasers in ophthalmology, *Int Ophthalmol* 17:297, 1993.

25. Uram M: Endoscopic cyclophotocoagulation in glaucoma management, *Curr Opin Ophthalmol* 11:19, 1995.

26. Hoskins HD Jr, Migliazzo C: Management of failing filtering blebs with the argon laser, *Ophthalmic Surg* 15:731, 1984.

27. Ticho U, Ivry M: Reopening of occluded filtering blebs by argon laser photocoagulation, *Am J Ophthalmol* 84:413, 1977.

28. Ticho U, Zauberman H: Argon laser application to the angle structures in the glaucomas, *Arch Ophthalmol* 94:61, 1976.

29. Van Buskirk EM: Reopening filtration sites with the argon laser, *Am J Ophthalmol* 94:1, 1982.

30. Dailey RA, Samples JR, van Buskirk EM: Reopening filtration fistulas with the neodymium-YAG laser, *Am J Ophthalmol* 102:491, 1986.

31. Praeger DL: The reopening of closed filtering blebs using the neodymium:YAG laser, *Ophthalmology* 91:373, 1984.

32. Cohn HC, and others: YAG laser treatment in a series of failed trabeculectomies, *Am J Ophthalmol* 108:395, 1989.

33. Kandarakis A, and others: Reopening of failed trabeculectomies with ab interno Nd:YAG laser, *Eur J Ophthalmol* 6:143, 1996.

34. Rankin GA, Latina MA: Transconjunctival Nd:YAG laser revision of failing trabeculectomy, *Ophthalmic Surg* 21:365, 1990.

35. Latina MA, Rankin GA: Internal and transconjunctival neodymium:YAG laser revision of late failing filters, *Ophthalmology* 98:215, 1991.

36. Grosskreutz C, and others: Cyclodialysis, *Int Ophthalmol Clin* 35:105, 1995.

37. Alward WL, and others: Argon laser endophotocoagulator closure of cyclodialysis clefts, *Am J Ophthalmol* 106:748, 1988.

38. Ormerod LD, and others: Management of the hypotonous cyclodialysis cleft, *Ophthalmology* 98:1384, 1991.

39. Bauer B: Argon laser photocoagulation of cyclodialysis clefts after cataract surgery, *Acta Ophthalmol Scand* 73:283, 1995.

40. Brooks AM, and others: Noninvasive closure of a persistent cyclodialysis cleft, *Ophthalmology* 103:1943, 1996.

41. Brown SV, Mizen T: Transscleral diode laser therapy for traumatic cyclodialysis cleft, *Ophthalmic Surg* 28:313, 1997.

42. Fellman RL, Starita RJ, Spaeth GL: Reopening cyclodialysis cleft with Nd:YAG laser following trabeculectomy, *Ophthalmic Surg* 15:285, 1984.

43. Harbin TS Jr: Treatment of cyclodialysis clefts with argon laser photocoagulation, *Ophthalmology* 89:1082, 1982.

44. Wise JB: Iris sphincterotomy, iridotomy, and synechiotomy by linear incision with the argon laser, *Ophthalmology* 92:641, 1985.

45. Fankhauser F, Swasniewska S, Klapper RM: Neodymium Q-switched YAG laser lysis of iris lens synechiae, *Ophthalmology* 92:790, 1985.

46. Flynn WJ, Carlson DW: Laser synechialysis to prevent membrane recurrence on silicone intraocular lenses, *Am J Ophthalmol* 122:426, 1996.

47. Simmons RJ, Deppermann SR, Dueker DK: The role of goniophotocoagulation in neovascularization of the anterior chamber angle, *Ophthalmology* 87:79, 1980.

PART VII

Surgical Principles

33

General Surgical Care

THE SURGICAL DECISION

The decision to operate on any eye is a serious one in which glaucoma surgeons confront two basic situations. The first is when the intraocular pressure (IOP) is quite high and the patient has pain, corneal edema, or rapid deterioration of vision. In this situation the patient can appreciate that his or her vision is immediately threatened and can understand the need for surgery with its attendant risks, discomfort, and inconvenience. The surgeon also understands this, and the decision to operate is clear.

The other situation is one in which the patient may not be experiencing any discomfort or visual impairment. This type of situation is more typical in patients with chronic open-angle glaucoma. In this situation the indication for surgery is a progressive or worrisome visual field loss or deterioration of the optic nerve, which the physician can recognize but the patient usually does not. The patient must subject adequate or even normal vision to a procedure that may worsen vision and thus decrease the ability to read, drive, watch television, or recognize family and friends. The surgeon faces the very real risk, from the patient's point of view, of ruining the vision rather than saving it.

It is important in this latter situation to remember that the goal of glaucoma therapy is to maintain good vision for the patient's lifetime. Thus to make the right recommendation to the patient, the surgeon must consider the life expectancy of the patient, the rate of disease progression, and the risks and benefits of other therapies. The surgeon must also weigh the surgical benefit (i.e., the likelihood that the surgery will be successful and prevent further visual loss) against the risks of surgical failure or complications.[1]

It is also important to remember that visual loss from damage to the optic nerve is irrevocable, whereas visual loss from the most common complications of glaucoma surgery (cataract or refractive change) can be corrected. Therefore the guiding principle in this situation must be to protect the optic nerve. For each patient, the physician must weigh the evidence of progressive nerve damage against the need for and likelihood of arresting that progression (Box 33-1).

PREOPERATIVE CARE

Nothing is more reassuring to a patient than to have complete confidence in his or her physician. Preparation of a patient for surgery begins with a careful and thorough history and physical examination by the ophthalmologist. The ophthalmologist must know the patient's medical history as well as his or her current physical status. Consultation with the primary care physician should be a routine part of the preoperative plan. It is important that the surgical decision be made in the context of the patient's whole life. Family, social, and work-related considerations are important in the patient's decision to proceed with surgery as well as in the patient's ability to follow the prescribed postoperative treatment plan. When outpatient or "come-and-go" surgery is performed rehabilitation takes place away from the traditional health care setting. Postoperative care is crucial in glaucoma surgical management. Every effort should be made to ensure that the patient is being discharged to an appropriately supportive environment.

Instructions to the Patient

The physician should tell the patient what to expect with the surgical experience, including a careful explanation of the expected rehabilitation and recovery period. Successful filtration surgery is of-

---

Box 33-1
Indications for Filtering Surgery

- Documented visual field and optic nerve damage, despite maximum tolerated medications and laser therapy, that threatens the patient's vision.
- Anticipated progressive damage (e.g., experience in the same or fellow eye that indicates the current course will lead to loss of vision) or intolerably high intraocular pressure (IOP). Medication failure because of ineffectiveness, intolerance, poor compliance, or complications.
- IOP that is high enough to place the future health of the optic nerve at significant risk. This pressure will differ dramatically, depending on the condition of the nerve and the patient's prior history. For example, if the patient has extensive fixation threatening field loss, pressures in or near the "normal" range may be too high for the nerve to tolerate. If the physician waits for further progression before operating, central vision may be lost.
- Dysfunctional ocular tissues (corneal edema or bullous keratopathy, pulsating central retinal artery).
- Combined with cataract procedure if there is borderline IOP control, advanced damage, or history of postoperative intraocular pressure rise in the fellow eye.

---

ten followed by a period of relative hypotony and poor vision, which may last from several days to a few weeks after the procedure. Patients can become needlessly demoralized during this period if they have not been properly counseled to expect that visual recovery will take time. A thorough explanation of potential complications is mandatory.

Physicians are now legally required to provide this information to obtain the patient's agreement to operate (informed consent). Patients must be warned that they may lose vision or even the eye. They may develop cataracts, infection, and hemorrhage. The risk of these complications for each patient should be estimated using the best available evidence and should be shared with the patient. It is best to give these data as ranges, simple ratios, or approximate percentages so that the patient can understand the risk. The surgery itself and the probability of success can be explained reassuringly so that the patient can develop realistic expectations. It is useful to emphasize the unfortunate fact that glaucoma surgery is rarely intended or expected to improve vision, but rather such surgery is performed in an attempt to protect the remaining vision. Patients who expect the operation to restore lost vision can be profoundly disappointed with a result that the surgeon views as completely successful.

It is important to explain to the patient that the local anesthetic will be momentarily painful but that the surgery itself is essentially painless. A patient thus prepared is more calm, less apprehensive, and more cooperative; preoperative sedation is more effective, and the surgery will go more smoothly for both the patient and surgeon.

Glaucoma patients are usually older and naturally prone to other diseases. A history of previous illnesses and a review of symptoms particularly related to the cardiovascular system are in order. Significant findings should be further evaluated by the appropriate physical examination or laboratory tests. Laboratory studies, radiography, electrocardiography, and other diagnostic tests should be ordered when indicated by these findings. Electrolyte levels, including potassium, may be altered, especially in patients using oral carbonic anhydrase inhibitors and thiazide diuretics.

Before the orders are written, the surgeon should question the patient about possible allergy to medications. The patient should take to the hospital any medications he or she routinely uses at home, including systemic medications as well as ophthalmic eyedrops and tablets, and should continue to use these on the same schedule as at home. Misplaced orders, closed pharmacies, and the overloaded workday for nurses too often result in delays in obtaining and administering new medications. Patients facing surgery are apprehensive, and their confidence in both the hospital and the surgeon can be shaken by the failure to receive promptly medication that they have been told is vital.

Outpatient Versus Inpatient Surgery

Outpatient surgery has been routine for cataract extraction since the early 1980s. Glaucoma surgery leaves a filtering wound that disrupts the integrity of the eye and, unlike cataract surgery, may leave the eye hypotonous and susceptible to injury from external pressure or Valsalva's maneuvers. Nevertheless, many patients have undergone successful and uncomplicated outpatient filtering surgery,[2] and many patients prefer not to stay in the hospital. We have been performing virtually all of our glaucoma surgeries on an outpatient basis since the mid-1980s. In many places, particularly the United States, health plans do not authorize overnight stays for routine glaucoma surgery.

Surgical arrangements should be tailored to each patient's needs. There may be cardiac, pulmonary, or other systemic problems that require hospitalization either before or after surgery. Hospitalization may be indicated if there is a history of a complication in the other eye, if the patient is one-eyed, or if there is risk of hemorrhage or other complication. Patients traveling from long distances may need to stay in a hotel or guest house for some portion of the preoperative or postoperative period. Although this is not as convenient as staying in the hospital, it is preferable to driving long distances for daily follow-up and is much less expensive than the hospital. Some hospitals with excess bed capacity have programs that allow outpatients to rent rooms without hospital services for rates similar to those charged at boarding houses. Others have programs in which patients from out of town are permitted to stay for free in the hospital the night before outpatient surgery. These programs are popular with patients and make the operating room less vulnerable to late arrivals or "no-shows."

Preoperative Medications

With the exception of the strong cholinesterase inhibitors, glaucoma medications should be continued until surgery. The cholinesterase inhibitors demecarium bromide (Humorsol) and echothiophate iodide (Phospholine) cause prolonged postoperative inflammation and possibly increase surgical bleeding.[3,4] A weaker miotic (e.g., pilocarpine) should be substituted for these drops 2 or 3 weeks before surgery if time permits.

The cholinesterase inhibitors also lower blood cholinesterase and pseudocholinesterase for weeks. Therefore adjunctive anesthetic agents such as succinylcholine may cause prolonged apnea. The anesthesiologist should be told of all drugs that have been taken recently by the patient.

Most systemic medications should be continued unless they have the potential to cause bleeding. Aspirin is one such medication and should be discontinued for 10 to 14 days before surgery if possible. A surprising number of patients fail to list aspirin among the medicines they are taking unless asked specifically. The ophthalmologist should consult with the treating physician for patients who are using coumadin or other antithrombotic therapy. Surgery can often be performed safely while the patient uses these agents; they do add risk, however, and it is better whenever possible to delay surgery until their effects can be reduced or stopped.

Preoperative sedation eases the patient's passage through the operating room. If an anesthesiologist is not in attendance, meperidine (Demerol) and hydroxyzine hydrochloride (Vistaril), each given in a dose of 0.5 to 1 mg/kg body weight, make an excellent combination of analgesic and tranquilizer. A wide variety of other perianesthetic agents have been used as well, and each physician should consult his or her own experience on this issue.

OPERATIVE CARE

The Operating Room

The patient should be the center of attention in the operating room and should be transferred to the operating table with care and positioned comfortably. A pillow under the knees often eases back strain. Conversation should be quiet and purposeful. A relaxed atmosphere is good, but the patient may find joking and laughter inappropriate.

Patient monitoring is simple and necessary. Devices that monitor pulse with appropriate alarm capability are commonly used. More sophisticated monitors that measure blood pressure and oxygen saturation and provide electrocardiographic tracings give more precise indications of patient status.

Cardiac arrest occurs in approximately 1 in 6000 patients receiving general anesthesia,[5] with a higher incidence in children and the elderly. The physician must therefore be familiar with resuscitation equipment, medications, and procedures. An anesthesiologist will monitor the patient and lead any resuscitation effort; if an anesthesiologist is not present, the surgeon is responsible.

Anesthesia

The choice of anesthesia depends on the patient. Children require general anesthesia, whereas most adults do well with preoperative sedation and local block. Most adults, however, prefer to receive something more.

Neuroleptanalgesic, ataractic, or dissociative anesthesia is provided by an anesthesiologist. The result is heavy sedation with analgesia, hypomobility, antiemesis, vasomotor stability, and emotional detachment. These anesthetics are usually provided intravenously using varying amounts and combinations of meperidine, hydroxyzine hydrochloride, phencyclidine, or fentanyl, all of which can be supplemented as needed throughout the procedure.

Retrobulbar local block is accomplished with lidocaine (Xylocaine) 2% to 4% either alone or combined with bupivacaine hydrochloride (Marcaine) 0.5% or 0.75% combined with hyaluronidase. An injection of 1.5 to 3 ml usually is adequate for most types of glaucoma surgery when supplemented with topical proparacaine or tetracaine drops instilled three or four times into the eye. Some surgeons prefer to use larger volumes of less-concentrated anesthetic agents.

Retrobulbar block is necessary in all patients who do not receive general anesthesia. An anesthesiologist can administer a small amount of pentobarbital or other short-acting agent intravenously immediately before the retrobulbar injection so the patient will not feel it. It is not necessary for the patient to be awake and cooperative to accurately inject retrobulbar anesthesia. O'Brien, van Lint, or Nadbath lid block traditionally has been given with the same solution, but this is not strictly necessary.

Equipment

A good surgical microscope providing magnification up to 25× is needed for procedures that require precise localization of Schlemm's canal (e.g., trabeculotomy). In most other situations 16× or 10× magnification is adequate for glaucoma surgery. Zoom controls add convenience.

Light from the microscope can damage the retina.[6,7] Even though many surgical glaucoma patients have miotic pupils, the surgeon should use the least amount of light that is adequate. The microscope should be angled so that light is not directed at the macula. A corneal cover, which is included in many surgical kits or can be fashioned during surgery from part of a Weckcel sponge, can help protect the retina during stages of the operation in which visualization of the anterior chamber is not necessary. Fine-quality instruments that are well maintained with sharp edges and delicate teeth reduce tissue trauma and surgeon frustration.

Cauterization is accomplished with a bipolar instrument, an erasure tip, or the unipolar tip, which should be adjusted to achieve hemostasis without charring. Although each system has advantages, we prefer the unipolar tip because of its precision and because it eases cauterization of the trabeculectomy site if bleeding occurs from the region of the ciliary body.

Swabs that leave debris (e.g., cotton-tipped applicators) should be avoided. Precut Weckcel swabs are effective. A variety of good suture material is available, and selection is often related to surgeon preference. The surgeon should generally use the least amount of suture that has the least amount of inflammatory stimulus. Cutting needles are preferred for the sclera. Nylon sutures, commonly 10-0 or 9-0, can be cut with the laser in the postoperative period if necessary. Some surgeons advocate finely tapered needles to create smaller needle tracts for conjunctival closure, especially when antimetabolites are used (see Chapter 36).

POSTOPERATIVE CARE

Activity

The trend toward outpatient ophthalmic surgery has resulted in earlier ambulation of patients. Earlier ambulation leads to more rapid systemic recovery, especially in elderly patients. As soon as the effects of sedation and anesthesia have subsided, ambulation can begin. Unless there has been excessive bleeding or the eye is left extremely hypotonous, there is little reason to restrict the patient to bed rest.

Because of visual limitations, one-eyed adults or those with poor vision in the unoperated eye may be kept hospitalized unless they strongly desire to go home and have a capable person there to care for them. Conversely, children may feel more secure at home, and parents may feel quite comfortable caring for them there.

Patients should refrain from vigorous activity and movements that cause a Valsalva's effect (e.g., straining, lifting, and bending) for the first week after filtering surgery. Reading causes rapid jerky eye movements, whereas watching television requires less eye motion. Looking out of the window while riding in a car can induce rapid saccades as sign posts, telephone poles, and other similar objects are tracked and released almost subconsciously. If patients must travel a great distance by car in the immediate postoperative period they may have less eye movement if they look straight ahead or keep their eyes closed.

Medications

With the exception of antithrombotic medication, systemic drugs should be continued after surgery. Because of the bleeding aspirin may induce, acetaminophen (Tylenol) should be taken to relieve pain.

Pain after glaucoma surgery is unusual. If pain is severe, the ophthalmologist should consider complications such as anterior or posterior hemorrhage, infection, or elevated IOP. Severe postoperative pain is an emergency and should be evaluated immediately by a member of the surgical team. Anxiety is responsible for much of the postoperative unrest. If reassurance is not adequate, a gentle tranquilizer such as diazepam (Valium) is better than sedation when the patient is recuperating at home.

Glaucoma medications should be continued in the unoperated eye. Fluctuations in IOP in the unoperated eye are common and may range several millimeters up or down during the weeks after surgery. Fluctuations are also seen in the untreated eye after laser trabeculoplasty and may be related to a central pressure-regulating mechanism. It may also be that the IOP is being measured more frequently and so physiologic or pathologic fluctuations are being seen.

Systemic aqueous suppressants such as carbonic anhydrase inhibitors (CAIs) reduce the flow of aqueous through the newly formed stoma in filtering surgery. The flow of aqueous inhibits scarring and helps form and maintain an adequate bleb. If possible, these drugs should be discontinued for at least several weeks postoperatively. Our current practice is to replace systemic CAIs with a topical CAI in the unoperated eye. If this is insufficient to maintain IOP control we begin to consider surgery in the unoperated eye rather than reinstituting systemic CAIs. In the postoperative setting we tend to reserve CAIs for patients who have had bilateral surgery and still failed to achieve adequate IOP control.

Management of the operated eye depends on the procedure performed. Generally, the eye is patched for the first 24 hours. Topical steroid drops, such as prednisolone 1% or dexamethasone 0.1%, will reduce inflammation and scarring. Dose frequency varies from once hourly to twice daily for the first week. Steroids are effective in reducing inflammation and should be used abundantly when necessary. Often the steroids are administered in combination with a broad-spectrum antibiotic. If so, the antibiotic usually can be discontinued after a week or so. Steroid drops often are continued for 2 to 3 weeks or until the eye is quiet. In some cases we continue using very–low-dose steroid drops for many weeks postoperatively. We always taper steroid drops rather than discontinuing them abruptly.

Some surgeons advocate systemic steroid therapy for patients in whom previous filtering surgery has failed or in those who have preexisting inflammation. In routine cases, systemic steroids appear to offer little advantage over topical therapy but do pose additional risk.[8]

REFERENCES

1. Watson PG: When to operate in open-angle glaucoma, *Eye* 1(Pt I):51, 1987.
2. Kimbrough RL, Stewart RH: Outpatient trabeculectomy, *Ophthalmic Surg* 11:379, 1980.
3. Abraham SV: Miotic iridocyclitis, *Am J Ophthalmol* 1(1):109, 1957.
4. Leopold IH: Ocular cholinesterase and cholinesterase inhibitors, *Am J Ophthalmol* 54:855, 1961.
5. Keenan RL, Boyan CP: Cardiac arrest due to anesthesia: a study of incidence and causes, *JAMA* 253:2373, 1985.
6. Irvine AR, Copenhagen DR: The focal nature of retinal illumination from the operating microscope, *Arch Ophthalmol* 103:549, 1985.
7. Irvine AR, Wood I, Morris BW: Retinal damage from the illumination of the operating microscope: an experimental study in pseudophakic monkeys, *Arch Ophthalmol* 102:1358, 1984.
8. Starita RJ, and others: Short- and long-term effects of postoperative corticosteroids on trabeculectomy, *Ophthalmology* 92:938, 1985.

34

Surgical Anatomy and Pathophysiology: Internal Flow Block Versus Outflow Block

SURGICAL ANATOMY

There is no more critical area in ophthalmic surgery than the transition zone at the corneoscleral junction known as the *limbus*. The limbus is the site of most glaucoma surgical incisions, with success or failure often depending on the accuracy of that incision. With a stereoscopic view through the operating microscope, the surgeon can assess where the iris would attach to the scleral wall beneath the overlying scleral shelf. Incision into the anterior chamber must be anterior to this attachment.

Conjunctiva and Tenon's Capsule

The conjunctiva and a very thin subconjunctival fascia extend from the fornices to the limbus. Tenon's capsule is the denser subconjunctival connective tissue that is continuous with the muscle sheaths. Both the fascia and the conjunctiva are more dense in young patients. Tenon's capsule tends to be thick in black patients. Both Tenon's capsule and the overlying conjunctiva can be quite thin and diaphenous in the elderly. Tenon's capsule is thickest in the fornices, becoming thinner as the limbus is approached. At the limbus, Tenon's capsule cannot be distinguished from the wispy subconjunctival connective tissue that inserts into the sclera just posterior to the limbus. Elevating this connective tissue from the sclera reveals a tiny ridge where the conjunctival epithelium merges with the corneal epithelium at the end of Bowman's membrane. This marks the anterior limit of the limbus (Fig. 34-1).

The necessity of removing a portion of Tenon's tissue during filtering surgery is controversial. The fact that the conjunctiva and Tenon's capsule combine near the limbus limits practical manipulation and removal of tissues in this crucial filter area. Additional destruction of Tenon's capsule away from the limbus predisposes the eye to a thin-walled flap and may increase fibrosis and scarring. The indications for removal come from clinical impressions and need further investigation.[1-7]

Blood Supply to the Anterior Segment

Conjunctival blood vessels are usually not troublesome unless the eye is congested. Tenon's capsule has no large vessels, and heavy bleeding occurs only when the unwary surgeon incising the fascia cuts into an underlying muscle. This complication usually occurs when the surgeon has become disoriented anatomically while developing a limbal-based conjunctival flap. The eye may have been distorted in one or another direction by the fixation sutures, and an incision thought to be in the quadrant between the muscles lands in or too near the muscle itself. This can be avoided by carrying incisions of the conjunctiva and Tenon's capsule down to the sclera in the quadrants between the muscles before completing the incision in the area of the muscle.

There are many tiny surface scleral vessels (Figs. 34-2 and 34-3). These vessels should be avoided in the reflection of the conjunctiva. Procedures that require scleral incisions can be preceded by light cautery to the area.

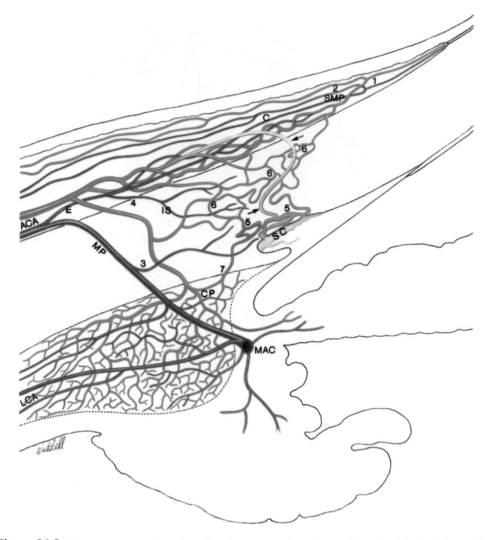

Figure 34-3   Drawing of a meridional section of the eye to show the blood supply of the limbal area. The *red areas* indicate arterial channels. An anterior ciliary artery *(ACA)* is divided to form an episcleral *(E)* and a major perforating *(MP)* branch. The episcleral branches produce episcleral, conjunctival *(C)*, and intrascleral *(IS)* nutrient vessels. The conjunctival vessels form the superficial marginal plexus of the cornea *(SMP)*. Two sets of vessels arise from the superficial marginal plexus: one *(1)* extends forward to form the peripheral corneal arcades; the other forms recurrent vessels *(2)* that run posteriorly to supply 3 to 6 mm of the perilimbal conjunctiva. The latter eventually anastomose with the recurrent conjunctival vessels from the fornices. The major perforating artery passes through the sclera to join the major arterial circle *(MAC)* of the iris. *(3)*, Point at which a branch from the major perforating artery passes forward to form the intrascleral arterial channels of the limbus. This region is often supplied by a vessel that arises directly from the anterior ciliary artery as an episcleral vessel *(4)*. The *blue areas* indicate venous channels. The major venous drainage from the limbus is into the episcleral veins, which then unite with the ophthalmic veins. The deep scleral venous plexus *(5)* is close to Schlemm's canal *(SC)*. An aqueous vein *(arrows)* arises from the deep scleral plexus and joins the episcleral veins. The intrascleral venous plexus *(6)* forms an extensive network in the limbal stroma. An important part of the drainage from the ciliary plexus *(CP)* is into the deep and intrascleral venous plexuses *(7)*. (From Hogan MJ, and others: *Histology of the human eye,* Philadelphia, 1971, Saunders.)

the surface of the globe at this point enters the chamber in the midtrabecular area of most wide-angled eyes but may be in the area of the angle recess or even in the ciliary body of an eye with a small anterior segment. Therefore it is necessary to bevel or angle incisions slightly toward the anterior chamber and to start the incision in a narrow-angled eye between the corneoscleral sulcus and the conjunctival reflection. The surgeon should be able to see clear corneal tissue after cutting the external scleral fibers if the incision is truly limbal.

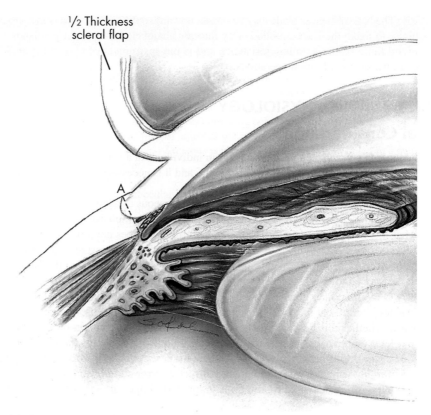

Figure 34-4   Beneath a flap of one half the scleral thickness, the blue line of the cornea extends more posteriorly. Note than an incision perpendicularly placed at this blue line *(A)* would pass posterior to the trabecular meshwork and Schlemm's canal and enter the eye at the insertion of the ciliary body. This must be kept in mind when trying to locate Schlemm's canal for trabeculotomy.

Fewer complications arise if an ab-externo or "scratch" incision is used. The same technique can be used for all glaucoma operations at the limbus. This results in safer, more accurate, and more successful surgery.

Incisions made parallel to the iris (shelved incisions) through the limbal tissues enter the anterior chamber well anterior to the iris insertion. Consequently, the incisions can safely begin farther posterior from the limbus than can a more nearly perpendicular ab-externo incision and still reach the anterior chamber in front of the trabecular meshwork. This is why many older texts advise incisions 2 mm behind the limbus. A perpendicular ab-externo incision in that position can go directly into the ciliary body, particularly in eyes with small anterior segments. The tragic results of this surgical error can be seen in the laboratory of ophthalmic pathology where enucleated eyes show intravitreal hemorrhage, lens dislocations, cataract, intravitreal fibroblastic proliferation with retinal separation, uveitis, and sympathetic ophthalmia.

Trabeculectomy and trabeculotomy procedures require a knowledge of the limbal area as it is approached through a scleral flap incision. Deeper landmarks may be confusing, and an unwary surgeon may miss Schlemm's canal while attempting trabeculotomy. The limbus appears more posterior if the dissected flap is thick because the corneal wedge tissue is exposed at a deeper level (Fig. 34-4). The color change from the white of the sclera to the bluish cast given off by the cornea adjoining the sclera is more distinct. The scleral spur is located at this junction, and just anterior to the scleral spur is Schlemm's canal. Experience is needed, however, to increase the skill of the surgeon in locating small structures in this critical area. Technique can be improved by performing surgery with the operating microscope on unused eyebank eyes.

Descemet's membrane does not cut like corneoscleral fibers. Like cellophane, this inner tissue resists cutting until an initial perforation has been made; then it splits easily. It is important to remember this point. Otherwise, the surgeon is tempted to push harder and harder to enter the anterior chamber, with the danger of damaging the iris and lens with sudden penetration. The depth of penetration is more readily controlled when cutting upward rather than pressing down toward the

REFERENCES

1. Ben Sira I, Ticho U: Excision of Tenon's capsule in fistulizing operations on Africans, *Am J Ophthalmol* 68:336, 1969.

2. Gorin G: Use of a thin conjunctival flap in limbosclerectomy, *Ann Ophthalmol* 3:258, 1971.

3. Kapetansky FM: Trabeculectomy, or trabeculectomy plus tenectomy: a comparative study, *Glaucoma* 2:451, 1980.

4. Kietzman B: Glaucoma surgery in Nigerian eyes: a five-year study, *Ophthalmic Surg* 7:52, 1976.

5. Maumenee AE: External filtering operations for glaucoma: the mechanism of function and failure, *Trans Am Ophthalmol Soc* 58:319, 1960.

6. Maumenee AE: *Mechanism of filtration of fistulizing glaucoma procedures.* In *Transactions of the New Orleans Academy of Ophthalmology Symposium on Glaucoma,* St Louis, 1981, Mosby.

7. Welsh NH: Failure of filtering operations in the African, *Br J Ophthalmol* 54:594, 1972.

8. Hogan MJ, Alvarado JA, Weddell JE: *Histology of the human eye,* Philadelphia, 1971, Saunders.

35

Factors Influencing the Outcome of Filtering Surgery

PATHOPHYSIOLOGY OF FILTERING BLEBS

It is remarkable that filtering procedures are ever successful! The postsurgical eye faces a daunting paradox: The conjunctival–Tenon's flap incision is expected to seal water-tight within the first few postoperative days; but the sclerostomy site and scleral flap, which may be only a couple of millimeters away, are supposed to remain open for many years. The protective mechanisms of the body are designed to reestablish the integrity of body cavities and to prevent such things as filtering blebs from forming. Why, then, is routine filtering surgery successful in the majority of cases? Many investigators believe that aqueous humor has properties that inhibit or modify the scar, allowing the bleb to become established.[1-9] Lack of fibroblast nutrients, collagenolytic activity, fibroblastic inhibitory activity, and mechanical flow characteristics have all been suggested as properties of aqueous humor that encourage bleb formation.

Studies of full-thickness filtering surgery in subhuman primates[3] have found failure of filtration resulting from closure of the sclerostomy site within 14 days by fibroblastic proliferation. Numerous studies in rabbits have reported bleb failure in 1 to 12 days after sclerostomy.[10-12] Many of these animals had large amounts of inflammation, even including hypopyon in some eyes. This finding indicates the potent wound-healing response of the eye to injury. Surgeons use a variety of techniques to modify this response.

In humans, the postoperative course of filtering surgery follows general patterns. The successful outcome usually demonstrates a reasonable bleb during the first week. If the anterior chamber is too shallow initially, it usually deepens by the second or third day after surgery. Cellular reaction in the anterior chamber should be minimal by the end of the first week. The bleb tends to become more localized in the second and third weeks, but it should not appear to have a wall around it. In fact at this point it should be difficult to determine precisely where the bleb ends; the borders should be obscure for weeks. By the end of about the first month, the bleb is well established and moderately diffuse, and the eye is quiet. The intraocular pressure (IOP) should approximate the level that it will maintain for the next several months. In most cases the ideal pressure is about 8 to 10 mm Hg. The bleb will gradually become less hyperemic and at 3 months should be well established with small microcysts visible on the conjunctival surface by slit-lamp examination.

Bleb appearance can differ dramatically from person to person. As time passes after a good initial result, however, the bleb usually develops into one of three types by (1) becoming more localized, with thinner walls and a more cystic structure (see Fig. 37-23); (2) becoming less vascular but maintaining its thickness and translucency (see Fig. 35-2, *C*); or (3) thickening and becoming more opaque. This last event indicates increased collagen content and is usually accompanied by a gradual increase in pressure.

Localization and thinning of the bleb wall can continue until the wall is perfectly transparent. Such blebs usually consist of multiple thin-walled, adjacent locules overlying the sclerostomy and appear to result from the interaction over time of large quantities of aqueous humor with the collagen of the bleb. A positive Seidel's test may demonstrate aqueous flow directly through the wall of such a bleb if gentle pressure is applied to the globe, indicating transconjunctival diffusion of aqueous.

Guarded filtering procedures are more likely to produce type 2 blebs, which are more desirable.

The bleb has no distinct margins and is translucent enough to see the outline of the underlying scleral flap. With fornix-based conjunctival flaps the filtration area may be fairly posterior and diffuse so that it is difficult to define much of a bleb at all, although effective pressure control indicates continual filtration.[13] Seidel's test is negative in such blebs, indicating that their function must be related at least in part to the absorption of aqueous, probably predominantly by the vessels and somewhat by lymphatics.[14] Clinically it appears that more of these blebs gradually thicken and fail over time.

Failure of filtration within 3 months of surgery can occur for a variety of reasons.[15,16] In reoperations, it is not uncommon to see total scarring of the bleb within 2 weeks. This is heralded by marked hyperemia and thickening of the conjunctiva, which can occur whether or not Tenon's capsule was excised.

A second course of failure is recognizable in the second or third postoperative week by the development of a wall around the bleb. This is first evident as a more prominent demarcation of the periphery of the bleb that becomes increasingly obvious until the bleb has the appearance of a single, relatively thick-walled cyst accompanied by a rise in the IOP. These blebs often begin to function if left alone, treated with gentle digital presure, or, if necessary to lower IOP, treated with aqueous suppressants.[17]

A third common cause of bleb failure follows occlusion of the sclerostomy as a result of internal blockage or oversuturing of the guarding flap. In these cases the bleb is not elevated and never forms. The eye may remain quiet, but the lack of aqueous flow allows the conjunctiva to scar to the episcleral tissue and the IOP rises. These eyes should be examined gonioscopically to determine the site of blockage. If the fistula is blocked internally, either by iris or by a ridge of sclera, it can often be reopened with laser[18-21] or with a modified goniotomy approach if laser is not available. If the internal opening is blocked by blood, fibrin, or viscoelastic material it can usually be managed by observation for a few days. If the blockage does not resolve spontaneously, gentle digital massage can be applied to elevate the bleb. If the blockage results from oversuturing of the sclerostomy flap, laser suture lysis should be used. A less frequent course of early failure occurs when a bleb that appears to be functioning well at 1 month continues to be mildly hyperemic and gradually scars down over the next few months.

INFLUENCING THE OUTCOME OF FILTERING SURGERY

Although specific modifications in surgical technique are often advocated, few controlled randomized studies are available to establish superiority of a particular modality. This is because it is virtually impossible to eliminate surgical variables or to mask the surgeon performing the procedure. Further, reported series tend to be based on large groups of patients operated on by very busy subspecialists. The results of these studies may be accurate, but they are not generalizable to either the average practitioner or the individual patient.

Modification of Technique

A few consistently important surgical principles are vitally important in filtration surgery. There should be minimal tissue trauma, careful hemostasis without damaging tissues, and the least amount of tissue invasion required for the purpose. Other than a greater lowering of IOP obtained with full-thickness surgery than with guarded filtration, there is little evidence in the literature to support the efficacy of one technique over another.[22-25]

Viscoelastic substances have been advocated by many surgeons to help retain the anterior chamber after filtering surgery.[26,27] Viscoelastic may be particularly useful in reducing the incidence of early wound leaks in filtering procedures performed with fornix-based conjunctival flaps. These substances may contribute to postoperative pressure rise, which can occasionally be severe. Opinions differ as to whether these substances have any influence on the ultimate outcome of the procedure.[28-31]

Study of the factors influencing outcome will lead to the development of new methods to improve success. However, many problems are involved in studying these factors. Although prospective, randomized studies are useful in making comparisons between gross differences in techniques, they require large numbers of patients to prove the advantages of subtle differences because it is nearly impossible for the same surgeon to perform an identical operation on two successive patients. The problems involved with large numbers of surgeons performing a technique with subtle variations becomes proportionately greater when considering all possible variations in preoperative, intraoperative, and postoperative care combined with the variety of patient characteristics included in the analysis. Therefore to proceed in this area we must follow those avenues that appear to have a major influence on outcome.

Patient Characteristics

Older patients tend to have better success with glaucoma filtering surgery[29,32-37] than do younger patients, but the reasons for this may not be related to age *per se*. Using modern surgical techniques, several authors have found success rates in young adults that are quite similar to those reported for older adults.[38,39] Sturmer and co-workers[40] found that the decrease in surgical success seen in younger patients in clinical practice was related to the presence of other established risk factors, such as trauma or prior surgery, rather than to age. The population of young adults with glaucoma severe enough to require surgery is apparently skewed toward higher-risk diagnoses. The effect of race remains unclear.[41-43] As with younger individuals, the poorer prognosis seen in black patients may be related to factors other than race.[35,44-51] It is an interesting clinical observation that the difference in outcome between two eyes of the same patient may be surprisingly large. This is probably the result of variations in technique but may also be due to unrecognized differences between eyes.[30]

Ocular Characteristics

Patients who are aphakic, have had prior surgery, or have neovascular glaucoma have lower success rates with filtering surgery[34,46,49,52-60]; patients with secondary glaucomas with preexisting peripheral anterior synechiae or inflammation also have poorer outcomes.[61] Glaucoma in patients who have had penetrating keratoplasties can be extremely difficult to control.[62-65] To make matters worse, successful glaucoma surgery can increase the risk of graft failure in some patients.[66] Posterior chamber pseudophakia improves the success rate of filtering surgery over aphakia, but outcome seems to be worse than in the previously unoperated eye with primary open-angle glaucoma. Pressure lowering in patients who undergo combined filtration and cataract surgery may be less than that in patients who undergo trabeculectomy alone.[67,68]

Chronic use of glaucoma medication alters the ocular state. Timolol, pilocarpine, and epinephrine impair the blood-aqueous barrier. Chronic use of topical medication increases the surgical reactivity of the conjunctiva.[68a] Anyone who performs cataract surgery on glaucoma patients recognizes the increased postoperative inflammatory response compared with that in "normal" cataractous eyes. This increased inflammatory response may interfere to some degree with bleb formation and causes some surgeons to advocate earlier surgery.[69,70] The inflammatory response can be diminished by discontinuing sympathomimetics for 1 month before surgery and treating the patient with a course of topical steroids.[71]

Wound Modulation

Wound Healing

After trauma, the wound-healing process[15,72,73] begins immediately with increased vascular permeability producing inflammatory exudate and edema, which give blood elements access to the wound (inflammatory stage) (Fig. 35-1). These blood elements clear the wound of debris by phagocytosis and enzyme activity, such as removal of damaged collagen by collagenase. They provide clotting and the stimulus for a variety of cell developments.

The fibroblastic proliferative stage intensifies after 12 to 24 hours, possibly as a result of mitogenic stimuli from platelets. The fibroblasts produce collagen, initially as monomers that undergo polymerization in the extracellular space. These collagen fibers serve as support for angiogenesis.

New vessels start as capillary buds that extend onto the collagen matrix. These vessels provide nutrients for more fibroblasts, which lay down more immature collagen, allowing further growth of the new vessels. This process continues until the wound is bridged by this fragile network of new vessels, usually occurring in a few days in a clean surgical wound.

In the next phase, connective tissue synthesis, at least 11 different enzymes participate in the production of at least 7 different forms of collagen. As this collagen is laid down, cross-linking and

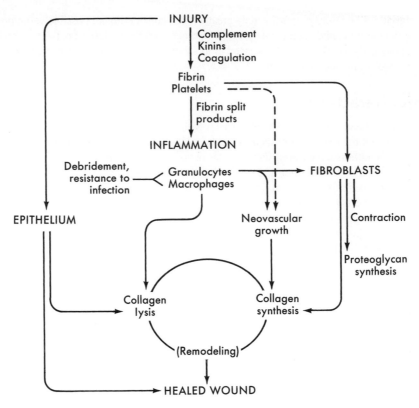

Figure 35-1   Schematic diagram of the sequence of events in wound healing. (Modified from Hunt TK, Van Winkle W Jr: *Fundamentals of wound management,* vol 1, 1976, Chirurgecom Press.)

contraction occur, producing the acute scar. Over time, the collagen is remodeled to more nearly approximate the characteristics of the original tissue. This can be quite accurate in some scleral wounds but will vary greatly depending on the size of the wound, the original tissue, and other factors.

In glaucoma filtering surgery it is the production, contraction, and remodeling of collagen that cause failure of most blebs. A number of factors can inhibit these processes, including marked malnutrition or protein depletion, hypoxia or wound ischemia,[74] zinc deficiency, diabetes mellitus, corticosteroids, nonsteroidal antiinflammatory drugs (NSAIDs), antimetabolites, and other pharmaceutic agents.[75,76]

Corticosteroids

When used in adequate amounts, antiinflammatory corticosteroids slow the rate of conjunctival epithelialization, angiogenesis, and collagen synthesis. Trabeculectomy success is improved by the topical use of these agents.[77-79] Their influence is greatest during the inflammatory phase of the first 3 days after injury. If administration is delayed until the fourth or fifth postoperative day, their effect is reduced. The effect of steroids is dose related, so that initial high doses should be tapered after a few weeks. There is no documented advantage of systemic versus local corticosteroid administration in glaucoma surgery, although some surgeons use systemic steroids in difficult cases.

The effect of corticosteroids on anterior segment inflammation is well documented.[2,80-84] Topical instillation every 15 minutes is more effective than is hourly administration or periocular injection. Hourly administration is more effective than is a four-times-daily dosage. Combined periocular injection with frequent topical administration may be the most effective route. For topical administration, the acetate base appears to be more effective; prednisolone acetate 1.0% is recommended by one source as the most potent.[85]

Steroids may cause postoperative IOP elevation even in some eyes with functioning filtering blebs. Discontinuation of the steroids may lower IOP.[86] This effect also occurs after trabeculectomy.

NSAIDs such as indomethacin and flurbiprofen also reduce inflammation.[75,87] These NSAIDs may be additive to the effect of corticosteroids in restoring the integrity of the blood-aqueous barrier after surgery.[85,88] Vitamin A can reverse the effect of steroids on wound healing.[89]

ANTIMETABOLITES

5-Fluorouracil

The intraoperative and postoperative use of 5-fluorouracil (5-FU) and mitomycin C has had a profound effect on surgical glaucoma management. This has been particularly noticeable in glaucomas that traditionally had a very poor surgical prognosis. 5-FU (Fig. 35-2) is a pyrimidine analogue that inhibits fibroblastic proliferation. As such it should be most effective in reducing scar formation during the first 14 days after injury, although it apparently can be effective when used well beyond that time. 5-FU has been used to prevent proliferative vitreoretinopathy after vitrectomy.[90-92]

In a pilot study using monkeys, subconjunctival injection of 5-FU maintained filtering blebs in six of eight eyes, whereas all control eyes failed to maintain a bleb.[93] Subsequent studies have demonstrated its efficacy as an adjunct to filtering surgery in a variety of difficult glaucomas in humans.[57,94-99] 5-FU is frequently given as a subconjunctival injection of 5 mg for several days immediately after filtration surgery, although other routes of administration have also been shown to be effective.[100,101] Animal studies indicate substantial aqueous and vitreous concentrations of 5-FU after either topical or subconjunctival administration.[102-104] The route of entry after either administration seems to be via the tear film through the cornea. In one animal study, topical administration resulted in greater corneal complications.[105]

The indications for use, dosage, and frequency of administration of 5-FU in glaucoma filtering surgery continue to evolve. 5-FU improves the success rate of filtering surgery in eyes with a poor prognosis, and many surgeons use it when operating on patients with aphakia, a history of prior failed filtering surgery, penetrating ocular trauma, inflammatory or neovascular glaucoma, or in other high-risk situations. Others have administered low-dose 5-FU in patients undergoing primary trabeculectomy with impressive results.[106,107]

Initial protocols advocated twice-daily subconjunctival injections of 5.0 mg of 5-FU in 0.5 ml of unpreserved normal saline solution injected via a 30-gauge needle 3 mm from the limbus and 180° from the filtering site beginning on the day of or day after surgery for a period of 7 days. This was followed by a single daily injection for another 7 days.[34] This regimen proved difficult for both patients and surgeons and led to corneal toxicity in an intolerably high percentage of cases. Good results have been obtained using less frequent administration.[108,109] Most surgeons today inject 0.1 ml (5 mg) of the commercially available solution rather than diluting it.

Early complications[110-112] with 5-FU are predominantly corneal. Corneal erosions may reach 6 to 8 mm in diameter but usually heal with little if any sequelae in a few weeks. Corneal ulceration has occurred. Conjunctival wound and suture tract leaks occur in about one third of patients. The incidence of such leaks is reduced by meticulous wound closure using tapered, noncutting needles. Absorbable sutures such as Vicryl (polyglactin) disintegrate before 5-FU–treated tissues have healed fully.

A host of serious complications have been associated with 5-FU. One series reported a 13% rate of nonexpulsive choroidal hemorrhages in aphakic patients.[34] Other complications, including endophthalmitis, hypotony maculopathy, malignant glaucoma, pupillary block, and late bleb leaks, have occurred more frequently in 5-FU–treated eyes than in eyes undergoing trabeculectomy without adjunctive 5-FU.[113-119] Punctal occlusion and cicatricial ectropion have been reported with systemic 5-FU administration.[120,121]

Because of the intensity of side effects, the inconvenience of twice-daily injections, and the effectiveness of lower doses of 5-FU, most surgeons titrate the dose to the clinical circumstances of the patient. Patients who are doing well may receive only three or four injections spaced several days apart. Patients whose blebs are failing may receive six or more injections over a period of several months.

Mitomycin C

Mitomycin C is an antineoplastic–antibiotic agent whose initial ophthalmic use was in the prevention of recurrences after pterygium excision.[122,123] Its success and favorable ocular toxicity profile

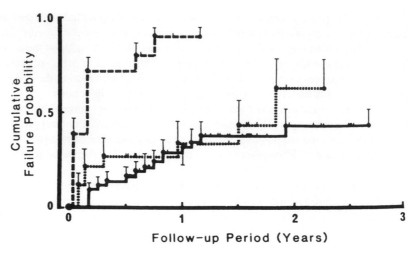

Figure 35-4 Life-table analysis of failure after trabeculectomy and primary open-angle glaucoma. The *solid line* represents the first trabeculectomy; the *dotted line* represents the second trabeculectomy; and the *dashed line* represents the third trabeculectomy. Failure was measured as a pressure level above 21 mm Hg with or without medication. The table clearly indicates that subsequent trabeculectomies have a higher probability of failure over time than do initial trabeculectomies. (From Shirato S, Kitazawa Y, Mishima S: *Jpn J Ophthalmol* 26:468, 1982.)

Box 35-1
Possible Definitions of "Success" and "Failure" After Filtering Surgery

Success

Intraocular pressure (IOP) <20 mm Hg without glaucoma medications

IOP <20 mm Hg with glaucoma medications

Stabilization of visual field without glaucoma medications

Stabilization of visual field with glaucoma medications

Stabilization of optic nerve without glaucoma medications

Stabilization of optic nerve with glaucoma medications

IOP reduced to 75% of preoperative levels without medications

IOP reduced to 75% of preoperative levels with medications

Failure

Further filtering surgery required to lower IOP

Further laser surgery required to lower IOP

The opposite of any of the above listed successes

Censored (excluded from the analysis)

Lost to follow-up, death

Underwent unrelated intraocular surgery (e.g., cataract surgery)

Other factors influencing outcome (e.g., trauma, other disease)

---

process for both patient and physician might be three IOPs measured in a masked fashion at least an hour apart within a time span not to exceed 1 month.

Should IOP be the only criterion for success? Progressive glaucoma is usually defined as visual field loss or optic nerve atrophy. If the main indication for surgery (or any treatment for that matter) is preservation of vision, shouldn't some measure of vision be a required part of the definition of success? The patient is certainly more interested in preservation of the visual field and optic nerve. Measurement of these variables also requires long and careful follow-up. Reproducibility of visual field examinations has improved with computerized perimetry, but marked fluctuation can exist. If stabilization of the visual field is to be documented, at least four (and preferably five) visual field examinations are needed to permit reasonable interpretation in light of such fluctuation, unless the change is extraordinary. Regression analysis of computerized perimetry results is feasi-

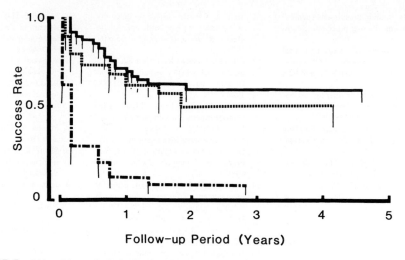

Figure 35-5 Life-table analysis indicating the probability of success using the same criteria as in Figure 35-4. This analysis technique provides more meaningful information than does the simple overall statement of percent success. (From Yamashita H, and others: *Jpn J Ophthalmol* 29:250, 1985.)

ble, useful, and proper in such situations. Similar treatment of optic nervc head change will soon be possible with computerized optic nerve analysis.

These are demanding tasks, but they will lead to a better understanding of how surgical intervention influences the outcome of glaucoma. This will allow ophthalmologists to modify techniques and the timing of treatments to better serve patients.

REFERENCES

1. Addicks EM, and others: Histologic characteristics of filtering blebs in glaucomatous eyes, *Arch Ophthalmol* 101: 795, 1983.
2. Bartley J, and others: Hemolytic complement activity in aqueous humor, *Arch Ophthalmol* 101:465, 1983.
3. Desjardins DC, and others: Wound healing after filtering surgery in owl monkeys, *Arch Ophthalmol* 104:1835, 1986.
4. Herschler J, Clafin AJ, Fiorentino G: The effect of aqueous humor on the growth of subconjunctival fibroblasts in tissue culture and its implications for glaucoma surgery, *Am J Ophthalmol* 89:245, 1980.
5. Kornblueth W, Tenenbaum E: The inhibitory effect of aqueous humor on the growth of cells in tissue cultures, *Am J Ophthalmol* 42:70, 1956.
6. Lutjen-Drecoll E, Barany EH: Functional and electron microscopic changes in the trabecular meshwork remaining after trabeculectomy in cynomologous monkeys, *Invest Ophthalmol Vis Sci* 13:511, 1974.
7. Maumenee AE: External filtering operations for glaucoma: the mechanism of function and failure, *Trans Am Ophthalmol Soc* 58:319, 1960.
8. Radius RI, Herschler J, Clafin A: Aqueous humor changes after experimental filtering surgery, *Am J Ophthalmol* 89: 250, 1980.

9. Teng CC, Chi HH, Katzin HM: Histology and mechanism of filtering operations, *Am J Ophthalmol* 47:16, 1959.
10. Bergstrom TJ, and others: The effects of subconjunctival mitomycin-C on glaucoma filtration surgery in rabbits, *Arch Ophthalmol* 109:1725, 1991.
11. Chi TS: Holmium laser sclerostomy via corneal approach with transconjunctival mitomycin-C in rabbits, *Ophthalmic Surg* 26:353, 1995.
12. Wang TH, and others: THC:YAG laser sclerostomy with mitomycin subconjunctival injection in rabbits, *J Ocul Pharmacol* 8:325, 1992.
13. Brincker P, Kessing SV: Limbus-based versus fornix-based conjunctival flap in glaucoma filtering surgery, *Acta Ophthalmol (Copenh)* 70:641, 1992.
14. Benedikt OP: Drainage mechanism after filtration, *Glaucoma* 1:71, 1979.
15. Skuta GL, Parrish RK: Wound healing in glaucoma filtering surgery, *Surv Ophthalmol* 32:149, 1987.
16. Vesti E: Filtering blebs: follow up of trabeculectomy, *Ophthalmic Surg* 24:249, 1993.
17. Richter CU, and others: The development of encapsulated filtering blebs, *Ophthalmology* 95:1163, 1988.
18. Latina M, and others: Experimental ab interno sclerotomies using a pulsed-dye laser, *Lasers Surg Med* 8:233, 1988.

19. Rankin GA, Latina MA: Transconjunctival Nd:YAG laser revision of failing trabeculectomy, *Ophthalmic Surg* 21: 365, 1990.
20. Latina MA, Rankin GA: Internal and transconjunctival neodymium:YAG laser revision of late failing filters, *Ophthalmology* 98:215, 1991.
21. Oh Y, Katz LJ: Indications and technique for reopening closed filtering blebs using the Nd:YAG laser: a review and case series, *Ophthalmic Surg* 24:617, 1993.
22. Blondeau P, Phelps CD: Trabeculectomy vs thermosclerostomy: a randomized prospective clinical trial, *Arch Ophthalmol* 99:810, 1981.
23. Lamping KA, and others: Long-term evaluation of initial filtration surgery, *Ophthalmology* 93:91, 1986.
24. Lewis RA, Phelps CD: Trabeculectomy v thermosclerostomy: a five-year follow-up, *Arch Ophthalmol* 102:533, 1984.
25. Spaeth GL, Poryzees E: A comparison between peripheral iridectomy with thermal sclerostomy and trabeculectomy: a controlled study, *Br J Ophthalmol* 65: 783, 1981.
26. Barak A, and others: The protective effect of early intraoperative injection of viscoelastic material in trabeculectomy, *Ophthalmic Surg* 23:206, 1992.
27. Wand M: Viscoelastic agent and the prevention of post-filtration flat anterior chamber, *Ophthalmic Surg* 19:523, 1988.

28. Alpar JJ: Sodium hyaluronate (healon) in glaucoma filtering procedures, *Ophthalmic Surg* 17:724, 1986.

29. D'Ermo F, Bonomi L, Doro D: A critical analysis of the long-term results of trabeculectomy, *Am J Ophthalmol* 88:829, 1979.

30. Levene RZ: Glaucoma filtering surgery: factors that determine pressure control, *Ophthalmic Surg* 15:475, 1984.

31. Wilson RP, Lloyd J: The place of sodium hyaluronate in glaucoma surgery, *Ophthalmic Surg* 17:30, 1986.

32. Beauchamp GR, Parks MM: Filtering surgery in children: barriers to success, *Ophthalmology* 86:170, 1979.

33. Cadera W, and others: Filtering surgery in childhood glaucoma, *Ophthalmic Surg* 15:319, 1984.

34. Heuer DK, and others: 5-Fluorouracil and glaucoma filtering surgery, *Ophthalmology* 93:1537, 1986.

35. Inaba Z: Long-term results of trabeculectomy in the Japanese: an analysis of life-table method, *Jpn J Ophthalmol* 26:361, 1982.

36. Shirato S, Kitazawa Y, Mishima S: A critical analysis of the trabeculectomy results by a prospective follow-up design, *Jpn J Ophthalmol* 26:468, 1982.

37. Sugar HS: Results and complications of limbal trephination and subscleral trephination (trabeculectomy), *Lasers Surg Med* 1:221, 1981.

38. Costa VP, and others: Primary trabeculectomy in young adults, *Ophthalmology* 100:1071, 1993.

39. Whiteside-Michel J, and others: Initial 5-fluorouracil trabeculectomy in young patients, *Ophthalmology* 99:7, 1992.

40. Sturmer J, and others: Young patient trabeculectomy: assessment of risk factors for failure, *Ophthalmology* 100:928, 1993.

41. Broadway D, and others: Racial differences in the results of glaucoma filtration surgery: are racial differences in the conjunctival cell profile important? *Br J Ophthalmol* 78:466, 1994.

42. McMillan TA, and others: Histologic differences in the conjunctiva of black and white glaucoma patients, *Ophthalmic Surg* 23:762, 1992.

43. Wilson MR: Posterior lip sclerectomy vs trabeculectomy in West Indian blacks, *Arch Ophthalmol* 107:1604, 1989.

44. Javitt JC, and others: Undertreatment of glaucoma among black Americans, *N Engl J Med* 325:1418, 1991.

45. Javitt JC: Preventing blindness in Americans: the need for eye health education, *Surv Ophthalmol* 40:41, 1995.

46. Bakker NJA, Manku SI: Trabeculectomy versus Scheie's operation: a comparative retrospective study in open-angle glaucoma in Kenyans, *Br J Ophthalmol* 63:643, 1979.

47. Merritt JC: Filtering procedures in American blacks, *Ophthalmic Surg* 11:91, 1980.

48. Miller RD, Barber JC: Trabeculectomy in black patients, *Ophthalmic Surg* 12:46, 1981.

49. Shin DH: Trabeculectomy, *Int Ophthalmol Clin* 21:47, 1981.

50. Stilma JS: Subscleral trepanation in the treatment of glaucoma, *Doc Ophthalmol* 44:121, 1977.

51. Thommy CP, Bhar IS: Trabeculectomy in Nigerian patients with open-angle glaucoma, *Br J Ophthalmol* 63:636, 1979.

52. Allen RC, Bellows R, Hutchinson T: Filtration surgery in treatment of neovascular glaucoma, *Ophthalmology* 89:1181, 1982.

53. Baerveldt G, Freedman J, Minckler D: Clinical experience with the single plate Molteno implant. Presented at the Ninetieth Annual Meeting of the American Academy of Ophthalmology, San Francisco, September 29-October 3, 1985.

54. Bellows AR, Johnstone MA: Surgical management of chronic glaucoma in aphakia, *Ophthalmology* 90:807, 1983.

55. Herschler J: Medically uncontrolled glaucoma in the aphakic eye, *Ann Ophthalmol* 13:909, 1981.

56. Herschler J, Agness D: A modified filtering operation for neovascular glaucoma, *Arch Ophthalmol* 97:2339, 1979.

57. Heuer DK, and others: 5-Fluorouracil and glaucoma filtering surgery. II. A pilot study, *Ophthalmology* 91:384, 1984.

58. Mills KB: Trabeculectomy: a retrospective long-term follow-up of 444 cases, *Br J Ophthalmol* 65:790, 1981.

59. Parrish R, Herschler J: Eyes with end-stage neovascular glaucoma: natural history following successful modified filtering operation, *Arch Ophthalmol* 101:746, 1983.

60. Schwartz PL, and others: Further experience with trabeculectomy, *Ann Ophthalmol* 8:207, 1976.

61. Portney GL: Trabeculectomy and postoperative ocular hypertension in secondary angle closure glaucoma, *Am J Ophthalmol* 84:145, 1977.

62. Foulks GN: Glaucoma associated with penetrating keratoplasty, *Ophthalmology* 94:871, 1987.

63. Gilvarry AM, and others: The management of post-keratoplasty glaucoma by trabeculectomy, *Eye* 3:713, 1989.

64. McDonnell PJ, and others: Molteno implant for control of glaucoma in eyes after penetrating keratoplasty, *Ophthalmology* 95:364, 1988.

65. Sherwood MB, and others: Drainage tube implants in the treatment of glaucoma following penetrating keratoplasty, *Ophthalmic Surg* 24:185, 1993.

66. Ficker LA, and others: Intraocular surgery following penetrating keratoplasty: the risks and advantages, *Eye* 4:693, 1990.

67. Naveh N, and others: The long-term effect on intraocular pressure of a procedure combining trabeculectomy and cataract surgery, as compared with trabeculectomy alone, *Ophthalmic Surg* 21:339, 1990.

68. Yu CB, and others: Long-term results of combined cataract and glaucoma surgery versus trabeculectomy alone in low-risk patients, *J Cataract Refract Surg* 22:352, 1996.

68a. Broadway DC, and others: Adverse effects of topical antiglaucoma medication. II. The outcome of filtration surgery, *Arch Ophthalmol* 112:1446, 1994.

69. Migdal C, Hitchings R: Primary therapy for chronic simple glaucoma: the role of argon laser trabeculoplasty, *Trans Ophthalmol Soc UK* 104:62, 1985.

70. Watson PG: When to operate in open angle glaucoma, *Eye* 1:51, 1987.

71. Broadway DC, and others: Reversal of topical antiglaucoma medication effects on the conjunctiva, *Arch Ophthalmol* 114:262, 1996.

72. Shoshan S: Wound healing, *Int Rev Connect Tissue Res* 9:1, 1981.

73. Skuta GL, Parrish RK II: Wound healing in glaucoma filtering surgery, *Surv Ophthalmol* 32:149, 1987.

74. Jonsson K: Tissue oxygenation, anemia, and perfusion in relation to wound healing in surgical patients, *Ann Surg* 214:605, 1991.

75. Costa VP: Wound healing modulation in glaucoma filtration surgery, *Ophthalmic Surg* 24:152, 1993.

76. Tahery MM, Lee DA: Review: pharmacologic control of wound healing in glaucoma filtration surgery, *J Ocul Pharmacol* 5:155, 1989.

77. Robinson DI, and others: Long-term intraocular pressure control by trabeculectomy: a ten-year life table, *Aust N Z J Ophthalmol* 21:79, 1993.

78. Roth SM, and others: The effects of postoperative corticosteroids on trabeculectomy and the clinical course of glaucoma: five-year follow-up study, *Ophthalmic Surg* 22:724, 1991.

79. Starita RJ, Fellman RL, Spaeth GL: Short- and long-term effects of postoperative corticosteroids on trabeculectomy, *Ophthalmology* 92:938, 1985.

80. Dunne JA, Travers JP: Double-blind clinical trial of topical steroids in anterior uveitis, *Br J Ophthalmol* 63:762, 1979.

81. Dunne JA, Travers JP: Topical steroids in anterior uveitis, *Trans Ophthalmol Soc UK* 99:481, 1979.

82. Leibowitz HM, Kupferman A: Anti-inflammatory medications, *Int Ophthalmol Clin* 20:117, 1980.

83. Okada M, Shimada K: Effects of various pharmacologic agents on allergic inflammation of the eye: the roles of chemical mediators in ocular inflammation, *Invest Ophthalmol Vis Sci* 19:176, 1980.

84. Yamaguchi H, Iso T, Iwata H: Ocular anti-inflammatory and systemic immunosuppressive effects of topically applied fluorometholene, *Jpn J Pharmacol* 29:87, 1979.

85. Leibowitz HM, Kupferman A: Drug interaction in the eye: concurrent corticosteroid-antibiotic therapy for inflammatory keratitis, *Arch Ophthalmol* 95:682, 1977.

86. Wilensky JT, Snyder D, Gieser D: Steroid-induced ocular hypertension in patients with filtering bleb, *Ophthalmology* 87:240, 1980.

87. Gwin TD, and others: Filtration surgery in rabbits treated with diclofenac or prednisolone acetate, *Ophthalmic Surg* 25:245, 1994.

88. Diestelhorst M, and others: The effect of argon laser trabeculoplasty on the blood-aqueous barrier and intraocular pressure in human glaucomatous eyes treated with diclofenac 0.1%, *Graefes Arch Clin Exp Ophthalmol* 233:559, 1995.

89. Hunt T, and others: Effect of cortisone and vitamin A on wound infections, *Am J Surg* 121:569, 1971.

90. Blumenkranz MS, Claflin A, Hajek AS: Selection of therapeutic agents for intraocular proliferative disease: cell culture evaluation, *Arch Ophthalmol* 102:598, 1984.

91. Blumenkranz MS, and others: Fluorouracil for the treatment of massive periretinal proliferation, *Am J Ophthalmol* 94:458, 1982.

92. Stern WH, and others: Fluorouracil therapy for proliferative vitreoretinopathy after vitrectomy, *Am J Ophthalmol* 96:33, 1983.

93. Greesel MG, Parrish RK II, Folberg R: 5-Fluorouracil and glaucoma filtering surgery.I. An animal model, *Ophthalmology* 91:378, 1984.

94. Egbert PR, and others: A prospective trial of intraoperative fluorouracil during trabeculectomy in a black population, *Am J Ophthalmol* 116:612, 1993.

95. Goldenfeld, and others: 5-Fluorouracil in initial trabeculectomy: a prospective, randomized, multicenter study, *Ophthalmology* 101:1024, 1994.

96. Taniguchi T, and others: Long-term results of 5-fluorouracil trabeculectomy for primary open-angle glaucoma, *Int Ophthalmol* 13:145, 1989.

97. Rockwood EJ, and others: Glaucoma filtering surgery with 5-fluorouracil, *Ophthalmology* 94:1071, 1987.

98. Ruderman JM, and others: A randomized study of 5-fluorouracil and filtration surgery, *Am J Ophthalmol* 104:218, 1987.

99. Five-year follow-up of the Fluorouracil Filtering Surgery Study: the Fluorouracil Filtering Surgery Study Group, *Am J Ophthalmol* 121:349, 1996.

100. Dietze PJ, and others: Intraoperative application of 5-fluorouracil during trabeculectomy, *Ophthalmic Surg* 23:662, 1992.

101. Mora JS, and others: Trabeculectomy with intraoperative sponge 5-fluorouracil, *Ophthalmology* 103:963, 1996.

102. Fantes FE, and others: Topical fluorouracil: pharmacokinetics in normal rabbit eyes, *Arch Ophthalmol* 103:953, 1985.

103. Rootman J, Ostry A, Gudauskas G: Pharmacokinetics and metabolism of 5-fluorouracil following subconjunctival versus intravenous administration, *Can J Ophthalmol* 19:187, 1984.

104. Rootman J, and others: Intraocular penetration of subconjunctivally administered 14C-fluorouracil in rabbits, *Arch Ophthalmol* 97:2375, 1979.

105. Heuer DK, and others: Topical fluorouracil. II. Postoperative administration in an animal model of glaucoma filtering surgery, *Arch Ophthalmol* 104:132, 1986.

106. Liebmann JM, and others: Initial 5-fluorouracil trabeculectomy in uncomplicated glaucoma, *Ophthalmology* 98:1036, 1991.

107. Ophir A, Ticho U: A randomized study of trabeculectomy and subconjunctival administration of fluorouracil in primary glaucomas, *Arch Ophthalmol* 110:1072, 1992.

108. Loane ME, Weinreb RN: Reducing corneal toxicity of 5-fluorouracil in the early postoperative period following glaucoma filtering surgery, *Aust N Z J Ophthalmol* 19:197, 1991.

109. Weinreb RN: Adjusting the dose of 5-fluorouracil after filtration surgery to minimize side effects, *Ophthalmology* 94:564, 1987.

110. Fluorouracil Filtering Surgery Study one-year follow-up: the Fluorouracil Filtering Surgery Study Group, *Am J Ophthalmol* 108:625, 1989.

111. Knapp A, and others: Serious corneal complications of glaucoma filtering surgery with postoperative 5-fluorouracil, *Am J Ophthalmol* 103:183, 1987.

112. Lee DA, and others: Complications of subconjunctival 5-fluorouracil following glaucoma filtering surgery, *Ophthalmic Surg* 18:187, 1987.

113. Altan T, and others: Hypotonic maculopathy after trabeculectomy with postoperative use of 5-fluorouracil, *Ophthalmologica* 208:318, 1994.

114. Hickey-Dwyer M, Wishart PK: Serious corneal complication of 5-fluorouracil, *Br J Ophthalmol* 77:250, 1993.

115. Risk factors for suprachoroidal hemorrhage after filtering surgery: the Fluorouracil Filtering Surgery Study Group, *Am J Ophthalmol* 113:501, 1992.

116. Patitsas CJ, and others: Glaucoma filtering surgery with postoperative 5-fluorouracil in patients with intraocular inflammatory disease, *Ophthalmology* 99:594, 1992.

117. Parrish R, Minckler D: "Late endophthalmitis": filtering surgery time bomb? *Ophthalmology* 103:1167, 1996 (editorial).

118. Ticho U, Ophir A: Late complications after glaucoma filtering surgery with adjunctive 5-fluorouracil, *Am J Ophthalmol* 115:506, 1993.

119. Wilson RP, Steinmann WC: Use of trabeculectomy with postoperative 5-fluorouracil in patients requiring extremely low intraocular pressure levels to limit further glaucoma progression, *Ophthalmology* 98:1047, 1991.

120. Caravella LP, Burns JA, Zangmeister M: Punctal-canalicular stenosis related to systemic fluorouracil therapy, *Arch Ophthalmol* 99:284, 1981.

121. Straus DJ, and others: Cicatricial ectropion secondary to 5-fluorouracil therapy, *Med Pediatr Oncol* 3:15, 1977.

122. Hayasaka S, and others: Postoperative instillation of low-dose mitomycin C in the treatment of primary pterygium, *Am J Ophthalmol* 106:715, 1988.

123. Singh G, and others: Mitomycin eye drops as treatment for pterygium, *Ophthalmology* 95:813, 1988.

124. Chen CW, and others: Trabeculectomy with simultaneous topical application of mitomycin-C in refractory glaucoma, *J Ocul Pharmacol* 6:175, 1990.

125. Jampel HD: Effect of brief exposure to mitomycin C on viability and proliferation of cultured human Tenon's capsule fibroblasts, *Ophthalmology* 99:1471, 1992.

126. Kitazawa Y, and others: Trabeculectomy with mitomycin: a comparative study with fluorouracil, *Arch Ophthalmol* 109:1693, 1991.

127. Palmer SS: Mitomycin as adjunct chemotherapy with trabeculectomy, *Ophthalmology* 98:317, 1991.

128. Pasquale LR, and others: Effect of topical mitomycin C on glaucoma filtration surgery in monkeys, *Ophthalmology* 99:14, 1992.

129. Hong C, and others: Effects of topical mitomycin C on glaucoma filtration surgery, *Korean J Ophthalmol* 7:1, 1993.

131. Ramakrishnan R, and others: Safety and efficacy of mitomycin C trabeculectomy in southern India: a short-term pilot study, *Ophthalmology* 100:1619, 1993.

132. Khaw PT, and others: Effects of intraoperative 5-fluorouracil or mitomycin C on glaucoma filtration surgery in the rabbit, *Ophthalmology* 100:367, 1993.

133. Lamping KA, Belkin JK: 5-Fluorouracil and mitomycin C in pseudophakic patients, *Ophthalmology* 102:70, 1995.

134. Prata JA Jr, and others: Trabeculectomy in pseudophakic patients: postoperative 5-fluorouracil versus intraoperative mitomycin C antiproliferative therapy, *Ophthalmic Surg* 26:73, 1995.

135. Skuta GL, and others: Intraoperative mitomycin versus postoperative 5-fluorouracil in high-risk glaucoma filtering surgery, *Ophthalmology* 99:438, 1992.

136. Skuta GL: Antifibrotic agents in glaucoma filtering surgery, *Int Ophthalmol Clin* 33:165, 1993.

137. Annen DJ, Sturmer J: Follow-up of a pilot study of trabeculectomy with low dosage mitomycin C (0.2 mg/ml for 1 minute): Independent evaluation of a retrospective nonrandomized study, *Klin Monatsbl Augenheilkd* 206:300, 1995.

138. Kitazawa Y, and others: Low-dose and high-dose mitomycin trabeculectomy as an initial surgery in primary open-angle glaucoma, *Ophthalmology* 100:1624, 1993.

139. Lee JJ, and others: The effect of low- and high-dose adjunctive mitomycin C in trabeculectomy, *Korean J Ophthalmol* 10:42, 1996.

140. Joos KM, and others: One-year follow-up results of combined mitomycin C trabeculectomy and extracapsular cataract extraction, *Ophthalmology* 102:76, 1995.

141. Munden PM, Alward WL: Combined phacoemulsification, posterior chamber intraocular lens implantation, and trabeculectomy with mitomycin C, *Am J Ophthalmol* 119:20, 1995.

142. Lederer CM Jr: Combined cataract extraction with intraocular lens implant and mitomycin-augmented trabeculectomy, *Ophthalmology* 103:1025, 1996.

143. Costa VP: Effects of topical mitomycin C on primary trabeculectomies and combined procedures, *Br J Ophthalmol* 77:693, 1993.

144. Jampel HD: Hypotony maculopathy following trabeculectomy with mitomycin C, *Arch Ophthalmol* 110:1049, 1992 (letter).

145. Higginbotham EJ, and others: Bleb-related endophthalmitis after trabeculectomy with mitomycin C, *Ophthalmology* 103:650, 1996.

146. Prata JA Jr, and others: Trabeculectomy with mitomycin C in glaucoma associated with uveitis, *Ophthalmic Surg* 25:616, 1994.

147. Mietz H, Krieglstein GK: Short-term clinical results and complications of trabeculectomies performed with mitomycin C using different concentrations, *Int Ophthalmol* 19:51, 1995.

148. Shields MB, and others: Clinical and histopathologic observations concerning hypotony after trabeculectomy with adjunctive mitomycin C, *Am J Ophthalmol* 116:673, 1993.

149. Yaldo MK, Stamper RL: Long-term effects of mitomycin on filtering blebs: lack of fibrovascular proliferative response following severe inflammation [published erratum appears in *Arch Ophthalmol* 111:1358, 1993], *Arch Ophthalmol* 111:824, 1993.

150. Cox DR: Regression models and life-tables, *S Roy Stat Soc Series B* 34:187, 1972.

151. Kaplan EL, Meier P: Nonparametric estimation from incomplete observations, *J Am Statist Assn* 53:457, 1958.

152. Yamashita H, and others: Trabeculectomy: a prospective study of complications and results of long-term follow-up, *Jpn J Ophthalmol* 29:250, 1985.

PART VIII

Surgical Procedures and Techniques

36

Surgery to Relieve Outflow Block: Filtering Procedures

GENERAL CONSIDERATIONS

If there is no internal flow block and intraocular pressure (IOP) remains too high despite maximally tolerated medical therapy, then surgery to relieve outflow block is needed. Most such procedures are designed to increase the flow of aqueous out of the eye, thus reducing IOP.

Laser trabeculoplasty to relieve outflow block is described in detail in Chapter 31. Laser trabeculoplasty is generally attempted before incisional surgery unless the IOP is very high or the optic nerve is severely damaged. Incisional surgery may also be selected before laser surgery in cases of normal-tension, inflammatory, traumatic, and developmental glaucoma, or in cases in which the angle is covered by synechiae or the cornea is clouded. Several studies have supported using filtration surgery as the initial therapy in routine open-angle glaucoma, citing better medium- and long-term visual outcome as one of the major benefits.[1,2] Although this remains an area of active debate,[3] there is widespread agreement that the individual circumstances of the patient must be evaluated before the appropriate initial therapy can be chosen.

Incisional surgery to relieve outflow block may create external filtration (e.g., trabeculectomy or full-thickness filtering procedures) or internal filtration (e.g., cyclodialysis), or it may essentially remove the trabecular meshwork from the outflow pathway (e.g., trabeculectomy and goniotomy). Regardless of the procedure used, the goal is to reduce the IOP to a level that will prevent further damage to the optic nerve but not reduce it so much as to cause problems from hypotony. The lowest IOP that can be tolerated by the eye is generally about 5 to 6 mm Hg. Below this level cataracts, choroidal elevation, macular swelling, optic nerve swelling, and refractive variations may occur.[4-6]

Traditionally, many surgeons try to lower the IOP below the "magic number" of 20 mm Hg because this number is given as one standard deviation above the mean IOP for the normal population. There is no evidence to support the notion that a specific protective effect is conferred on glaucoma patients whose pressure is simply reduced to 20 mm Hg or lower. Some studies indicate that more severely damaged nerves may require pressures below 16 mm Hg if damage is to be stopped.[7,8] Although evidence supporting the notion that a specific pressure level is safe for all patients is lacking, there is ample evidence to suggest that lowering the IOP in glaucoma patients slows the rate of visual field loss. Some of the most compelling evidence in this regard comes from a series of studies on surgery in patients with normal-tension glaucoma.[9,10] Rather than choosing a specific target pressure, these studies used a targeted percentage pressure reduction as the therapeutic goal.

Full-thickness procedures generally provide lower pressures for a longer time than do guarded filtration procedures such as trabeculectomy.[11-13] However, such procedures also have a higher complication rate in most surgeons' hands. Efforts continue to achieve better pressure control with fewer complications using the guarded approach, mostly via pharmacologic modifications of wound healing and manipulations of flap closure using releasable sutures or laser suture lysis (LSL).

EXTERNAL FILTRATION SURGERY

The goal of external filtration is to create a new drainage pathway that allows aqueous to pass from the anterior chamber into the subconjunctival space. There the fluid either is absorbed into the conjunctival blood vessels or lymphatics or, if the bleb is thin-walled, passes directly across the conjunctiva into the tear layer.[14-17]

Filtering surgery requires an opening through the scleral wall at the limbus. The surgeon makes this opening much larger than the 15-μm diameter hole that (theoretically) is adequate for all aqueous flow out of the eye[18] because the healing process works to reduce the ultimate or effective size of the opening. Indeed, the healing process often obliterates the opening entirely. A larger initial opening, however, does not ensure success and may in fact lead to higher failure and complication rates. These rates increase because initial hypotony causes production of secondary aqueous, which contains the ingredients required for accelerated wound healing and may reduce the flow of aqueous humor through the sclerostomy. This causes the episcleral surface to scar down around the sclerostomy and close it.

Early postoperative hypotony is to be avoided when possible. The ideal procedure would lower IOP to 8 to 10 mm Hg immediately and keep it there. The collagenolytic activity of pure aqueous passing through the sclerostomy would modify the conjunctiva, converting it to an acellular matrix that easily transports the aqueous. If the aqueous contains protein and serum as a result of hypotony, healing is accelerated rather than retarded and the outcome may be poor.

There are two basic types of external filtration procedures: guarded and full-thickness.

Guarded Procedures

When the filtering sclerostomy is protected from excessive flow either by partially closing it with a scleral flap or by suturing techniques, it is described in terms such as *guarded, protected, subscleral,* or *partial-thickness filtration surgery.* The advantage of such techniques is that the initial egress of aqueous from the anterior chamber is retarded, which reduces the incidence of postoperative flat chambers.[19] Additionally, such maneuvers may reduce the incidence of hypotony and suprachoroidal hemorrhage.

Decreasing the incidence of postoperative hypotony and flat chamber appears to reduce inflammation, peripheral anterior synechiae, and cataract formation as well. Guarded filtration procedures may also reduce the long-term success rate of the surgery and prevent attainment of the very low pressures that seem desirable in advanced glaucoma or normal-tension glaucoma.[12]

Guarded procedures with or without antimetabolites are generally preferred except under unusual circumstances. There are a number of guarded filtering techniques, of which trabeculectomy and its variations are the most popular.

Full-Thickness Procedures

Procedures such as thermal sclerostomy, posterior or anterior lip sclerectomy, or Elliott's trephination have no guard over the external surface of the sclerostomy other than the conjunctiva and Tenon's capsule. These procedures are labeled *full-thickness filtration surgery.* Such procedures may be preferable if very low pressures are desired (e.g., in normal-tension glaucoma) or if guarded filtration surgery has failed.[20] They usually require a limbal-based conjunctival flap because of high aqueous outflow in the early postoperative period.

RESULTS OF EXTERNAL FILTRATION SURGERY

External filtration surgery achieves reasonable IOP lowering in 65% to 85% of adults, depending on the condition of the eye, the use of antimetabolites, the healing tendencies of the eye, and the skill with which the surgery is performed. This success rate may be increased to over 90% if eyes in which antiglaucomatous medication use was resumed are included.

It is difficult to compare surgical results because of variations in techniques and definitions of success. In a prospective, randomized study of the differences between thermal sclerostomy and trabeculectomy, however, Blondeau and Phelps[11] reported IOPs less than 22 mm Hg in 65% of thermal sclerostomies and 76% of trabeculectomies followed up for 5 years. When medications were added, the success rates rose to 91% for the eyes treated with thermal sclerostomy and 94% for those treated with trabeculectomy. Pressures tended to be somewhat lower in eyes undergoing thermal sclerostomy, but visually significant cataracts occurred three times more often and hypotony twice as often with thermal sclerostomy.[11] Thinner blebs were also more frequent with thermal scle-

scleral incision. A short radial relaxing incision can be made at one or both ends of the flap if exposure is restricted or if particularly wide exposure is needed to insert a seton or valve.

Closure of this flap is usually done with a wing suture at each end of the flap drawn tightly enough so that the cut edge of the flap is held snugly against the corneoscleral junction. Mattress-type sutures can be used in the center of the cut edge of the flap if necessary to reduce leakage. Careful closure with mattress sutures may be done without the wing suture if the sutures extend to the edge of the conjunctival flap. A careful running suture may also be used (Figs. 36-4 and 36-5).

Initial comparisons recognized no difference in success between fornix- and limbus-based flaps.[21-23] A later study of difficult cases showed a higher failure rate with fornix-based flaps compared with limbus-based flaps,[24] but as always surgical technique and differences between cases may have had a significant effect on the outcome.

Excision of Tenon's Capsule

Some researchers have suggested that excision of Tenon's capsule in young people, in African-Americans, or in people who require reoperations may enhance filtration success.[25-28] Evidence for this is not conclusive. If excision of Tenon's capsule is desired, the dissection can be eased by in-

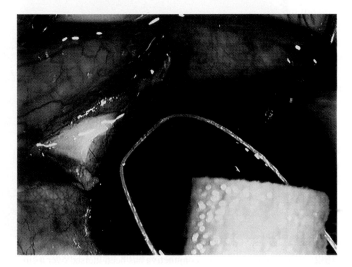

Figure 36-4   Running 10-0 Prolene closure of Tenon's portion of a conjunctival flap.

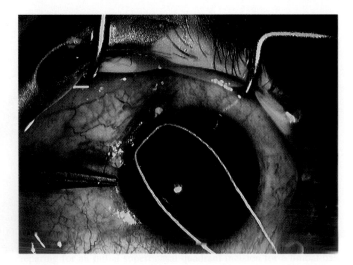

Figure 36-5   Winged conjunctival closure (in this case after Tenon's closure).

jecting BSS between the capsule and conjunctiva. Because of the chance of a buttonhole or other problems associated with excising Tenon's capsule, many surgeons have abandoned this step in favor of using antimetabolites in these cases.[29]

GUARDED FILTRATION PROCEDURE

Trabeculectomy

Trabeculectomy, with its many modifications, is the most commonly used guarded filtration procedure. Cairns[30] introduced the modern-day trabeculectomy in the 1960s. It was initially believed that aqueous escaped through the cut ends of Schlemm's canal, but it subsequently became obvious that the major effect of the surgery occurred via filtration of aqueous into the subconjunctival space.[31] The reduced incidence of hypotony and flat anterior chambers made trabeculectomy attractive to glaucoma surgeons.

Indications

Trabeculectomy has become the standard glaucoma procedure, with excellent results for most forms of open-angle and chronic angle-closure glaucoma. Aphakic, inflammatory, traumatic, and other secondary forms of uncontrolled glaucoma also are treated by trabeculectomy; success rates are good when wound-healing retardants are used,[32-34] although success rates tend to be lower than in uncomplicated cases. Trabeculectomy can be combined with cataract extraction under a variety of circumstances. Before the routine use of posterior chamber lenses with extracapsular cataract extraction or phacoemulsification, combined cataract extraction–filtering procedures were rarely indicated. Modern techniques have broadened the indications[35,36] for combining these procedures, however, and many surgeons report excellent results.[37-40]

Technique

The first procedure is usually performed superiorly and slightly nasally to preserve the temporal area of the eye for future cataract extraction. In aphakic or pseudophakic glaucoma, the surgical area selected should have minimal conjunctival scarring. This can be determined by attempting to move the anesthetized conjunctiva with an instrument or by injecting BSS under the conjunctiva. If the conjunctiva is tightly adherent to the globe, another site should be selected.

The region of the sclera planned for the scleral flap is cauterized (Fig. 36-6) to reduce bleeding and the need for later cautery, which shrinks the scleral flap. Excessive cauterization should be avoided, however. Cauterization can be done with wetfield cautery or with a microdiathermy instrument. Microdiathermy offers the advantage of pinpoint cauterization, which is useful when cauterizing individual vessels during the early parts of the procedure and when controlling occasional

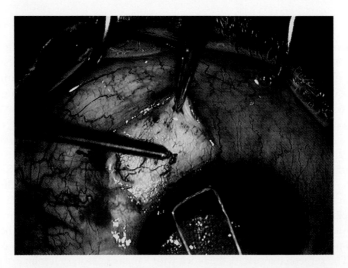

Figure 36-6   Unipolar cautery to a scleral bleed in preparation for developing a scleral flap.

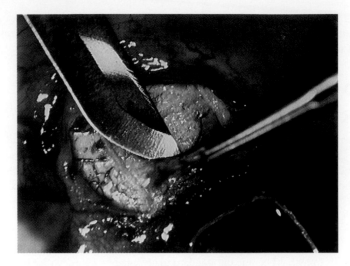

Figure 36-7   Scleral flap.

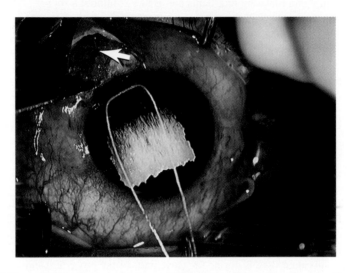

Figure 36-8   Mitomycin C–soaked sponge *(arrow)* being removed from the subconjunctival space after 3 to 5 minutes of scleral contact.

worrisome hemorrhage from the ciliary body or deep sclera after excising the trabeculectomy specimen. The scleral flap is usually one third to one half the scleral thickness, rectangular or triangular in shape, and hinged anteriorly at the limbus (Fig. 36-7). Antimetabolites may be administered before or after the scleral flap is developed, but always before any opening is made into the anterior chamber (Fig. 36-8). It is useful to place a self-sealing paracentesis at the temporal horizontal (i.e., 9 or 3 o'clock position) limbus using a super-sharp blade after preparing the scleral flap but before otherwise entering the globe (Fig. 36-9). The paracentesis site can be used to fill the eye with viscoelastic before taking the trabeculectomy specimen or for re-forming the chamber at the end of the procedure. It can also be used to re-form a flat anterior chamber with BSS or viscoelastic during the first postoperative week or so. After the scleral flap is extended past the limbus into the cornea and the paracentesis site has been made, the anterior chamber is entered under the flap (Fig. 36-10) and a block of tissue approximately 1 to 1.5 mm anteroposterior by 3 to 4 mm wide is removed just anterior to the scleral spur. Removal of the trabeculectomy block over or behind the scleral spur appears not to improve the success of the procedure and increases the risk of hemorrhage.

The surgeon may excise the block with Vannas scissors, a trephine, a scleral punch, or thermal cautery (Fig. 36-11). The success rate of these approaches is similar. A peripheral iridectomy should

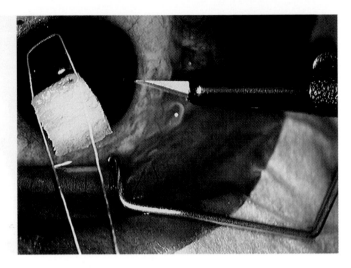

Figure 36-9   Paracentesis with a super-sharp blade.

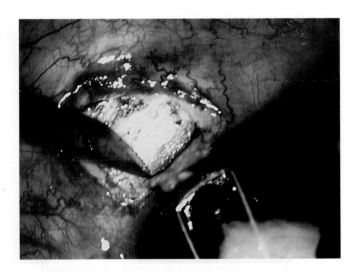

Figure 36-10   The site of the trabeculectomy specimen is outlined.

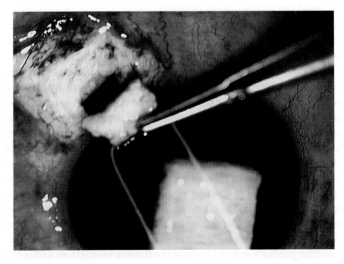

Figure 36-11   A rectangular block of tissue has been excised.

Sclerectomy

The scleral tissue to be excised is always the limbal tissue, but the ab externo incision must be varied, depending on whether the sclerectomy is to be performed on the anterior or posterior lips of the incision.

Posterior Lip Sclerectomy

In posterior lip sclerectomy, the ab externo incision is placed just behind the point of reflection of the conjunctiva in the anterior limbus. It is beveled forward somewhat more so than for other procedures. The length of the incision must be at least 3 to 4 mm to permit the punch to slide easily under the back lip of the incision. Among the many instruments available for this purpose, the Kelley, Descemet, Walser, or Gass punches have seen broad acceptance. With these punches, the cutting blade can be inserted into the anterior chamber through a small incision. One or two 1-mm bites placed side by side are adequate. This opening must be inspected carefully. Not infrequently the outer sclera is excised, but the punch slips off before the internal limbal tissues are excised, and a full-thickness opening is not made. As in the trephine operation, the specimen removed provides opportunities for studying the pathology, histology, and electron microscopic appearance of freshly excised trabecular meshwork in glaucomatous eyes. After sclerectomy, the iris usually prolapses into the opening. If it does not, it should be grasped gently by forceps and a peripheral iridotomy performed. Closure of the conjunctival incision is as previously described.

Anterior Lip Sclerectomy

In anterior lip sclerectomy, the ab externo incision must be placed back at the corneoscleral sulcus to permit removal of the tissue between the incision and the conjunctival reflection. Otherwise, the procedure is the same. Scissors also can be used to excise the 0.5-mm semicircle of tissue. Buttonholing of the conjunctival flap while cutting out the scleral fragment is the principal danger in anterior lip sclerectomy. Most surgeons prefer the posterior lip technique.

Trephination

Corneoscleral trephination is a difficult procedure for surgeons who perform it only occasionally. Disastrous errors can occur during surgery, such as misplacement of the trephine, buttonholing of the flap, injury to the lens or ciliary body, and incomplete removal of the corneoscleral button. The large opening produced by trephination invites hypotony, flat anterior chamber, and incarceration of intraocular tissue, particularly in the crowded segment of narrow-angle eyes. Although similar complications can occur with other operations, they are less frequent and more easily avoided. In patients who require full-thickness procedures, punch sclerectomy is generally simpler and probably safer for surgeons who perform trephination infrequently.

Iridencleisis

Iridencleisis is rarely, if ever, used today. The technique is described briefly here for historical completeness.

An ab externo incision is placed at the corneoscleral sulcus and beveled forward slightly toward the anterior chamber. The entrance into the anterior chamber is approximately 2 to 3 mm in length. If only one pillar is to be incarcerated, the surgeon pulls the iris out until the pupillary margin is visible and then runs de Wecker scissors under the iris to its base to perform a complete vertical iridotomy beside the forceps. The iris is then wedged firmly in the incision and dropped. With a double-pillar iris incarceration, the assistant should grasp the iris beside the surgeon's forceps. The radial iridotomy is similarly completed between the two forceps, and the pillars are incarcerated in opposite edges of the incision.

SETON OPERATIONS

Setons[77-82] are synthetic devices used in glaucoma surgery to maintain a patent drainage fistula. Horsehair, silk, metal sutures, tantalum mesh, tubes of gold, platinum, polyethylene, collagen and silicone, Gelfilm, and acrylic plates have all been used in various ways. Most have initial success, but fibrosis around the tube or plate reduces long-term success.

The Molteno Implant

In 1969 Molteno[83] established the idea of connecting a tube from the anterior chamber to a drainage field provided by an acrylic plate.[83-86] Similar to the concept of a drainage field for a house, this concept recognizes that the fluid must not only escape from the confines of the anterior chamber but also must be carried away by providing a large area that can absorb it. The acrylic plate guarantees that the bleb will not be less than the area of the plate.

Molteno also recognized that the device's outflow was too great in the immediate postoperative period, resulting in prolonged initial hypotony with its undesirable sequelae. He addressed this problem by modifying the procedure to implant the plate first to allow it to become encapsulated.[84] Six weeks later, the tube was introduced into the anterior chamber to allow the aqueous to drain into the immature fibrovascular sac surrounding the plate. The sac provides a controlled absorption membrane for the aqueous. A fairly spectacular regimen of antifibrosis therapy, including systemic nonsteroidal antiinflammatory agents; colchicine as a mitotic inhibitor; and topical atropine, epinephrine, and steroids was used to prevent excessive fibrosis of the sac. An absorbable Vicryl ligature or a nylon suture that could be cut with a laser has recently been used around the tube to allow single-stage insertion with delayed aqueous outflow into the sac.[87-89]

Results

Molteno and others have had initial success with a single plate form of this device in a variety of serious forms of glaucoma.[83-86,90-93]

Technique

The Molteno drainage device can be inserted via a limbal-type conjunctival incision 8 mm posterior to the limbus or by a peritomy incision of the conjunctiva. If a peritomy incision is used, a radial relaxing incision is usually required at one end of the peritomy to allow positioning of the drainage plate over the equator of the globe. The plate has suture holes on its anterior edge for suturing the plate to the sclera with a 6-0 nonabsorbable suture. Fixation of the plate helps prevent subsequent migration of the tube out of or further into the anterior chamber. The plate should be positioned well posterior to the insertion of the rectus muscles. If a double-plate implant is used, a plate is positioned in each quadrant. The tube connecting the two plates was designed to pass under the intervening muscle, but in practice this is often quite difficult to achieve and the tube can pass over the muscle. If a single-stage procedure is to be performed, the tube connecting the plate to the anterior chamber is placed under a half-thickness scleral flap approximately 6 mm wide and 8 mm long, hinged at the limbus much like a trabeculectomy scleral flap. The tube itself should be carefully measured so that after insertion it will extend at least 2 mm into the anterior chamber. Less extension than this may allow the tube to retract out of the anterior chamber postoperatively.

The tube is introduced into the anterior chamber via a paracentesis tract created with a 23-gauge needle passed through the junction of the scleral flap and the limbus at an angle that suspends the tube in the middle of the anterior chamber. The scleral flap is then sutured over the tube to hold it in place and act as a barrier to its external erosion. In the single-stage operation, many surgeons try to prevent the excessive initial outflow of aqueous by ligating the tube with a 5-0 or 7-0 Vicryl suture.[85] This suture dissolves in 3 to 4 weeks, opening the tube and establishing aqueous drainage into the sub-Tenon's sac that is developing around the plate. An 8-0 nylon suture can be used for the same purpose, but it must be lysed with a laser to establish flow.

If a two-stage procedure is used, the tube is simply turned aside and sutured onto the sclera. In 5 to 6 weeks, after the drainage sac has developed, the area is reexposed and the tube positioned in the anterior chamber as described previously. No ligature is required in the two-stage procedure.

Schocket Procedure

Schocket and co-workers[94,95] introduced a variation of the Molteno concept that involves shunting of aqueous via a tube to an encircling band. Results with the Schocket implant are similar to those with the Molteno implant, with some authors reporting slightly higher complication or reoperation rates.[96-100]

A 30-mm long Silastic tube with an internal diameter of 0.30 mm is sutured inside the groove of a #20 silicone band, leaving 15 mm of the tube extending from the band. The encircling band is sutured to the sclera, 10 to 12 mm from the limbus and beneath the four rectus muscles, with 5-0

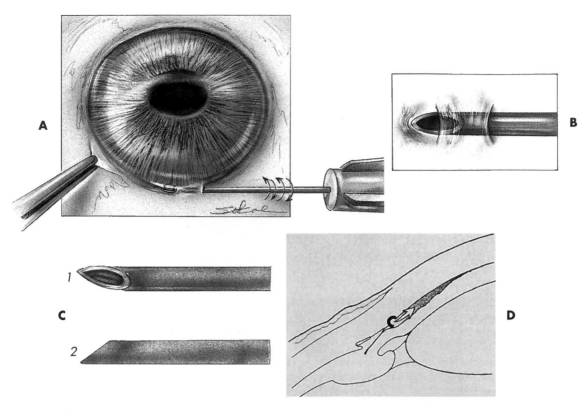

Figure 37-9   **A,** A disposable 30-gauge needle can be used to penetrate the cornea of even a hypotonous eye by gently rotating the tip back and forth. **B,** The bevel should face the surgeon as the tip is passed through the cornea until the tip can just be seen to move the iris. **C,** The tip is then rotated (*1* to *2*) so that **(D)** air can be injected into the anterior chamber through the beveled portion of the needle even though the full tip is not yet in the anterior chamber.

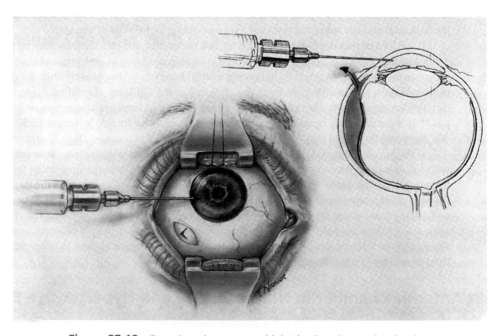

Figure 37-10   Posterior sclerostomy and injection into the anterior chamber.

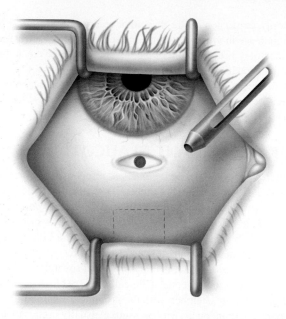

Figure 37-11 Dellaporta technique for choroidal drainage. After a conjunctival incision is made 4 mm from the limbus at the 6 o'clock position over the pars plana (and anterior to the inferior rectus muscle), a 1-mm trephine is used to remove a divot of sclera, with great care taken to avoid penetrating the underlying uveal tissue. The divot of sclera can be removed after the drainage of fluid or be lightly sutured into place. (From Lieberman MF: *Complications of glaucoma surgery.* In Charlton J, Weinstein G, editors: *Ophthalmic surgery complications,* Philadelphia, 1995, Lippincott–Raven.)

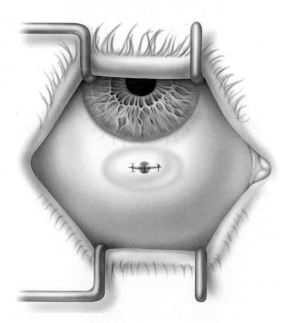

Figure 37-12 Dellaporta technique. After a watertight closure of the conjunctival wound (e.g., using 9-0 Vicryl suture), a dependent bleb forms from the persistent egress of fluid through the 1-mm trephine hole. Uveal prolapse is rarely seen, and the drainage of fluid, activated by the extraocular movements, can sometimes persist for several days, thus reducing the tendency for recurrent accumulation of suprachoroidal effusion. (From Lieberman MF: *Complications of glaucoma surgery.* In Charlton J, Weinstein G, editors: *Ophthalmic surgery complications,* Philadelphia, 1995, Lippincott–Raven.)

plete iridectomy, expansion of the choroid or enlargement of the suprachoroidal space by blood or effusion, an increase in vitreous volume caused by blood or effusion, or the misdirection of aqueous. If an iridectomy is not present or patent, one should be created immediately either by laser or, if necessary, incisional surgery.

If a patent iridectomy exists, there are two common causes of flat chamber with normal or high IOP after glaucoma surgery: ciliary block (e.g., aqueous misdirection syndrome, malignant glaucoma) and suprachoroidal hemorrhage (SCH).

CILIARY BLOCK (MALIGNANT GLAUCOMA)

The term *ciliary block* or *malignant glaucoma* refers to a spectrum of atypical angle-closure glaucomas that share several essential features.[29] Other terms have been proposed for this condition, many of which purportedly point to the underlying pathophysiology. These terms include *aqueous misdirection* or *hyaloid block glaucoma* and *posterior aqueous entrapment*. Historically this condition was commonly appreciated as a complication of a filtering procedure in eyes with preexisting angle-closure glaucoma or shallow anterior chambers.

There is good agreement in the literature about several essential features of this condition, but other features are more controversial. Clinically, ciliary block glaucoma is suspected in the presence of a grade 2 or 3 shallow chamber, with the prominent shallowing of the peripheral and central anterior chambers simultaneously. The pressure is usually higher than expected; in the early postoperative period it may simply be between 15 and 20 mm Hg despite the appearance of what would seem to be an otherwise adequate bleb; in other cases the pressure can be quite high indeed.

To diagnose ciliary block glaucoma, it is essential to eliminate the possibility of pupillary block; hence a patent iridectomy must be established before this diagnosis can be considered. Sometimes the diagnosis is made only in retrospect, after evaluating the eye's response to several interventions. For example, cycloplegics can be curative of malignant glaucoma and miotics can be exacerbative. If surgical intervention is necessary, disrupting the hyaloid face or collapsing the vitreous is usually curative.

Other aspects that are sometimes seen with ciliary block glaucoma include the rarity of spontaneous resolution—and hence its "malignant" designation. It is usually bilateral in predisposition, and it is often worsened by conventional glaucoma surgery such as iridectomy or filtration procedures. The clinical presentation of ciliary block glaucoma is similar to that of other conditions, notably angle-closure glaucoma with ciliary choroidal detachment.[30] For example, some authors have observed the accumulation of fluid in the suprachoroidal space in some cases of ciliary block glaucoma,[29,31] and this has been confirmed by ultrasonic biomicroscopy.[32] Other situations that may overlap with the appearance of ciliary block glaucoma include eyes that have undergone cataract extraction, with or without lens implantation, with sequestration of aqueous behind the iris plane. These conditions have been referred to as "iridovitreal block"[33] and "retrocapsular aqueous misdirection."[34]

The pathophysiologic sequence of ciliary block glaucoma is thought to be as follows.[35,36] After some initiating event (e.g., shallowing of the chamber during trabeculectomy) there is cause for misdirection of the aqueous to circulate into or behind the vitreous body. This apparently leads to an alteration of the vitreous volume and its compaction, with a cycle of increasing vitreous swelling and reduced conductivity of aqueous anteriorly. The enlarging vitreous body is unable to exchange aqueous across the hyaloid face at the junction of the zonules, vitreous face, and ciliary processes. This progressive vitreal engorgement results in shallowing both axially and peripherally in the anterior chamber, with increasing apposition of the peripheral iris into the angle, setting up a further cycle of angle-closure glaucoma.

The management of ciliary block glaucoma is straightforward. It is important to eliminate the possibility of pupillary block glaucoma by verifying or creating a patent iridectomy. Miotic medications should be discontinued, and vigorous cycloplegia as well as the use of topical steroids should be instituted. Other agents to reduce aqueous production, such as topical α-agonists or β-blockers, carbonic anhydrase inhibitors, or osmotic agents, can be used to reduce the pressure. A waiting period of approximately 5 days has been advised with this intensive medical regimen to see if there is resolution, with as many as half of the cases resolving during this interval.[37]

In the event that surgical intervention is necessary, either a needle aspiration of vitreous through the pars plana[38] or pars plana vitrectomy[39] will usually be curative in phakic eyes (Fig. 37-13). Eyes that have cataract extraction—with or without a lens implant—and a retained posterior capsule offer a less complicated intervention: direct incision of the hyaloid face using the neodymium:yttrium-aluminum-garnet (Nd:YAG) laser.[40,41] In this presentation with a retained posterior capsule (Fig. 37-14), it is necessary to sequentially eliminate pupillary block, retrocapsular block, and hyaloid block by respectively lasering through the iris, posterior capsule, and hyaloid face.[29] In the acapsular eye (e.g., aphakia) (Fig. 37-15), hyaloidectomy centrally and peripherally can be undertaken with the Nd:YAG laser or with incisional surgery.

Vigorous surveillance is still necessary in these eyes because recurrent cases of ciliary block glaucoma have been reported, especially after vitreous aspiration or vitrectomy, which may not have been sufficiently anterior in the phakic eye to interrupt the obstruction of the hyaloid face. In rare cases it is necessary to sacrifice the lens to access the hyaloid itself. Chronic atropine drops may

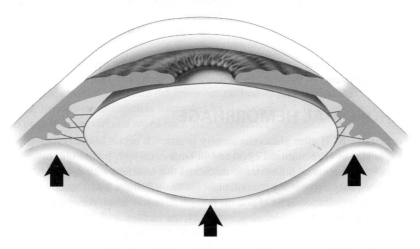

Figure 37-13 Phakic malignant glaucoma. With the sequestration of aqueous within the vitreous body, there is compression of the anterior chamber both axially and peripherally *(arrows)*, causing central shallowing of the chamber with forward movement of the lens and peripheral angle closure. (From Lieberman MF: *Complications of glaucoma surgery.* In Charlton J, Weinstein G, editors: *Ophthalmic surgery complications,* Philadelphia, 1995, Lippincott–Raven.)

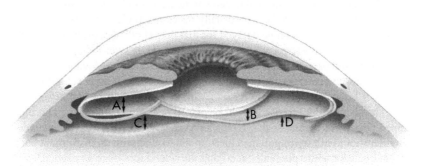

Figure 37-14 Capsular malignant glaucoma. In the presence of a posterior capsule with a posterior-chamber intraocular lens there are multiple sites in which aqueous can be sequestered, and these sites must be sequentially eliminated: *(A)* aqueous pockets between the iris and anterior capsule, *(B)* pockets within the capsular bag and lens implant, *(C)* pockets between the posterior capsule and hyaloid face, and *(D)* aqueous trapped within the vitreous cavity behind an intact hyaloid face. (From Lieberman MF: *Complications of glaucoma surgery.* In Charlton J, Weinstein G, editors: *Ophthalmic surgery complications,* Philadelphia, 1995, Lippincott–Raven.)

Table 37-1

Causes and Management of Intraoperative Flat Anterior Chamber

Condition	Causes	Management
Scleral contraction	Young eyes usually with relatively high intraocular pressure	Secure the wound as best possible; administer atropine
Choroidal expansion	Hemangioma (e.g., Sturge-Weber syndrome); effusion (nanophthalmos)	Recognize choroidal elevation; secure the wound; perform posterior sclerotomy that *does not* perforate choroid (for drainage of subchoroidal fluid); administer atropine
Suprachoroidal hemorrhage	Rare in phakic eyes unless it is buphthalmic	Recognize vitreous loss; secure the wound; perform posterior sclerotomy over choroidal elevation area to drain blood; administer atropine
Ciliary block (malignant glaucoma)	Absence of choroidal elevation; anterior chamber flattens and eye firms as balanced salt solution is injected into the anterior chamber	Secure the wound; confirm the absence of choroidal expansion or suprachoroidal hemorrhage; perform vitrectomy or aspiration 3 mm posterior to the limbus; inject air into the anterior chamber; administer atropine

Modified from Hoskins HD Jr, Migliazzo CV: *Filtering surgery for glaucoma. Focal points 1986: clinical modules for ophthalmologists,* vol 4, mod 9, San Francisco, 1986, American Academy of Ophthalmology.

After a few days, as the IOP returns to preoperative levels, the anterior chamber will re-form and the choroidal mass will subside. This phenomenon probably results from arteriolar communications to the choroidal hemangioma. When IOP falls below the arteriolar pressure level of approximately 30 mm Hg, there is not enough resistance to keep the hemangioma from expanding, creating a serious dilemma for both the surgeon and the patient (see the section on Sturge-Weber syndrome in Chapter 20).

Ciliary block glaucoma may occur during surgery when BSS injected into the anterior chamber is inadvertently diverted into the vitreous cavity and the chamber becomes shallow while the eye becomes firm. One may close the trabeculectomy flap securely and try to re-form the chamber through a paracentesis opening. If this fails, 0.5 to 1.0 ml of liquified vitreous should be removed through a sclerostomy positioned 3 mm posterior to the limbus. If the chamber then cannot be re-formed with BSS, viscoelastic substance or a large air bubble should be placed into the anterior chamber to maintain it. Atropine and topical steroids should be used frequently in the early post-operative period. The eye should be observed carefully for recurrence of the ciliary block if the atropine is discontinued.

HYPHEMA

Hemorrhage may accompany any intraocular procedure, particularly in the first 3 to 5 postoperative days. Bleeding is usually from the iris, anterior ciliary body, or corneoscleral wound, producing a hyphema that commonly subsides without intervention. Activities must be restricted, and a protective eye shield should be worn during the critical follow-up period. Knowing the patient's general medical condition or medications in use is helpful because they may affect vascular conditions and further management. Evacuation of the hyphema is rarely necessary. If the hyphema remains for several days or increases, laser photocoagulation of localized hemorrhaging may be possible through a clear portion of the anterior chamber. Rarely, the incision area must be reentered to apply wetfield cautery to the bleeding site. Clot lysis, with prompt resolution of the hyphema, can be effected with intracameral or subconjunctival administration of tissue plasminogen activator[60-63] or urokinase.[64]

Large Hyphema

Very rarely, the surgeon will encounter a large, clotted hyphema postoperatively. This is usually associated with some other precipitating factor such as the use of salicylates or other clotting inhibitors, trauma, inflammation, or rubeosis iridis. Its management must be tailored to the particular situation. High pressure can be relieved by periodically depressing the posterior lip of the sclerostomy or of the paracentesis incision if one exists.

Clot removal from the anterior chamber can be accomplished with a vitrectomy instrument but will almost certainly cause a cataract.[65] Repeated drainage and irrigation of the anterior chamber via a 2-mm paracentesis incision is a less traumatic approach if intervention is required.[66] Here too the use of intracameral fibrinolytic agents, (e.g., tissue plasminogen activator or urokinase) may be useful.

Late hyphema is rare; it is usually the result of a small capillary or vein in the filtration site that ruptures during Valsalva's maneuvers. If the site of bleeding can be visualized gonioscopically, it can be cauterized with argon laser. Failing that, a single application of cryotherapy over the area of the bleeding site may stimulate scarring and closure of the vessel, though occasionally at the cost of scarring the filtration site.

INTRAOCULAR INFECTION

Fortunately, infection is a rare complication after glaucoma surgery. As with any intraocular procedure, infections can occur in the early postoperative period but may also be seen months to years later when a filtering bleb is present.[67-70] After filtering surgery, all patients should be thoroughly informed about the symptoms and signs of infection, including pain, reduced vision, and purulent discharge; patients should be instructed to contact an ophthalmologist immediately if these symptoms occur. Intensive self-medication with sterile antibiotic eyedrops may be begun while awaiting ophthalmologic evaluation. If infection is even suspected, smears and cultures should be obtained from the lids, conjunctiva, and filtering bleb.

The presence of a bleb in general and of antimetabolite use in particular are major risk factors for intraocular infection. Other risk factors include myopia, thin-walled blebs with leaks, the presence of releasable sutures, concurrent upper respiratory infection, and blebs located at the inferior limbus.[71-75] Onset of infection can be anywhere from the first few days to up to 20 years later.[72] Both of the most commonly used antimetabolites, mitomycin C and 5-FU, have seemingly increased the frequency of postoperative endophthalmitis—to estimates as high as a 2.0% incidence.[71,74,76-79]

An important distinction has been made between bacterial infection confined to the bleb with limited anterior chamber reaction ("blebitis") and infection that penetrates into the vitreous cavity (classic endophthalmitis).[80,81] Blebitis is more likely to respond promptly to intensive antibiotic treatment; it can be treated in an outpatient setting[82]; and it has a more favorable visual outcome than does diffuse intraocular infection.[81,83,84] *Staphylococcus* and *Streptococcus* species account for approximately half of the culture-positive organisms.

When hypopyon is present, fluid for culture should be obtained from the anterior chamber and vitreous. Antibiotics should be initiated while the specific causative organism is determined at the laboratory. Vitreous aspiration with intraocular injection of antibiotics is necessary if the posterior segment is involved.[85]

SYMPATHETIC OPHTHALMIA

Sympathetic ophthalmia may arise 2 weeks to many years after any form of glaucoma surgery, but it is more common after procedures that involve intentional or unintentional iris or ciliary body incarceration or after ciliary body destruction with either cryotherapy or transscleral laser.[86-91] An incidence of 0.08% has been estimated after glaucoma operations.

Although rare, sympathetic ophthalmia is severe enough that ophthalmologists should be alerted to its symptoms and signs to make the diagnosis. Symptoms and signs include photophobia, blurred vision, and redness first in the traumatized eye and then in the fellow eye. Keratitic precipitates, iris nodules, and anterior chamber flare and cell are part of the granulomatous uveitis. Dalen-Fuchs nodules form in the peripheral fundus and appear ophthalmoscopically as yellow-white spots. Fundus fluorescein angiography has characteristic patterns that establish the correct diagnosis. A thorough evaluation is advised to establish the correct diagnosis, which then requires aggressive

acute situation, Nd:YAG and argon lasers can be used to disrupt these membranes and reestablish filtration.[95,130]

The use of antimetabolites is the most important single advance in reducing the frequency of bleb scarification. Technically, perioperative corticosteroid eyedrops are antimetabolites that powerfully interrupt the normal inflammatory cascades[131] and whose use has proven to contribute to successful glaucoma filtration.[132] (The role of preoperative subconjunctival steroids and the use of the antimetabolites 5-FU and mitomycin C are fully discussed in Chapter 35.)

REOPERATION AFTER FAILED FILTRATION

Revision of Encysted Bleb

If a bleb continues to either scar or encapsulate so there is gradual loss of IOP control despite medical therapy, massage, or suture manipulation, reoperation becomes necessary. Needling of the bleb may be successful at the slit-lamp or in a minor surgery setting; full surgical revision is sometimes required.[133]

Needling of Failed Blebs

Slit-Lamp or Minor Surgery Setting

The Pederson needling technique[123] was originally described for encapsulated blebs but has been found to be useful with failing blebs long after surgery, and even when nearly flat.[134] If undertaken on one or two occasions and augmented with 5-FU injections, full reoperation can often be avoided.[135]

With the patient sitting at the slit lamp or supine under a microscope, the ocular area is cleansed with an iodine preparation and a wire lid speculum is placed using sterile technique. With the eye looking downward, the surgeon inserts a short ¾-inch 25-gauge needle attached to a 3-ml syringe with lidocaine 1% approximately 10 mm away from and tangential to the limbus. While carefully monitoring the needle tip, the conjunctiva surrounding the bleb is ballooned. The surgeon continues to advance the needle up to one edge of the scarred capsule, at the bleb margin, and carefully penetrates the bleb. A gentle sweeping motion is used to engage and lyse fibrotic strands; small amounts of additional solution can be injected to further expand the bleb as it becomes more free. In pseudophakic or aphakic eyes, the needle can even perforate into the anterior chamber at the site where the trabeculectomy stoma presumably is. After a bleb has been raised, the needle is withdrawn and the minute conjunctival entry wound can be closed either with a quick touch of a battery cautery tip or with a 10-0 nylon purse-string suture (Fig. 37-19). This can then be combined with the use of subconjunctival 5-FU injections[135] (Fig. 37-20) or mitomycin C to enhance filtration.[136]

Operating Room Setting

Following is the surgical technique performed in the operating room (Fig. 37-21). This technique is also useful when there is a preexisting superior bleb that requires "refreshing," usually in conjunction with a temporally performed cataract/lens implantation. After local conjunctival anesthesia or retrobulbar block, the conjunctiva surrounding the encysted bleb is elevated with Xylocaine 1% containing 1:100,000 epinephrine (for hemostasis) injected through a 27- or 30-gauge needle introduced into the conjunctiva 12 to 15 mm from the bleb site. Either a short 25-gauge needle or a needle knife (e.g., Ziegler blade) is then introduced at the same location and passed through the fibrous capsule of the bleb. The eye will usually soften at this point, and subsequent maneuvers must be performed carefully to prevent damage to the globe or external perforation of the bleb wall. The knife should be passed across the bleb, incising the opposite wall and then the blade swept superiorly to open the bleb superiorly into the subconjunctival space. If the bleb wall is very dense, this upward sweep may not be possible and multiple stab incisions must suffice. The conjunctival entry point may be closed with 9-0 or 10-0 suture on a tapered needle if the wound leaks excessively.

An alternate method is to approach the bleb from the original limbal-based flap incision, carrying this forward until the thickened cystic wall is encountered. The wall is penetrated, and scissors are used to incise both lateral edges of the wall to the limbus. The conjunctiva is then closed. This allows free flow of aqueous peripheral to the cyst wall, which hopefully will not readhere to the episclera.

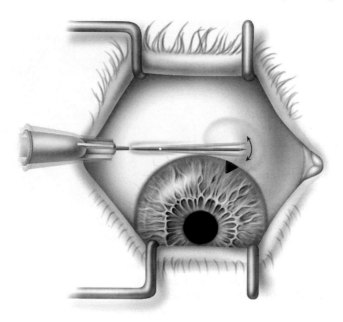

Figure 37-19 Pederson needling. A 25-gauge needle is inserted approximately 8 to 10 mm from the failing bleb, and the subconjunctival tissue is ballooned with lidocaine 1%. After entry into the bleb, the episcleral fibrosis is lacerated with a sweeping motion using the sharp edge of the subconjunctival needle. Magnification by an operating microscope or loupe is advised to avoid unintentional perforation of the bleb. (From Lieberman MF: *Complications of glaucoma surgery.* In Charlton J, Weinstein G, editors: *Ophthalmic surgery complications,* Philadelphia, 1995, Lippincott–Raven.)

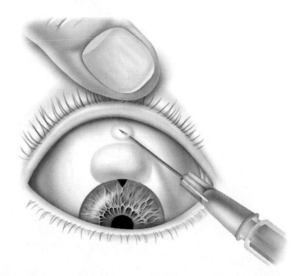

Figure 37-20 5-Fluorouracil (5-FU) injection. After the successful lysing of the bleb scar, evidenced by an obvious reduction of intraocular pressure, an injection of 5-FU can be given. With a tuberculin syringe containing 0.2 ml of 5 mg/ml solution of 5-FU and a 30-gauge needle, a small bleb is raised with 0.15 ml (7.5 mg) injected above the true filtering site. (From Lieberman MF: *Complications of glaucoma surgery.* In Charlton J, Weinstein G, editors: *Ophthalmic surgery complications,* Philadelphia, 1995, Lippincott–Raven.)

Excision of the cyst can be performed by approaching the bleb via the limbal incision, carefully dissecting conjunctiva away from the intact cyst until the conjunctiva is freed to the limbus. The cyst then can be excised in its entirety and the conjunctiva closed (Fig. 37-22).

In either of these latter two revisions, the sclerostomy opening can be modified if needed. In this situation, the sclerostomy usually is adequate as evidenced by a brisk flow of aqueous. Bleed-

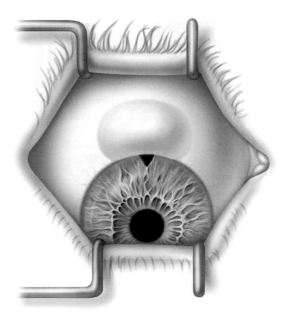

Figure 37-27 Surgical bleb reduction. With retrobulbar administration of anesthesia in the operating room, the excessive bleb can be viewed at the operating microscope. (From Lieberman MF: *Complications of glaucoma surgery.* In Charlton J, Weinstein G, editors: *Ophthalmic surgery complications,* Philadelphia, 1995, Lippincott–Raven.)

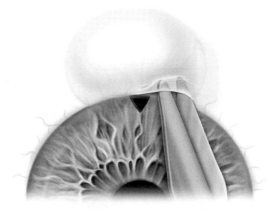

Figure 37-28 Surgical bleb reduction. A fornix-based conjunctival flap is prepared at the base of the excessive bleb. (From Lieberman MF: *Complications of glaucoma surgery.* In Charlton J, Weinstein G, editors: *Ophthalmic surgery complications,* Philadelphia, 1995, Lippincott–Raven.)

tive involves inserting of a piece of Tenon's capsule beneath the bleb (see Fig. 37-1). The Tenon's tissue is sutured directly into the undersurface of the fistula to plug the fistula.

If these strategies do not work, more extensive bleb revision is required. A sliding flap of conjunctiva is made accessible by either undermining the subconjunctival space toward the fornix with blunt-tipped scissors to mobilize available conjunctiva downward or by making a parallel vertical incision into the upper cul-de-sac and pulling it over the bleb area (Figs. 37-27 through 37-32). If the bleb surface continues to leak or is necrotic, the bleb tissue is excised. If the scleral flap appears incontinent, the stoma can be tamponaded with a freehand partial-thickness autologous or donor scleral graft,[6,141] with a partial-thickness piece of host sclera, or with donor fascia lata.[142] A groove incision is made in the superficial corneal tissue at the limbus. The flap is sutured into this groove and to adjacent conjunctiva with running 10-0 nylon. The flap must not be stretched too tautly or it will retract.

Although such extensive surgical disruption of the bleb can lead to unwanted scarring, the ma-

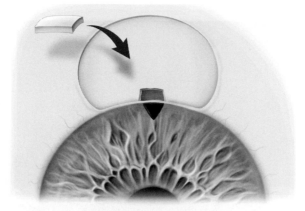

Figure 37-29   Surgical bleb reduction. After removal of the offending bleb structure, the episclera is exposed and the stoma of the original trabeculectomy is evaluated. Sometimes, with the use of antimetabolites such as mitomycin, the scleral flap may have "melted away" (as illustrated here), necessitating the use of a donor or host scleral patch graft that is hand-cut and sutured as a secondary trabeculectomy flap. (From Lieberman MF: *Complications of glaucoma surgery.* In Charlton J, Weinstein G, editors: *Ophthalmic surgery complications,* Philadelphia, 1995, Lippincott–Raven.)

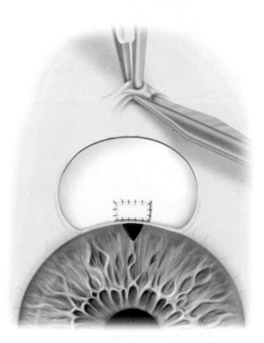

Figure 37-30   Surgical bleb reduction. Once the scleral graft is secured above the trabeculectomy ostium, a relaxing incision can be made peripherally to mobilize the conjunctiva to be drawn toward the limbus. (From Lieberman MF: *Complications of glaucoma surgery.* In Charlton J, Weinstein G, editors: *Ophthalmic surgery complications,* Philadelphia, 1995, Lippincott–Raven.)

jority of refashioned blebs maintain adequate IOP control with or without medication.[141,143] Nevertheless, as much adjacent limbal tissue as possible should be spared for future surgery if needed.

Because of the risk of perforating or infecting a thin-walled bleb, rigid contact lenses are avoided in such eyes;[67] soft lenses may be used with special caution. Since even the value of prophylactic intraoperative antibiotics to prevent endophthalmitis after cataract surgery remains controversial,[144-147] it is not surprising that there is even less evidence for prophylactic antibiosis in the presence of thin-walled blebs. Because of the risk of overgrowth of resistant species of bacteria and the irritating properties of the drops, many authorities prefer not to use them.[138,148] Rather, pa-

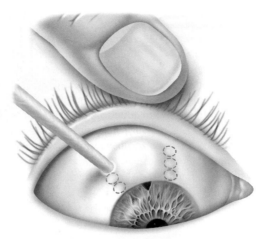

Figure 37-37 Chemical bleb reduction. A wooden applicator is dipped into a supersaturated solution of trichloroacetic acid and carefully applied in several rows surrounding the exuberant bleb, with care taken to avoid leakage of the chemical onto the corneal surface. The bleb surface itself is usually avoided. Light chemical blanching and whitening is seen after a few seconds of application. This technique may be uncomfortable for the patient, and topical atropine and patching are often useful. (From Lieberman MF: *Complications of glaucoma surgery.* In Charlton J, Weinstein G, editors: *Ophthalmic surgery complications,* Philadelphia, 1995, Lippincott–Raven.)

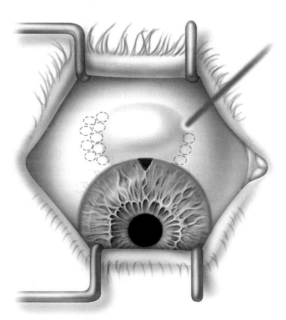

Figure 37-38 Argon laser bleb treatment. With the patient under topical anesthesia, foci of bleb leakage (or the margins of large blebs, as illustrated here) can be lightly coagulated with an argon laser, using a large spot size and minimal energy. Topical dyes, such as fluorescein or rose bengal, may enhance the thermal absorption. (From Lieberman MF: *Complications of glaucoma surgery.* In Charlton J, Weinstein G, editors: *Ophthalmic surgery complications,* Philadelphia, 1995, Lippincott–Raven.)

Argon laser energy can be delivered to the surface of a conjunctival bleb that has been stained by swabbing it with methylene blue dye (Fig. 37-38). Laser settings of 400 to 700 mW with a 500-μm spot size applied for 0.2 to 0.5 second will shrink the surface of the bleb. Because bleb perforation has occurred with this technique, it should be used with caution in blebs pretreated with antimetabolites, which may fail to heal spontaneously

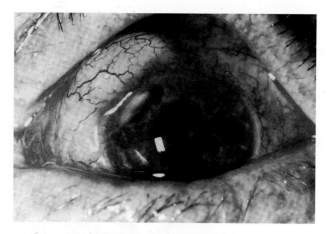

Figure 37-39 Dellen adjacent to a bleb. A large bleb after filtering surgery prevents the tear film from reaching that area of the cornea. Spontaneous healing is the rule.

Dellen

If a bleb is markedly elevated at the limbus, the lid cannot spread tears over the adjacent cornea, and dellen form (Fig. 37-39).[157] These dellen are almost always self-limited and may be palliated with ointment, frequent eyedrop application, or nonsteroidal antiinflammatory drops. Steroid drops may be contraindicated because they retard corneal surface healing; vascularization of the base in fact precedes healing.[158] Cryotherapy over the bleb adjacent to the dellen has been effective.

HYPOTONOUS MACULOPATHY

One complication of hypotony may occur early or late, within hours or days, after the reduction of IOP. Although reported many decades ago during the advent of full-thickness filtering procedures,[159] hypotonous maculopathy was later described as a specific syndrome[160] and is being appreciated in large numbers today. This situation has been extensively reported in filters augmented both with 5-FU[161,162] and mitomycin C.[163-165] It is characterized by persistent hypotony (usually defined as IOP less than 5 mm Hg) for many weeks after surgery, with decreased visual acuity.[166] Funduscopic examination reveals no specific macular edema but rather choroidal wrinkling behind the macula leading to the appearance of choroidal folds—particularly well seen on red-free photography. Subsequent series have identified two risk factors associated with hypotonous maculopathy and loss of vision: high myopia and age (patients younger than 50 years of age).[167,168] These factors may relate to decreased scleral rigidity in the area of the posterior pole and tendency towards collapse in the presence of low IOP. Low pressure alone is not incompatible with good visual acuity.[167,169]

Although it has been established that there is a slight decrease in the axial length of the eye after trabeculectomy without the use of antimetabolite (on the order of 0.27 mm),[170] eyes with hypotonous visual loss often require vigorous intervention to reduce the apparent effect of a collapsed posterior pole. By and large, nonsurgical interventions (e.g., soft contact lenses, bleb size reduction by cryotherapy,[164] or autologous blood injections[171,172] [Fig. 37-40]) are inconsistently effective. Tightly resuturing the scleral flap and elevating the IOP for the short term offer the most expeditious return of visual function and retention of IOP control.[168,173,174] Occasionally more extensive surgery, such as vitrectomy with intraocular gas, is required.[175] Avoidance of hypotony altogether with the primary surgery is, of course, the optimal procedure; surgical technique modifications with this goal in mind have been described.[176]

When IOPs are consistently brought above the level of 6 mm Hg, a return of visual function is seen in most eyes. It sometimes takes 8 to 24 months until restoration to within 1 or 2 Snellen lines of the preoperative acuity is achieved, albeit with some persistent metamorphopsia. Return of vision is faster with higher postrepair IOPs.

17. Liebmann J, and others: Management of chronic hypotony after glaucoma filtration surgery, *J Glaucoma* 5:210, 1996.

18. Fourman S: Management of cornea-lens touch after filtering surgery for glaucoma [see comments], *Ophthalmology* 97:424, 1990.

19. Hill RA, and others: Use of a symblepharon ring for treatment of over-filtration and leaking blebs after glaucoma filtration surgery, *Ophthalmic Surg* 21:707, 1990.

20. Melamed S, and others: The use of glaucoma shell tamponade in leaking filtration blebs, *Arch Ophthalmol* 104:201, 1986.

21. Ruderman JM, Allen RC: Simmon's tamponade shell for leaking filtration blebs, *Arch Ophthalmol* 103:1708, 1985.

22. Spurny RC, and others: *Shell tamponade technique.* In Thomas JV, Belcher CD, Simmons RJ, editors: *Glaucoma surgery,* St Louis, 1992, Mosby.

23. Zalta AH, Wider RH: Closure of leaking filtering blebs with cyanoacrylate tissue adhesive, *Br J Ophthalmol* 75:170, 1991.

24. Fiore PM, and others: The effect of anterior chamber depth on endothelial cell count after filtration surgery, *Arch Ophthalmol* 107:1609, 1989.

25. Smith DL, and others: The effect of glaucoma filtering surgery on corneal endothelial cell density, *Ophthalmic Surg* 22:251, 1991.

26. Hoskins HD Jr, Migliazzo C: *Filtering surgery for glaucoma. Focal points 1986: clinical modules for ophthalmologists,* vol 4, module 9, San Francisco, 1986, American Academy of Ophthalmology.

27. Spurny RC, Thomas JV: *Choroidal tap and anterior chamber re-formation.* In Thomas JV, Belcher CD, Simmons RJ, editors: *Glaucoma surgery,* St Louis, 1992, Mosby.

28. Dellaporta A: Scleral trephination for subchoroidal effusion, *Arch Ophthalmol* 101:1917, 1983.

29. Lieberman MF: *Diagnosis and management of malignant glaucoma.* In Higginbotham EJ, Lee DA, editors: *Management of difficult glaucomas: a clinician's guide,* Boston, 1994, Blackwell Scientific.

30. Fourman S: Angle-closure glaucoma complicating ciliochoroidal detachment, *Ophthalmology* 96:646, 1989.

31. Luntz MH, Rosenblatt M: Malignant glaucoma, *Surv Ophthalmol* 32:73, 1987.

32. Trope GE, and others: Malignant glaucoma: clinical and ultrasound biomicroscopic features, *Ophthalmology* 101:1030, 1994.

33. Shrader CE, and others: Pupillary and iridovitreal block in pseudophakic eyes, *Ophthalmology* 91:831, 1984.

34. Karim F, and others: Mechanisms of pupillary block (in reply), *Arch Ophthalmol* 106:167, 1988.

35. Epstein DL, and others: Experimental perfusions through the anterior and vitreous chambers with possible relationships to malignant glaucoma, *Am J Ophthalmol* 88:1078, 1979.

36. Quigley HA: Malignant glaucoma and fluid flow rate, *Am J Ophthalmol* 89:879, 1980.

37. Yaqub M, and others: *Malignant glaucoma.* In El Sayyad F, and others, editors: *The refractory glaucomas,* New York, 1995, Igaku-Shoin.

38. Simmons RJ, Thomas JV: *Surgical therapy of malignant glaucoma.* In Thomas JV, Belcher CD, Simmons RJ, editors: *Glaucoma surgery,* St Louis, 1992, Mosby.

39. Lynch MG, and others: Surgical vitrectomy for pseudophakic malignant glaucoma, *Am J Ophthalmol* 102:149, 1986.

40. Epstein DL, and others: Neodymium-YAG laser therapy to the anterior hyaloid in aphakic malignant (ciliovitreal block) glaucoma, *Am J Ophthalmol* 98:137, 1984.

41. Halkias A, and others: Ciliary block (malignant) glaucoma after cataract extraction with lens implant treated with YAG laser capsulotomy and anterior hyaloidotomy, *Br J Ophthalmol* 76:569, 1992.

42. Chu T: *Expulsive and delayed suprachoroidal hemorrhage.* In Charlton J, Weinstein G, editors: *Ophthalmic surgery complications,* Philadelphia, 1995, Lippincott-Raven.

43. Brubaker RF: Intraocular surgery and choroidal hemorrhage, *Arch Ophthalmol* 102:1753, 1984.

44. Cantor LB, Katz JL, Spaeth GL: Complications of surgery in glaucoma: suprachoroidal expulsive hemorrhage in glaucoma patients undergoing intraocular surgery, *Ophthalmology* 92:1266, 1985.

45. Frenkel REP, Shin DH: Prevention and management of delayed suprachoroidal hemorrhage after filtration surgery, *Arch Ophthalmol* 104:1459, 1986.

46. Givens K, Shields MB: Suprachoroidal hemorrhage after glaucoma filtering surgery, *Am J Ophthalmol* 103:689, 1987.

47. Gressel MG, Parrish RK II, Heuer DK: Delayed non-expulsive suprachoroidal hemorrhage, *Arch Ophthalmol* 102:1757, 1984.

48. Ruderman JM, Harbin TS, Campbell DG: Postoperative suprachoroidal hemorrhage following filtration procedures, *Arch Ophthalmol* 104:210, 1986.

49. Wheeler TM, Zimmerman TJ: Expulsive choroidal hemorrhage in the glaucoma patient, *Ann Ophthalmol* 19:165, 1987.

49a. Maumenee AE: Acute intraoperative choroidal effusion, *Am J Ophthalmol* 100:147, 1985.

50. Fluorouracil Filtering Surgery Study Group: Risk factors for suprachoroidal hemorrhage after filtering surgery, *Am J Ophthalmol* 113:501, 1992.

51. Speaker MG, and others: A case-control study of risk factors for intraoperative suprachoroidal expulsive hemorrhage, *Ophthalmology* 98:202, 1991.

52. Spaeth GL: Suprachoroidal hemorrhage: no longer a disaster, *Ophthalmic Surg* 18:329, 1987.

53. Abrams GW, and others: Management of postoperative suprachoroidal hemorrhage with continuous infusion air pump, *Arch Ophthalmol* 104:1455, 1986.

54. Davison JA: Vitrectomy and fluid infusion in the treatment of delayed suprachoroidal hemorrhage after combined cataract and glaucoma filtration surgery, *Ophthalmic Surg* 18:334, 1987.

55. Franks WA, Hitchings RA: Injection of perfluoropropane gas to prevent hypotony in eyes undergoing tube implant surgery, *Ophthalmology* 97:899, 1990.

56. Reynolds MG, and others: Suprachoroidal hemorrhage: clinical features and results of secondary surgical management, *Ophthalmology* 100:460, 1993.

57. Shihab ZM, Kristan RW: Recurrent intraoperative choroidal effusion in Sturge-Weber syndrome, *J Pediatr Strabismus* 20:250, 1983.

58. Bellows AR, and others: Choroidal effusion during glaucoma surgery in patients with prominent episcleral vessels, *Arch Ophthalmol* 97:493, 1979.

59. Hoskins HD Jr, Hetherington J, Shaffer RN: Developmental glaucoma: therapy, *Proceedings of New Orleans Academy Ophthalmology Glaucoma Symposium,* St Louis, 1980, Mosby.

60. Szymanski A: Sclerectomy under a clot in surgical treatment of glaucoma, *Mater Med Pol* 19:278, 1987.

61. Richards DW: Intracameral tissue plasminogen activator to treat blocked glaucoma implants, *Ophthalmic Surg* 24:854, 1993.

62. Piltz JR, Starita RJ: The use of subconjunctivally administered tissue plasminogen activator after trabeculectomy, *Ophthalmic Surg* 25:51, 1994.

63. Lundy DC, and others: Intracameral tissue plasminogen activator after glaucoma surgery: indications, effectiveness, and complications, *Ophthalmology* 103:274, 1996.

64. WuDunn D: Intracameral urokinase for dissolution of fibrin or blood clots after glaucoma surgery, *Am J Ophthalmol* 124:693, 1997.

65. Diddie KR, Dinsmore S, Murphree AL: Total hyphema evacuation by vitrectomy instrumentation, *Ophthalmology* 188:917, 1981.

66. Belcher CD III, Brown SV, Simmons RJ: Anterior chamber washout for traumatic hyphema, *Ophthalmic Surg* 16:475, 1985.

67. Bellows AR, McCulley JP: Endophthalmitis in aphakic patients with unplanned filtering blebs wearing contact lenses, *Ophthalmology* 88:839, 1981.

68. Christensen L, Robinson PJ: Late infection of filtration blebs, *Trans Pacific Coast Oto-ophthalmol Soc* 44:95, 1963.

69. Freedman J, Gupta M, Bunke A: Endophthalmitis after trabeculectomy, *Arch Ophthalmol* 96:1017, 1978.

70. Hattenhauer JM, Lipsich MP: Late endophthalmitis after filtering surgery, *Am J Ophthalmol* 72:1097, 1971.

71. Wolner B, and others: Late bleb-related endophthalmitis after trabeculectomy with adjunctive 5-fluorouracil, *Ophthalmology* 98:1053, 1991.

72. Phillips WB, and others: Late onset endophthalmitis associated with filtering blebs, *Ophthalmic Surg* 25:88, 1994.

73. Burchfield JC, and others: Endophthalmitis following trabeculectomy with releasable sutures, *Arch Ophthalmol* 114:766, 1996 (letter).

74. Greenfield DS, and others: Endophthalmitis after filtering surgery with mitomycin, *Arch Ophthalmol* 114:943, 1996.

75. Rosenberg LF, Siegfried CJ: Endophthalmitis associated with a releasable suture, *Arch Ophthalmol* 114:767, 1996 (letter).

76. Katz LJ: *Endophthalmitis*. In Sherwood MB, Spaeth GL, editors: *Complications of glaucoma surgery,* Thorofare, NJ, 1990, Slack.

77. Ticho U, Ophir A: Late complications after glaucoma filtering surgery with adjunctive 5-fluorouracil, *Am J Ophthalmol* 115:506, 1993.

78. Higginbotham EJ, and others: Bleb-related endophthalmitis after trabeculectomy with mitomycin C, *Ophthalmology* 103:650, 1996.

79. Parris R, Minckler D: "Late endophthalmitis": filtering surgery time bomb? *Ophthalmology* 103:1167, 1996 (editorial).

80. Ashkenazi I, and others: Risk factors associated with late infection of filtering blebs and endophthalmitis, *Ophthalmic Surg* 22:570, 1991.

81. Ciulla TA, and others: Blebitis, early endophthalmitis, and late endophthalmitis after glaucoma-filtering surgery, *Ophthalmology* 104:986, 1997.

82. Chen PP, and others: Outpatient treatment of bleb infection, *Arch Ophthalmol* 115:1124, 1997.

83. Brown RH, and others: Treatment of bleb infection after glaucoma surgery, *Arch Ophthalmol* 112:57, 1994.

84. Kangas TA, and others: Delayed-onset endophthalmitis associated with conjunctival filtering blebs, *Ophthalmology* 104:746, 1997.

85. Dhaliwal R, Meredith T: *Endophthalmitis*. In Charlton J, Weinstein G, editors: *Ophthalmic surgery complications,* Philadelphia, 1995, Lippincott-Raven.

86. Edward DP, and others: Sympathetic ophthalmia following neodymium:YAG cyclotherapy, *Ophthalmic Surg* 20:544, 1989.

87. Brown SV, and others: Sympathetic ophthalmia following Nd:YAG cyclotherapy, *Ophthalmic Surg* 21:736, 1990 (letter).

88. Lam S: High incidence of sympathetic ophthalmia after contact and noncontact neodymium:YAG cyclotherapy, *Ophthalmology* 99:1818, 1992.

89. Harrison TJ: Sympathetic ophthalmia after cyclocryotherapy of neovascular glaucoma without ocular penetration, *Ophthalmic Surg* 24:44, 1993.

90. Singh G: Sympathetic ophthalmia after Nd:YAG cyclotherapy, *Ophthalmology* 100:798, 1993 (letter; comment).

91. Bechrakis NE, and others: Sympathetic ophthalmia following laser cyclocoagulation, *Arch Ophthalmol* 112:80, 1994.

92. Traverso CE, and others: Focal pressure: a new method to encourage filtration after trabeculectomy, *Ophthalmic Surg* 15:62, 1984.

93. Kane H, and others: Response of filtered eyes to digital ocular pressure, *Ophthalmology* 104:202, 1997.

94. MacRae SM, Van Buskirk EM: Late wound dehiscence after penetrating keratoplasty in association with digital massage, *Am J Ophthalmol* 102:391, 1986.

95. van Buskirk EM: Reopening filtration sites with the argon laser, *Am J Ophthalmol* 94:1, 1982.

96. Ticho U, Ivry M: Reopening of occluded filtering blebs by argon laser photocoagulation, *Am J Ophthalmol* 84:413, 1977.

97. Kurata F, and others: Reopening filtration fistulas with transconjunctival argon laser photocoagulation, *Am J Ophthalmol* 98:340, 1984.

98. Dailey RA, and others: Reopening filtration fistulas with the neodymium-YAG laser, *Am J Ophthalmol* 102:491, 1986.

99. Cohn HC, and others: YAG laser treatment in a series of failed trabeculectomies, *Am J Ophthalmol* 108:395, 1989.

100. Rankin GA, Latina MA: Transconjunctival Nd:YAG laser revision of failing trabeculectomy, *Ophthalmic Surg* 21:365, 1990.

101. Latina MA, Rankin GA: Internal and transconjunctival neodymium:YAG laser revision of late failing filters, *Ophthalmology* 98:215, 1991.

102. Wilson RP, Lloyd J: The place of sodium hyaluronate in glaucoma surgery, *Ophthalmic Surg* 17:30, 1986.

103. Glasser DB, Matsuda M, Edelhauser HF: A comparison of the efficacy and toxicity of and intraocular pressure response to viscous solutions in the anterior chamber, *Arch Ophthalmol* 104:1819, 1986.

104. Anmarkrud N, and others: A comparison of Healon and Amvisc on the early postoperative pressure after extracapsular cataract extraction with implantation of posterior chamber lens, *Acta Ophthalmol Scand* 74:626, 1996.

105. Henry JC, Olander K: Comparison of the effect of four viscoelastic agents on early postoperative intraocular pressure, *J Cataract Refract Surg* 22:960, 1996.

106. Hutz WW, and others: Comparison of viscoelastic substances used in phacoemulsification, *J Cataract Refract Surg* 22:955, 1996.

107. Kanellopoulos AJ, and others: Comparison of topical timolol gel to oral acetazolamide in the prophylaxis of viscoelastic-induced ocular hypertension after penetrating keratoplasty, *Cornea* 16:12, 1997.

108. Vesti E, Raitta C: A review of the outcome of trabeculectomy in open-angle glaucoma, *Ophthalmic Surg Lasers* 28:128, 1997.

109. Kolker AE, and others: Trabeculectomy with releasable sutures, *Trans Am Ophthalmol Soc* 91:131, 1993.

110. Kolker AE, and others: Trabeculectomy with releasable sutures, *Arch Ophthalmol* 112:62, 1994.

111. Hsu CT, Yarng SS: A modified removable suture in trabeculectomy, *Ophthalmic Surg* 24:579, 1993.

112. Johnstone MA, and others: A releasable scleral-flap tamponade suture for guarded filtration surgery, *Arch Ophthalmol* 111:398, 1993.

113. Maberley D, and others: Releasable "U" suture for trabeculectomy surgery, *Ophthalmic Surg* 25:251, 1994.

114. Lieberman MF: Suture lysis by laser and goniolens, *Am J Ophthalmol* 95:257, 1983 (letter).

115. Hoskins H Jr, Migliazzo C: Management of failing filtering blebs with the argon laser, *Ophthalmic Surg* 15:731, 1984.

116. Tomey KF: A simple device for laser suture lysis after trabeculectomy, *Arch Ophthalmol* 109:14, 1991 (letter).

117. Mandelkorn RM, and others: A new argon laser suture lysis lens, *Ophthalmic Surg* 25:480, 1994 (letter).

118. Ritch R: A new lens for argon laser suture lysis, *Ophthalmic Surg* 25:126, 1994.

119. Temel A, Sayin I: An inexpensive visualization method for laser suture lysis, *Arch Ophthalmol* 114:1301, 1996 (letter).

120. Lieberman MF: Diode laser suture lysis following trabeculectomy with mitomycin, *Arch Ophthalmol* 114:364, 1996 (letter).

121. Asamoto A, and others: A retrospective study of the effects of laser suture lysis on the long-term results of trabeculectomy, *Ophthalmic Surg* 26:223, 1995.

122. van Buskirk EM: Cysts of Tenon's capsule following filtration surgery, *Am J Ophthalmol* 94:522, 1982.

123. Pederson JE, Smith SG: Surgical management of encapsulated filtering blebs, *Ophthalmology* 92:955, 1985.

124. Sherwood MB, and others: Cysts of Tenon's capsule following filtration surgery: medical management, *Arch Ophthalmol* 105:1517, 1987.

125. Richter CU, and others: The development of encapsulated filtering blebs, *Ophthalmology* 95:1163, 1988.

126. Ophir A: Encapsulated filtering bleb. A selective review: new deductions, *Eye* 6:348, 1992.

127. Ophir A, Ticho U: Encapsulated filtering bleb and subconjunctival 5-fluorouracil, *Ophthalmic Surg* 23:339, 1992.

128. Costa VP, and others: Needling versus medical treatment in encapsulated blebs: a randomized, prospective study, *Ophthalmology* 104:1215, 1997.

129. Scott DR, Quigley HA: Medical management of a high bleb phase after trabeculectomies, *Ophthalmology* 95:1169, 1988.

130. Kurata F, Krupin T, Kolker AE: Reopening filtration fistulas with transconjunctival argon laser photocoagulation, *Am J Ophthalmol* 98:340, 1984.

131. Fankhauser F: *Wound healing in glaucoma filtering surgery,* Amsterdam/New York, 1992, Kugler Publications.

132. Starita RJ, and others: Short- and long-term effects of postoperative corticosteroids on trabeculectomy, *Ophthalmology* 92:938, 1985.

133. Cohen JS, and others: Revision of filtration surgery, *Arch Ophthalmol* 95:1612, 1977.

134. Gillies WE, Brooks AM: Restoring the function of the failed bleb, *Aust N Z J Ophthalmol* 19:49, 1991.

135. Ewing RH, Stamper RL: Needle revision with and without 5-fluorouracil for the treatment of failed filtering blebs, *Am J Ophthalmol* 110:254, 1990.

136. Mardelli PG, and others: Slit-lamp needle revision of failed filtering blebs using mitomycin C, *Ophthalmology* 103:1946, 1996.

137. Lieberman MF, Ewing RH: Drainage implant surgery for refractory glaucoma, *Int Ophthalmol Clin* 30:198, 1990.

138. Kanski JJ: Treatment of late endophthalmitis associated with filtering blebs, *Arch Ophthalmol* 91:339, 1974.

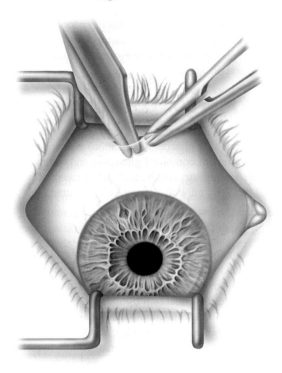

Figure 38-1   *Phacoemulsification + IOL + trabeculectomy + mitomycin C.* Preparation of a limbus-based conjunctival flap approximately 8 mm from the superior limbus, with dissection of conjunctiva and Tenon tissue anteriorly to expose the superior 6 mm of the limbal tissue. A 7-0 Vicryl traction suture to the clear cornea is used to spare unnecessary perforation of the superior conjunctiva. (From Lieberman MF: *Complications in glaucoma surgery.* In Charlton J, Weinstein G, editors: *Ophthalmic surgery complications,* Philadelphia, 1990, Lippincott-Raven.)

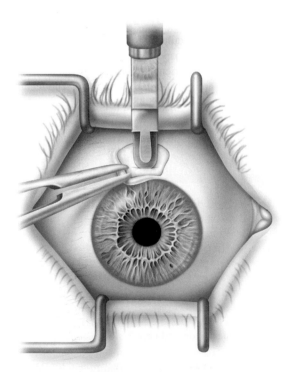

Figure 38-2   Preparation of a standard phacoemulsification scleral tunnel, which is approximately 2 mm from the limbus surface posteriorly, 3.5 mm in width, and at a depth of one half the scleral thickness. (From Lieberman MF: *Complications in glaucoma surgery.* In Charlton J, Weinstein G, editors: *Ophthalmic surgery complications,* Philadelphia, 1990, Lippincott-Raven.)

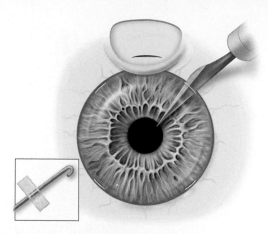

Figure 38-3 If the pupil fails to dilate, four Prolene transcorneal iris retractors (inset) can be used. (The retractor shafts are available as either metal or suture material, with rectangular sleeves of soft silicone.) Creation of four separate paracentesis "stab wounds" with a 15° sharp blade anterior to the limbal vessels and with each insertion 90° apart allows placement of the retractors. (From Lieberman MF: *Complications in glaucoma surgery.* In Charlton J, Weinstein G, editors: *Ophthalmic surgery complications,* Philadelphia, 1990, Lippincott-Raven.)

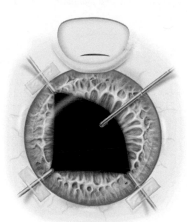

Figure 38-4 Introduction of transcorneal iris retractors. Each hook is introduced to grasp the pupillary edge and pull it peripherally to the limbus. The large, square pupil is secured by sliding the clear plastic sleeves forward along the shaft of the retractor up to the limbus itself. (From Lieberman MF: *Complications in glaucoma surgery.* In Charlton J, Weinstein G, editors: *Ophthalmic surgery complications,* Philadelphia, 1990, Lippincott-Raven.)

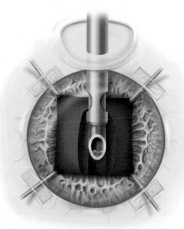

Figure 38-5 With the enlargement of the pupil, a standard phacoemulsification can proceed, with capsulorrhexis and cataract removal. The superior iris is sometimes "tented" between the two superior iris refractors; care is necessary to avoid trauma to the superior iris both when entering the eye and when intracamerally manipulating the phacoemulsification unit. (From Lieberman MF: *Complications in glaucoma surgery.* In Charlton J, Weinstein G, editors: *Ophthalmic surgery complications,* Philadelphia, 1990, Lippincott-Raven.)

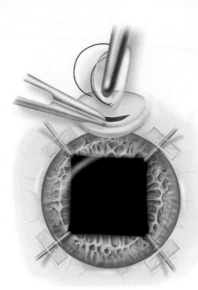

Figure 38-6 After completion of the irrigation and aspiration of the lens, the scleral tunnel can be enlarged horizontally in preparation for foldable lens implantation. (From Lieberman MF: *Complications in glaucoma surgery.* In Charlton J, Weinstein G, editors: *Ophthalmic surgery complications,* Philadelphia, 1990, Lippincott-Raven.)

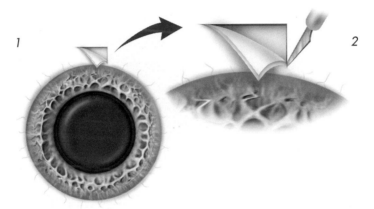

Figure 38-7 After placement of the posterior chamber lens implant in the capsular bag, the surgeon converts the phacoscleral tunnel (1) into a nonstandard trabeculectomy flap. This is simply fashioned by making a radial cut (2) from the corner of the scleral tunnel anteriorly to the limbus itself. (From Lieberman MF: *Complications in glaucoma surgery.* In Charlton J, Weinstein G, editors: *Ophthalmic surgery complications,* Philadelphia, 1990, Lippincott-Raven.)

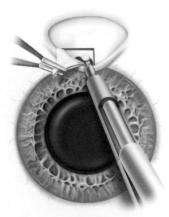

Figure 38-8 At the phacoemulsification site at the limbus, a Descemet's punch is used to fashion the trabeculectomy stoma, which is approximately 2 × 2 mm in size. (From Lieberman MF: *Complications in glaucoma surgery.* In Charlton J, Weinstein G, editors: *Ophthalmic surgery complications,* Philadelphia, 1990, Lippincott-Raven.)

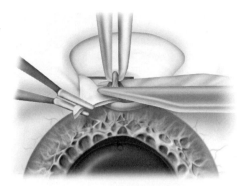

Figure 38-9 A basal peripheral iridectomy is performed at the site of the trabeculectomy. (From Lieberman MF: *Complications in glaucoma surgery.* In Charlton J, Weinstein G, editors: *Ophthalmic surgery complications,* Philadelphia, 1990, Lippincott-Raven.)

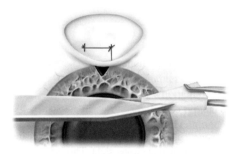

Figure 38-10 After suturing the phacoemulsification wound with one 10-0 nylon suture at the corner and an optional suture along the length of the bed of scleral tunnel, the surgeon prepares for the placement of the antimetabolite (either mitomycin C or 5-fluorouracil). A sponge that is one half the thickness of the triangular cellulose is cut parallel to the surface of the sponge (shown here), and this triangular element is again cut so that the triangular sides are approximately 4 to 5 mm in length. The sponge fragment is then saturated with the antimetabolite, using a few drops delivered via syringe and a small needle. (From Lieberman MF: *Complications in glaucoma surgery.* In Charlton J, Weinstein G, editors: *Ophthalmic surgery complications,* Philadelphia, 1990, Lippincott-Raven.)

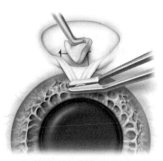

Figure 38-11 The saturated cellulose sponge fragment is carefully placed over the trabeculectomy flap, with care taken to lift the Tenon's tissue and overlying conjunctiva on top of the saturated sponge but to avoid contact between the conjunctival wound edge and the sponge. Exposure of the antimetabolite to the wound depends on several factors but is approximately 1 to 5 minutes depending on the concentration and antimetabolite chosen. (From Lieberman MF: *Complications in glaucoma surgery.* In Charlton J, Weinstein G, editors: *Ophthalmic surgery complications,* Philadelphia, 1990, Lippincott-Raven.)

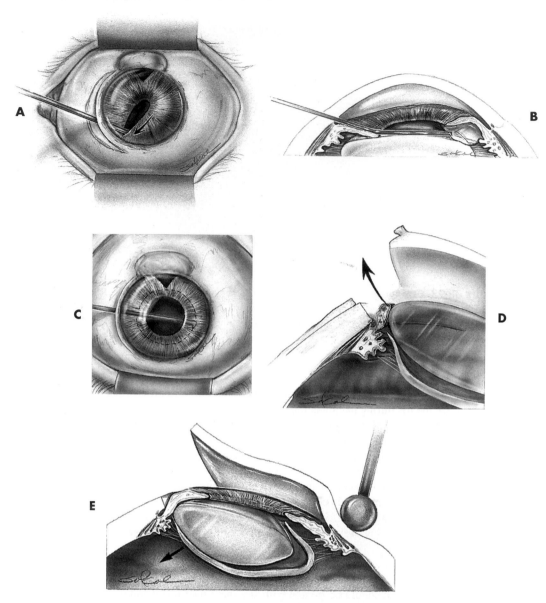

Figure 38-24   Temporal ECCE in presence of superior preexisting bleb. **A,** After making an initial fornix-based flap, a stab incision is made. A microspatula is used to stretch the pupil and break any existing synechiae. **B,** Viscoelastic material is injected under the iris to stretch the pupil and elevate the iris from the anterior capsule. **C,** The capsulotomy is done behind the iris. It should be done slowly with minimal trauma to the posterior surface of the iris. **D,** In an eye with a well-dilated pupil, the nucleus slides easily past the pupillary margin. **E,** A miotic pupil tends to trap the nucleus behind the iris. Excessive pressure may force the nucleus posteriorly *(arrow)* and rupture the zonules.   *Continued*

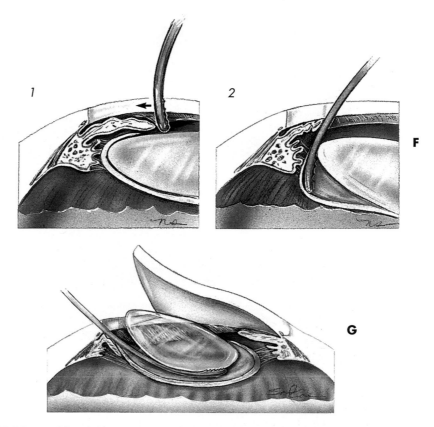

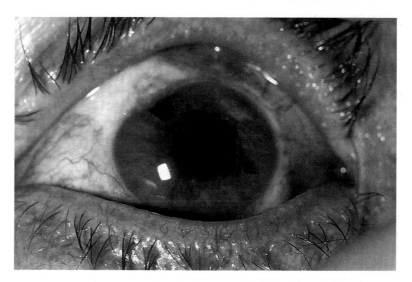

Figure 38-24, cont'd **F,** A curved irrigating vectus, such as the one designed by Simcoe, retracts the iris *(1)* and slips behind the nucleus *(2).* **G,** The vectus is then slid beneath the nucleus to facilitate its delivery.

Figure 38-25 This patient had an upper nasal temporal extraction through a miotic pupil to preserve the filtering bleb. Five sphincterotomies were performed. Even so, small pupillary tears between the sphincterotomies can be seen. The laxity of the temporal iris allowed a small amount of pupillary capture to occur even though posteriorly angled haptics were used. This capture was not evident until 2 weeks after surgery.

REFERENCES

1. Russell-Eggitt IM, and others: Relapse following goniotomy for congenital glaucoma due to trabecular dysgenesis, *Eye* 6:197, 1992.

2. Walton DS: *Goniotomy.* In Thomas JV, Belcher CD, Simmons RJ, editors: *Glaucoma surgery,* St Louis, 1992, Mosby.

3. Catalano RA, and others: One versus two simultaneous goniotomies as the initial surgical procedure for primary infantile glaucoma, *J Pediatr Ophthalmol Strabismus* 26:9, 1989.

4. Mandal AK: Current concepts in the diagnosis and management of developmental glaucomas, *Indian J Ophthalmol* 41:51, 1993.

5. Mandal AK, and others: Mitomycin C-augmented trabeculectomy in refractory congenital glaucoma, *Ophthalmology* 104:996, 1997.

6. Quigley H: Childhood glaucoma: results with trabeculotomy and study of reversible cupping, *Ophthalmology* 89:219, 1982.

7. Luntz M: The advantages of trabeculotomy over goniotomy, *J Pediatr Ophthalmol Strabismus* 21:150, 1984.

8. Martin BB: External trabeculotomy in the surgical treatment of congenital glaucoma, *Aust N Z J Ophthalmol* 17:299, 1989.

9. Anderson DR: Trabeculotomy compared to goniotomy for glaucoma in children, *Ophthalmology* 90:805, 1983.

10. Gregersen E, Kessing S: Congenital glaucoma surgery before and after the introduction of microsurgery: results of "macrosurgery" 1943-1963 and of microsurgery (trabeculotomy/ectomy) 1970-1974, *Acta Ophthalmol* 55:422, 1977.

11. deLuise V, Anderson D: Primary infantile glaucoma (congenital glaucoma), *Surv Ophthalmol* 28:1, 1983.

12. Akimoto M, and others: Surgical results of trabeculectomy ab externo for developmental glaucoma, *Arch Ophthalmol* 112:1540, 1994.

13. Shrader CE, Cibis GW: *External trabeculotomy.* In Thomas JV, Belcher CD, Simmons RJ, editors: *Glaucoma surgery,* St Louis, 1992, Mosby.

14. Beck AD, Lynch MG: 360 Degrees trabeculotomy for primary congenital glaucoma, *Arch Ophthalmol* 113:1200, 1995.

15. Shaffer RN: Prognosis of goniotomy in primary infantile glaucoma (trabeculodysgenesis), *Trans Am Ophthalmol Soc* 80:321, 1982.

16. Shaffer RN, Hoskins HD Jr: Montgomery lecture: goniotomy in the treatment of isolated trabeculodysgenesis (primary congenital [infantile] developmental glaucoma), *Trans Am Ophthalmol Soc UK* 103:581, 1983.

17. Hoskins HD Jr, and others: *Developmental glaucoma: therapy, Proceedings of the New Orleans Academy of Ophthalmology Glaucoma Symposium,* St Louis, 1980, Mosby.

18. Litinski SM, and others: Operative complications of goniotomy, *Trans Am Acad Ophthalmol Otolaryngol* 83:78, 1977.

19. Hoskins HD Jr, Hetherington J Jr, Shaffer RN: Surgical management of the inflammatory glaucomas, *Perspect Ophthalmol* 1:173, 1977.

20. Kanski JJ, McAllister JA: Trabeculodialysis for inflammatory glaucoma in children and young adults, *Ophthalmology* 92:927, 1985.

21. Williams RD, and others: Trabeculodialysis for inflammatory glaucoma: a review of 25 cases, *Ophthalmic Surg* 23:36, 1992.

22. Campbell DG, Vela A: Modern goniosynechialysis for the treatment of synechial angle-closure glaucoma, *Ophthalmology* 91:1052, 1984.

23. Sharpe ED, and others: *Goniosynechialysis.* In Thomas JV, Belcher CD, Simmons RJ, editors: *Glaucoma surgery,* St Louis, 1992, Mosby.

24. Benson MT, Nelson ME: Cyclocryotherapy: a review of cases over a 10-year period, *Br J Ophthalmol* 74:103, 1990.

25. Devreese M, and others: Cyclocryotherapy in primary glaucoma: intraocular pressure reducing effects and complications, *Bull Soc Belge Ophthalmol* 241:105, 1991.

26. Suzuki Y, and others: Transscleral Nd: YAG laser cyclophotocoagulation versus cyclocryotherapy, *Graefes Arch Clin Exp Ophthalmol* 229:33, 1991.

27. Mora JS, and others: Endoscopic diode laser cyclophotocoagulation with a limbal approach, *Ophthalmic Surg Lasers* 28:118, 1997.

28. Chen J, and others: Endoscopic photocoagulation of the ciliary body for treatment of refractory glaucoma, *Am J Ophthalmol* 124:6, 787, 1997.

29. Brown S, and others: *Cyclocryosurgery.* In Thomas JV, Belcher CD, Simmons RJ, editors: *Glaucoma surgery,* St Louis, 1992, Mosby.

30. Geyer O, and others: The mechanism of intraocular pressure rise during cyclocryotherapy, *Invest Ophthalmol Vis Sci* 38:1012, 1997.

31. Hennekes R, Belgrado G: Cyclocryotherapy as an alternative treatment for primary glaucoma, *Bull Soc Belge Ophthalmol* 244:169, 1992.

32. Harrison TJ: Sympathetic ophthalmia after cyclocryotherapy of neovascular glaucoma without ocular penetration, *Ophthalmic Surg* 24:44, 1993.

33. Biswas J, Fogla R: Sympathetic ophthalmia following cyclocryotherapy with histopathologic correlation, *Ophthalmic Surg Lasers* 27:1035, 1996.

34. Hoskins HD Jr: Neovascular glaucoma: current concepts, *Trans Am Acad Ophthalmol Otolaryngol* 78:330, 1974.

35. al-Faran MF, al-Omar OM: Retrobulbar alcohol injection in blind painful eyes, *Ann Ophthalmol* 22:460, 1990.

36. Birch M, and others: Retrobulbar phenol injection in blind painful eyes, *Ann Ophthalmol* 25:267, 1993.

37. Singh OS, Simmons RJ: *Cyclodialysis.* In Thomas JV, Belcher CD, Simmons RJ, editors: *Glaucoma surgery,* St Louis, 1992, Mosby.

38. Burgess SE, and others: Treatment of glauco high-intensity focused ultrasound, *Ophthalmology* 93:831, 1986.

39. Coleman DJ, and others: Therapeutic ultrasound in the treatment of glaucoma: II. Clinical applications, *Ophthalmology* 92:347, 1985.

40. Coleman DJ, and others: Therapeutic ultrasound, *Ultrasound Med Biol* 12:633, 1986.

41. Yablonski M, and others: Use of therapeutic ultrasound to restore failed trabeculectomies, *Am J Ophthalmol* 103:492, 1987.

42. Wilensky JT: Staphyloma formation as a complication of ultrasound treatment in glaucoma, *Arch Ophthalmol* 103:508, 1985 (letter).

PART IX

Present Status and
Future Approaches